Child maltreatment

Child maltreatment
Theory and research on the causes and consequences of child abuse and neglect

Edited by

DANTE CICCHETTI
University of Rochester

and

VICKI CARLSON
Washington University, St. Louis

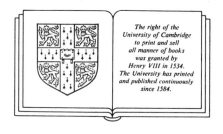

The right of the
University of Cambridge
to print and sell
all manner of books
was granted by
Henry VIII in 1534.
The University has printed
and published continuously
since 1584.

CAMBRIDGE UNIVERSITY PRESS

Cambridge

New York   Port Chester   Melbourne   Sydney

Published by the Press Syndicate of the University of Cambridge
The Pitt Building, Trumpington Street, Cambridge CB2 1RP
40 West 20th Street, New York, NY 10011, USA
10 Stamford Road, Oakleigh, Melbourne 3166, Australia

First published 1989
Reprinted 1990

Printed in the United States of America

Library of Congress Cataloging-in-Publication Data

Child maltreatment : theory and research on the causes and
consequences of child abuse and neglect / edited by Dante Cicchetti
and Vicki Carlson.
p.   cm.
Includes bibliographies and index.
ISBN 0-521-36455-8
1. Child abuse.   2. Child neglect.   I. Cicchetti, Dante.
II. Carlson, Vicki.
[DNLM: 1. Child Abuse.   WA 320 C53487]
RC569.5.C55C47   1989
616.85'82 – dc19   88-38174

British Library Cataloguing in Publication applied for

ISBN 0-521-36455-8 hardback
ISBN 0-521-37969-5 paperback

Contents

v

Contents

Contributors

J. Lawrence Aber
Barnard College
Columbia University

Mary D. S. Ainsworth
University of Virginia

Joseph P. Allen
Harvard University

Douglas Barnett
Mt. Hope Family Center
University of Rochester

Jay Belsky
Pennsylvania State University

Karen G. Braunwald
Westwood Lodge Hospital
Westwood, Massachusetts

Daphne Blunt Bugental
University of California at Santa
  Barbara

Ann W. Burgess
University of Pennsylvania School
  of Nursing

Vicki Carlson
Washington University School of
  Medicine

Dante Cicchetti
Director, Mt. Hope Family
  Center
University of Rochester

David B. Connell
Harvard Medical School and Abt
  Associates

Patricia M. Crittenden
Mailman Center for Child
  Development
University of Miami

Howard Dubowitz
University of Maryland Medical
  School

Byron Egeland
University of Minnesota

Martha Farrell Erickson
University of Minnesota

ix

Norma Deitch Feshbach
Department of Education and
Graduate School of Education
University of California at Los
    Angeles

James Garbarino
Erikson Institute
Chicago, Illinois

Jeanne Giovannoni
School of Social Welfare
University of California at Los
    Angeles

Nancy W. Hall
Yale Bush Center in Child
    Development and Social Policy
Yale University

Carol R. Hartman
Boston College School of Nursing

Charles R. Henderson, Jr.
Cornell University

Joan Kaufman
Yale Bush Center in Child
    Development and Social Policy
Yale University

Mario Kelly
University of Nebraska

Dorothy Otnow Lewis
New York University School of
    Medicine and
Yale University Child Study Center

Jeffrey Lewis
University of California at Santa
    Barbara

Karlen Lyons-Ruth
Harvard Medical School

Catherine Mallouh
New York University School of
    Medicine

Susan Madith Mantyla
Graduate School of Education
University of California at Santa
    Barbara

Edward Mueller
Boston University

Carolyn Moore Newberger
The Children's Hospital
Boston, Massachusetts

Eli Newberger
Harvard Medical School
Cambridge, Massachusetts

David L. Olds
University of Rochester Medical
    Center

Robert Pianta
Institute of Clinical Psychology
University of Virginia

Michael Rutter
MRC Child Psychiatry Unit
Institute of Psychiatry, London

Nancy Silverman
Boston University

Judith G. Smetana
Graduate School of Education and
    Human Development
University of Rochester

Elizabeth J. Susman
College of Health and Human
    Development
Pennsylvania State University

Penelope K. Trickett
The Chesapeake Institute and
National Institute of Mental
    Health

Joan Vondra
Mt. Hope Family Center
University of Rochester

Victoria Webb
New York University School of
    Medicine

Kathleen M. White
Boston University

Edward Zigler
Yale Bush Center in Child
    Development and Social Policy
Yale University

David Zoll
Harvard Medical School

Preface

Child maltreatment is a complex, insidious problem that, although predominant in impoverished families (Pelton, 1978), cuts across all sectors of society. The American Association for Protecting Children (1986) tallied 1,727,000 reports of suspected child maltreatment in 1984. Forty-two percent of these reports were substantiated. A national survey reported that 10.7 percent of parents admitted to having perpetrated a "severe violent act" against their child in the previous year (Straus and Gelles, 1986) and prevalence rates of sexual abuse have been estimated to be as high as 62 percent for girls and 31 percent for boys (Dubowitz, 1986). The economic and human costs of maltreatment in American society are astronomical. It is likely that billions of dollars are spent in treatment and social service costs and lost in lessened productivity for a generation of maltreated children (Dubowitz, 1986). The human costs are a litany of psychological tragedies. Maltreated children suffer from poor peer relations, cognitive deficits, and low self esteem among other problems; moreover, they tend to be more aggressive than their peers, as well as having behavior problems and psychopathology (see Aber and Cicchetti, 1984, for a review). The emotional damage due to maltreatment may last a lifetime.

History documents that the problem of child maltreatment has existed since the beginning of civilization (Ariès, 1962; Radbill, 1968; Ross, 1980). Unfortunately, our understanding of the etiology, intergenerational transmission, and developmental sequelae of this pervasive social problem largely has been the result of relatively recent systematic inquiry. Until a generation ago, modern society had refused to recognize the scope and gravity of child maltreatment. In fact, prior to the 1960s, many sectors of our society (e.g., medical personnel) failed even to acknowledge its existence (Dubowitz and Newberger, this volume; see also Nelson, 1984, for an important and insightful chronicling of the forces responsible for mobilizing societal interest in child abuse).

xiii

It was apparently not until 1961 that these efforts had a clear impact among the medical community (Cicchetti, Taraldson, and Egeland, 1978; Lynch, 1985). Alarmed by the increasing number of children with nonaccidental injuries being admitted to pediatric clinics, C. Henry Kempe and his colleagues conducted a symposium on child abuse at the annual national meeting of the American Academy of Pediatrics. In an effort to underscore the seriousness of the problem, Kempe and his colleagues, in an influential article published in the *Journal of the American Medical Association,* coined the term "battered child syndrome" (Kempe, Silverman, Steele, Droegemueller, and Silver, 1962). As a direct result of this paper, a dramatic increase in legislative activity ensued, resulting in the establishment of mandated child abuse reporting laws for all 50 states before the year 1970. Moreover, at about this same time, a heightened sensitivity to the needs of children began to emerge, reflecting a contemporary ethos increasingly concerned about the rights of the disadvantaged sectors of our society. Regional centers for retarded children, Project Head Start, and Medicaid were all initiated during this era (Dubowitz and Newberger, this volume). Furthermore, during the past two decades, the legal status of children has changed considerably (Koocher, 1976; Polier, 1975; Rodham, 1973; Wald, 1975) and children are now seen as having a right to the fulfillment of their developmental needs (Alvy, 1975; Derdeyn, 1977; Goldstein, Freud, and Solnit, 1973). It is clear that the problem of child maltreatment is considered an important issue, worthy of both scientific and policy analysis. The enactment of the legislation supporting the creation of the National Center on Child Abuse and Neglect provides testimony to this assertion.

Despite the positive consequences of the yeoman efforts of Kempe and his colleagues, a number of unfortunate negative ramifications ensued. The adoption of the term "battered child syndrome" connoted a psychologically disturbed parent-as-perpetrator model of child abuse (Parke and Collmer, 1975). This narrow etiological view of helpless infants and children being battered maliciously by psychiatrically ill parents (Spinetta and Rigler, 1972; Steele and Pollock, 1968) virtually absolved society of any responsibility for the occurrence of child abuse (Alvy, 1975). In addition, the treatment prescriptions emanating from this medicalization and legalization of child abuse focused on supplying treatment for the abusing parent without stressing the need to provide concomitant intervention for the abused child (Cicchetti et al., 1978).

During the 1970s, the laws mandating the reporting of child abuse were changed. The Child Abuse Prevention and Treatment Act of 1974 expanded the definition of child abuse to encompass emotional injury, neglect, parental deprivation of medical services, and factors deleterious to children's moral development (Aber and Zigler, 1981; Dubowitz and Newberger, this volume; Giovannoni, this volume; Wald, 1975, 1976). This broadened definition of child abuse contributed to the belief that not all abusing parents set out with the intention to destroy their helpless offspring.

Increasingly, broader social factors (e.g., societal attitudes, structures, and stressors; persistent poverty) were implicated as playing causal roles in child maltreatment (Garbarino, 1976; Garbarino and Gilliam, 1980; Gil, 1970; Pelton, 1978). As the etiological models became less focused on parental psychopathology as the cause of child abuse, increased attention was paid to the prevention of child abuse and to the research and treatment of maltreated children (Kempe and Helfer, 1972; Kempe and Kempe, 1978; Martin, 1976). Because careful analyses of the foster care system of the United States demonstrated significant problems (Children's Defense Fund, 1979; Fanshel and Shinn, 1972; Gruber, 1978; Mnookin, 1973), efforts were made to keep children at home whenever possible. The work of Jane Knitzer and her colleagues is exemplary among these studies. They brilliantly documented and analyzed the dangerous tendency for temporary foster care to become permanent – much to the detriment of the child, who would often develop more soundly and happily living with an abusive parent than with a series of foster parents (Children's Defense Fund, 1979). As a result of such investigations, growing numbers of clinicians advocated that the entire family be treated in maltreatment cases (Cicchetti et al., 1978; Kempe and Kempe, 1978).

In recent years, two new theoretical viewpoints on child maltreatment have been introduced: the ecological model (Belsky, 1980) and the transactional model (Cicchetti and Rizley, 1981). These models are significant because both are explicitly developmental in their orientation to the causes, intergenerational transmission, and sequelae of maltreatment. The influence of developmental theorizing in the field of child maltreatment has resulted in the formation of appropriately complex etiological models and a rich framework for conceptualizing the effects that maltreatment has upon adaptive and maladaptive ontogenetic processes.

Empirical research on the cognitive, linguistic, socioemotional, and social-cognitive sequelae of child maltreatment is a very recent phenomenon. In addition to the contributions they can make to the formulation of an integrative developmental theory, studies of the sequelae of maltreatment are very important for enhancing the quality of clinical, legal, and policy making decisions for maltreated children (Aber and Zigler, 1981; Cicchetti and Aber, 1980; Juvenile Justice Standards Project, 1977). Decisions concerning such issues as whether to report a child as maltreated, whether to remove a child coercively from the home, how to develop services to meet the specific psychological needs of maltreated children, and how to evaluate these service efforts would all benefit from a solid and sophisticated

database on the developmental sequelae of maltreatment (Aber and Cicchetti, 1984; Cicchetti et al., 1978; Wald, 1975; Wald, Carlsmith, Leiderman
and Smith, 1983).

In a review and critique of the available research on the social, emotional,
and cognitive developmental consequences of maltreatment, Aber and Cicchetti (1984) highlighted some of the methodological inadequacies of the
initial studies. Before the late 1970s, the vast majority of research conducted
on the developmental consequences of maltreatment was theoretical, cross-
sectional, and often severely flawed conceptually and methodologically (e.g.,
no control groups; improperly matched comparison samples; inappropriate
measures; little or no attention paid to the child's developmental status during data analyses; and "non-blind" experimenters and coders assessing the
children's functioning). Because most of this research was atheoretically
conceived and adevelopmentally executed and interpreted, these studies
primarily presented a great deal of unintegrated data on the clinical problems, social difficulties, and poor school performance of maltreated children
(see Aber and Cicchetti, 1984). Not surprisingly, the conclusions emanating
from these various reports often contained apparently contradictory information (e.g., maltreated children are described as: hypervigilant or less perceptive, aggressive or withdrawn, etc.). Thus, in the absence of an overarching developmental theory, it was difficult to make definitive statements
about the social, emotional, and cognitive consequences of maltreatment.
Moreover, the lack of a sound theory to guide the research programs made
it difficult to put the findings from even the well-designed studies to scientific or practical use.

Within the past decade, influenced by the emergence of increasingly
sophisticated developmental models of maltreatment (Belsky, 1980; Cicchetti and Rizley, 1981; Garbarino, 1977), theory and research on the consequences of child maltreatment have improved significantly. The exemplary theoretical and empirical work that has been included in this volume
documents the major gains that have occurred. We believe that the results
of this work will have important implications for practitioners and researchers alike. When maltreatment is viewed within the context of a normal
developmental perspective (Cicchetti, this volume) and takes into account
the multifaceted nature of maltreatment, interventions may be appropriately timed and guided (Cicchetti and Toth, 1987; Cicchetti, Toth, and
Bush, in press). Moreover, preventive efforts will be better informed and
increasingly likely to succeed (Kaufman and Zigler, in press; Olds and Henderson, this volume).

We would like to acknowledge the grants we received from the Founda-
tion for Child Development Young Scholars Program, the John D. and
Catherine T. MacArthur Foundation on Early Childhood, the National
Institute of Mental Health (R01–MH37960–01), the National Center on

Child Abuse and Neglect (90–C–1929), the Spencer Foundation, and the William T. Grant Foundation in support of our research on the Harvard Child Maltreatment Project. We wish to thank the staff of the Harvard Child Maltreatment Project for their dedication and for all of their valuable contributions, most notably J. Lawrence Aber, Douglas Barnett, Marjorie Beeghly, Judy Bigelow, Karen Braunwald, Ann Churchill, Wender Coster, Michelle Gersten, Joan Kaufman, Carolyn Reider, Karen Schneider-Rosen, Miriam Wetzel, and, especially, Carol Kottmeier. In addition, we are grateful to the officials and especially to the social workers of the Massachusetts Department of Social Services and of the Massachusetts Society for the Prevention of Cruelty to Children for their dedicated effort in serving maltreated children and families and for their commitment to making our university–state government collaboration work. We would also like to thank the families who have participated in our studies. We have learned a great deal from their willingness to share personal and sometimes painful information with us and are committed to seeing the results of empirical work in the area of child maltreatment translated into successful policy and intervention on their behalf. Finally, we wish to acknowledge the superb work of Susan Milmoe and Helen Wheeler at Cambridge University Press. Their support and patience have played a major role in the development of this book.

Each of us would like to add several personal acknowledgments here. Dante Cicchetti would like to thank all of his colleagues at the Mt. Hope Family Center, especially Douglas Barnett, Jan Gillespie, Laura McCloskey, Jody Todd Manley, Sheree Toth and Joan Vondra. Furthermore, Dante would like to acknowledge the Rochester Monroe County Department of Social Services, the New York State Department of Social Services, and the New York State Department of Special Education for their commitment to providing high quality services to maltreated children and their families and for the invaluable support that they provide to the Mt. Hope Family Center. In particular, Dante would like to thank Diane Larter, Gabriel Russo, Katherine Sosin, and Michelle Cournoyer Walsh. Additionally, Dante would like to acknowledge the support received from the United Way Agency of the Greater Rochester area. Finally, Dante wishes to acknowledge the generous support of the A. L. Mailman Family Foundation, the Smith Richardson Foundation and the Spunk Fund, Inc.

Thanks also are extended to his friends and colleagues, Drs. J. Lawrence Aber, Jules Bemporad, Byron Egeland, Norman Garmezy, Kenneth Kaplan, Paul Meehl, Ping Serafica, Alex Siegel, Alan Sroufe, Bonnie Taraldson, Sheree Toth, and Edward Zigler for their intellectual and emotional support over the years. Furthermore, Dante would like to thank Victoria Gill for the superb help she has provided in typing and organizing this work. Lastly, Dante would like to extend his most special thanks to his parents, Dolores and Eugene, his grandparents, Josephine and George Butch, his sisters, Candace and Eugenia, his son, Justin, and to Dorothy Dittman, Heidi Mitke, and Jennifer White. Through different pathways, each has contributed immeasurably to his personal and professional growth.

Vicki Carlson would like to add her thanks to Drs. Elizabeth Bates, Inge Bretherton, Eugene Gollin, and Lee Robins for their encouragement and wise direction, and to her family for their invaluable and enduring support.

Dante Cicchetti
Vicki Carlson

References

Aber, J. L., and Cicchetti, D. (1984). Socioemotional development in maltreated children: An empirical and theoretical analysis. In H. Fitzgerald, B. Lester, and M. Yogman (Eds.), *Theory and research in behavioral pediatrics,* Vol. II. New York: Plenum.

Aber, J. L., and Zigler, E. (1981). Developmental considerations in the definition of child maltreatment. *New Directions for Child Development, 11,* 1–29.

Alvy, K. T. (1975). Preventing child abuse. *American Psychologist, 30,* 921–928.

American Association for Protecting Children (AAPC) (1986). *Highlights of Official Child Neglect and Abuse Reporting 1984.* Denver, CO: The American Humane Association.

Ariès, P. (1962). *Centuries of childhood.* New York: Vintage Books.

Belsky, J. (1980). Child maltreatment: An ecological integration. *American Psychologist, 35,* 320–335.

Children's Defense Fund (1979). *Children without homes: An examination of public responsibility to children in out-of-home care.* Washington, DC: Children's Defense Fund.

Cicchetti, D., and Aber, J. L. (1980). Abused children–abusive parents: An overstated case? *Harvard Educational Review, 50,* 244–255.

Cicchetti, D., and Rizley, R. (1981). Developmental perspectives on the etiology, intergenerational transmission, and sequelae of child maltreatment. *New Directions for Child Development, 11,* 31–55.

Cicchetti, D., Taraldson, B., and Egeland, B. (1978). Perspectives in the treatment and understanding of child abuse. In A. Goldstein (Ed.), *Perspectives for child mental health and education.* New York: Pergamon.

Cicchetti, D., and Toth, S. (1987). The application of a transactional risk model to intervention with multi-risk maltreating families. *Zero to Three, 7,* 1–8.

Cicchetti, D., Toth, S., and Bush, M. (in press). Developmental psychopathology and incompetence in childhood: Suggestions for intervention. In B. Lahey and A. Kazdin (Eds.), *Advances in clinical child psychology.* New York: Plenum.

Cicchetti, D., Toth, S., Bush, M. A., and Gillespie, J. F. (1988). Stage-salient issues: A transactional model of intervention. *New Directions for Child Development,* No. 39, 123–145.

Derdeyn, A. 91977). Child abuse and neglect: The rights of parents and the needs of their children. *American Journal of Orthopsychiatry, 47,* 377–387.

Dubowitz, H. (1986). *Child maltreatment in the United States: Etiology, impact and prevention.* Background paper prepared for the Congress of the United States, Office of Technology Assessment.

Fanshel, D., and Shinn, E. G. (1972). *Dollars and sense in the foster care of children: A look at cost factors.* New York: Child Welfare League of America.

Garbarino, J. A. (1976). A preliminary study of some ecological correlates of child abuse: The impact of socioeconomic stress on mothers. *American Journal of Orthopsychiatry, 47*, 372–381.

Garbarino, J. (1977). The human ecology of child maltreatment: A conceptual model for research. *Journal of Marriage and the Family, 39*, 721–732.

Garbarino, J., and Gilliam, G. (1980). *Understanding abusive families.* Lexington, MA: Lexington Press.

Gil, D. B. (1970). *Violence against children: Physical child abuse in the United States.* Cambridge, MA: Harvard University Press.

Goldstein, J., Freud, A., and Solnit, A. (1973). *Beyond the best interests of the child.* New York: Free Press.

Gruber, A. R. (1978). *Children in foster care.* New York: Human Science Press.

Juvenile Justice Standards Project (1977). *Standards relating to abuse and neglect.* Cambridge, MA: Ballinger.

Kaufman, J., and Zigler, E. (in press). The prevention of child maltreatment: Programming, research, and policy. In D. Willis, E. Holden, and M. Rosenberg (Eds.), *Child abuse prevention.* New York: Wiley.

Kempe, C. H. and Helfer, R. E. (1972). *Helping the battered child and his family.* Philadelphia: Lippincott.

Kempe, C. H., Silverman, F. N., Steele, B. B., Droegemueller, W., and Silver, H. K. (1962). The battered child syndrome. *Journal of the American Medical Association, 181*, 17–24.

Kempe, R., and Kempe, C. H. (1978). *Child Abuse.* London: Fontana/Open Books.

Koocher, G. P. (Ed.) (1976). *Children's rights and the mental health professions.* New York: Wiley–Interscience.

Lynch, M. (1985). Child abuse before Kempe: An historical literature review. *Child Abuse and Neglect, 9*, 7–15.

Martin, H. P. (Ed.) (1976). *The abused child: Multidisciplinary approach to developmental issues and treatment.* Cambridge, MA: Ballinger.

Mnookin, R. (1973). Foster care: In whose best interest? *Harvard Educational Review, 43*, 599–638.

Nelson, B. (1984). *Making an issue of child abuse.* Chicago: University of Chicago Press.

Parke, R. D. and Collmer, C. W. (1975). Child abuse: An interdisciplinary analysis. In E. Mavis Hetherington (Ed.), *Review of child development research,* Vol. V, 509–590.

Pelton, L. (1978). Child abuse and neglect: The myth of classlessness. *American Journal of Orthopsychiatry, 48*, 608–617.

Polier, J. W. (1975). Professional abuse of children: Responsibility for the delivery of services. *American Journal of Orthopsychiatry, 45*, 357–362.

Radbill, S. X. (1968). A history of child abuse and infanticide. In R. E. Helfer and C. H. Kempe (Eds.), *The battered child.* Chicago: University of Chicago Press.

Rodham, H. (1973). Children under the law. *Harvard Educational Review, 43*, 487–514.

Ross, C. (1980). The lessons of the past: Defining and controlling child abuse in the United States. In G. Gerbner, C. Ross, and E. Zigler (Eds.), *Child abuse: An agenda for action.* New York/Oxford: Oxford University Press.

Spinetta, J. J. and Rigler, D. (1972). The child-abusing parent: A psychological review. *Psychological Bulletin, 77*, 296–304.

Steele, B. F., and Pollock, C. B. (1968). A psychiatric study of parents who abuse infants and small children. In R. E. Helfer and C. H. Kempe (Eds.), *The battered child.* Chicago: University of Chicago Press.

Straus, M. A., and Gelles, R. J. (1986). Change in family violence from 1975–1985. *Journal of Marriage and the Family, 48*, 465–479.

Wald, M. S. (1975). State intervention on behalf of neglected children: A search for realistic standards. *Stanford Law Review, 27*, 985–1040.

Wald, M. S. (1976). State intervention on behalf of neglected children: Standards for removal of children from their homes, monitoring the status of children in foster care, and termination of parental rights. *Stanford Law Review, 28,* 625–706.

Wald, M. S., Carlsmith, J., and Leiderman, P. H. (1988). *Protecting abused/neglected children: A comparison of home and foster placement.* Stanford, CA: Stanford University Press.

Wald, M. S., Carlsmith, J., Leiderman, P., and Smith, C. (1983). Intervention to protect abused and neglected children. In M. Perlmutter (Ed.), *Minnesota Symposium on Child Psychology,* Vol. 16. Hillsdale, NJ: Erlbaum.

Part I

History and definition

1 Definitional issues in child maltreatment

Jeanne Giovannoni

To begin a book such as this with a chapter on defining child maltreatment is at once an indication that the definition of the very subject of the book is problematic and that these problems can be resolved. If such resolution were not possible then how could the research reported in subsequent chapters have been accomplished? In this chapter we look at the evidence that a construct of child maltreatment exists, the problematic nature of its definition, and the potential resolutions of those problems.

Child development scholars engaged in work on child maltreatment confront a situation wherein the subject of their inquiry has been defined by others for a variety of reasons in a number of different arenas. All of the contributors to this book have faced one or more of the following issues in formulating and executing their work and in interpreting the results:

> How widely or narrowly should definitions of child maltreatment be drawn? What are the subcategories that should be included in the construct? Some of the most common are physical abuse, neglect, sexual abuse, and emotional abuse. Other less frequently used but legitimate subtypes include moral/legal issues and educational neglect.
> Definitions of maltreatment will vary depending upon the reasons for which they are needed and the uses to which they will be put; when these conflict, how can choices be made among the resultant (conflicting) definitions?
> Does the issue of parental (or perpetrator) intention play a major role in definitions, and should it?
> Are there universal viewpoints or definitions that transcend history and culture or is child maltreatment only defined relative to time and place?
> Although the sources of child abuse definitions are most often social policy and practice, child development researchers have come to need operational criteria for their work. How well do definitions derived for policy and intervention purposes serve as research definitions?
> How do definitions of child maltreatment shift and change for children of different ages and developmental levels?

3

How can child development research and theory better inform definitions of the construct?

It is the intent of this chapter to provide a context for addressing these questions by examining the historical development of the complex issues in defining child maltreatment, the current status of extant definitions, research devoted to definitional issues, and the implications of all of these for child development research and theory.

We begin with an overview of the evolution of child maltreatment as a social problem, including its enunciation in social policy through institutional responses and legislation, and an examination of the influences of key professions – social work, medicine, and law – on the definitional issues that have emerged. Next, we assess the present status of definitions, both in statutes and the interpretation of those statutes and in the professional literature of the key professions. Research directly relevant to definitions is then examined. The implications of the extant definitional issues for child-development research and alternative resolutions to those issues are then explored. Finally, we deal with the relationship between child development theory and definitions of maltreatment and the potential contributions it can make to the refinement of the construct of maltreatment.

Throughout the chapter the term "maltreatment" is intended to cover the wide range of behaviors and conditions that can be subsumed under the term, such as physical and emotional abuse, neglect, and sexual abuse – indeed, the spectrum covered in the following chapters. Further, though not strictly limited to maltreatment engendered in the family rather than that perpetrated by individuals unrelated to the child, because of the special social policy implications of societal intervention into family life for definitions of maltreatment, familially engendered maltreatment serves as the primary referent in the issues examined.

Evolution of child maltreatment as a social problem

However else child maltreatment might be defined, or for whatever purposes, it is a matter of social policy, one defined for purposes of designating a social problem, a problem worthy of and amenable to social intervention. Over the past 150 years child maltreatment has emerged as a social problem with a complex of sociolegal mechanisms to deal with it. In this section, we examine first the origins of the recognition of child maltreatment, the social institutions that spawned that recognition, and the development of statutory responses to it, including its definition. Next, we look at the development of professional orientations to child maltreatment in social work, medicine, and law and the influences of these orientations on the definitions of the problem and institutional responses.

The institutional core

The identification of child maltreatment as a social problem and the development of social and legal mechanisms to deal with it began in the United States in the nineteenth century. To be sure, analogs of present-day statutes can be found dating back to Colonial times, in local mandates that proscribed particular parental behaviors as being contrary to the community norms and enabling local and religious authorities to intervene into errant families (Morgan, 1966). Our present-day social institutions and statutes, however, had their origins in the early nineteenth century.

The rapid social changes that occurred at this time broke up extended families as many moved from rural areas or from other countries to American cities in search of economic advancement. The economic changes that came with industrialization, the disruptions to families, child labor in factories, and the growth of working and poverty classes, especially in large urban centers, actually increased child suffering, making it increasingly visible to the empowered individuals who became advocates of reform. At first, maltreated children were not singled out for special attention but subsumed into efforts to correct errant and destitute children. In the first half of the nineteenth century, social reformers, many with a strong religious bent, translated their concerns about the moral development of children growing up in the impoverished families of the urban slums into the establishment of institutions to care for such children, chiefly juvenile reformatories and orphanages (Abbott, 1938). It is instructive to note that the earliest treatment of choice was removal of the maltreated child from the abusing family.

In a sense, it might be said that the institutions to deal with these children came first and the legislation enabling public authorities to commit children to them and to allocate public resources for their keep in them came later. State statutes in the latter part of the century followed those enacted earlier at the local level. These statutes were designed to deal with "dependent" children (i.e., children dependent on the state for their care and subsistence), and to this day state laws under which abused and neglected children are handled are to be found in the states' civil codes dealing with "dependent" children.

Legislative actions. The first legislative definitions of abused children had the function of categorizing their situations as ones that brought them under the purview and protection of the dependent child statutes. Generally speaking, these laws identified three categories of parental failure toward children: (1) endangering the morals of their children or allowing others to do so; (2) exhibiting morally reprehensible behavior themselves; and (3) endangering the life and health of children (McCrea, 1910). Notably, the focus of these laws was not so much on the condition of the children as on their parents' failure. And the public concern seemed to be not so much for the immediate suffering of the children but rather for the long-range impact on their moral development into law abiding citizens.

Once identified as dependent, such children were not accorded any special treatment because of abuse or neglect. They were treated as were the vast majority of dependent children (those who were destitute because their parents were dead or could not support them); for the most part, removed to orphanages and foster homes or, until child labor was outlawed, apprenticed or indentured (Folks, 1902). For decades this remained the case, the only change being that, as in-home public relief programs for destitute children and their families expanded, the majority of dependent children became those so categorized because of abuse or neglect rather than destitution. The first legal definitions of abuse and neglect, then, had the purpose of designating situations where states and public authorities had the right to intervene. Beyond that, there was nothing of note about the children, their parents, or their treatment.

The rise of the SPCC. One social institution, created in 1874, did focus specifically on mistreated children – The Society for the Prevention of Cruelty to Children. The SPCC was organized in New York City by the leadership of the Society for the Prevention of Cruelty to Animals after the uncovering of the plight of a child beaten by her stepmother – a child who under existing statutes could not be removed from the woman until she was proven guilty (Robin, 1982). The growth of the organization was rapid. By 1900 there were 161 such organizations either exclusively for children or combined with the protection of animals (McCrea, 1910). In 1877 these societies for children had been incorporated into a national organization: the American Humane Association. The present-day successor of the original Society for the Prevention of Cruelty to Children is the American Association for Protecting Children, a division of the American Humane Association.

For eighty years this organization was the vanguard of distinguishing child abuse as a special and distinct social problem. At first, its various local chapters functioned as a quasi-law-enforcement agency, much as the animal protection agents did, investigating situations of abuse, presenting evidence to and advising courts on dispositions. Equally important, they and the national organization played a strong advocacy role, pressing for legislation that would enable authorities to intervene in situations of maltreatment. In states that relied on existing criminal statutes against "carnal knowledge" and "assault and battery," they pressed for and got legislation specific to children in the criminal statutes and the child dependency laws (Carstens, 1914). In effect, they pressed for expanding the boundaries of the legal definitions of "child abuse."

Their influence in the development of ideas about child abuse derived not only from their role as social advocates, but also through their function as a direct service agency (McCrea, 1910). The initial focus as a law-enforcement agency gradually shifted to a social service function. This may in part have been due to changes in the external environment of the organization.

The establishment of the Juvenile Court and the professionalization of social work. In the early part of the twentieth century the Juvenile Court was established, along with its social service arm – probation. This court, by design both a court of law and a social-service agency, became responsible for the judicial management of "dependent" children and "delinquent" children, and consequently for abused and neglected children under the statutes. Probation officers took on investigatory responsibilities as well as the management and service functions for families and children under the Juvenile Court's jurisdiction. In some cities the local SPCCs performed these functions, but the pattern was by no means uniform (Abbott, 1938).

The other influence that prevailed at the turn of the century was the development of social work as a professional entity – a profession with specialized training and specialized functions and identity. Until that time, many social work endeavors had been indistinguishable from law enforcement, on the one hand, and from charitable good works, on the other. Whatever the impact of these influences, it is clear that the SPCCs took on the character of social work agencies. As early as 1910 (ten years after the establishment of the first Juvenile Court), C. C. Carstens exhorted his colleagues to take on and serve those families of children "whose circumstances are, each week, that the family is left to itself, becoming worse, but which are not yet so bad that court action is advisable or possible" (quoted in McCrea, 1910, p. 153).

This preventive orientation of the SPCCs was slow in evolving, but as decades passed it became the dominant one. In effect, what was created was a parallel definition that constituted situations of abuse and neglect. The statutory delineations continued to exist, but these definers were demarcating an area outside them. In part, they were doing it for the same reason – as a rationale for social intervention and the allocation of social resources. Their interventions were to be distinguished from other charitable organizations, such as family agencies, who also sought to render social work interventions into families' lives. But the objects of such intervention were deemed to be in a special category by themselves. Thus, "abusive and neglectful families" could be distinguished from those served by other social agencies, and the particular ones of concern could be distinguished along a spectrum of families whom the statutes recognized as deserving of court intervention.

Although technically private charitable organizations, the local SPCCs and the national organization, The American Humane Association, can be

considered as enunciators of public social policy. Not only is their legiti-
mation as social agencies dependent upon recognition through public social
policy, their exercise of authority without restraint at the local level is also
a public mandate. So how The American Humane Association and its local
constituents defined child abuse can indeed be considered as a matter of
public social policy. Indeed, it was through their work that the concept of
"professional authority" was developed, not an authority derived from specific legislation but rather community sanction of particular professionals to
intrude on family life without judicial or other legal sanctions, when circumstances of abuse or neglect were susepcted (De Schwainitz and De Schwainitz, 1964).

Evolution of the construct of child maltreatment

Social work refinement. Various professionals within the Humane Association and elsewhere contributed to the definition of child abuse. They
worked on the refinement of designating subcategories – such as neglect as
an act of omission as distinct from abuse as an act of commission. They
further distinguished the realms of a child's life imposed upon by these acts
– the physical and the emotional (Mulford, 1958; Young, 1964). More than
that, however, they contributed to the distinction of child abuse and neglect
as diagnostic entities, situations largely demarcated by parental behavior,
with assumed noxious consequences for their children. In addition, they
proposed formulations of possible etiologies of the parental behavior and
delineated prescriptions for their correction. In 1955 an American Humane
Association publication gave the following definition of child protective
services, a definition that at once captures the designation of the problem,
its etiology, and its corrective:

A specialized casework service to neglected, abused, exploited or rejected children.
The focus of the service is preventive and nonpunitive and is geared toward rehabilitation through identification and treatment of the motivating factors which
underlie the problems. (de Francis, 1955: p. 2)

Through its social advocacy role, the American Humane Association had
influenced the legislative definitions. Through its national leadership and
the practitioners in its constituent agencies, another element was added to
the definitional process – that of professional judgment, judgment made
outside the judicial process and not dependent on the legislative interpretation. Further, with the emphasis on prevention there was an assumption
that abusive and neglectful situations could be predicted and identified
before they were sufficiently manifest to warrant judicial intervention. In
time a professional literature developed that conceptualized these indicators, subtypes, and treatment methods (Kadushin, 1980; Sandusky, 1964).

Until the late 1950s both the definition and the management of child abuse and neglect remained largely the province of the legal and social service systems. Some behaviors were proscribed in criminal statutes and handled through the criminal justice system. A broader spectrum was defined in the dependent child provisions of the civil codes, interpreted by juvenile court personnel, and largely managed through its probation services. Paralleling and complementing these structures, the private social agencies of the AHA and a small but growing number of public child welfare agencies dealt with families independently as adjuncts or alternatives to probation services (AHS, 1967).

In spite of the many thousands of families and children processed through these systems over the years, there was little public awareness of the problem and certainly nothing national in scope beyond the immediate circle of the cadres of professionals concerned.

The "battered child": medical definitions. In the early 1960s this public unawareness changed as a new group of definers came into focus. Led by Dr. C. Henry Kempe of the University of Colorado Medical School, a movement was launched to bring to public consciousness the plight of "the battered child" (Kempe, Silverman, Steele, Droegemueller, and Silver, 1962). Kempe and his colleagues, notably Dr. Ray Helfer (1974), brought about dramatic changes in a few short years. First, they redefined the century-old social problems of child abuse as a medical diagnosis (Newberger and Bourne, 1978). The initial concern was the "battered child," a relatively narrowly defined entity, the diagnosis of which had been made possible through radiological techniques that could detect old bone fractures. But it was not long before this relatively circumscribed phenomenon was broadened to include, in Helfer's words, "physical, nutritional and emotional abuse, one of the most common maladies of the young child" (1974, p. 25). Through their clinical observations and research, Kempe and his colleagues expanded the medical diagnosis to include symptomatic indicators to be found resident both in children and in their abusing parents, etiologic precipitants, and ameliorative treatment modalities. While mindful that both the legal and social service systems also played a part in the management of the problems, they saw such roles as largely secondary, subsidiary to the diagnosis and treatment of a medical phenomenon (Helfer, 1974).

The impact of Kempe and his colleagues went beyond their immediate medical professional circles. They spurred a campaign to have each state pass a law requiring physicians to report cases of child abuse. These efforts to bring the problem of the "battered child" to the attention of state legislators also brought it into public consciousness. In a sense their efforts did not simply redefine the social problem of child abuse as a medical entity; they defined a new problem with the attendant stimulus to do something about it. The campaign for reporting-laws was enormously successful in its short range aim, for within a few years every state had passed such a law (Antler, 1978). But the impact was more widespread and long-lasting. In the public arena – again led by these pediatricians – a new federal agency, the National Center on Child Abuse and Neglect, was created within the United States Children's Bureau. Since its inception, the resources distributed through this Center have been used to expand public awareness through voluntary and community organizations, as well as to conduct research into various facets of the problems and to fund demonstration projects to elucidate and improve the management and treatment of the problem. Largely through these efforts, child abuse has become a common household word.

The legal profession. These developments have not been without controversy, a principal source of which has emanated from the legal profession. (The essence of the controversy is detailed in the next section.) Just as medicine had always been peripherally involved in the treatment of specific cases of child abuse, so lawyers had always been involved in court cases (Katz, 1971). However, their involvement escalated in the early 1970s as juvenile court procedures became more adversarial in nature and concerns for due process forced the recognition of errant parents' rights to counsel. Beyond the legal profession's involvement at the individual case level, there has also been a professional movement to clarify and justify the legal and judicial standards by which situations of child abuse and neglect can be justly and fairly defined.

In sum, over the last one hundred and fifty years child abuse – "cruelty," "neglect," "unfit parents," the "battered child" – has emerged, persisted, and been defined and redefined as an American social problem. Beginning with social and religious reformers of the nineteenth century, various professions and social institutions have emerged as concerned participants in the definition of the problem and in its management. Each has brought its own perspective to the task, conditioned by the particular functions of that profession or institution. Thus, at various times child abuse has been defined in statutes, by judges interpreting those statutes, by social workers intervening in the problem, by medical practitioners managing a medical entity, or by lawyers assuring legal rights.

Present status of definitions

Given this multiplicity of definers, what can be said about their definitions, and what can be said about the agreement among them? Any definition is a classification. It is a means by which some phenomenon or set of events can be set apart from others because its members share commonalities that nonmembers do not share. A strong definition possesses two characteristics:

First, it must delineate a class that can be distinguished from other phenomena and events; second, it must provide criteria under which a specific event can be accurately judged to belong within that class. How do the present definitions of child abuse measure up against these criteria? In answering that question, we look first at some of the available definitions of child abuse, and then at the evidence about their utility.

The vagueness of statutes. In the previous discussion of the historical development of child abuse as a social problem little was said about the actual words used in the various definitions. Although developed at different times and for different purposes, they all share a commonality: They are vague. They are particularly vague in setting the boundaries, even in abstract terms, about what is encompassed and what is not. Typical phrases in the laws (not only the early laws, but also the present ones, including all three sets of laws: the criminal, dependency, and reporting statutes) include such phrases as: "a home or suitable place of abode," "an unfit place by reason of neglect, cruelty, depravity, or physical abuse," "mental suffering," "endangering health," and "failure to maintain a reasonable degree of interest, concern or responsibility for the child's welfare." Were these not vague enough, child dependency statutes – those that empower courts to curtail or terminate parental custody – will almost invariably contain a catchall phrase such as "or any other care necessary for his well-being." This same vagueness is shared by the criminal and the reporting laws in referring to child maltreatment. Criminal statutes, for example, may be quite specific as to what constitutes various degrees and kinds of sexual abuse, but also include phrases such as "or inflicts mental injury." Some reporting laws are quite restrictive and designate as a reportable event the "willful infliction of physical injury," whereas others have sweeping phrases such as "or otherwise interfere with the child's general welfare." Whether in a given state or across state lines, what is encompassed by "maltreatment" varies in the three different kinds of statutes. This is understandable, since each is legislated for a different purpose: Criminal statutes define a criminal act for purposes of prosecution, dependency statutes designate a category of children who may be made wards of the court, and reporting laws bring situations to the attention of responsible authorities. Nonetheless, given these variations in definition, there is no possible assumption that a given set of situations defined under one law will share commonalities with those defined under a different one either in the same state or across state borders.

Interpreting the statutes. The vagueness of the legal definitions is not the only problematic aspect of such definitions. In fact, there is controversy about the utility and desirability of that very vagueness. Many judges oppose the elimination of the catchall phrases because it would "tie their hands" in some individual situations where they think they should properly take protective action (Institute of Judicial Administration, 1977).

There is also controversy about what the standards should be in interpreting the laws. In the 1970s, within the legal profession, an effort was made to rectify the vagueness of definitions and the absence of standards. The Juvenile Justice Standards Project, cosponsored by the American Bar Association, recommended elimination of the terms "neglect" and "abuse" in dependency statutory definitions, suggesting in their place a new term – "endangered child." The proposed definition of an endangered child specified a child suffering from one of six kinds of harm. The standard proposed referred to observable and serious consequences for each of the six kinds of harm. For example, the criteria of "parental negligence" would have been limited to such situations where the neglect had resulted or was likely to result in physical injury. Similarly "sexual abuse" would have been limited to cases where the child was "seriously harmed physically or emotionally" (Institute of Judicial Administration, 1971).

These proposed changes in the statutes and judicial standards were never adopted by the Bar Association and none have subsequently been enacted. The failure to adopt them was largely the result of judicial opposition to the restrictiveness imposed by the criterion of the consequences for the child, regardless of the parental act and the seriousness of those consequences. The definitions of child maltreatment in the legal system thus remain ambiguous and controversial. Notably, however, the controversy is not over *what* constitutes serious consequences for children or abusive and neglectful parental behavior, but rather over what consequences and behaviors the terms *should* encompass for purposes of legitimating the exercise of legal and judicial authority.

If this is the state of affairs in the legal arena, what is the status of definitions in the other professional arenas, namely the medical and the social service? Here, as with the laws, we have a spectrum of specificity and a wide range in the dimension utilized in making definitions.

Medical definition. In medicine, the purpose of a definition is to make a diagnosis; a diagnosis, encompassing more than the delineation of a disease entity, includes an etiology and a suggested course of treatment. Some medical diagnoses are relatively straightforward in establishing the boundaries of the "disease," although less clear with respect to the etiology or the treatment.

Most hospitals today will have some diagnostic category that circumscribes physical injury of children. "Nonaccidental traumas" is a common one. Likely to be considered a form of child neglect, and specifically mentioned in some statutes, is the diagnosis of "failure to thrive." As a type of maltreatment, this diagnosis originated within pediatrics. With respect to nosology, identification of such cases is fairly clear, designating children whose development is deficient in relation to established norms and/or whose physical condition may be incompatible with viability and growth. What is less clear about "failure to thrive" is its etiology. Such a diagnosis might be made in the case of a child who exhibits the deficits, but where no known cause of the deficits can be established. Thus, while "failure to thrive" is an established medical diagnosis, there is some possibility that cases so classified may in fact not all share the same etiology. The conditions of the children may be the same, but the precipitants of those conditions may not be. To be considered a form of maltreatment, definitional criteria must depend on these precipitating factors.

Within the specialties of pediatrics, family medicine, and pediatric psychiatry, a growing literature based on clinical observation and empirical research has developed systematizing diagnostic indicators of various conditions that can be classified as "maltreatment" (Newberger and Bourne, 1978). Within that literature, however, there is some evidence of controversy that would reflect on the reliability of diagnoses. Of principal concern here is not the recognition of symptoms in children in making the diagnoses, but rather the recognition of symptoms in the actual or potential perpetrator of maltreatment. Some have maintained, for example, that maternal behavior and life histories can be utilized as reliable diagnostic indicators and predictors of child abuse and neglect. Others have abandoned the effort to establish certain maternal characteristics or mother–child interactions as useful clinical diagnostic indicators because they simply do not find any that reliably distinguish between the abusive and neglectful and the nonabusive and neglectful (Starr, 1982). The issue as to which maternal characteristics and mother–child interactions, if any, can serve as diagnostic indicators of abuse and neglect remains controversial (Bittner and Newberger, 1982).

It should be noted here that when physicians make diagnoses reflective of maltreatment, or synonymous with a subcategory of maltreatment, they often act in dual roles. This is certainly true of those situations mandated by law as reportable. On the one hand, physicians act as medical diagnosticians; on the other, the treatment to be invoked by their diagnoses is not solely a medical but also a social and legal one. The social and legal consequences may, and in fact do, deter some clinicians from making a diagnosis that would invoke them (Nagi, 1977; Sanders, 1972; Silver, Barton, and Dublin, 1967). There are some circumstances in which, although the physicians may make a medical diagnosis such as improper feeding or under- or over-nourishment, they will not classify the situation as one of maltreatment or neglect, simply because they do not think the situation warrants social or legal intervention. On the one hand, they diagnose as medical experts, but on the other, they define maltreatment as laypersons.

What can perhaps best be said about definitions of maltreatment as medical diagnoses is that they are presently in a state of development. Some categories, such as "failure to thrive," do approximate disease entities that can be diagnosed by trained clinicians. Others, including "non-accidental trauma" and "neglect," call not only for the medical judgments of trained clinicians but also for social judgments about whether given conditions and situations warrant social and legal as well as medical intervention. Such judgments are not made on the basis of medical knowledge alone, but also involve the social values of the reporting physician (Gelles, 1979). Hence, medical definitions of maltreatment can be expected to vary from practitioner to practitioner and from hospital to hospital, and these definitions share the same ambiguities as those observed for legal definitions. Given the same set of facts, one clinician might diagnose maltreatment and another might not.

Social service definitions. Finally, let us look at the state of definitions of maltreatment in the social-service arena. We refer here to that particular aspect of social welfare concerned with the identification of maltreatment as a social welfare function, not to social services geared toward amelioration. In some respects these are inseparable; treatment and service prescriptions are both tied to definition and to etiologic suppositions. In the past, the primary profession involved has been social work, as we noted in our earlier discussion of the historical development of the management of child maltreatment. But today, the professional boundaries are blurred, and certain members of clinical psychology, psychiatry, and other counseling professions consider themselves expert in the treatment of some aspect of child maltreatment. In many jurisdictions they also are likely to be mandated reporters of child abuse and neglect. Indeed, the most highly promulgated response to child maltreatment, even to its identification, is an interdisciplinary one. But those engaged in the treatment of cases once identified do not play a primary role in the identification and labeling of those cases. Rather, they come into the picture after the other actors in the definitional process have played their parts.

The emergence of professionals as experts in the treatment of particular kinds of maltreatment does play an important role in the definitional process, if perhaps a symbolic one. The development of specialized treatments for special problems reinforces the concept that the particular problem categories are distinct entities, separable from others, and, just as with a medical diagnosis, accompanied by a particular etiology and dynamic that is amenable to a particular treatment modality. Whether all or even most of the largely mental health practitioners who treat maltreating families, or particular categories of them, do in fact orient their treatment in a way different from that accorded to those with other identified problems, such as school phobia or behavioral disorders, is not known.

The role played by social service professionals in investigation and identification of maltreatment is more germane to a discussion of definitional issues than is their treatment role. Earlier in our historical review we described the importance of the American Humane Association as a social-service agency contributing to definitions of maltreatment that transcended the legal ones, definitions intended to categorize a spectrum of maltreatment suitable for social agency intervention, but not for court action. Since that time, during the 1970s, public social services have replaced court probation agents as the primary receivers and investigators of reports and complaints of maltreatment and their personnel regularly make recommendations for disposition to the courts (Giovannoni and Becerra, 1979). Because this is now the case, social service identification is guided by the same state laws that guide court intervention. Hence, the need for the addition of extralegal parameters to the definition of maltreatment has been obviated. There has been a dwindling in the professional literature of efforts to establish such definitions or to refine the original ones. In effect, in the last ten years, child maltreatment has been firmly ensconced as a social problem within the purview of the social services and efforts to establish it as such have become redundant.

It is instructive, however, to look at the definitions of maltreatment that have been formulated within the social services arena. They are very like medical diagnostic categories in that they circumscribe situations assumed to be discrete – such as child neglect, emotional abuse, emotional neglect, and physical abuse – not only in the situations described but in the precipitants or etiology of those situations. Unlike some medical diagnoses, however, they do not circumscribe a disease entity with a specific cause and sequelae. Rather, in these definitions the consequences for children are seen to exist along a spectrum, one which concerns the child's development. At the upper level there is optimal development; at the threshold of the categories of maltreatment there is essential or normal development.

These are some examples: Polansky, Hally, and Polansky (1975, p. 5) defined "child neglect" as "a condition in which a caretaker . . . fails to provide one or more of the ingredients deemed essential for developing a person's physical, intellectual and emotional capacities." Similarly, the Child Welfare League of America (1973, p. 5) described a child deserving of protective services as one who is not provided with "the love, care, guidance and protection a child requires for healthy growth and development." Both definitions, and others like them, would then include under the rubric of maltreatment parental behaviors that are anticipated to interfere with long-range development as well as ones where such developmental deficits are already manifest. Certainly such a definitional approach is in direct conflict with that promulgated by members of the legal profession, who would define maltreatment not in relation to the upper limits of optimal development, but at the much lower threshold of "endangerment."

We have looked thus far at the historical development of the emergence and definition of child maltreatment as a social problem and at the status of the definitions promulgated by the various participants in its present definition. There is evidence that boundaries of these definitions at the conceptual level are vague and somewhat amorphous and that the criteria suggested for establishing the fit of an individual case under a given definition are ambiguous and in conflict both across and within the involved disciplines. We now look at the available research evidence about the impact of these ambiguities and conflicts on the definition of categories of maltreatment and the identification of individual cases within these categories.

Research relevant to definitional issues

Although research directly focused on definitional issues has been limited, several pieces of work indicate that there is controversy and disagreement among definers. First, there is research on differential responses and reporting practices with actual cases among official definers. Next, there is opinion survey research that has examined the effects of factors extraneous to the mistreatment on definition within members of the same profession. Finally, there is research that has surveyed definitional agreement across professions.

Differential reporting and responses to actual cases

Some work has been done examining actual reports of child abuse and neglect that has implications for assessing both the level of agreement among definers and the variables that might influence decisions to label a case officially that transcend or interact with the actual maltreatment. Carr (1979) examined 2,989 reports made in Florida between 1971 to 1977. Regardless of the seriousness of the reported maltreatment, reports made by professionals were more likely to be validated than those made by private individuals. Groeneveld and Giovannoni (1977) examined 2,400 reports of child abuse and neglect contributed by five states to the American Humane Association. Validation was related to the interactions of the kind of maltreatment reported, the source of the report, and the recipient of the report. Most likely to be validated were reports of physical injury made by law enforcement personnel to a law enforcement agency. Least likely to be validated were reports of neglect made by private individuals to departments of social services.

The most comprehensive data indicative of definitional dispute and problems among those who could contribute to the categorization of cases of maltreatment comes from the National Study of the Incidence and Severity of Child Abuse and Neglect, funded by the National Center on Child Abuse and Neglect and implemented by the U.S. Department of Health and

Human Services (1981). The object of this research was to establish incidence rates of maltreatment across the nation. Most germane to our discussion is not the incidence rates themselves, but study findings incidental to that major purpose. Through a multistage national sampling procedure, the National Incidence study collected data on cases reported to Child Protective Services (CPS) and on cases not so reported but identified (according to specified study criteria and definitions) by other law enforcement, health, and social welfare agencies. We have here data on a sample of cases (those with a potential for being labeled as "maltreatment") reported to child protective services and a sample not so reported, without such a chance. Inclusion of the unreported cases in the study was an attempt to get at the "real" incidence of maltreatment. Within both the reported and the unreported cases a distinction is made between those that met the research definitions employed by the study and those that did not. The study definitions covered a wide range of maltreatment situations, including physical and sexual abuse, as well as physical, emotional, and educational neglect. The criteria for inclusion – the study definition – was stringent, one where the mistreating behavior "caused foreseeable and avoidable injury or impairment to a child or materially contributed to unreasonable prolongation or worsening of an existing injury or impairment." (U.S. Department of Health and Human Services, 1981, p. 6.)

In a portion of the analysis the study delineates several categories of cases within the entire definitional process. The first consists of those within the reported and not reported cases that were submitted, whether they did or did not meet study criteria. The second includes those reported cases that were or were not "substantiated" by the receiving CPS agency. And the final category, among the unsubstantiated, includes the subcategories of reasons why they were not. Following are the results.

First, among the cases reported to CPS, the study estimates the rate of reporting to be 17.8 children per 1,000 per year. Given an estimated substantiation rate of 42.7, that national estimate drops to 7.6 children per 1,000 per year substantiated by CPS agencies as victims of child abuse or neglect. The variation in substantiation rates among reporters can in part be taken as an indication of differences between key actors in the definitional process. Private individuals accounted for nearly half of the reports to CPS, but only about a third of these reports were substantiated. The major professional report sources were educational, law enforcement, and medical sources (36% of reports), but their substantiation rate, while higher than that of private individuals, was only 53%. The reasons given for lack of substantiation can reflect differences in perception about the definitions of maltreatment and about the functions of child protective services. The largest proportion of the unsubstantiated were rated as "allegation invalid." This might or might not reflect different perceptions, but since many reporting

laws mandate reporting if there is "suspicion," it would not be an indication of definitional difference. One category of reasons does suggest a disparity: "Not serious enough." Surprisingly, this was the largest single category of unsubstantiated cases among the reports, not from private individuals but from law enforcement and educational sources – 39%. Among medical sources of unsubstantiated reports, 52% were found by CPS to be "invalid" and 29% to be "not serious enough." The notion that a given set of cases identified as warranting CPS intervention by one group of definers – the reporters, including professionals – might not be considered "serious enough" by other definers empowered to give that intervention – CPS social workers – underscores the definitional issues in making relative judgments. These cases were all considered to be "valid" cases of maltreatment; the disagreement was around the relative seriousness of the maltreatment as a criterion for intervention.

Aside from differences in perception among individual professional definers, systemic factors also seemed to be related to the substantiation of reports. Substantiation rates were found to vary on an urban–rural dimension. Rural counties were estimated to have the highest incidence of substantiated reports (9.7 children per 1,000) and suburban the lowest (4.5 children per 1,000). Within the urban–surburban–rural categories, counties with relatively high rates of reporting tended to substantiate lower proportions of their reports than those with relatively low rates of reporting. The investigators hypothesized that agency resources and service capabilities establish the upper boundary on the number of cases that can be handled by individual agencies and that substantiation rates are more likely to reflect such constraints than the actual extent of child abuse or neglect in the community. The work by Groeneveld and Giovannoni (1977) on five states' reports contributes data to support this hypothesis. When the data from the 48 counties in the five states were aggregated, correlations were found between the rates of substantiation and the ratio of each county's welfare needs to welfare expenditures. Counties with a favorable ratio were more likely to generate a large volume of reports but to substantiate a significantly lower proportion. Those with a less favorable ratio generated fewer reports but substantiated a larger volume. This suggests that the level of a county's resources will influence not only substantiation rates but also reporting behavior itself.

A second part of this data from the National Incidence study reflects on the homogeneity of cases under the rubric "substantiated," those deemed to warrant intervention. When the sample of substantiated cases was screened according to the study criteria, only 44.5% passed the screening. The study criteria, as noted, were quite stringent. CPS intervention of some kind might well have been warranted within the proper scope of CPS functions and still not meet evidence of study criteria of "injury or impairment." Still, the data do indicate the heterogeneity among a sample of cases considered suitable for intervention.

The design of the study aimed at getting at the true incidence of maltreatment. Cases that had not been reported to CPS were collected from other investigatory agencies (law enforcement, public health, and probation) and from other social and health agencies (hospitals, schools, social agencies, and mental health facilities). These cases were submitted to the study and screened according to the criteria. A much higher percentage of these – 65.1% – met the study criteria. This was to be expected, because the study criteria were the only ones used in submitting these unreported cases to the study. Although this was so, the large proportion of cases that were submitted and did not meet the criteria may indicate the difficulty of fitting specific cases into a definition of maltreatment, even one so circumscribed as this one. Again, the element of relative judgments comes into focus and the reliability of those judgments is called into question.

The National Incidence Study report does not explain why those agencies that submitted new cases had not reported them to CPS. It does give comparative data on the characteristics of the reported and unreported cases. Two features stand out: the ages of the children and the kinds of maltreatment. Sixty percent of the children under age 6 who met the study criteria had been reported, whereas 78% of such children aged 12–17 had not been reported. Less than 25% of the cases designated as "emotional abuse," "emotional neglect," or "educational neglect" had been reported. Keeping in mind that all of the children among the unreported cases were "known" to one of the participating agencies, what we may have here is evidence that the boundaries between "maltreatment" and other problems, such as those dealt with by mental health practitioners or probation and truant officers, may be blurred and overlapping. Thus, it would appear that some definitions of some kinds of maltreatment in fact do not clearly delineate a class of events that can be unambiguously distinguished from those encompassed by other classifications, including classes of other social problems.

The conclusions of this study on the final estimates of the incidence of child maltreatment give evidence of wide variations introduced into the definitional process by the actual and potential definers. Yearly national incidence estimates based only on CPS substantiated cases that met study criteria calculated 3.4 children per 1,000. When cases submitted by other investigatory agencies are included, this figure rises to 4.6 per 1,000. And when cases submitted by other agencies are included, the national estimate is 10.5 cases per 1,000, or 652,000 children per year. This, the authors point out, is a very conservative estimate dependent upon their sampling procedures and criteria. Other estimates have ranged from 1,000,000 to 6,000,000 children per year. It may well be that pursuit of a single, national incidence figure is a vain effort. The only answer to how many children are maltreated annually may be "It all depends on to whom you are talking and what they are talking about."

Opinion survey research

Definitional disparities within professions. It would be wrong to leave the impression that the official labeling of cases of maltreatment and the observable variation in such labeling is due solely to differences in definitions of maltreatment. Opinion surveys indicate that disparities exist even among members of the same profession and that these are related to factors extraneous to the maltreatment itself. The disparities make sense if we keep in mind that the purpose of official designation is to take official action. Such action includes both interfering in family life and allocating social resources to alleviate the problems. Hence, considerations other than the actual incidents of maltreatment come sensibly into play. These include the conditions under which the maltreatment took place and the behavior and attitudes of the maltreating parents in relation to the agents of intervention. Beyond these, several other variables extraneous to the maltreatment situation have been examined. Investigators have explored a variety of factors that might impinge on definitions and perceptions of child maltreatment. These include work setting, community variables, professional discipline, and mitigating circumstances beyond the actual maltreatment.

Billingsley (1964; see also Billingsley, Giovannoni, and Purvine, 1969) conducted three surveys that examined the effects of work setting and community variables on the perceptions of members of the same profession. Using vignettes intended to describe various neglect and abuse situations, he inquired into social workers' perceptions of the causes and recommended treatment for each of the hypothetical situations. If it can be assumed that professionals' perceptions of the cause of and suitable treatment for a problem will influence their actions in disposing of it, Billingsley's work will have relevance to definition in the sense of official labeling. Different perceptions of a problem can influence what systems are sought for resolution and hence how problems might be officially labeled. In the first study (1964), he compared the responses of social workers in a private child protective agency with those working in a family counseling agency. Responses from workers in the family agency indicated that they perceived both cause and treatment of the situations to be psychological in nature, whereas those in the protective agency responded in much more socially oriented terms. In a related work, Billingsley compared the responses of social workers in specialized child protective units in public welfare agencies with those in generalized service units. He inquired about their perceptions of the proper kind of dispositions in hypothetical abuse and neglect vignettes. Responses differed on the dimension of a legalistic versus a therapeutic intervention, e.g., provide counseling and environmental supports versus seek court intervention. Protective service workers significantly more frequently elected the therapeutic and generalized services workers the legalistic intervention option.

Billingsley et al. (1969) also investigated the effects of community variables in a similar survey of social workers in public social services. Using indexes such as the amount of welfare expenditures and the degree of autonomy of welfare administrators, he divided the communities studied into "repressive" or "supportive" ones. Using the same vignette technique, he found workers in the repressive communities to be more legalistic in their responses and those in the supportive ones more therapeutically oriented.

This attitudinal work would seem to complement the findings on the effects of systemic variables on child maltreatment report validation described earlier. Thus, Billingsley's opinion surveys and the data on substantiation rates do suggest that both work setting and community systems variables influence the perception and definition of child abuse and neglect.

Surveys of physicians indicate that in making a diagnosis of child abuse or neglect they are influenced by the intentions of the parents and by their social and economic circumstances. Gelles (1977) reported that in his survey of 157 physicians, 97% agreed that malnutrition was child abuse when the situation was presented to them as willfully inflicted, but only 16% so classified a situation of malnutrition when it was described as due to parental ignorance.

In this same survey Gelles reported that 5% stated that race and ethnicity of a caretaker were so important in making a diagnosis that they could file a child abuse report based on these characteristics alone. Turbett and O'Toole (1980) studied the attitudes of 76 pediatricians by presenting them with a set of vignettes, each describing a situation potentially classifiable as child abuse and in each of which three factors were systematically varied: the socioeconomic status of the caretaker, the ethnicity of the caretaker, and the severity of injury to the child. They found an interactive effect of these variables on the pediatricians' recognition of child abuse. In the presence of severe injuries black children were nearly twice as likely to be seen as victims of child abuse than were children described as white. Similarly, children described as lower class whites were more likely to be seen as abused than were upper class white children depicted as suffering the same major injury.

These findings indicate that physicians, like social workers, are apt to be influenced by factors extraneous to the maltreatment itself in making a diagnosis and in reporting situations so diagnosed.

Interprofessional perceptions. Several investigations have been made of differences in perceptions of maltreatment attributable to professional and disciplinary affiliations. The data on substantiations of reports from various disciplines as well as the variations in definitions and criteria espoused in the literature of different professional groups would suggest that professionals do have discrepant perceptions of child maltreatment. The work done using survey techniques bears out these disagreements but also points to some substantial areas of relative consensus.

One of the earliest studies was done by Boehm (1962) who surveyed 1,400 community leadership groups' perceptions of child neglect. Included were lawyers, physicians, social workers, educators, nurses, clergy, and business managers. Boehm used vignettes and asked respondents to indicate the kind of intervention they would employ in such situations, ranging from nonintervention to coercive intervention. Social workers, clergy, nurses, and teachers were significantly more likely to perceive a need for intervention than were lawyers or business managers.

Boehm explained her findings as a reflection of differences in the respective groups' work settings: The former work in bureacratized settings, whereas the work of the latter is organized along entrepreneurial lines. Those with an entrepreneurial orientation, she posited, were most likely to adhere to values of individual freedom, legal rights, and minimal intervention into family matters.

Gelles (1977) used a similarly diverse group of 476 respondents, presenting them with 13 different circumstances and asking if they considered each to be "child abuse." The harms to the children depicted were similar – physical injury and malnutrition – but the depictions varied on a dimension of willfulness of the perpetrator. For example, willful physical injury was varied with injury due to poor housing. Overall, Gelles found relatively high agreement among the respondents when the conditions presented were "willful." Responses were much more widely discrepant when mitigating circumstances were introduced. Gelles did not report consistent findings of disagreement by discipline, but was of the opinion that the general level of disagreement that he found did not augur well for consistent and reliable definition across disciplines in actual practice.

Lena and Warkov (1978) surveyed 558 respondents, including judges, nurses, social workers, and teachers. They presented respondents with six conditions identical to those used by Gelles and asked which of these conditions evoked the term "child abuse." They also presented the respondents with nine possible causes, ranging from immaturity to sadism. They used factor analysis in interpreting their data and reported substantial commonalities. Two different kinds of phenomena were identified by all of the professionals as constituting "child abuse," "neglect," and "physical abuse." These causes were dualized as "psychological rejection" and "uncontrollable behavior." The authors concluded that there is substantial homogeneity among professionals as to what constitutes "child abuse."

Our own work (Giovannoni and Becerra, 1979) covered a much more extensive range of acts that might be considered as maltreatment than any of the above. Opinions about these acts were surveyed among a sample of 313 professionals and 1065 lay or general population respondents. The professionals included lawyers, police officers, and social workers, all engaged in identifying and handling maltreatment as part of their work, and a sample of pediatricians, all mandated to report child abuse. We report first on the study of professionals.

The technique used was the presentation of vignettes to respondents, who were asked to rate each depicted action on a scale from one to nine as to the seriousness of the act for the welfare of the child. Among professionals the child was described as being seven years old. The vignettes were constructed so that 78 depicted only parental or caretaker behaviors in 14 hypothetical areas. For each of the 78 a companion vignette was composed that depicted not only the action but also a consequence for the child. For example, a stem vignette read, "The parent banged the child's head against the wall while shaking him by the shoulders." With the added consequence, the vignette read, "The parent . . . shoulders. The child suffered a concussion." Vignettes were constructed for 14 hypothetical categories of maltreatment, including physical injury, emotional maltreatment, parental sexual immorality, nutritional neglect, and lack of supervision. Within each category an attempt was made to depict acts of varying seriousness.

Respondents were presented with a random sample of the vignettes (78 with and 78 without consequences served as the base pool of vignettes from which the sample presentations of 60 were drawn). Each respondent was asked to rate each vignette as to the seriousness for the welfare of the child. Respondents were not asked to classify the acts as abuse or neglect, only to rate the seriousness of each. Four questions were posed in the analysis of the professionals' ratings. The results are reported here for each of the questions, all of which were intended to answer the question, "How do professionals define child maltreatment?"

What effects did the addition of a consequence have on ratings? Are some acts considered as serious maltreatment regardless of the consequences for the child? (Here it should be noted that although the vignettes within a given category were designed to capture relative seriousness, this was not so with the consequences. Rather, these were composed with the simple intent that the consequence be one likely to occur as a result of the act described.) For virtually all of the groups of professional ratings, the addition of a consequence increased the seriousness rating. There were some exceptions – namely among the pediatricians, where the addition of the consequence decreased the rating, no doubt indicating their professional expertise in delineating the relative seriousness of various physical conditions for children. The general pattern, however, was that although the addition of a consequence increased the seriousness rating, it did not distort the relative rating given to any particular vignette. This suggests that specific parental actions can be judged, at least as to their relative seriousness, apart from the consequences for the children. Notice of the consequences increases the rating, but does not disrupt the pattern of ratings.

What was the extent of agreement among respondents as to the absolute and relative seriousness of specific incidents of maltreatment? Each profession's ratings of all 78 vignettes were compared. Statistical analyses tested the particular combinations of professionals who did agree and those who deviated in the ratings of each vignette. Overall, the police and social workers were the ones most often in agreement (73% of the time) and both tended to rate the incidents as more serious than did either the pediatricians or the lawyers. The lawyers were most often in disagreement with all others (about 45% of the time), and they definitely tended to rate the incidents as less serious. Pediatricians' overall ratings tended to fall in the middle, but were much more often in agreement with police and social workers than were the lawyers (pediatricians 40%, lawyers 13% of the time). Thus, with respect to the absolute ratings of the seriousness of these wide-ranging acts of maltreatment, there was significant and extensive disagreement. There also was considerable agreement between particular professional groups. Although the disagreement was considerable, it was not random.

Our next questions concerned the professionals' perceptions of underlying commonalities of the specific incidents. The vignettes themselves had been hypothesized to fall into 14 categories of behaviors. Using the ratings, we posed the question, "Do professionals perceive common categories of maltreatment?" The answer was clearly, "Yes, they do." A principal components factor analysis of the ratings was interpreted to result in 9 categories of maltreatment. In general, the items that had been hypothesized as falling into common categories were amazingly similar to those derived from the professionals' ratings. Seven of the original categories remained virtually intact with the exception of one or two items. The major divergence from the original categories was the merging of those subcategories that dealt with the physical neglect of children – i.e., nutrition, medical care, clothing, and hygiene. In the analysis these emerged as a single factor within which all items had the commonality of failing to provide for some aspect of children's physical needs.

Thirteen of the original vignettes failed to correlate with any of the derived categories. These are interesting to note because they may illustrate professionals' perceptions of the boundaries of child maltreatment. These 13 vignettes dealt either with very extreme or bizarre behavior, such as locking a child in a room for years, or with marginal environments such as overcrowding and disreputable neighborhoods.

Do professionals agree on the relative seriousness of specific incidents of child maltreatment? In both the analysis of separate vignettes and a comparison of the relative rankings of the average ratings of the categories of maltreatment, there was considerable agreement among the professional groups. In rank order by mean ratings for each, the nine categories were as follows: physical abuse, sexual abuse, fostering delinquency, lack of supervision, emotional maltreatment, alcohol/drug use, failure to provide physical necessities, education neglect, and deviant parental mores. There was some slight variation for one or another professional grouping in this ordering of their rankings, but the overall patterning was essentially the same.

These data do suggest that professionals are not at such loggerheads about the definition of child maltreatment as might be supposed. Very crucially, they do see underlying commonalities among different kinds of actions, and they agree on the relative seriousness of these common sets of maltreatment subcategories. They do disagree on the valuations that are put on specific incidents and on given categories. What this suggests is that professionals dealing with maltreatment in their work do agree on what they see and share a common perception of what is or potentially is child maltreatment. They differ in the social valuations that they put on specific types of maltreatment. This does not suggest definitional chaos. Particularly from the standpoint of researchers, it is possible to select populations that have been exposed to similar sets of conditions and that can be recognized by professionals as having shared characteristics. The differing social valuations can be handled. What is important is that operational definitions of maltreatment can be formulated. Research consumers may agree or disagree as to whether the definitions do constitute maltreatment or, if they do, how serious that maltreatment is, but they can do so on a sound and objective basis of fact. That professionals disagree, particularly professionals who perform different functions in the overall official designation of cases for intervention, does not mean that the ultimate definitions are either idiosyncratic or random. They do indeed have meaning.

Public opinion. Having reviewed research on professionals' concepts of maltreatment, we should note what is known about the general populations. The data previously reviewed on the reporting of child abuse and the substantiation of these reports suggest that the lay population may be somewhat at odds with the professionals. It also suggests that the general public is a salient definer of maltreatment. The majority of reports come from them and the majority of their reports are not substantiated. Despite speculations in the literature that child maltreatment is somehow related to a greater tolerance for abuse or neglect among some population groups, particularly lower income and ethnic minorities, all evidence is to the contrary, both that noted about the sources of reports and that available from survey research.

Polansky et al. (1981) surveyed 57 working-class and 58 middle-class mothers. Using his Childhood Level of Living scale as a basis, he asked these respondents to rate each of the 214 items on a scale ranging from "should be reported to legal authorities" to "excellent care." Polansky's scale is intended to capture child neglect and hence does not deal with physical or sexual abuse. It also includes descriptions of optimal child care and thus might be considered to tap the outer edges of the boundaries of maltreatment. The interclass comparisons of their sample respondents revealed startling similarities and it was concluded that despite differences in education and other socioeconomic indicators the mothers in the respondent groups were indeed homogeneous in their evaluations of basic elements in child care.

The same vignettes reported in our study of professionals conducted in Los Angeles were used with a randomly selected area household sample of the general population and similar analyses were performed. The lay population overall rated all vignettes as more serious than did the professionals. Factor analyses of their ratings indicated that, although they did not make as fine a distinction as did the professionals among subtypes of maltreatment, they did indeed see separate categories. Analyses of their ratings yielded five categories rather than the nine derived from the professionals. The major difference was a commingling of items dealing with basic physical, educational, and emotional aspects of child care. Physical abuse, sexual abuse, lack of supervision, and drug usage were similar to the professionals'. Most interesting about the general population survey were the marked ethnic and social class differences in the perceptions of the relative seriousness of different kinds of child maltreatment. Again, as with the professionals, the lay populations made distinctions as to subtypes and as to the relative seriousness ascribed to the subtypes. They differed by ethnic group, within ethnic group, and by social class in the relative valuations placed on the seriousness of the different subtypes. In general, black respondents, regardless of social class, rated matters pertaining to supervision and basic child care as more serious than did other respondents. Hispanic respondents rated as more serious matters pertaining to sexual abuse and sexual mores, and these differences from other ethnic groups were more pronounced within the Hispanic population. English-speaking and less well educated respondents rated these matters as even more serious than did their better educated English-speaking counterparts. Among white respondents, lower education and income was also related to ratings of greater seriousness.

These data would certainly suggest that child maltreatment is not something that is of concern or understanding only to professionals. Indeed, if anything, they may bespeak a greater concern among lay people, albeit one that differs in specifics by ethnicity and social class.

If nothing else, these data speak to the complexity of the impact of both social class and ethnicity on perceptions of child maltreatment. The notion that the labeling of maltreatment by white middle-class professionals is simply an imposition of their values on lower-class people who are not white is clearly an overly simplistic one. Certainly both social class and culture influence perceptions of deviant child rearing just as they do ideas about normal or acceptable care. However, in the face of what we presently know, great caution must be used in making any generalizations about the content and direction of those inferences with reference to any group.

Implications for research and theory

We have seen that the definition of child maltreatment in its various forms of child abuse and neglect has emerged and persisted as a lay term and has been adopted and defined in various ways by different professions. Through social policies, child maltreatment has been established as a social problem, and a diverse set of social institutions have emerged to manage it. Only recently have policymakers and practitioners looked to the social and behavioral scientists and to child development specialists for enlightenment and understanding of the problems they have identified. With rare exceptions, such as failure to thrive, phenomena have first been identified as harmful to children by scientists and then defined into policy as maltreatment. Child development researchers and theoreticians have thus been asked to study and explain phenomena that have not emerged or been identified out of their own body of knowledge.

The demands made by the policymakers and practitioners have been far reaching: to find the cause, to predict the occurrence, to find methods of prevention, and to prescribe techniques of amelioration. Rarely have these demands sought to refine definitions or to clarify standards and criteria for making individual case designations, whether the criteria be "endangerment," "essentials for development," or "optimal development." Ambiguity surrounds the concepts of the nature of the problem in public policy definition and the locus of child maltreatment in the array of social problems addressed by public policy. This is evident in the variety of public funding sources for research: a child welfare agency, the National Center of Child Abuse and Prevention; a mental health agency, the National Institute of Mental Health; and a law enforcement agency, the National Center on Crime and Delinquency.

This pattern of events is not unusual. It is, in fact, typical of the application of the social and behavioral sciences to the solution of social problems. The study of "juvenile delinquency" has followed an identical course. It was first identified as a separate category of criminal behavior by social reformers who sought special and more lenient treatment for errant children. It was only after this designation was made in social policy that sociologists and then psychologists sought to understand this special class of children, not this special class of criminals. And over the decades the statutory definitions both of "juvenile" and of "delinquent" have changed. A more recent example concerns the attention being paid to "teenage pregnancy and parenthood."

What are the implications of this state of affairs for the conduct of child development research and theory in child maltreatment? What are the implications for the advancement of child development knowledge and for the relationship between child development research and theory and the formulation and implementation of public social policy? We look first at definitions of maltreatment in the conduct of research and then at issues in the conceptualization of maltreatment in theoretical development.

Research implications

What are the options available to the child development investigator engaged in studying some facet of child maltreatment in defining the populations to be studied? There would seem to be at least three. The first is the acceptance of definitions made by official agencies, child protective services, and the courts. The second is to ignore such official designations and to create one's own definitions or criteria for selecting and designating study samples and populations. The third is to employ a combination of both approaches. We look at the relative advantages and disadvantages of each within the context of the different research purposes that are undertaken.

We must first note, however, that the vantage points of researchers vary. Some will be operating from positions totally outside of and unrelated to official agencies or clinical settings where cases of child maltreatment are identified and handled. Frequently this is the case with university based investigators or those in independent research organizations and foundations. Others may be in clinical settings, such as hospitals, where designations of maltreatment are ongoing or where maltreated children and their parents may be under treatment. And some may actually be a part of the official labeling systems attached to Child Protective Services and the courts, such as clinical psychologists. The options available to each of these three vantage points will vary, as will the access to potential study populations, and all options will be conditioned by the purposes and methods of the research.

Reliance on officially designated cases. As could easily be anticipated from the foregoing discussion on the ambiguity and controversy that surrounds the definitions of maltreatment, sole reliance on official designation as the definition of study populations is fraught with problems. First of all, the official designation is the result of a negotiated process. Some cases are observed and not reported, some are reported and not acted upon, and some make it through to the stage of official designation. Although we know something of the facts that enter into the screening-out process in this negotiation, and something about the attitudes and opinions of the participants in it, we do not know how these forces affect the designation of any given set of cases. Second, what constitutes the actual maltreatment that has occurred – in officially designated cases – is given in only the grossest terms: "physical abuse," "neglect," "sexual abuse," "emotional abuse." No indication of relative seriousness is given, and no indication of combinations of different types of maltreatment is explored. The most that can be assumed is that a case designated as "neglect" had no known manifestations of physical abuse, although even this cannot be certain, because the case may be so designated for purposes of disposition when there is evidence to prove the neglect but not the physical abuse. Whether one is undertaking the research to investigate the effects of maltreatment or to predict it on the basis of earlier observed parental characteristics, the fuzziness of definition of such crucial independent or dependent variables does not augur well for the research outcomes. We have presented some evidence that factors extraneous to the given maltreatment situation may play a part in official designation. These may include social class biases among the definers but, more importantly, they may also reflect factors totally extraneous to the given maltreatment situation, such as the level of available resources to manage cases in relation to the demand for such resources.

The implications of these potential definitional problems are twofold. One relates to the heterogeneity of a given population selected by these criteria and the other to the generalizability of the results of research so designed. With respect to generalizability, the most one can do is to hope that a sample of cases drawn from one system are like cases drawn from any other system. The previously reported data on systemic variation in the substantiation of cases indicates there may well be limitations here, but there is simply no way of knowing the extent of those limitations. When research results on cases drawn from different populations are similar, this is not a problem. When they differ, however, the degree of variation due to sampling alone cannot be estimated. With respect to the heterogeneity issue, the problem is straightforward. One simply runs a strong risk of a Type II error due to the unknown and therefore uncontrolled variance introduced by the population selection process. This is so whether maltreatment is considered as the dependent, intervening, or independent variable. If the aim of the study is prediction, using official designation as the dependent variable is subject to all of the capriciousness noted. If populations of children are selected with the assumption that they have undergone some form of maltreatment, the potentially wide variations in their actual experiences may militate against finding significant differences between their developmental progress and that of children assumed not to have undergone such experiences.

Finally, there is the probability that factors resident in the parents and children but extraneous to the maltreatment may play a part in official designation – factors such as race and social class, willingness to seek or accept help, and aggressiveness in resisting outside interferences. It is possible to control for the former, less so for the latter. In any case, these extraneous variables, although they may be of paramount interest to the sociologist studying deviance, are simply a source of extraneous variance to the child development investigator.

In essence, then, we have two types of overlapping problems that face investigators who rely solely on official designations for the selection of populations of mistreating parents or mistreated children: uncontrolled systemic variations in the designation, and uncontrolled variance in the populations under study. The former limits the generalizability of the results and their comparability to the population drawn for the particular study conducted. The latter, the heterogeneity problem, militates against positive findings and the validation of potentially useful and accurate theoretical formulations. When either or both situations prevail, the resulting research will fail to inform correctly and thus expand our understanding of child maltreatment.

Definitions made by researchers. The second resource for investigators is simply to eschew any reference to official designation and to construct their own definitions. The major problem here is whether the study populations or the parental behaviors selected for study have any meaning as maltreatment outside the purviews of the research setting. Although such studies are perfectly respectable endeavors within the field of child development, their utility and validity in enhancing our understanding of maltreatment as it is used in enunciating public policy is highly questionable. Indeed, such research definitions may be the purest in a scientific sense, but that very purity may render them inapplicable outside the research setting or, worse yet, inappropriate to the policy setting, should they be so used.

Again, keeping in mind that the policy need is for guidelines and criteria for taking action, we must especially question the use of research that investigates maternal behaviors without relevance to the developmental impact on children, or that investigates maternal behavior as a potential contributor or intervening variable in the precipitating circumstances of effects on children that might be considered as maltreatment.

Such research clearly has its place in enhancing understanding. However, if the research itself is included under the rubric of research on "maltreatment" only on the basis of the researchers' definition of maltreatment, there is the danger that the results themselves might be added to the ongoing definitions. For example, research on bonding and attachment insofar as it might be considered to reflect maltreatment must be treated very cautiously.

Should the failure to "bond" be considered as maltreatment in and of itself or as an intervening variable that, in concert with other factors, may eventuate in maltreatment? This is a very crucial question. But if mothers who never have had a chance to demonstrate how they will take care of their babies are labeled through the child development literature as "maltreating" or as "neglectful," the circumventing of the crucial evidence may indeed have a noxious effect on the understanding of maltreatment. The effects may be indirect, but nonetheless forceful. Child development research can be very influential simply on the basis of who the investigators were and the significance of their research. Two examples are paramount.

First, there is Bowlby's (1969) classic report on institutionalized children in World War II. There is scarcely an essay on "child neglect" that does not refer to that work as testimony to the extreme consequences of "neglect." If anything, Bowlby's work should be considered a classic in research on institutional neglect, and in fact it has had a profound impact on institutional practices, but it is also used to bolster pleas that more resources be devoted to ameliorating and apprehending parental neglect.

The second example concerns the work of Goldstein, Freud, and Solnit reported in *Beyond the Best Interests of the Child* (1979). This work has had a profound effect on policies related to the management of maltreated children. Yet, in fact, none of the documentation reported in the book involved such children. Its application to situations of abuse and neglect was promulgated by the authors' extrapolation to these situations. Nonetheless, the concept that the most profound impact on a child's psychological well-being comes from separation from the "psychological parent" has had a direct impact on establishing criteria for defining child maltreatment (i.e., the criteria for the least detrimental course of action is that remaining in the situation of maltreatment would be more detrimental to the child than would separation from its psychological parents).

No implication is being made here that child development research should be constrained in any way by social and legal institutions outside its purview. Child development investigators must research whatever variables they see fit – maternal deficiency, developmental lags in children, cognitive stimulation of preschoolers, and so forth. The problem arises when they label such research as dealing with maltreatment. They cannot be held responsible for extrapolations others make from their research, but they can be held responsible when their research, labeled as maltreatment investigation, is used in policy formulation and implementation, even if the outcomes of those policies were never their intent.

One problem with research on child maltreatment in which the investigators rely solely on their own definitions, without any reference to official designation of cases, is in the utility of such research findings for populations so designated. There is the noted danger of misapplication and the corresponding possibility that potentially useful findings will not be applied to such populations because extrapolations cannot be made based on the idiosyncratic definitions. These problems, however, can be mitigated if the investigators use specific operational definitions of the maltreatment they are studying (see next section). For example, if they are trying to predict the occurrence of "neglect," there are clear behavioral indicators of what constitutes the predicted neglect, such as "not feeding," "leaving alone," or "not talking to." With clear operational definitions there is greater potential for transferability, or at least informed judgment about applicability. Of course, this is also true in comparing results across studies. Without such operational definitions, it is just as problematic to compare research findings across studies in which investigators have defined their own populations as it is to compare studies that rely solely on officially designated but otherwise undefined populations.

There may also be practical and even legal reasons why research based only on investigators' definitions may be problematic. When studying reportable conditions of maltreatment, the investigators may be liable to statutory mandates to report such cases. This is apt to be especially true of those in clinical settings, where even if the investigator might not be mandated to report, the institutions might be.

Combined definitional approaches. A third option to the resolution of research definitions is a combination of the official designation and the researcher's own. Essentially, this entails seeking cases out of officially designated populations and subjecting them to independent measures. This method may be used in predictive studies, follow-up studies, and cross-sectional laboratory results.

In a predictive study, official designation might be utilized as one measure of the dependent variable – maltreatment of some specified kind – and the investigator can then develop a second index to measure the specifics and severity of the maltreatment. The same or similar measures might be utilized with the nonidentified portions of the sample as further checks on the occurrence of the maltreatment and on the validity of the final classifications used in analysis. Cases among the officially designated that do not meet the criteria specified in the measurement could be culled. A similar approach can be used in selecting cases for laboratory observation or in other designs investigating the sequelae of maltreatment, familial interaction, or maternal characteristics. The combined approach has been used in some of the studies reported in this book. It has the advantage of circumventing the ambiguities that surround the identification of maltreatment by agencies, clarifying types of maltreatment and degrees of severity. This advantage should make measurement of the variability in maltreatment optimally robust and reduce extraneous variance. Further, it has the advantage over idiosyncratic definitions of being more appropriately generalizable to other populations.

There is another reason why this combined approach is desirable, one that is more ethically bounded than research oriented. The children and their families who pass through our protective agencies and courts really are the reasons for the public interest and the public investment in research. That the research so generated should have direct applicability to their situations seems only just. Orienting research toward these populations seems more prudent as well as more useful in policy formulation.

Theoretical implications

What should be the relationship between child development research and theory and the social problem of child maltreatment? What kinds of contributions can child development knowledge make toward the definitional issues that persist in social policies and among institutions that manage the problem? There are at least two ways in which such a contribution might be made. The first is in the provision of objective information about the effects of maltreatment on children. The second, even more important, way is through continuing clarification of the concept itself and the development of empirically based theory.

Child development knowledge and definitional objectivity

Social and legal definitions of child maltreatment are and will remain matters of social value judgments. Rationales for intervention will continue to be based on the negotiated compromises of a complex array of interests. In this sense, there can be no definition of maltreatment outside of a given social context. This does not mean, however, that the information on which such judgments are to be made cannot be objectively based. Providing such information is a fundamental contribution child development research can make at a descriptive level. It is certainly possible to improve the basis on which definitions are made and decisions about intervention are implemented.

The more that is known about the consequences, immediate and long-range, of specific situations of maltreatment, the more informed the judgments that can be made about appropriate interventions. There is much to be learned but, as the research reported in this book indicates, strong beginnings have been achieved. Describing and measuring the effects of known maltreatment on children can serve as the basis for making judgments, whether the criteria be "endangerment" or "less than optimal development." The relative seriousness of the consequences may remain subjective social judgments, but those judgments cannot be made without knowledge of the consequences. Relative judgments may still be made about the importance of various aspects of children's development – cognitive, physical, and emotional – but the information has to be there first. Hence, a crucial role for the child development researcher is really that of an independent assessor.

Insofar as the research investigators are independent of and outside the definitional process, they need not be bound by the criteria employed by that process in making their judgments. Very crucially, they can select the consequences to be studied and measured, and in so doing enlarge the picture of the total consequences of maltreatment and thus proactively influence its definitions. A broken bone due to physical attack may be a useful operational definition of child abuse but, from the standpoint of children, the consequences may be far more extensive, just as the experience itself, in its totality, reaches far beyond the broken arm. The bruise or red welt that may not be considered "serious" enough to be classified as child abuse may, from the standpoint of the child recipient's total experience, have a value virtually identical to that of the child with a broken arm. Thus, although child development research and accumulated knowledge may bring more objectivity to our existing definitions of child maltreatment and currently designated harms by describing and measuring their consequences on the children's development, they can actually do much more. The ultimate purpose of defining maltreatment is to protect children against it. The definitions should logically be child-centered. But, of necessity, adults must make the definitions. Perhaps the most important contribution the child development investigator can make is to explore fully, from the standpoint of children and their development, the range of the consequences of the maltreatment so defined, whether these consequences be of concern to the adults or not. In this we might come to develop definitions that are more fully child-centered than those we now have.

Child development theory and the construct of child maltreatment

Beyond mere definition there is a continuing need to clarify and expand the construct of maltreatment. The definitions we have reviewed are complex. Indeed, part of the definitional confusion stems from the failure to distinguish the component parts of the definitions. Situations of maltreatment are designated in part by parental or caretaker behaviors and the resulting effects of those behaviors on children. The ultimate purpose of social intervention into maltreatment is presumably to protect children. It follows that the ultimate criteria should then rest on the harm done to children, whether measured by a standard of endangerment or by less than optimal development. But no such designation can be made without reference to the parental behavior that is assumed to have provoked the harm. Hence there are two social judgments that must be made: one about the parental behavior and the other about the effects on the children. What most definitions omit, however, is the idea that the effects on children are not a direct result of the parental behavior; rather, the effects – the ultimate criteria of maltreatment – are the results of an interaction between the child and the parental behavior. At the most obvious level there is the age of the child. Parental behavior might result in effects that could be classified as maltreatment when directed toward a child of a certain age, but not when directed toward an older child. Although these considerations may be implicit in child maltreatment definitions, none make them explicit. Judgments must thus be made on the basis of some implied though unstated norms. Indeed, it is here that child development knowledge must play a crucial role. Certainly it is the primary domain of child development to describe and elucidate which parental behavior, in interaction with which child characteristics, is likely to produce consequences harmful to children. Such understanding goes far beyond the present approach to defining maltreatment through a cataloging of parental behaviors and a cataloging of undesirable effects on children, either or both of which are assumed to be noxious enough to warrant social intervention. Hence, child development research and the theory derived from it have a major role to play in the exploration of the kinds of interactions that produce effects that might be considered maltreatment.

It is here that there may be a mutuality of interest between the study of maltreatment and child development theory. Basic ethics preclude the kind of experimentation with children that could test hypotheses about the kinds of parental behaviors that might be variables in such interactions. But the study of children and families where such behaviors have been or are occurring makes it possible to investigate them. This is one reason why, in the previous section on research definitions, it was urged that study populations be drawn from officially designated cases rather than from independent populations that might or might not approximate the conditions that maintain among the officially designated ones. Until recently, child development research has had little or nothing to say about the effects on children of maltreatment or of deviant or potentially noxious parental behavior, perhaps because it has been limited to explorations within the normal range. The boundaries of maltreatment begin somewhere at the outer edges of that normal range.

In any field where investigation has been limited, so also has related theory. In the case of child maltreatment, the most profound contribution that child development can make is in formulating theory. Objective measures of the effects of various parental behaviors on children can tell us which behaviors seem to have which effects on children. But these correlational data do not tell us why they do – only well formulated, empirically based theory can do that. The chapters that follow are intended to fill that gap between child development research and theory and our understanding of child maltreatment.

References

Abbott, Grace. *The Child and the State,* Vol. 1. Chicago: University of Chicago Press, 1938.

Antler, Stephen. Child abuse: an emerging social priority. *Social Work, 23* (January 1978): 58–61.

American Humane Association (AHS). *Child Protective Services in the United States: A Nation-wide Survey.* Denver, 1967.

Billingsley, Andrew. The role of the social worker in a child protective agency. *Child Welfare 43* (1964): 472–92, 497.

Billingsley, A., Giovannoni, J. M., and Purvine, M. E. *Studies in Child Protective Services.* Mimeographed, 1969.

Bittner, Stephen and Newberger, Eli H. "Pediatric Understanding of Child Abuse and Neglect" in Newberger, E. (Ed.), *Child Abuse.* Boston: Little Brown, 1982, pp. 137–158.

Boehm, Bernice. An assessment of family adequacy in protective cases. *Child Welfare, 41* (1962): 10–16.

Bowlby, John. *Attachment and Loss Volume 1: Attachment.* London: Penguin, 1969.

Carr, A. Social worker response to the status of those reporting child maltreatment: a study of multiple gatekeeping. Unpublished manuscript, 1979.

Carstens, C. C. The laws for child protection. In S. M. Lindsay (Ed.), *Legislation for the Protection of Animals and Children.* New York: Columbia University, 1914.

Child Welfare League of America. *Standards for Child Protective Service.* Rev. ed. New York: Child Welfare League of America, 1973.

De Francis, Vincent. *The Fundamentals of Child Protection.* Denver: American Humane Association, 1955.

De Francis, Vincent, and Lucht, Carroll L. *Child abuse legislation of the 1970s.* Denver: American Humane Association, 1967.

De Schwainitz, Elizabeth, and De Schwainitz, Karl. The place of authority in the protective service function of the Public Welfare Agency. *Child Welfare, XIIII* (1964): 286–291.

Folks, Homer. *The Care of Destitute, Neglected and Delinquent Children.* New York: Macmillan, 1902.

Gelles, Richard. *Problems in Defining and Labeling Child Abuse.* Paper presented to the Study Group on Problems in the Prediction of Child Abuse and Neglect. Wilmington, DE, June 27, 1977.

Gelles, R. J. Community agencies and child abuse: labeling and gatekeeping. In R. Gelles (Ed.), *Family Violence.* Beverly Hills, CA: Sage Publications, 1979, pp. 55–72.

Giovannoni, Jeanne M., and Becerra, Rosena M. *Defining Child Abuse.* New York: The Free Press, 1979.

Goldstein, Joseph, Freud, Anna, and Solnit, Albert. *Beyond the Best Interests of the Child.* New York: Free Press, 1973. (Revised 1979)

Groeneveld, L. G., and Giovannoni, J. M. Variations in child abuse reporting: the influence of state and county characteristics. Mimeographed. The disposition of child abuse and neglect cases. *Social Work Research and Abstracts, 13* (Summer 1977): 36–47.

Helfer, Ray E. The responsibility and role of the physician. In Ray E. Helfer and C. Henry Kempe (Eds.), *The Battered Child.* Chicago: University of Chicago Press, 1974.

Institute of Judicial Administration, American Bar Association Juvenile Justice Standards Project. *Standards Relating to Abuse and Neglect.* Tentative draft. Cambridge: Ballinger, 1977.

Kadushin, Alfred. *Child Welfare Services.* New York: Macmillan, 1980.

Katz, Sanford. *When Parents Fail: The Law's Response to Family Breakdown.* Boston: Beacon Press, 1971.

Kempe, C. Henry, Silverman, Frederic N., Steele, Brandt F., Droegemueller, William, and Silver, Henry K. The battered child syndrome. *Journal of the American Medical Association, 181* (1962): 4–11.

Lena, H. F., and Warkov, S. Occupation perceptions of the causes and consequences of child abuse/neglect. *Medical Anthropology, 2* (Winter, part 1, 1978): 1–28.

McCrea, Roswell C. *The Humane Movement.* New York: Columbia University Press, 1910. (Reprinted by McGrath Publishing Co., College Park, MD)

Morgan, Edmund S. *The Puritan Family.* New York: Harper & Row, 1966.

Mulford, R. M. *Emotional Neglect of Children: A Challenge to Protective Services.* Denver: Children's Division, American Humane Association, 1958.

Nagi, Saad Z. *Child Maltreatment in the United States.* New York: Columbia University Press, 1977.

Newberger, Eli H., and Bourne, Richard. The medicalization and legalization of child abuse. *American Journal of Orthopsychiatry, 4* (Vol. 48, October, 1978): 593–607.

Polansky, Norman, Hally, D., and Polansky, N. F. *Profile of Neglect: A Survey of the State of Knowledge of Child Neglect.* Community Services Administration, Social and Rehabilitation Services, Department of Health, Education, and Welfare, 1975.

Polansky, Norman A., Chalmers, Mary Ann, Buttenwieser, Elizabeth, and Williams, David P. *Damaged Parents: An Anatomy of Child Neglect.* Chicago: University of Chicago Press, 1981.

Robin, Michael. Historical introduction sheltering arms: The roots of child protection. In Newberger, E. (Ed.), *Child Abuse.* Boston: Little Brown and Company, 1982, pp. 1–21.

Sanders, R. W. Resistance to dealing with parents of battered children. *Pediatrics, 50* (December 1972): 853–57.

Sandusky, Annie L. Protective services. In *Encyclopedia of Social Work.* New York: National Association of Social Workers, 1964.

Silver, L. B., Barton, W., and Dublin, C. C. Child abuse laws: Are they enough? *Journal of the American Medical Association, 194* (Jan. 9, 1967): 65–68.

Starr, Raymond H., Ed. *Child Abuse Prediction: Policy Implications.* Cambridge, MA: Ballinger Publishing Company, 1982.

Turbett, J. P., and O'Toole, R. *Physician's Recognition of Child Abuse.* Paper presented at the annual meeting of the American Sociological Association, New York, 1980.

U.S. Department of Health and Human Services. *Study Findings: National Study of the Incidence and Severity of Child Abuse and Neglect.* DHHS Publication No. (OHDS)81–30325: Washington, DC, 1981.

Young, Leontine R. *Wednesday's Children: A Study of Child Neglect and Abuse.* New York: McGraw-Hill, 1964.

2 Physical child abuse in America: past, present, and future

Edward Zigler and Nancy W. Hall

Introduction

Although the problem of child maltreatment is not a new one, the systematic study of this phenomenon began in the relatively recent past. Since the early 1960s this topic has been much discussed and debated, with controversies existing on every issue from definition to treatment. One reason is that child abuse is a concern of workers in a variety of fields, including pediatrics, psychology, psychiatry, education, law, social work, theology, and government. Workers in all these disciplines have contributed to the mosaic of ideas, opinions, and empirical findings that represent what we understand – and much of what we have yet to understand – about the maltreatment of children.

In this chapter we will begin with an overview of child abuse as a historical phenomenon. Definitional issues and the concurrent problem of determining the incidence of child maltreatment will then be considered, as will several etiological theories. Then we will review evidence on the correlates of child maltreatment, and also evaluate the validity of popular notions and myths about child abuse. Finally, we will examine the societal context in which child abuse occurs, and conclude with a number of recommendations for further research and for treatment approaches.

Child maltreatment throughout history

The history of child maltreatment is at once very long and very short. The systematic study of this phenomenon is relatively new, but the maltreatment of children is at least as old as recorded history. Most of the evidence we have today indicates that child abuse is on the rise (Cohn, 1983). If we take a broader, historical perspective, however, it would appear that there has been a marked improvement in the treatment of children over the ages (Ariès, 1962; Helfer and Kempe, 1968).

Throughout history, children worldwide have been subjected to domination, murder, abandonment, incarceration, mutilation, beatings, and forced labor – to name but a few examples from the litany of child maltreatment. It is important that we acknowledge the historical *context* of these phenomena, and recognize that many things that seem to us today to be brutal and senseless were entirely in keeping with their contemporary ethos (Ross, 1980). Some practices, in fact, such as the use of infanticide as a population control measure in certain cultures, were necessary for the strength and survival of the community. Others seem, even in light of the prevailing philosophy of their time, to be unnecessary and damaging. In any case, understanding the past manifestations of child maltreatment and the ideas that supported or promoted them may lend to our understanding of the present context of child maltreatment.

Ancient history: child abuse in biblical times

The Bible alludes frequently to infanticide. The most famous examples of the widespread killing of children were those ordained by the pharaoh at the time of the birth of Moses and by Herod when the birth of Jesus was foretold to him. The latter became itself the grounds for child beatings at a much later time, as this massacre was commemorated during the Middle Ages by the whipping of children on Innocents' Day. Ritual sacrifice of children is also recorded in the Bible. In Jericho 7:32 we read of "the valley of slaughter," Hinnon, the burning valley in which children were sacrificed to the god Moloch and from which is derived the classical conception of hell as a burning pit. The kings Solomon and Manasseh sacrificed children there; King Ahaz, we read, "burnt incense in the valley of the son of Hinnom and burnt his children in the fire" (2 Chron. 28:3).

Another biblically documented form of child sacrifice that persisted long after biblical times is recorded in the story of Jericho. Joshua's curse against any who might aspire to rebuild the walls of that unhappy city was that "he shall lay the foundation thereof in his firstborn, and in his youngest son shall set up the gates of it" (Josh. 6:26). And, in fact, Hiel the Bethelite "in his days did . . . build Jericho: he laid a foundation thereof in Abiram, his firstborn, and set up the gates thereof in his youngest son, Segub, according to the word of the Lord, which he spoke by Joshua the son of Nun" (1 Kings 16:34). This practice of interring live newborns in the foundations of buildings and bridges is recorded in a variety of sources across centuries and cultures (Bakan, 1971; Radbill, 1974). Archaeological explorations of biblical-era Canaanite dwellings have revealed jars of infant bones in the foundations (Potter, 1949). In seventeenth-century Europe this practice, though officially outlawed, still prevailed; children were found to have been buried in the dikes of Oldenburg and in the foundations of London Bridge. This grisly story inspired the children's rhyme, "London Bridge." In India, the practice prevailed until this century, when it was outlawed by the British government (Stern, 1948).

Nor were other ancient civilizations free from the spectre of child abuse. Besides Egypt and India, infanticide was routinely practiced and condoned in ancient Greece, Rome, Arabia, and China. Seneca, Plato, and Aristotle all urged the destruction of defective newborns, although Plato urged more lenience than did Aristotle in the upbringing of those children who lived past infancy. Defective children, female infants, the children of the poor, or those born into large families were routinely put to death. In Rome, the *Patria Potestas* gave a father complete power over a son, and the Laws of Justinian boasted that "the legal power which we have over our children is peculiar to Roman citizens, for no other men have the power over their children that we have" (Lee, 1956). The Roman Laws of the Twelve Tables actually forbade the rearing of a child with a defect or deformity. In every way the child was a possession of the father, who had the legal right to sell his child into slavery, mutilate him to make him an effective beggar, castrate him, and, of course, kill him at any time.

In many cultures, breathing upon a child, feeding it, or even picking it up were symbols that it was to be allowed to live and that its life was to be protected by law. In Egypt, the midwife prayed for the soul to come and join the newborn, but the child could be killed immediately after birth without penalty (Helfer and Kempe, 1968). Athenian infants found wanting by their parents were exposed and left to die; some of these were found and sold into slavery. Spartan children were examined and appraised, not by their parents but by the local elders, who had the power to cast unacceptable children off of Mt. Taggetus into a canyon (Sorel, 1984). Scandinavian fathers also had the power of life or death over their newborns; only if the father deigned to take the child up into his arms could it be fed and baptized. Otherwise, the child was killed or exposed. This practice was not limited to ancient times, as it persisted as a legal right until 1731 in Sweden and as late as the 1850s in Norway and Denmark (Werner, 1917).

Europe: the Middle Ages to the industrial revolution

Children did not fare any better during the Middle Ages. Widespread poverty made children an economic liability, and they were frequently abandoned, sold, or, as in Roman times, mutilated, their limbs amputated or deformed, to make them more piteous and effective beggars. A medieval heretical sect of monks, the Boni Homines, engaged in a ritual in which a purposefully injured child was passed from man to man, the legend being that the child's soul would pass to that man in whose hands it died (Krappe, 1965). In Scotland, the practice of burying a live child with the grain crop in hopes of obtaining a good harvest gave rise to the folk song, "John Barleycorn" (Krappe, 1965).

Detailed histories of the European school system are replete with tales of the beatings and abuses heaped upon the young scholars by their masters. Ariès (1962), in a comprehensive account of discipline practices in the schools, theorizes that after the fifteenth century, beatings took on a new tone. Prior to this time, corporal punishment was framed as having a pious and monastic austerity. As time passed, however, violence against students became imbued with a sense of bestiality and brutal humiliation. English schools of the sixteenth and seventeenth centuries were referred to as "places of execution" (Watshon, 1908, in Ariès, 1962). Montagu, writing at this time of his experiences at Eton, tells us,

> From Powles I went, to Aeton sent
> To learne straightwayes the Latin Phrase
> Where fiftie three stripes given to me once I had.
> (Tusser, 1560, in Ariès, 1962)

The birch rod had become the symbol of education. Although beating or birching was at first applied to very young or poor students only (in lieu of the fines charged to others for infractions of the academic rules), by the seventeenth century "scholastic punishment" (Ariès, 1962) was applied to children and youths of all social levels and ages. Even in the Jesuit schools, in which the Fathers themselves were prohibited from administering corporal punishment, students were beaten by "correctors" chosen from their own ranks. It is not likely that receiving a beating from the hands of one's schoolmates was any more pleasant than receiving one from a schoolmaster.

More recent times brought little respite from the pall of physical abuse of children. The industrial revolution brought relief from hard labor for many, but it ushered in a new age of darkness for the children of the lower classes. Even very young children were forced to work long hours at backbreaking tasks in the worst conditions. Very often they were beaten, shackled, starved, or dipped in cold water barrels, either to make them work or as punishment for not working hard enough. Working in very hot or very cold factories (depending on the time of year and the type of industry) with dangerous machinery, they were exposed to the hazards of occupational injuries and disease. A common occupation for young boys of this period was that of chimney sweep, and many succumbed at an early age to "chimney sweep's disease," cancer of the testicles. Bone deformities were another common result of spending many hours in the tight chimneys (Hanway, 1785).

Infants sent out to wetnurses – a common practice when there were many children, when the mother was in poor health, or when the father objected to nursing interfering with his sexual relationship with his wife – often died of disease or neglect or were killed outright by their nurses after the fee had been accepted (Kessen, 1965; Shorter, 1975; Stone, 1977). Midwives helped newborns out of the world as well as into it, accepting payment to surreptitiously kill unwanted infants. "Burial clubs," the first insurance agencies, became sources of income for parents who insured their child, murdered it, and collected sometimes as much as eight times as much as the premium they had paid (Radbill, 1974).

The beginnings of child advocacy

There have certainly been intermittent voices of reason and restraint in the treatment of children. Jews, Christians, and Muslims have long been commanded by religious law not to commit infanticide. Tertullian spoke out against the killing of children, as did the emperors Constantine, Valens, Theodosius, and many others. The ancient Egyptian code of Hammurabi specified that if a woman should murder her newborn child, her breast must be amputated (Garrison, 1965). The Roman emperor Tiberius ordered the death penalty in Carthage for the sacrifice of children by worshippers of Moloch. Plutarch and Erasmus decried child maltreatment, and Thomas More emphasized the dim view he took of the harsh physical discipline of children by beating his own daughters with peacock feathers (Ariès, 1962).

The establishment of hospitals and orphanages for abandoned children and orphans began as early as the second century A.D., when the empress Faustina established a foundation to save female infants from destruction (Garrison, 1965). Her successes were short-lived, but similar efforts were more effective. In the thirteenth century, Pope Innocent III sponsored the building of foundling homes to care for the illegitimate children left in the wake of the Crusades. The Council of Nicea, in 325, established *brephotrophia* – asylums for children – and some hundred years later the Council of Vaison commended the care of abandoned children to the church. Later, Russian empress Catherine II ordered the construction of children's institutions, and many others sprang up throughout Europe (Radbill, 1974). Conditions at many of these were little better than the original homes of the children, but as the beginnings of the establishment of social policies for children they were of great importance.

Henry II of France, in 1556, and, somewhat later, King James I of England, passed laws against concealing the birth of a child, a common practice that abetted the undetected murder of children (Radbill, 1974). The French child advocate, Theophile Roussel, was instrumental of the passage, in 1874, of the *loi Roussel*, which protected infants sent out to nurse. Five years later, a similar law was passed in France for the protection of abandoned or abused children (Ariès, 1962). In Germany, infanticide was so common in the eighteenth century that Frederick the Great made it a crime punishable by drowning.

The mid-nineteenth century ushered in the age of the romanticization of childhood as a time of innocence, best typified in Rousseau's *Emile*. Even so, child murder was still so prevalent in England that a select committee of the House of Commons had to be appointed to look into the phenomenon, and as late as 1890 an encyclopedia entry describes infanticide as a persistent problem in Europe (Encyclopaedia Britannica, 1890).

Recognition: child maltreatment in the last century

Although it was not the first child abuse case to come to the attention of the American authorities, the story of Mary Ellen marks the real beginning of the recognition of child maltreatment in the U.S. In 1874, no child protection agency existed to handle the case of 8-year-old Mary Ellen Wilson, whom a New York City social worker discovered chained, beaten, and starved by her adoptive parents. Because there were no laws at the time that specifically addressed the abuse of children by their caretakers, the New York Police Department refused to take action. It was only through the intervention of Henry Berg, founder of the Society for the Prevention of Cruelty to Animals (and not, as is widely held, through the actions of the SPCA itself) that the case was brought to trial. Mary Ellen was placed by the court in an orphanage, and her adoptive mother incarcerated for one year. Widespread publicity of the case, including detailed newspaper accounts of Mary Ellen's rescue and the dramatic trial, led to the founding of the Society for the Prevention of Cruelty to Children in 1875. The late nineteenth century witnessed the formation of many other child protection agencies, foundling hospitals, and charity homes for abandoned or abused children (Bremner, 1971).

Despite this long history, child abuse as an area of scientific and sociological inquiry is a relatively new phenomenon. A paper presented to the Medical Society of London in the late nineteenth century (West, 1888) described the case of a family with five children, four of whom had been treated for mysterious thickenings of the arm and leg bones. What would today most likely be recognized as evidence of child abuse was at that time dismissed as the early stages of rickets. In the 1940s, advances in pediatric radiology made possible the detection of cases of subdural hematomata frequently seen in children brought to hospitals for treatment of fractures of the long bones (Caffey, 1946). Caffey's seminal paper made little mention of the possible causes of such fractures. Although Caffey briefly considered "intentional ill-treatment of the infant," he added that "evidence was inadequate to prove or disprove this point" (p. 172). By the late 1950s, other radiologists were corroborating Caffey's findings (Wooley and Evans, 1955), and ascribing the injuries to "traumatic origins," but it was not until Kempe and his colleagues described what they called the "battered child syndrome" (Kempe, Silverman, Steele, Droegemueller, and Silver, 1962) that parents and other caretakers began to be held responsible for these injuries. Since the time of these pioneer articles this area of study has evolved and grown, and workers have matured beyond the days of the "battered child syndrome" typology to embrace more sophisticated and subtle approaches to the problem.

This is not to say, however, that the area of child abuse as a field of medical, psychological, and sociologic inquiry is free of nonobjective and emotional overtones. Indeed, the field is still heavily influenced by "[m]yth and ... mystique" (Gerbner, Ross, and Zigler, 1980, p. vii), preconceived notions and fallacies that are still widely held and propagated, even by professionals in this field, despite lack of empirical support. Child maltreatment is an emotionally laden topic even for health professionals and social scientists who are confronted by it daily. Emotional responses to child abuse run the gamut from anger and moral outrage to hysteria and revulsion. Zigler (1980) suggests three reasons why child abuse elicits such responses from us. First, our own underlying dependency needs make us feel insecure and threatened by the idea that a small and helpless person is being mistreated by someone larger and stronger. Second, such behavior is antithetical to that of millions of parents whose relationships with their children are mutually satisfying and nonabusive; child maltreatment seems to these parents foreign and perverse. Finally, many who still hold that there is a parental instinct in human beings cannot reconcile this notion with what would appear to be a very basic form of aggression against children.

This emotional response to the problem of child abuse, coupled with a dearth of sound empirical evidence, has led to the birth and perpetuation of a host of myths about child abuse. Among the most strongly held, and ill-founded, beliefs about child abuse are the following:

> *The notion of intergenerational transmission of abusive behavior.* In its purest and most dogmatic form, this entails the idea that abused children will grow up to be child abusers themselves, and, conversely, that all child abusers were themselves mistreated when they were children.
> *The "them" versus "us" ideology.* This idea, held perhaps as a defense against what seems to most people to be a monstrous phenomenon, allows us to distance ourselves from our stereotype of a child-maltreating individual by proposing that all child abusers are basically "different" from other parents.
> *Socioeconomic biases.* It has long been widely held that child abuse is a phenomenon of the lower socioeconomic classes and is more often associated with nonwhites than whites. In its simplest form such a bias embraces the idea that child abuse is a practice endemic to only certain socioeconomic groups.

In the course of this paper we will examine the evidence for and against each of these concepts, explore how they arose, and discuss the ramifications of their continuation for research as well as for treatment.

What is child abuse?

A major dilemma facing modern workers is the lack of a widely accepted definition or set of definitions to describe child abuse. The seriousness of this void must not be underestimated, for the practical ramifications are many. The definition of child abuse will affect how cases are classified, how placement decisions are made, how eligibility for social and legal services is determined, and how the abusers and the abused child will be viewed by others and by themselves. To give just a hint of the complexities involved, we might ask whether the definition of abuse should focus on the child/ outcome or perpetrator/intent aspect of a given case. Before pondering this loaded question, load it further with Parke's (1977) suggestion that the definition must also address "the antecedents, form and intensity of the response, the extent of the injury, and the role and status of agent and victim" (p. 184). We realize immediately that the ultimate definition of abuse will not be a short, concise sentence that students will highlight in their textbooks or workers will recite from memory.

A range of definitions

The many definitions of child abuse that have been proposed can be arranged in a continuum from very narrow to rather broad. The narrowest definitions include only intentional and severe physical abuse. One state law, for example, lists specific actions considered to be abusive, including "skin bruising, malnutrition, burns, etc." (Giovannoni and Becerra, 1979, p. 7). Such a definition may even exclude sexual abuse unless the child is physically injured as a result. A broader definition would include not only overt action intended to injure a child, but also cases of neglect. For example, Gil described the physical abuse of children as "the intentional, nonaccidental use of physical force or intentional, nonaccidental acts of omission, on the part of a parent or other caretaker interacting with a child in his care, aimed at hurting, injuring, or destroying that child" (1970, p. 6).

The broadest definitions of child abuse and neglect are those that include anything that interferes with the child's optimal development. For example, the Child Welfare League of America defines abuse as the denial of "normal experiences that produce feelings of being loved, wanted, secure and worthy" and exposure "to unwelcome and demoralizing circumstances" (Giovannoni and Becerra, 1979, p. 88). Other broad definitions might include as abusive parents those who knowingly allow their child to be chronically truant from school, who fail to maintain sanitary conditions in the home,

who do not conform to mainstream sexual mores, or who encourage or fail
to discourage their children in delinquent or harmful acts such as theft or
substance abuse. Inherent in such broad definitions is the notion that abuse
may be a relative rather than an absolute concept (Parke, 1977). Again quoting the Child Welfare League:

Community standards for child care reflect public attitudes and different views
among different groups regarding what is essential for the child and what jeopardizes
his or her well-being and future development. What may be considered neglect or
abuse in one community, or for one group of children, may not be so considered in
another. (Giovannoni and Becerra, 1979, p. 159)

It is clear that a democracy cannot have different standards for different
citizens. Child abuse is such a complex phenomenon, however, that professionals might be aided by the use of different definitional sets for various
purposes. In this regard, social worker David Gil distinguished between conceptual and operational definitions of child abuse. Each state, for instance,
has three sets of child abuse definitions and laws: One set concerns the mandated reporting of all known cases of abuse; another is part of the civil code
and concerns placement decisions; and the third, a criminal law, sets forth
the standards for criminal abuse and neglect. Unfortunately, many of these
laws are vague and confusing, and there is very little consistency from one
state to the next (Giovannoni and Becerra, 1979). Nor is there any real
agreement at the federal level: the Child Abuse Prevention and Treatment
Act, first enacted in 1974,[1] has polarized Congress over the issue of how to
define child abuse. This act, PL 93–247, now broadly defines child abuse as
the "physical or mental injury, sexual abuse, negligent treatment, or maltreatment of a child under the age of eighteen by a person who is responsible
for the child's welfare under circumstances which indicate that the child's
health or welfare is threatened thereby."

One thing that is clear, however, is that any definitions of child abuse will
be firmly imbedded in the political and philosophical ethos of a given society. As Giovannoni and Becerra (1979) point out, definitions must necessarily arise from what is consensually agreed in that society to be acceptable
– or nonacceptable – child rearing practice. But, they ask, "if the issues that
surround the definitions of child abuse and neglect are basically value issues,
especially ones of conflicting values, can they be resolved in any rational
way?" (p. 5). They then go on to propose that such issues can be resolved,
but only through empirical investigation. Giovannoni and Becerra's work
involved presenting a wide range of vignettes about child abuse, differing
with respect to area (medical care, adequacy of clothing, physical punishment, etc.), to over 300 lawyers, social workers, police, and pediatricians, to
see whether some consensus might be reached on what constituted abuse
and on how different levels of severity were perceived. Their results indicate
that, although there is some agreement within these professional groups,

very little consensus exists *across* groups with regard to what is viewed as abusive, or with respect to the perceived severity of those abuses. Such an outcome illustrates the significance of one's values, training, and cultural-political milieu in defining abuse.

It also emphasizes the concept that child abuse is not a homogeneous phenomenon (Cicchetti and Rizley, 1981) but a range of phenomena. Differences exist with respect to a number of factors: the nature of the abusive act(s), the perpetrator, the circumstances leading up to the abuse, the sequelae of the abuse, etc. Some have found it useful to think of each of these as categories containing discrete units (e.g., deliberately burning a child would be thought of as qualitatively distinct from injuring a child in the course of an overzealous disciplinary spanking). Others (Zigler, 1980) have found it useful to view child abuse as existing on a continuum of caretaking practices, ranging from competent, loving care to murder. Behaving as a skilled, caring parent, bruising a child accidentally while disciplining her, and murdering a child would all be viewed as different points on the same hypothetical line.

Developmental perspective

Another element is added to the definitional dilemma with the argument that we must take a developmental perspective when looking at, defining, and acting to ameliorate the effects of child abuse (Aber and Zigler, 1981). Regardless of whether we employ a legal definition, a research-oriented definition, or a medical definition, the conceptualization of the child as a changing, developing system must be maintained. Over the course of his development, the child's relationship with the world and with his parents – and the way in which stimuli are perceived and assimilated by the child, regardless of whether they are physical, cognitive, or social–emotional in nature – is affected by developmental changes in the child. For a parent to physically abuse an infant, whose attachments to significant adults are in a crucial stage of development, will have far different effects on him, and on the family, than will the same incident if it involves a ten-year-old or a teenager, for whom growing independence from the family is a salient developmental issue. Similarly, it is likely that the events and variables leading up to the abusive incident will differ with the developmental level of the child and the family. A new mother, unsure of her ability to care for her highly dependent infant and unaware of what to expect from herself and her child, is faced with a very different circumstance than is the father of three school-aged children who seem to him to be "into everything." An abusive behavior that is expressed in one of these cases will necessarily be fundamentally different from any that may occur in the other. And although we will not deal (in this chapter) with the consequences of abuse, it is easy to see that the child will perceive abuse very differently at different developmental stages, and will play very different roles in any legal or medical proceedings that follow as a result of abuse, depending on that child's developmental level. Workers in the field of child abuse study would do well to consider this issue when attempting to establish working definitions of abuse.

The extent of the problem

The lack of consensus on the definition of child abuse has compounded the problems involved in determining its incidence. Estimates of the extent of child abuse in this country range from 200,000 to 4 million cases annually, a range that is accounted for by differences in sampling method, source of data, and, of course, demographers' definitions of abuse. Such disparate estimates make it impossible to determine the severity of the problem of child abuse and to allocate effectively the resources to combat it.

The most widely accepted incidence figures are those prepared by the National Committee for the Prevention of Child Abuse (Cohn, 1983), which estimates that over 1 million children are "seriously abused" (p. 1) and 2,000 to 5,000 abuse-related deaths occur in the United States each year. In other words, it believes that 2 to 2.5 percent of the families in this country engage in physical child abuse. Other researchers take a more conservative approach to estimating the incidence of abuse, stating that "no reliable data are available on either the local or national level" (Uviller, 1980, p. 151) and urging caution in attempts to identify and label cases of child abuse. Available figures on the incidence of physical child abuse undoubtedly reflect only a portion of the actual cases, with several factors accounting for this underestimation (Parke and Lewis, 1981). Despite legislated mandates that have increased the level of reporting, many cases do not reach the books of the central registries in each state. The failure to uncover episodes of abuse is caused by the breakdown of one or more of three processes essential to the accurate determination of the incidence rate. First, there is often *failure to detect* injury caused by abuse. Hospital or clinic "shopping" by parents – that is, utilization of different health care facilities instead of obtaining all of a child's care from one place – hinders medical personnel from recognizing repeated or chronic injuries and makes it more likely that a parent-inflicted injury will pass for an isolated accident. Further, many parents do not seek immediate medical care for their abused child at all, whereas others delay treatment. Physicians may find radiologic evidence of healed or healing fractures, old scar tissue, subdural hematomata, or other disturbing signs, such as low hematocrit readings, some time after the injury occurred. Because any of these can be symptomatic of abuse as well as accidental injury or legitimate illness, it is often impossible to determine with certainty the cause of the problem. In very young children, certain types of injury may escape detection because of the nature of infant physiology. From birth to about 3 years of age, much of a child's cartilage is radiolucent, that is, so translucent that injuries to these areas are radiologically invisible and are therefore extremely difficult to detect (Kempe et al., 1962). Unless there is concurrent visible evidence of bruising or osteopathic anomalies (fractures, dislocations, etc.) such an injury may go unnoticed.

A second problem that contributes to the unreliability of statistics on child abuse is a *failure to recognize* abuse as the cause of a victim's injuries. One reason for this is a reluctance on the part of medical personnel to consider abuse as a diagnosis, particularly for middle- and upper-income families. This bias accounts for a great deal, though not all, of the class differences in reporting (Pelton, 1978). Another factor contributing to the failure to recognize abuse is again the definitional dilemma. A doctor must have in mind some idea of what does and what does not constitute abuse before labeling the etiology of an injury.

Finally, even after an injury has been detected and recognized as the result of abuse or neglect, there may be a *failure to report the case to the appropriate agency.* In a study of 267 abuse or neglect-related child deaths in Texas, Anderson, Ambrosino, Valentine, and Lauderdale (1983) report that fewer than 25 percent of the families studied had ever come to the attention of the state's child protective services agencies. Becker (in Light, 1973) reported that, of 3,000 cases brought to the attention of the New York Central Registry in one year, only eight had been reported by physicians. Here, too, the social class of the family and their degree of familiarity to the health professional may play a part in whether the incident will be reported (McPherson and Garcia, 1983). Some physicians worry that fear of such a report will keep parents from seeking medical care for their child in the future. Others may feel that, in what they deem to be "mild" or non-life-threatening cases of abuse, the negative consequences of the reporting process may outweigh any benefits that could be derived from filing such a report.

In this regard, Solnit (1980) has discussed the negative consequences that can follow from incautious or overzealous reporting of incidents believed to be related to child abuse. He argues persuasively that indiscriminate reporting violates family privacy and spreads too thinly the available services by applying them "regardless of whether it is effective or appropriate" (p. 144). Moreover, the label "child abuse" can exacerbate the stress already afflicting the family, resulting in further abuse. In considering the consequences of reporting, many professionals apparently deem it best to handle a possible abuse situation themselves, or to take a "wait and see" attitude while attempting to keep a watchful eye on the family involved.

A nationwide survey by Gil (1970) reveals a prevailing attitude that offers profound insight into why many cases of abuse go unreported. When Gil asked participants in this survey whether they thought a child could be injured while in the care of a parent or other adult, 58 percent of the respondents replied in the affirmative. Twenty-two percent indicated that they thought themselves capable of injuring a child in their care, and 16 percent reported that at some time they had in fact come close to doing so. In light of these statistics, it would seem that people may be reluctant to become involved in an abuse case, feeling some empathy with the abusing parent. Still others may refuse to report a case of abuse because of what they believe to be the parent's "right" to govern the treatment of his or her child (Zalba, 1971). This finding indicates that the historical tendency to view one's children as one's property still persists to some extent (Rodham, 1973).

Our dilemma is clear, but the best solutions are not so readily apparent. Steps must be taken to ensure that the rights of families are protected while we do our best to assess the incidence and impact of child maltreatment. As Solnit (1980) recommends, services to support children and families *must* be commensurate with the stresses that charges, inquiries, and labeling will inevitably bring.

Correlates of child abuse

A number of studies have attempted to uncover the factors associated with child abuse in order to piece together a profile of the "typical" case. Such studies generally conclude that there is no typical abused child and no particular family type at risk for involvement in abuse. There are, however, certain characteristics that have been found to occur with somewhat greater regularity than others.

The most ambitious study of its kind was carried out by Gil (1970), who collected data from central registries in all 50 states, Washington, D.C., Puerto Rico, and the Virgin Islands for the years 1967 and 1968. (When interpreting these results, it is important to bear in mind the problems of validity associated with statistics supplied by central registries, as discussed earlier in this chapter.) Although this study has been criticized (Spinetta and Rigler, 1972) mainly because Gil identifies child abuse with poverty and underestimates the incidence of abuse, it nevertheless remains one of the most comprehensive examinations of demographic correlates of abuse. When it is combined with the results of similar studies (e.g., Anderson, Ambrosino, Valentine, and Lauderdale, 1983; Junewicz, 1983), some understanding emerges of the factors associated and not associated with child abuse.

The abused child

Although the findings differ from study to study, it seems clear that age, sex, and birth order of the child are related to the incidence of abuse. Kempe et al. (1962) found that children under 3 were overrepresented in samples of abused children. Gil (1970) found that 13.8% of all cases involved children under 1 year; 75% of the reported cases involved children over 2, and nearly half of these children were older than 6. Seventeen percent were teens. Over 20% involved children 3 to 5 years old. Age distributions were not significantly different for any race. Slightly more than half of the children involved were boys, except in the teenage groups, where girls accounted for almost two-thirds of the reported cases.

Although infants in general are only slightly overrepresented, there is considerable evidence (Gil, 1970; Parke and Collmer, 1975; Zigler, 1976) that premature babies, low birthweight babies (Klein and Stern, 1971), and young children with problems such as hyperactivity (Parke, 1977), cerebral palsy (Diamond and Jaudes 1983), and mental retardation (Zigler, 1980) are at an elevated risk of abuse. Having an infant in one of these categories is undoubtedly very stressful for parents (Bakan, 1971): financial burdens may be great and certain behaviors of these children, such as feeding disturbances or the aversive cry of a premature baby (Frodi, 1981; Lester, 1984), have been found to be especially irritating. Increased stress may also contribute to the greater rates of abuse for children born of unwanted pregnancies (Kempe et al., 1962).

Most research indicates that abused children tend to come from relatively large families. Although only 20% of families in the United States today have four or more children, they account for 40% of the cases of abuse (Zigler, 1976). An early study by Young (1964) reveals even more dramatic findings: Only 20% of 180 abusing families studied had fewer than three children; 37% had between six and 12. Light's research (1973) yields similar findings not only for the United States but also for New Zealand and, to a lesser extent, for England. The smallest percentages of abusing families in all of these studies were those having only one child. (Anderson et al., 1983, found a smaller than average family to be associated with abuse-related deaths, but this is an exceptional finding.)

Oftentimes one child in a family is singled out for abuse while his or her siblings are treated well (Bakan, 1971; Parke, 1977). Bakan described this as a vicious cycle in which, for instance, an unattractive child, targeted for abuse by parents, becomes more alienated and unattractive with repeated abuse, and as a result is subjected to still more ill treatment. Frequently the youngest child is the one singled out for abuse (Zigler, 1976).

Abusing adults

Gil (1970) also reviewed the characteristics of the perpetrators of abuse and the circumstances under which it occurs. Mothers (or "mother substitutes") were found to be responsible for 47.6% of the abuse cases researched, while

39.2% of the incidents involved fathers or father substitutes. This would appear to be consistent with Gelles's (1980) finding that females are more likely to use physical violence against children than are males. Note, however, that no father resided in over 29% of the homes involved in Gil's survey; when a male head-of-household was present he was responsible for the abuse two-thirds of the time. Anderson et al. (1983) reported this figure to be 50%. This even split between male and female abusers is also seen when taking into account all perpetrators, including relatives and unrelated adult caretakers – Gil found females to be responsible for the abuse in 51% of the cases and males in about 48%. Because children generally spend the vast majority of their time with females, however, such data may actually indicate that women are less likely to victimize children than are men.

Ninety percent of abusive incidents take place in the child's own home (Bronfenbrenner, 1974, in Garbarino, 1976). Two and 2.5 percent, respectively, occurred in public places or in the home of an unrelated perpetrator such as a neighbor. Gil cites as highly typical the situation in which a child was temporarily left with a boyfriend or other unrelated male while the mother shopped or went to work. Over 17% of the episodes of abuse reviewed in his study occurred under these circumstances. Although there were no significant increases in reporting during any particular month or any one day of the week, there are variations in time of day. The greatest percentage of incidents clustered between the hours of 3 and 6 P.M. (when children return from school and the busy dinner hour gets underway) and 6 and 9 P.M. (when both children and adults are weary from the day). In 12.9% of the reports the perpetrator of abuse was intoxicated. Other researchers (Junewicz, 1983; Kempe and Kempe, 1978; Newberger and Daniel, 1979; Rosenfeld and Newberger, 1979), have also noted a correlation between substance abuse and child abuse.

Intergenerational transmission of abuse

The childhood histories of abusive parents have been a focus of concern ever since the landmark Kempe et al. paper of 1962. Kempe and his colleagues reported that many parents of abused children had been abused themselves during childhood. This notion has been reiterated so often (Bleiberg, 1965; Curtis, 1963; Friedrich and Wheeler, 1982; Fontana, 1968; Parke, 1977; Steele and Pollock, 1968; Tuteur and Glotzer, 1966) that one review of this literature boldly concludes that one "basic factor in the etiology of child abuse draws unanimity: Abusing parents were themselves abused or neglected, physically or emotionally, as children" (Spinetta and Rigler, 1972, p. 298). The theory of the "intergenerational transmission" of abuse has gained the status of being treated as fact, even in some psychology textbooks. This theory, however, has never been adequately substantiated, and there is mounting evidence to the contrary – evidence showing that the "cycle of abuse" can be, and frequently is, broken. Gil's study revealed that only about 11% of abusing parents were themselves the victims of abuse. Other workers (Dubanoski, 1981; Gelles, 1979a, 1979b; Gelles and Cornell, 1985; Giovannoni and Billingsley, 1970; Hunter and Kilstrom, 1979; Morris, Gould, and Matthews, 1964; C. Newberger, 1982; Oliver and Taylor, 1971) have proposed caveats suggesting that much of the intergenerational research is limited in its applicability. Kaufman and Zigler (1987), in a cogent analysis of the development of the theory of intergenerational transmission, note that the research in this area is flawed in several significant ways. The majority of the material on intergenerational transmission is derived from theoretical papers, isolated case study reports, data drawn from agency records on special populations, clinical interviews, and self-report questionnaires completed by the parents of children who had already been identified as having been abused (Altemeier, O'Connor, Vietze, Sandler, and Sherrod, 1982; Galdston, 1965; McHenry, Girdany, and Elmer, 1963). Most of what we have been given to understand about the parents of abused children, therefore, has been derived retrospectively from biased samples. Little attempt has been made, until recently, to identify parents who, though abused themselves as children, *do not* abuse their own children. When Hunter and Kilstrom (1979), for instance, employed a prospective rather than a retrospective technique, they found that 82 percent of the parents they followed who had themselves been abused were able to break the cycle of abuse. Similar results were obtained by Egeland and Jacobvitz (1984), who found that even in what might traditionally be considered a sample of parents at high risk for abusing their children, 70 percent were able to avoid doing so. In both the Egeland and Jacobvitz and the Hunter and Kilstrom studies, parents who refrained from abusive behavior were found to have many characteristics in common that differentiated them from the abusive parents in these studies. Nonabusive parents were found to have more extensive and readily available social supports, fewer life stresses, healthier babies, and, in the Hunter and Kilstrom study, less ambivalent feelings about their pregnancies and their babies. In both studies, abusive parents who had come to terms with their history of abuse – that is, those who were able to admit what their parents had done and who were appropriately angry about it – were more likely to refrain from abusing their own children than were those parents who were still attempting to deny what had happened or who had formed idealized images of their abusing parents.

Cicchetti and Rizley (1981) remind us that parental history is not a simple, unitary dimension that will determine absolutely whether or not a parent goes on to abuse. They propose a model in which a variety of factors interact to determine caregiving outcome. Among these are type of abuse, potentiating factors (those which increase the likelihood of abuse), and compensatory factors, such as those identified by Hunter and Kilstrom as being characteristic of nonabusing parents. Cicchetti and Rizley also emphasize the importance of conducting prospective research in this area whenever possible to maximize the likelihood of being able to compare a variety of histories and caregiving outcomes. Only by including both parents with and without histories of having been abused and studying both those who do and who do not abuse their children will we be able to compare families in which abuse and non-abuse are transmitted intergenerationally, as well as those in which caregiving style, with respect to abuse, changes from one generation to the next – those families in which "the cycle is broken."

We can conclude from the newer models of research on intergenerational transmission of abuse, and from the results that are beginning to be available, that earlier researchers were premature in their conclusion that the transmission of abusive behavior from one generation to the next is inevitable. It is likely (Kaufman and Zigler, 1987) that the actual number of families in which the transmission of abuse occurs is fewer than one in three. This is a far cry from the 100 percent rate of transmission in which an earlier generation of researchers believed. Most importantly, we have much to learn from these new models about the variables that strengthen families and that might be valuable in the prevention of abuse.

Abusing families

In interpreting Gil's data on the characteristics of families involved in abuse, it is important to remember that they describe families involved in cases *that get reported to central registries.* There is, therefore, a very real possibility that statistics regarding ethnicity, education, and occupation are biased in favor of white and middle- to upper-class families. Abusing families were unremarkable in most respects. Parents in these groups tended to be young, but not disproportionately so. Nearly half of them were between 20 and 30 years old, and fewer than 10% were younger than 20. Educational level was generally low: Fewer than 20% of the mothers and approximately 35% of the fathers were high school graduates. One striking finding was that, of the fathers and father-substitutes featured in these reports, only 52% were steadily employed throughout the year prior to the filing of the report; at the time of the abuse incident the unemployment rate for this group was 11.8%, although the national rate for the same year was only 3.2%. Over 37% of the families were receiving some form of public assistance at the time of the incident. Household income for these families was also much lower than the national average. In 1968 the rate of abuse reports for white families was 6.7 per 100,000, and 21 per 100,000 for nonwhites. No religious group was significantly under- or overrepresented among these families. Both Gil

(1970) and Kempe et al. (1962) found in their samples a high rate of divorce and marital separation. Over 29% of the families identified by the Gil study were headed by single mothers, but this statistic is difficult to interpret for a society in which the number of single-parent households has since soared. Although no other researchers have reached a similar conclusion, Kempe and Kempe suggest that some two-parent homes may be more abusive than single-parent families:

Child abuse is indeed a family affair. In our experience single parents are rather less abusive than couples, which is surprising because one would think that a spouse would provide support in the face of crisis. In fact a spouse who is not supportive is worse than no spouse at all when it comes to childrearing. (1978, p. 23)

Abuse in society

Nicholas Hobbs (1980) called child abuse "a swatch from the fabric of a violent and abusing society" (p. 280), and socioecological theorists echo this charge. They emphasize the increasingly violent nature of our society and our tolerance of violence by pointing to evidence of the following sort:

In 1980 there were 23,000 murders committed in the United States.
The National Association for Better Broadcasting estimated that the average child, from the ages of 5 to 15, would watch the violent destruction of more than 13,400 persons on television (Sabin, in Cline, 1974, p. 115).
Prizefighters earn millions for a single fight, yet teachers in our children's schools are fortunate if they can earn $18,000 a year.

Why do these situations happen in America? Our social ethos is such that we are conditioned to strike out at those who trouble or frustrate us. We are socialized, however, to control and suppress our violent impulses except under certain socially sanctioned settings, such as the sports arena (Kuttner, 1983), but have gone so far as to institutionalize violence so that it is pervasive throughout our schools, our legal systems, and our homes. Consider this statement from the chief of police in Kansas City, Missouri: "We must send this very definite message to people who might commit violence. That we as a society will deal with it very harshly. Because by dealing with it harshly we are reinforcing the belief that this kind of conduct is wrong" (McNamara, 1976, in Zigler, 1976, p. 200). Yet the human aggression literature suggests that an unavoidable consequence of harshness and violence is an escalated level of harshness and violence.

Human aggression

Seymour Feshback points out (1980) that humans differ from other animals in their use of aggression. In most animals, intraspecies aggression serves only as a display, as symbolic combat to establish dominance over females or territory, and is not ultimately destructive. In the contests of bison or bighorn sheep, for example (Barash, 1977), the submitting animal will signal his defeat by lowering his head and turning away. The aggression is thus terminated, usually without serious injury to either animal. In humans, however, either such stimuli are lacking or our responses to them have become less sensitive over the course of evolution (Lorenz, 1966).

Berkowitz (1975) described two major types of human aggression: that which arises from emotional excitation and that which, although intended to hurt, primarily stems from a desire to achieve "some other, non-aggressive goal" (p. 219). An example of the latter type, which Berkowitz refers to as "non-angry aggression," is the violent or destructive behavior of a teen who hopes to win peer approval. Another example is a parent who attempts to discipline a child by physical means but quite unintentionally causes the child injury.

Several factors influence whether a reaction to a particular stimulus (for instance, a child's persistent cry) will be aggressive. The frustration level of the hearer, for instance, will have an impact on whether aggression is likely to be the response (although, as Berkowitz 1973, notes, the classic frustration–aggression hypothesis no longer has as many adherents as once it did). The perceived intentionality of a frustrating act is also a mediating factor, as is the perception of the status of the instigator of frustration (S. Feshbach, 1980; Newberger and Cook, 1983). Feshbach also reports that threats to one's self-esteem – for example, to a parent's self-concept – are powerful elicitors of aggression. All of this suggests that education for parenting may help in the control or modification of abusive behavior. Imitation of non-aggressive models and training in alternative methods of dealing with a child's undesirable behavior can help a parent control aggressive impulses (S. Feshbach, 1980). As Feshbach notes, however, aggressive tendencies are so firmly rooted in human society that the ultimate control of the child abuse problem lies in changing our societal attitudes towards and acceptance of aggression as an appropriate mechanism for problem solving.

Corporal punishment at home. The following statistics hint at the extent of the use of corporal punishment in the American home:

> 93% of all parents practice some form of corporal punishment (Gil, 1970).
> One survey (Parke and Collmer, 1975) revealed that 25% of mothers spank their infants in the first six months of life; nearly half spank their babies by the end of the first year.
> Straus, Gelles, and Steinmetz (1979) found that 52% of a group of adolescents had been physically punished or threatened with physical punishment during their senior year in high school.
> A survey by Viano (in Park & Collmer, 1975) revealed that 66% of teachers, police, and clergy expressed approbation for striking a child with the hand; 10% condoned physical punishment with belts, brushes, and straps.

A statement by another authority figure, a Connecticut school superinten-
dent, echoes the message of the Kansas police chief in the context of parental
responsibility:

I give fair warning, unless parents – all parents – once again take control of and
responsibility for their children's behavior, expect the problems of discipline in the
schools and unrest in society to grow ... the greatest single need is for parents to
reinstill in their children a basic respect for authority and a realization that laxity in
parental discipline, as is presently the case, can only have one result – chaos in society. ... The seed doesn't fall very far from the tree. Show me a kid in trouble in
school and I will show you a home where discipline is lacking. (cited in Zigler, 1976,
p. 200)

The warning of this prominent school official is a strong illustration that
American culture not only condones but actively encourages parents to use
physical punishment with children.

It is small wonder then that corporal punishment in the home is responsible for over 60 percent of the child abuse in America (Gil, 1970; Zigler and
Hall, 1984). The scenario that accounts for most cases of child abuse is that
of the parent who sets out to discipline a child and ends up hurting him or
her. Parents often injure children when they are unable to control their anger
or to gauge their own strength. Usually they are unaware of a child's physical
vulnerabilities, not knowing that even a hard shaking can cause brain damage in a young child. Parents are often shocked by the tragic outcome of their
well-intentioned desire to discipline their children. The villain here is certainly not the child, nor is it the parent trying hard to raise the child. The
real villain is the society that promotes the use of corporal punishment.

Many scholars (N. Feshbach, 1980; Gelles, 1973; Gil, 1970; Reid, 1983;
Zigler, 1980) maintain that child abuse will continue to be a problem in this
country as long as corporal punishment remains an acceptable form of discipline. Cultures in which the physical punishment of children is rare – for
example, Sweden, Finland, China (Sidel, 1972), Japan, Tahiti (Levy, 1969),
the Arapesh communities of New Guinea (Mead, 1937) – have very low
rates of child abuse (Belsky, 1980; Gil, 1970; Rogers, 1979). Yet it seems
unlikely that corporal punishment of children in this country will ever be
officially designated as a crime, as it is in Sweden (Commission on Children's Rights, 1978). The 1977 Supreme Court decision legalizing spanking
in American schools merely set an official seal of approval on what was
already taken for granted in America: that the legal rights of children are
different from, and inferior to, those of any other group of people in this
country (Rodham, 1972). Children are the only people in America whom it
is legal for an adult to strike (Zigler and Hunsinger, 1977).

Corporal punishment at school. The use of physical methods of punishment
in schools has been officially outlawed in many countries, ranging in size
from China and the U.S.S.R. to Luxembourg and Quatar (Reitman, Foll-

man, and Ladd, 1972). The only European nations that still sanction corporal punishment in schools are Britain and the Republic of Ireland (N. Feshbach, 1980). The United States, however, has upheld the right of school authorities to act *in loco parentis* in meting out physical punishment (several states, including New Jersey, Maine, Hawaii, and Massachusetts, are exceptions). In some cases, the school's rights even supersede those of parents. In the Supreme Court case of *Baker v. Owen* (1975), the court upheld the school's right to use corporal punishment on an elementary school boy, in spite of his mother's written instructions that they not do so.

As we see it, corporal punishment in American schools should be legally abolished for several compelling reasons. The American Civil Liberties Union (Reitman et al., 1972, p. 36) stated that using "physical violence on school children is an affront to democratic values and [an] infringement of individual rights," and the authors concur. Secondly, the use of corporal punishment in a classroom is counterproductive and has never been demonstrated to be effective. Research indicates (albeit indirectly) that learning is actually deterred by the teacher's use of punishment (Bongiovanni, 1977), and that children exposed to corporal punishment behave more aggressively (Feshbach and Feshbach, 1971).

Finally, corporal punishment in the schools can lead to the same outcome as corporal punishment in the home: injury to a child. In the incident that led to the Supreme Court case of *Ingraham v. Wright* (1977), a junior high school boy who had responded too slowly to a teacher's instructions was held by two teachers and beaten more than 20 times with a 2-foot-long wooden paddle, resulting in a hematoma that required medical treatment and over 2 weeks' absence from school. The Court held that this did *not* constitute cruel and unusual punishment, nor, according to the ruling, did it violate the boy's right to due process of law. Although school incidents probably constitute a small percentage of the reported abuse cases each year, this setting for physical discipline stands out as a public showcase. Parents not only see that this form of violence against children is acceptable in our society, but children learn that violence is an appropriate tool for problem solving. If we wish to combat child abuse now and in the future, it is imperative that teachers be trained in and encouraged to use nonviolent methods of disciplining students. Prerequisite to real improvement will have to be widespread recognition and greater acceptance of the idea that children are *entitled* to protection from maltreatment. Although this might seem self-evident and inherently reasonable, the courts and educational institutions in this country have yet to be fully swayed.

Other settings. Corporal punishment and maltreatment in our nation's day care settings (Keyserling, 1972) and in facilities for mentally retarded and mentally ill persons (Blatt, 1980; Blatt and Kaplan, 1966) are common and within the boundaries of legality. Lax standards for some of these settings may set the stage for illegal abuses as well. To illustrate, in day care facilities in the United States, many of which are unlicensed, conditions vary tremendously. One reason is that there are no federal regulations and state standards are widely disparate and frequently inadequate (Young and Zigler, 1986). In the state of Florida, for instance, a 16-year-old high school drop-out can be assigned as the sole caretaker of as many as eight infants. Providing adequate safeguards for these children in the face of emergencies is impossible under such conditions. Providing adequate attention, stimulation, and sanitary care for the children is just as unlikely, and the potential for caregiver stress increases the likelihood of physical abuse. Of course, many day care facilities are excellent, but too many others are characterized by overcrowding, low staff-to-child ratios, unsanitary conditions, and inadequately trained and supervised caregivers. In such nonoptimal settings, physical abuse is almost inevitable.

The etiology of child abuse

Theoretical perspectives on the causes and correlates of child abuse are many and varied, though it is possible to classify the major schools of thought into groups according to their focus. These involve whether the explanation and treatment approach centers on the parent, the parent–child dyad, or other persons or groups as agents of influence.

Psychiatric approach

The earliest etiological model of child abuse stemmed from a psychiatric orientation. This model, which is still widely used, focuses on the parent or other adult as the perpetrator of abuse. Underlying this approach is the notion that the abuser is in some way pathological or is suffering from some form of mental illness. There has been an enormous amount of work done in an attempt to substantiate this position empirically (see Parke and Collmer, 1974, for a review of this literature) but findings remain mixed. Although Gill (1970) reported that 46 percent of his sample of abusers manifested "marked mental and/or emotional deviation" (p. 128), this is a much higher figure than that cited by other researchers. Kempe and Kempe (1978), for example, set at 10 percent the group of parents who could be labeled as psycho- or sociopathological. Junewicz (1983) cited the presence of "mentally ill patients" as one possible contributor to child abuse, but gave this situation no more weight than four other antecedent conditions. Blumberg (1974, in Parke and Collmer, 1975, p. 519) noted that "psychosis is very rarely a factor in child abuse" and that disturbed parents make up "only a very small fraction of the total."

There are several serious dangers inherent in the psychiatric approach to child abuse. It follows from the basic assumptions of this theory that it should be possible to identify a potentially abusive parent; Kempe has been the most outspoken but not the only advocate of this position (Helfer and Kempe, 1968, 1976; Kempe and Helfer, 1972; Kempe and Kempe, 1978; Kempe et al., 1962; Milner, Gold, Ayoub, and Jacewitz, 1984). The possibility for error here is great, as is the potential for harm to the parent and family unnecessarily labelled "at risk for child abuse." There is nothing inherently useful in making up lists of "potential child abusers," and such action can do great damage. It is essential to remember that the risk of child abuse in the general population is actually low, not much more than 2 percent. We cannot say what effect the labeling itself would have on the family; it seems unlikely that there would be any positive results of such a measure (Solnit, 1980).

The psychiatric approach sets up a dichotomy between "them" (the abusers), and "us" (nonabusers). It is helpful to recall here Gil's survey data (1970), which indicated that nearly 60 percent of the people interviewed felt that it was conceivable that an adult might injure a child. These respondents were not psychotic or sociopathic, nor are most of the people who maltreat children. But by believing abusers to be "crazies," remedial and preventive efforts are directed away from the general population, where abuse is most likely to occur.

When child abusers are assumed to be mentally ill or emotionally deviant, the appropriate treatment would be psychotherapy or counseling. This type of treatment is usually both lengthy and expensive. With over one million children being abused every year, this course of action is impractical at best. The numbers are such that there are simply not enough mental health professionals or facilities to treat all of even the grossest cases of abuse by this method (Ross and Zigler, 1983).

Social approach

The psychiatric model is an example of what Newberger and Newberger (1982) call a "unitary" theory, or one in which the cause of child abuse is thought to be a single agent. The group of theories that come under the social–ecological heading are "interactive," that is, they combine the influences of several mutually affective forces. Basic to these theories is the idea that social stresses, working in interaction with certain aspects of the cultural milieu and with family dynamics, build up until they result in an outbreak of aggression in the form of child abuse. Unlike the psychiatric model, the social or social stress models focus on the parents' and the families' interactions with society and the resulting pressures on the families, rather than implying that some defect or deficit inheres within the parent. Representative models of this type are those described by Garbarino (1976, 1982) and Gil (1970). In Gil's study, for example, 59 percent of the abuse cases were associated with "mounting stress on perpetrator due to life circumstances" (p. 129).

Other researchers have also emphasized the role of stress in child abuse (Garbarino, 1983; Gaudin and Pollane, 1983; Milner et al., 1984; Newberger, Reed, Daniel, Hyde, and Kotelchuck, 1977; Rosenberg and Repucci, 1983). When this stress is not mitigated by social support networks, the stressed parents are socially isolated (Garbarino, 1982; C. Newberger, 1982; Richmond and Janis, 1980; Zigler, 1980). They seldom have close ties with neighbors or extended family (Young, 1964) and they usually do not participate in any community organizations (Giovannoni and Billingsley, 1970; Kempe and Kempe, 1978; Parke and Collmer, 1975). A thought-provoking finding comes from Lenoski's report (1974, cited in Park and Collmer, 1975) that abusive parents were over seven times more likely to have unlisted phone numbers than nonabusive parents. The causes of isolation and stress can often be found in a family's social and environmental context. For instance, Gil (1970) found a positive relationship between mobility and child abuse within a family. High levels of child abuse in military families thus may be connected to the transience that is often associated with employment in the armed services (James, Furukawa, James, and Mangelsdorf, 1984). Families who move a lot do not have the support or assistance of their extended family, nor do they appear to establish the social bonds that could serve the same function.

Economic factors, such as loss of a job, cuts in pay (or increases in financial obligations), and dissatisfaction with one's job, are also frequently associated with child abuse. The fact that abuse rates are higher among the lower economic classes (reporting biases notwithstanding), where economic stresses are presumed to be greater, would seem to substantiate this theory. Financial difficulties may even have some role in the increased risk of abuse associated with the birth of a new baby (Parke, 1977), particularly if the situation is complicated by expensive health problems, prematurity, or the departure of one parent from the work force.

The treatment approach that stems from sociological theories of child abuse involves the use of support systems to reduce social stress and isolation. Examples of some support mechanisms will be discussed in the final section of this chapter.

Developmental approach

A new and promising approach to understanding abusing parents is based on the cognitive–developmental theory of C. Newberger and Cook (1983). Founded on the work of Kohlberg, Gilligan, and Selman, this theory posits that parenting attitudes and behaviors follow a pattern of stages similar to those described by Piaget. Focusing on issues revolving around the parent's perception of the "child as a person," of "child-rearing rules," and "interpersonal responsibility and connections in the 'parental role'" (p. 414), Newberger and Cook describe four levels of "parental awareness." In order of increasing cognitive sophistication, these involve egotistic, conventional, individualistic, and analytic orientations toward the parent–child relationship. The significance of this theory is best described in the authors' own words:

Analyses suggest that the cognitive foundations for understanding the child and the parental role are built through a process which unfolds developmentally throughout childhood and into adulthood. What the developmental model offers . . . is an orientation toward the natural process of adaptation to the vicissitudes of relationships, in which levels of competence – and not simply islands of pathology – can be identified. (p. 522)

The developmental approach of Newberger and Cook shares certain features with the interactive model of child abuse advanced by Ross and Zigler (1983). This interactive formulation posits that child abuse is the product of environmental stressors acting upon individuals with particular psychological makeups. Newberger and Cook treat stages of parenting in isolation and imply that an individual could be at a low stage in regard to parental skills while being at relatively high stages in other realms of functioning. Zigler and Ross adopt a more orthodox approach to cognitive-developmental theorizing, viewing the individual's developmental stage as a pervasive determinant of behavior across all of the individual's functioning.

The basic assumption in this theory is that the final stage of development or maturity achieved varies across individuals. Within this individual differences approach to cognitive-developmental theorizing there must be individuals whose maturity is characterized by lower developmental forms. When such individuals encounter stress, their methods of coping should also be characterized by mechanisms characteristic of the immature person – unmodulated, striking out. Indeed, considerable evidence now exists to indicate that child abuse is a response more common in individuals whose total lives are characterized by inadequacy and immaturity (Polansky, Chalmers, Buttenweiser, and Williams, 1981). What must be emphasized is that abusive behaviors are not in and of themselves pathological. They represent the reactions of normal individuals who are dealing with the environment with the mechanisms dictated by their developmental level. Thus the Ross and Zigler formulation suggests not a pathological difference between abusers and nonabusers, but a developmental maturational difference.

The relevance of developmental thought to the phenomenon of child abuse may be seen in work on the action–thought dimension in human behavior. Developmental theorists of both psychoanalytic (Freud, 1952; Hartmann, 1952; Kris, 1950; Rapaport, 1951) and nonpsychoanalytic persuasion (Lewin, 1936; Piaget, 1951; Werner, 1948) have suggested that primitive, developmentally early behavior is marked by immediate, direct, and unmodulated responses to external stimuli and internal need states. In contrast, higher levels of maturation are characterized by the appearance of indirect, ideational, conceptual, and symbolic or verbal behavior patterns. Thus, developmental psychology suggests that a shift in emphasis from action to thought is an expression of the maturational sequence.

The action–thought parameter (Zigler and Glick, 1986; Phillips and Zigler, 1961) leads to certain predictions concerning the relationship between behavior and maturity level, including the presence of abusive acts in a person's behavioral repertoire. Simply put, those at a higher maturational level will have interactions with children and others that are expressed in words and thoughts. Parents at a lower developmental level will, essentially, act before they think. Their interactions with their children will be characterized by impulsivity and direct action, including abusive acts when they are angry, frustrated, or highly stressed.

Ecological approach

Perhaps the most successful attempt to date to integrate the various components contributing to child abuse is represented by Belsky's ecological model (1980). Drawing heavily from Bronfenbrenner's ecological approach to the study of child development (1979), Belsky describes a system of nested, interactive levels that contribute to the development of behaviors, including abusive ones. Bronfenbrenner's original theory postulated three such spheres: He divides the "ecological space" (Belsky, 1980, p. 321) of the person or persons being studied into micro-, macro-, and exosystems. Belsky's framework incorporates into this ecological system the work of Burgess (1978) and Tinbergen (1951), both of whom propose that any behavior may be approached from a number of different levels of analysis. These include the historical and behavioral background of the action in question, the immediate antecedents thereof, and the sequelae.

The model that results from Belsky's synthesis of these materials makes available to us a comprehensive framework for the understanding of behaviors – in this case, of child abuse. The model proposes four levels of interactive, mutually nested spheres of influence: (a) the level of ontogenic development, (b) the microsystem, (c) the exosystem, and (d) the macrosystem. We will briefly review what each of these spheres represents, and how studies that fall under each area contribute to our understanding of the causes of child abuse.

Ontogenics. Ontogenic development is concerned with what the abuser brings to the situation. This includes such factors as parental history, the parent's developmental level, feelings toward the child, understanding of

child development, and parental mental health. We have already reviewed
in some detail the evidence for and against the intergenerational transmission of child abuse. Despite our conclusion that being abused as a child is
not a necessary and sufficient cause for becoming an abusive parent, it is
clear that the parents' own rearing history, the style of parenting to which
they were exposed, and their own conceptions of their childhood and their
parents contribute significantly to the way they view and practice childrearing (Altemeier, O'Connor, Vietze, Sandler, and Sherrod, 1982; Egeland and
Jacobvitz, 1984; Kempe et al., 1962; Hunter and Kilstrom, 1979; Main and
Goldwyn, 1984). As we saw in the previous section, the parents' own developmental level contributes heavily to their style of interaction with their
child (Newberger and Cook, 1983; Polansky et al., 1981; Ross and Zigler,
1983). Similarly, researchers have found that parents' understanding of
child development, of what may appropriately be expected of a child at a
given age, is related to whether or not they engage in abusive behaviors.
Parents who have unrealistically high expectations of their child are more
likely to abuse than are parents who have a good understanding of the
sequence of child development (Young, 1964).

The microsystem. A second factor contributing to behavior involves the
immediate environment of the child. Examples include the nature of the
family setting, child health, child temperament, family size, the nature of
the spousal relationship, and immediate antecedent incidents that may all
trigger an instance of physical abuse. The findings reviewed earlier in this
chapter indicate that certain child characteristics have been implicated in
abuse: Prematurity (Gil, 1970; Parke and Collmer, 1975), low birthweight
(Klein and Stern, 1971), aversive cry related to neurological problems
(Frodi, 1981; Lester, 1984), and hyperactivity (Parke, 1977) have all been
found to be related to increased incidence of physical abuse. Emotionally
unsatisfying spousal relationships (Morris and Gould, 1963) or spousal relationships in which the child is viewed as intrusive (Bakan, 1971) may also
contribute to increased likelihood of abuse.

The exosystem. It is essential that we view children and families as existing
within a broader system. Imbedded within extended families, the community, and the economic structure, families are influenced by all of these and
others. Much research links the world of work with child abuse. Unemployment, whether through increased economic hardship or loss of esteem and
power, has been found to be a common factor in child abuse (Gil, 1970;
Young, 1964), as has lack of job satisfaction (McKinley, 1964, cited in Parke
and Collmer, 1975). Numerous researchers have indicated that isolation of
the family from social supports, neighborhood networks, extended families,
and so on is a major contributor to child abuse (Bakan, 1971; Kempe, 1973;

Garbarino, 1982; Hunter and Kilstrom, 1979; Newberger et al., 1977; Parke and Collmer, 1975; Richmond and Janis, 1980; Zigler, 1980). Kempe (1973) emphasized the importance of such support systems by calling them a "lifeline" on which the parent can rely during times of stress. In the absence of this support, the unrelieved stress is likely to contribute to abuse.

The macrosystem is the "outmost" layer of influence that interacts with the three other spheres. This consists of, as Belsky says, "the larger cultural fabric in which the individual, the family, and the community are inextricably interwoven" (1980, p. 328). Into this category fall societal attitudes toward violence in general, societal expectations about child discipline in the home and at school, and the level of overall violence in the country and in the community. As we have noted, violence in the U.S. can be regarded only as very high (Gil, 1970; Hobbs, 1980; Zigler, 1976) and corporal punishment is the rule rather than the exception (Gil, 1970; Parke and Collmer, 1975; Straus et al., 1979). In this atmosphere, the physical punishment and abuse of children is to be expected, and is even, whether overtly or implicitly, condoned.

The essence of the ecological model is not simply in the cumulative or additive effects of each of these systems, but in their mutual interaction. Belsky stresses the nested nature of this framework: Every system works on every other one, here contributing to the increased likelihood of abuse, there providing a buffer or stress that may help to prevent it. Only when we consider all of these factors in and of themselves *and* as they interact can we understand the totality of the phenomenon that is physical child abuse.

Systems for intervention

A multidisciplinary approach

As we have already indicated, child abuse is not a heterogeneous, unitary phenomenon on which all workers take the same perspective. The empirical research of Giovannoni and Becerra (1979) demonstrates vividly the significant differences between professional groups asked to rate the seriousness of a series of abuse vignettes. Pediatricians, taking a medical model approach, may view certain behaviors as more or less serious, according to their training and the information available to them. Police officers, on the other hand, may identify as abusive situations that arouse little or no anxiety in physicians. The same may be said of the social workers and lawyers in the Giovannoni and Becerra study, or of teachers, day care workers, journalists, clinical psychologists, and developmental specialists. Each of these groups will have a unique perspective on the issue of physical child abuse, and within each group more individual differences will exist. Workers from each of these backgrounds will bring a different approach to the study of child abuse, and each will have different ideas about the identification and control of child abuse. It is realistic to assume that none of these has the whole picture but that, instead, input from many different disciplines will combine to form the most comprehensive, most useful approach to the problem of child abuse (Rotatori, Steckler, Fox and Green, 1984; Zigler and Hall, 1984).

Some efforts will focus specifically on child abuse (Parents Anonymous, for instance); others will address particular problems that contribute to violence toward children. Treatment for substance abusers and parent education efforts are examples of this type of approach. General efforts to improve the social ecology of our nation's families constitute a third orientation toward understanding and treating child abuse.

As we have noted, the first step in the right direction is already being made. It is essential that we continue to strive toward understanding all facets of child abuse. We have come a long way since the 1960s, when abusing parents were uniformly characterized as pathological monsters, and children were believed to be passive recipients of abusive behaviors. Now we understand that all members of a family – and, most likely, influences from beyond the circle of the family – play their roles in child abuse. But further research, further work is necessary. Health practitioners, members of the legal system, teachers, psychologists, law enforcement workers, and the media all have their roles to play in furthering our understanding of child abuse and in enhancing preventive efforts.

We must make appropriate use of existing facilities and social agencies for the identification and treatment of child abuse, but we must also lobby for the funding of additional facilities. Learning to make use of existing social networks in our communities is essential. Schools and churches must get involved, not in hunting down child abusers, but in making available the information that might help to prevent abuse and in providing support to families in which abuse has already occurred. Employers can act, as some already have, to enhance family life and relieve stress by upholding policies that promote day care, flex-time, and paid infant care leaves (Zigler and Muenchow, 1983). "Gatekeeper figures" such as school officials, clergy, and doctors in each community must be educated and kept informed, so that they in turn will be part of the education process.

Education for parenting

Professionals involved with child abuse are virtually unanimous in their call for parent education and training programs, not only to teach effective parenting skills, but also to help parents and parents-to-be know what to expect in the course of a child's development. Knowledge about children could certainly help to prevent many cases of abuse, from that of the mother who spanks her 6-month-old infant for soiling his diaper, to the parents who injure the legs of their 5-month-old son by attempting to teach him to walk (Kempe et al., 1962), to the college-educated couple whose efforts to produce a "super baby" by bombarding their child with cognitively inappropriate stimuli frustrate both the child and the parents and increase feelings of stress and inadequacy in the parents. Further, parents must be trained in effective disciplinary alternatives to physical punishment (N. D. Feshbach, 1980; S. Feshbach, 1980; Reid, in press). Children also should be trained in parenting, beginning in elementary school and continuing through high school. Such long-range planning is designed to enhance family-oriented attitudes, responsible family planning, and appropriate expectations regarding child and family life (Herzig and Mali, 1980).

The media can play a crucial role in the education of the general public and can be used in two important ways (Ross and Zigler, 1980). First, both print and broadcast media can be used to rally public support for child abuse policies and programs. Second, the communications industry can help to improve public awareness of child abuse: what it is, what it isn't, and what can be done to combat it. A program of 30- or 60-second television spots similar to the "Bicentennial Minute" feature that aired throughout 1976 or the "FYI" health features of the 1980s would be an efficient way of reaching large numbers of parents with brief, easy to assimilate bits of practical information. Such features should be informative rather than threatening; we must strive for sensitivity in our utilization of the communications networks.

Family support systems

Family support projects are springing up throughout the United States (Yale Bush Center, 1984) and addressing a variety of issues, including child abuse. An excellent example is the Ounce of Prevention program in Illinois, whose method of providing family support has been very effective in controlling child abuse and attenuating the influence of other negative social indicators. Another valuable early intervention program, Yale University's "Children's House" (Provence and Naylor, 1983) was only funded for a brief time and is no longer in operation. Follow-up assessments of the participating families revealed striking improvements in the kinds of factors that have been correlated with child abuse, such as family size, spacing of children, and maternal education. Moreover, evaluations show that these programs are actually cost-saving over time. Clearly, the family support movement has promising implications for child abuse prevention.

We must also promote services designed to support and educate families in nonoptimal situations: Groups such as Parents Anonymous, crisis nurseries where parents can leave a child for up to 24 hours to break a cycle of escalating violence, day care facilities, homemaker aids, Foster Grandparents' services, and any buddy system or means of relieving stress and isolation can make a difference in the incidence of child abuse (Kempe and Helfer, 1972). Social and community groups can act to coordinate and evaluate the services available in each community (Gray, 1984; National Council of Jewish Women, 1978).

Medical providers, as well as social service personnel, have an essential role in the primary prevention of child abuse. Their most vital function is to educate the public regarding family planning issues and then to make contraceptive services available to all those who desire them. Unwanted babies are more often the targets of abuse than are welcome babies, and abuse is more likely where there are too many babies. When childbirth occurs, Newberger and Newberger (1982) suggest that the delivery process be "humanized," and that fathers be included. These steps could strengthen family bonds at a time that, even at its most joyous, can be extremely stressful.

Adequate prenatal care is another cost-effective intervention. Maternal and child health programs, intensive prenatal care programs for teenagers and other high-risk mothers, and nutrition programs such as WIC (free food program for women, infants, and children) can offset the financial expenditure that might otherwise be required later and in larger amounts to fund remedial health programs. And, as we have seen, unhealthy, premature, and low birthweight babies are at greater risk for child abuse than are healthy, full-term infants. Educational programs for parents whose child is in one of these higher risk groups would help them form realistic expectations of what their child will be like and boost their self-confidence in dealing with a special-needs baby. Such families may also benefit, as would families in which abuse has already occurred, from visits by parent or homemaker aides. Being paired with other families with same-age babies would also provide relief from feelings of social isolation, give the parents someone with whom to share advice, crisis child care, and support. Finally, further research in this area is urgently needed. The research dollars allocated by the 1974 Child Abuse Prevention and Treatment Act were insufficient for mounting the sound studies that will help us to answer the questions we have raised about the nature of child abuse. Two areas in particular have yet to be adequately investigated. First, we must begin to evaluate the services currently being provided to families in trouble. In order to provide the most efficient and cost-effective services possible, it is crucial that we understand which among our treatment models are successful, and what makes them so. Second, we must investigate the long-term consequences of child abuse (Newberger,

Newberger, and Hampton, 1983). What are the cognitive, developmental, behavioral, emotional, and medical sequelae of having been abused? Only thorough, longitudinal research can tell us, and we must make this a priority if we are to help those who have been maltreated as well as those who may be in the future.

Conclusions

It has been less than a quarter of a century since Kempe and his colleagues identified the "battered child syndrome," and since then we have raised as many questions regarding the phenomenon of child abuse as we have answered. We do know that we can no longer view the field as Kempe did in 1962: The "them versus us," the "bad abusers versus the good non-abusers," model must be relegated to history. Anyone is a potential child abuser, regardless of social class or child-rearing history. With rare exceptions, the child abuser is not "sick," but troubled and isolated, as much a victim as the child. We also know more about the sociological factors implicated in the physical abuse of children. No longer do we believe that being poor "causes" child abuse. Rather, the social stresses and the scant educational, economic, and social network resources that so often accompany poverty in America are the variables that contribute to an increased likelihood of abuse. Finally, increased sophistication in our research in this area has enabled us to move beyond the idea that child abuse is necessarily transmitted from generation to generation. Further work in this area will contribute more to our understanding of the factors that protect families against engaging in abusive behaviors. It is time for a change in attitude on the part of all workers involved with child abuse. We must be supportive rather than punitive, compassionate instead of judgmental. More harm than good can come from applying self-righteous labels to families involved in abuse.

The problem of child abuse is not one that can be addressed in isolation. Although it is a problem that virtually everyone abhors, children's needs are still not a high priority among this nation's social policymakers. The wealthiest nation in the world is home not only to children who are physically abused, but also to children who are neglected, who are hungry, who receive inadequate medical and dental care, and who lack someone to give them responsible day care. America is home to infants who die because of inadequate prenatal and postnatal care. Despite this sad litany, there are steps that can be taken to solve the problems of children in the United States, including those of child abuse. We have the means in our possession to do so, but no progress will be made until we make the needs of children a social and financial priority. The magnitude of these issues is great, but we cannot allow that to be an excuse for inaction.

Note

1. Child Abuse Prevention and Treatment Act of 1974 (1974). Public law 92–247, *U.S. Statutes at Large*, 88, 4–8.

References

Aber, L. J., and Zigler, E. (1981). Developmental considerations in the definition of child maltreatment. In R. Rizley and D. Cicchetti (Eds.), *Developmental Perspectives on Child Maltreatment* (pp. 1–29). San Francisco: Jossey-Bass.

Altemeier, W., O'Connor, S., Vietze, P., Sandler, H., and Sherrod, K. (1982). Antecedents of child abuse. *Journal of Pediatrics, 100*, 823–829.

Anderson, R., Ambrosino, R., Valentine, D., and Lauderdale, M. (1983). Child deaths attributed to abuse and neglect: An empirical study. *Children and Youth Services Review, 5,* 75–89.

Ariès, P. (1962). *Centuries of childhood: A social history of family life.* New York: Alfred A. Knopf.

Bakan, D. (1971). *Slaughter of the innocents: A study of the battered child phenomenon.* San Francisco: Jossey-Bass Publishers.

Baker v. Owen (1975). 395 F. Supp. 294, 96 S. Ct. 210.

Barash, D. P. (1977). *Sociobiology and behavior.* New York: Elsevier Press.

Belsky, J. (1980). Child maltreatment: An ecological integration. *American Psychologist, 35,* 320–335.

Berkowitz, L. (1973). Control of aggression. In B. M. Caldwell and H. N. Ricciuti (Eds.), *Review of child development research.* Volume 3: Child development and social policy. Chicago: University of Chicago Press.

Berkowitz, L. (1975). *A survey of social psychology.* Hinsdale, IL: Dryden Press.

Blatt, B. (1980). The pariah industry: A diary from purgatory and other places. In G. Gerbner, C. Ross, and E. Zigler (Eds.), *Child abuse: An agenda for action.* New York: Cambridge University Press.

Blatt, B., and Kaplan, F. (1966). *Christmas in purgatory: A photographic essay on mental retardation,* 2nd. ed. Boston: Allyn and Bacon.

Bleiberg, N. (1965). The neglected child and the child health conference. *New York State Journal of Medicine, 65,* 880–1885.

Bongiovanni, A. (1977). A review of research on the effects of punishment: Implications for corporal punishment in the schools. In J. Wise (Ed.), *Proceedings conference on corporal punishment in the schools: A national debate.* Washington, D.C.: National Institute of Education. NIE p–77–0079.

Bourne, R. (1979). Child abuse and neglect: An overview. In R. Bourne and E. Newberger (Eds.), *Critical perspectives on child abuse.* Lexington, MA: Lexington Books.

Bremner, R. H. (Ed.) (1971). *Children and youth in America: A documentary history.* Vol II: 1866–1932. Cambridge, MA: Harvard University Press.

Bronfenbrenner, U. (1979). *The ecology of human development.* Cambridge, MA: Harvard University Press.

Burgess, R. (1978). Child abuse: A behavioral analysis. In B. Lakey and A. Kazdin (Eds.), *Advances in child clinical psychology.* New York: Plenum Press.

Caffey, J. (1946). Multiple fractures in the long bones of infants suffering from chronic subdural hematoma. *American Journal of Roentgenology, 56* (2), 163–173.

Cicchetti, D., and Rizley, R. (1981). Developmental perspectives on the etiology, intergenerational transmission, and sequelae of child maltreatment. In R. Rizley and D. Cicchetti (Eds.), Developmental perspectives on child maltreatment. *New Directions for Child Development, 11.*

Cline, V., (Ed.) (1974). *Where do you draw the line?* Provo, UT: Brigham Young University Press.

Cohn, Anne H. (1983). *An approach to preventing child abuse.* Chicago: National Committee for the Prevention of Child Abuse.

Commission on Children's Rights (1978). *Barnesratt: On forbud not aga.* Stockholm: Swedish Department of Justice.

Curtis, G. (1963). Violence breeds violence – perhaps. *American Journal of Psychiatry, 120,* 386–387.

Diamond, L. J., and Jaudes, P. K. (1983). Child abuse in a cerebral palsied population. *Developmental Medicine and Child Neurology, 35,* 169–174.

Dubanoski (1981). Child maltreatment in European- and Hawaiian-Americans. *International Journal of Child Abuse and Neglect, 5,* 457–465.

Egeland, B., and Jacobvitz, D. (1984). Intergenerational continuity of parental abuse: Causes and consequences. Presented at the Conference on Biosocial Perspectives in Abuse and Neglect. York, Maine.

Encyclopaedia Brittanica (1890). 9th edition, Vol. 13.

Feshbach, N. D. (1980). Corporal punishment in the schools: some paradoxes, some facts, some possible directions. In G. Gerbner, C. J. Ross, and E. Zigler (Eds.), *Child abuse: An agenda for action.* New York: Oxford University Press, 204–224.

Feshbach, N. D., and Feshbasch, S. (1971). Children's aggression. *Young Children, 26,* 364–377.

Feshbach, S. (1980). Child abuse and the dynamics of human aggression and violence. In G. Gerbner, C. J. Ross, and E. Zigler (Eds.), *Child abuse: An agenda for action.* New York: Oxford University Press, 48–62.

Fontana, V. J. (1968). Further reflections on maltreatment of children. *New York State Journal of Medicine, 68,* 2214–2215.

Freud, A. (1952). The mutual influences in the development of ego and id: Introduction to the discussion. *Psychoanalytic Studies of the Child, 7,* 42–50.

Friedrich, W., and Wheeler, K. (1982). The abusing parent revisited: A decade of psychological research. *The Journal of Nervous and Mental Disease, 170,* 577–587.

Frodi, A. (1981). Contribution of infant characteristics to child abuse. *American Journal of Mental Deficiency, 85,* 341–349.

Galdston, J. (1965). Observations on children who have been physically abused and their parents. *American Journal of Psychiatry, 122,* 440–443.

Garbarino, J. (1976). A preliminary study of some ecological correlates of child abuse: The impact of socioeconomic stress on the mother. *Child Development, 47,* 178–185.

Garbarino, J. (1982). Healing the wounds of social isolation. In E. H. Newberger (Ed.), *Child abuse.* Boston: Little, Brown, 25–55.

Garbarino, J. (1983). What we know about child maltreatment. *Children and Youth Services Review, 5,* 3–6.

Garrison, F. H. (1965). Abt–Garrison history of pediatrics. In I. A. Abt (Ed.), *Pediatrics,* Vol. I. Philadelphia: W. B. Saunders.

Gaudin, J. M., and Pollane, L. (1983). Social networks, stress and child abuse. *Children and Youth Services Review,* 91–102.

Gelles, R. J. (1973). Child abuse as psychopathology: A sociological critique and reformulation. *American Journal of Orthopsychiatry, 43,* 611–621.

Gelles, R. J. (1979a). *Family violence.* Beverly Hills, CA: Sage.

Gelles, R. J. (1979b). Violence toward children in the United States. In R. Bourne and E. H. Newberger (Eds.), *Critical perspectives on child abuse.* Lexington, MA: Lexington Books.

Gelles, R. J. (1980). Violence in the family: A review of research in the seventies. *Journal of Marriage and the Family, 42,* 873–885.

Gelles, R. J. (1982). Child abuse and family violence: Implications for medical professionals. In E. H. Newberger (Ed.), *Child abuse.* Boston, MA: Little, Brown.

Gelles, R. J., and Cornell, C. P. (1985). *Intimate violence in families. Family studies text services.* Vol. 2. Beverly Hills: Sage.

Gerbner, G., Ross, C., and Zigler, E. (Eds.). (1980). *Child abuse: An agenda for action.* New York: Oxford University Press.

Gil, D. (1970). *Violence against children: Physical child abuse in the United States.* Cambridge, MA: Harvard University Press.

Giovannoni, J., and Becerra, R. (1979). *Defining child abuse.* New York: The Free Press.

Giovannoni, J., and Billingsley, A. (1970). Child neglect among the poor: A study of parental adequacy in families of three ethnic groups. *Child Welfare, 49,* 196–204.

Gray, E. (1984). *What have we learned about preventing child abuse? An overview of the "Community and minority group action to prevent child abuse and neglect" program.* Chicago: National Committee for Prevention of Child Abuse.

Hanway, J. (1785). *A sentimental history of chimney sweepers.* London.

Hartmann, H. (1952). Mutual influences in the development of ego and id. *Psychoanalytic Studies of the Child, 7,* 9–30.

Helfer, R., and Kempe, E. (Eds.). (1968). *The battered child.* Chicago: University of Chicago Press.

Helfer, R., and Kempe, C. (1976). *Child abuse and neglect: The family and the community.* Cambridge, MA: Ballinger Publishing.

Herzig, A. C., and Mali, J. L. (1980). *Oh, boy! Babies.* Boston, MA: Little, Brown.

Hobbs, N. (1980). Knowledge transfer and the policy process. In G. Gerbner, C. J. Ross, and E. Zitler (Eds.), *Child abuse: An agenda for action.* New York: Oxford University Press.

Hunter, R. S., and Kilstrom, N. (1979). Breaking the cycle in abusive families. *American Journal of Psychiatry, 136,* 1320–1322.

Ingraham versus *Wright* (1977). 430 S. Ct. 651.

James, J. J. Furukawa, T. P., James, N., and Mangelsdorf, A. D. (1984). Child abuse and neglect reports in the United States Army Central Registry. *Military Medicine, 149,* 205–206.

Junewicz, W. J. (1983). A protective posture toward emotional neglect and abuse. *Child Welfare, 62,* 243–252.

Kaplan, S. J., and Zitrin, A. (1983a). Psychiatrists and child abuse. I. Case assessment by protective services. *Journal of the American Academy of Child Psychiatry, 22,* 253–256.

Kaplan, S. J., and Zitrin, A. (1983b). Psychiatrists and child abuse. II. Case assessment by hospitals. *Journal of the American Academy of Child Psychiatry, 22,* 257–261.

Kaufman, J., and Zigler, E. (1987). Do abused children become abusive parents? *American Journal of Orthopsychiatry, 57*(2), 186–192.

Kempe, C. (1973). A practical approach to the protection of the abused child and rehabilitation of the abusing parent. *Pediatrics, 51,* 804.

Kempe, C., and Helfer, R. (1972). *Helping the battered child and his family.* Philadelphia, PA: J. B. Lippincott.

Kempe, R., and Kempe, C. H. (1978). *Child abuse.* Cambridge MA: Harvard University Press.

Kempe, C., Silverman, F., Steele, B., Droegmueller, W., and Silver, H. (1962). The battered child syndrome. *Journal of the American Medical Association, 181,* 17–24.

Kessen, W. (1965). *The child.* New York: Wiley.

Keyserling, M. D. (1972). *Windows on day care.* New York: National Council of Jewish Women.

Klein, M., and Stern, L. (1971). Low birth weight and the battered child syndrome. *American Journal of the Disabled Child, 122,* 15–18.

Krappe, A. H. (1965). *The science of folklore.* London: Methuen.

Kris, E. (1950). Notes on the development and on some current problems of psychoanalytic child psychology. *Psychoanalytic Studies of the Child, 5,* 34–62.

Kuttner, R. E. (1983). Is child abuse a human instinct? *International Journal of Social Psychiatry, 29,* 231–233.

Lee, R. W. (1956). *The elements of Roman law.* London: Sweet and Maxwell.

Lester, B. M., (1984). A bisocial model of infant crying. In L. Lipsitt and C. Collier (Eds.), *Advances in infancy research: Monographs in infancy,* Vol. 3.

Levy, R. I. (1969). On getting angry in the Society Islands. In W. Candill and T. Y. Lin (Eds.), *Mental health research in Asia and the Pacific.* Honolulu: East-West Center Press.

Lewin, K. (1936). *Dynamic theory of personality.* New York: McGraw Hill.

Light, R. (1973). Abused and neglected children in America: A study of alternative policies. *Harvard Educational Review, 43,* 556–598.

Lorenz, K. (1966). *On aggression.* New York: Harcourt, Brace, & World.

Main, M., and Goldwyn, R. (1984). Predicting rejection of her infant from mother's representation of her own experiences: A preliminary report. *International Journal of Child Abuse and Neglect, 8,* 203–207.

McHenrey, T., Girdany, B. R., and Elmer, E. (1963). Unsuspected trauma with multiple skeletal injuries during infancy and childhood, *Pediatrics, 31,* 903–908.

McPherson, K. S., and Garcia, L. R. (1983). Effects of social class and familiarity on pediatrician's responses to child abuse. *Child Welfare, 62,* 387–393.

Mead, M. (1937). The Arapesh of New Guinea. In M. Mead (Ed.), *Cooperation and competition among primitive peoples.* New York: McGraw Hill.

Milner, J. S., Gold, R. G., Ayoub, C. E., and Jacewitz, M. M. (1984). Predictive validity of the Child Abuse Potential Inventory. *Journal of Consulting and Clinical Psychology, 52,* 879–884.

Morris, M. G., and Gould, R. W. (1963). Role reversal: A necessary concept in dealing with the battered child syndrome. In Child Welfare League of America (Ed.), *The neglected/battered child.* New York: Child Welfare League of America.

Morris, M. G., Gould, R. W., and Matthews, P. J. (1964). Toward prevention of child abuse. *Children, 11,* 55–60.

National Council of Jewish Women (1978). *Innocent victims: NCJW manual on child abuse and neglect programs.* New York: Justice for Children Task Force.

Newberger, C. M. (1982). Psychology and child abuse. In E. H. Newberger (Ed.), *Child abuse.* Boston, MA: Little, Brown.

Newberger, C. M., and Cook, S. (1983). Parental awareness and child abuse: A cognitive–developmental analysis of urban and rural samples. *American Journal of Orthopsychiatry, 53,* 512–524.

Newberger, C. M., and Newberger, E. (1982). Prevention of child abuse: Theory, myth and practice. *Journal of Preventive Psychiatry, 1,* 443–451.

Newberger, E. and Daniel, J. (1979). Knowledge and epidemiology of child abuse: A critical review of concepts. In R. Bourne and E. Newberger (Eds.). *Critical perspectives on child abuse.* Lexington, MA: Lexington Books.

Newberger, E., Newberger, C. M., and Hampton, R. (1983). Child abuse: The current theory base and future research needs. *Journal of the American Academy of Child Psychiatry, 22,* 262–268.

Newberger, E., Reed, R., Daniel, J., Hyde, J., and Kotelchuck, M. (1977). Pediatric social illness: Toward an etiologic classification. *Pediatrics, 60,* 178–184.

Oliver, J. E., and Taylor, A. (1971). Five generations of ill-treated children in one family pedigree. *British Journal of Psychiatry, 119,* 473–480.

Parke, R. (1977). Socialization into child abuse: A social interactional perspective. In J. L. Tapp and J. F. Levine (Eds.), *Law, justice, and the individual in society.* New York: Holt, Rinehart, and Winston.

Parke, R., and Collmer, C. (1975). Child abuse: An interdisciplinary analysis. In M. Hetherington (Ed.). *Review of child development research,* Vol. 5, Chicago: University of Chicago Press, 509–590.

Parke, R. D., and Lewis, N. G. (1981). The family in context: A multilevel interactional analysis of child abuse. In R. W. Henderson (Ed.). *Parent–child interaction – theory, research prospects.* New York: Academic Press.

Pelton, L. (1978). Child abuse and neglect: The myth of classlessness. *American Journal of Orthopsychiatry, 48,* 608–617.

Phillips, L., and Zigler, E. (1961). Social competence: The action–thought parameter and vicariousness in normal and pathological behaviors. *Journal of Abnormal and Social Psychology, 63,* 137–146.

Piaget, J. (1951). Principal factors in determining evolution from childhood to adult life. In D. Rapaport (Ed.), *Organization and pathology of thought.* New York: Columbia University Press, 154–175.

Polansky, N. A., Chalmers, M. A., Buttenweiser, E., and Williams, D. P. (1981). *Damaged parents; An anatomy of child neglect.* Chicago: University of Chicago Press.

Potter, C. F. (1949). Infanticides. In M. Leach (Ed.), *Dictionary of folklore, mythology, and legend,* Vol. 1. New York: Funk & Wagnalls.

Provence, S., and Naylor, A. (1983). *Working with disadvantaged parents and their children.* New Haven, CT: Yale University Press.

Radbill, S. (1974). A history of child abuse and infanticide. in R. Helfer and C. H. Kempe (Eds.), *The battered child* (2nd ed.). Chicago, Ill: University of Chicago Press.

Rapaport, D. (1951). Toward a theory of thinking. In D. Rapaport (Ed.), *Organization and pathology of thought.* New York: Columbia University Press, 689–730.

Reid, J. B. (1983). *Final report: Child abuse: Developmental factors and treatment.* Grant No. 7 RO1 MH 37938, NIMH 4, U.S. Ph.S.

Reid, J. B. (in press). Social-interactional patterns in families of abused and nonabused children. In C. Zahn Waxler, M. Cummings, and M. Radke-Yarrow (Eds.), *Social and biological origins of altruism and aggression.* New York: Cambridge University Press.

Reitman, A., Follman, J., and Ladd, E. (1972). *Corporal punishment in the public schools: The use of force in controlling behavior.* New York: American Civil Liberties Union.

Richmond, J. B., and Janis, J. (1980). Child health policy and child abuse. In G. Gerbner, C. J. Ross, and E. Zitler (Eds.), *Child abuse: An agenda for action.* New York: Oxford University Press, 281–292.

Robin, M. (1982). Sheltering arms: The roots of child protection. In E. H. Newberger (Ed.), *Child abuse.* Boston, MA: Little Brown, 1–24.

Rodham, H. (1973). Children under the law. *Harvard Educational Review, 43,* 487–514.

Rogers, J. A. (1979). Child abuse in humans: A clinician's view. In M. Reite and N. G. Caine (Eds.), *Child abuse: The nonhuman primate data.* New York: Alan R. Liss.

Rosenberg, M. S., and Repucci, N. D. (1983). Abusive mothers' perceptions of their own and their childrens' behavior. *Journal of Consulting and Clinical Psychology, 51,* 674–682.

Rosenfeld, A., and Newberger, E. (1979). Compassion versus control: Conceptual and practical pitfalls in the broadened definition of child abuse. In R. Bourne and E. Newberger (Eds.), *Critical perspectives on child abuse.* Lexington, MA: Lexington Books.

Ross, C. (1980). The lessons of the past: Defining and controlling child abuse in the United States. In G. Gerbner, C. Ross, and E. Zigler (Eds.), *Child abuse: An agenda for action.* New York: Oxford University Press.

Ross, C., and Zigler, E. (1980). An agenda for action. In G. Gerbner, C. Ross, and E. Zigler (Eds.). *Child abuse: An agenda for action.* New York: Oxford University Press, 293–304.

Ross, C., and Zigler, E. (1983). Editorial. Treatment issues in child abuse. *Journal of the American Academy of Child Psychiatry, 22,* 305–308.

Rotatori, A. F., Steckler, S., Fox, R. A., and Green, H. (1984). A multidisciplinary approach to assessing the abused youngster. *Early Child Development and Care, 14,* 93–108.

Shorter, E. (1975). *The making of the modern family.* New York: Basic Books.

Sidel, R. (1972). *Women and child care in China.* New York: Hill & Wang.

Solnit, A. (1980). Too much reporting, too little service: Roots and prevention of child abuse. In G. Gerbner, C. Ross, and E. Zigler (Eds.). *Child abuse: An agenda for action.* New York: Oxford University Press, 135–146.

Sorel, N. C. (1984). *Ever since Eve: Personal reflections on childbirth.* New York: Oxford University Press.

Spinetta, J. J., and Rigler, D. (1972). The child abusing parent: A psychological review. *Psychological Bulletin, 77*, 296–304.

Steele, B. F., and Pollock, D. (1968). A psychiatric study of parents who abuse infants and small children. In R. E. Helfer and C. H. Kempe (Eds.). *The battered child.* Chicago, IL: University of Chicago Press, 103–148.

Stern, E. S. (1948). The Medea complex: The mother's homicidal wishes to her child. *The Journal of Mental Sciences, 94*, 324–325.

Stone, L. (1977). *The family, sex, and marriage in England 1500–1800.* New York: Harper & Row.

Straus, M., Gelles, R., and Steinmetz, S. (1979). *Behind closed doors: Violence in the American family.* Garden City, N.Y.: Anchor/Doubleday.

Tinbergen, N. (1951). *The study of instinct.* London: Oxford University Press.

Tuteur, W., and Glotzer, J. (1966). Further observations on murdering mothers. *Journal of Forensic Sciences, 11*, 373–383.

Uviller, R. (1980). Save them from their saviors: The constitutional rights of the family. In G. Gerbner, C. Ross, and E. Zigler (Eds.). *Child abuse: An agenda for action.* New York: Oxford University Press, 147–155.

Werner, H. (1948). *Comparative psychology of mental development.* (Rev. ed.). Chicago: Follett.

Werner, O. H. (1917). *The unmarried mother in German literature.* New York: Columbia University Press.

West, S. (1888). Acute periosteal swelling in several young infants of the same family, probably rickety in nature. *British Medical Journal, 1*, 856.

Wooley, P., and Evans, W. (1955). Significance of skeletal lesions of infants resembling those of traumatic origin. *Journal of the American Medical Association, 15*, 539–543.

Yale Bush Center in Child Development Social Policy (1984). *Programs to strengthen families: A resource guide.* Chicago, IL: Yale University and the Family Resource Coalition.

Young, K., and Zigler, E. (1986). Infant and toddler day care: Regulation and policy implications. *American Journal of Orthopsychiatry, 56*, 45–55.

Young, L. (1964). *Wednesday's children: A study of child neglect and abuse.* New York: McGraw Hill.

Zalba, S. R. (1971). Battered children. *Transaction, 8*, 58–61.

Zigler, E. (1976). Controlling child abuse in America: An effort doomed to failure? In D. Adamovicz (Ed.). *Proceedings of the first national conference on child abuse and neglect.* Atlanta: Department of Health, Education, and Welfare.

Zigler, E. (1980). Controlling child abuse: Do we have the knowledge and/or the will? In G. Gerbner, C. Ross, and E. Zigler (Eds.). *Child abuse: An agenda for action.* New York Oxford University Press, 3–34.

Zitler, E. (1983). Understanding child abuse: A dilemma for policy development. In E. Zigler, S. L. Kagan, and E. Klugman (Eds.). *Children, families and government: Perspectives on American social policy.* New York: Cambridge University Press, 331–352.

Zigler, E., and Glick, M. (1986) *A developmental approach to adult psychopathology.* New York: Wiley.

Zigler, E., and Hall, N. (1984). Child abuse: Using multidisciplinary research to improve measurement and control. (Contract No. 1287-4464). Washington, D.C.: National Academy of Sciences.

Zigler, E., and Hunsinger, S. (1977). Supreme Court on spanking: Upholding discipline or abuse? *Society for Research in Child Development. Newsletter*, Fall.

Zigler, E., and Muenchow, S. (1983). Infant day care and infant care leaves: A policy vacuum. *American Psychologist, 38*, 91–94.

3   Pediatrics and child abuse

Howard Dubowitz and Eli Newberger

Introduction

In 1962 pediatricians were instrumental in bringing the "battered child syndrome" (Kempe, Silverman, Steele, Droegemueller, and Silver, 1962) to professional and public attention. Pediatricians are responsible for the health and welfare of children, and must therefore play an important role in addressing the immense problem of child maltreatment. In this chapter, we trace the development of pediatric involvement in the realm of child abuse and neglect, examine the principles and dilemmas of current practice, and explore potential roles.

Course of pediatric involvement and thinking

Radiologists have a maxim: "You see what you look for, and you look for what you know." For many years physicians have taken care of injured children, but until recently the likelihood that a proportion of those injuries were inflicted appears not to have been considered. Somehow, alternate explanations were found. Today, the major incidence studies of child maltreatment show it to be a phenomenon of epidemic proportions (Straus, Gelles, and Steinmetz, 1980; American Humane Association, 1985; Straus and Gelles, 1986), and pediatricians play a central role in the assessment, diagnosis, and care of maltreated children. A brief historical sketch of how this involvement has developed places current medical practice in perspective.

Before Kempe

Child abuse is not new. Although incidence data have only been assembled in recent years, it is evident that child abuse dates back at least to the beginning of recorded human history (Lynch, 1985; De Mause, 1974). And yet, there is no mention of child abuse in the medical literature until the middle of the twentieth century. How might this be explained?

The rights of children and the duties of parents were viewed in the past very differently from today (Ariès, 1962; De Mause, 1974). Children enjoyed few rights, and society invested immense trust in parents to raise their children as they saw fit. It is not that long ago that children were seen as the property of their parents, particularly their fathers. In addition, colonial America was heavily influenced by religious teaching on child raising, with its "spare the rod, spoil the child" philosophy (Tucker, 1974). Taking the child's perspective or considering the civil rights of children were just not issues of the day. In this context it is not difficult to understand how child maltreatment would not be identified as a problem.

Sexual mores in different cultures at different times reveal a broad range of views, many of which would today be considered sexual abuse. Ancient Egyptian royalty married their siblings to maintain the purity of their royal blood. In contrast, the powerful incest taboo in Viennese society in the early part of this century apparently dissuaded Freud from his seduction theory of neurosis (Masson, 1984). It is only in the last decade that sexual issues in the United States have been addressed with relative ease, and this has contributed to the discovery of the pervasive sexual abuse of children.

During the latter part of the nineteenth century, the field of social work was becoming increasingly involved with family problems, including child maltreatment. Physicians, in contrast, adhered primarily to a biomedical model – germs were being identified, vaccines and antibiotics developed, and scant attention was paid to the social contributors of health and illness. Given that narrow view, it is understandable that the possibility of a parent inflicting an injury upon a child was simply overlooked – or perhaps denied. Despite the romantic notion of the close relationship between the old-time family practitioner and his patients, it is probable that matters of child rearing or family conflict were not seen as issues for the doctor. If physicians avoided broaching such topics regarding family life, and families did not seek help from them to address these problems, it is not surprising that domestic strife and violence would pass undetected.

The first detectable movement in physician consciousness of abuse occurred in 1946 when a pediatric radiologist, Caffey, speculated as to how infants incurred multiple fractures in association with intracranial bleeds (Caffey, 1946). He gently raised the possibility of neglect or abuse as the cause. Several years later, specific bone injuries were attributed to abuse by a parent or guardian (Silverman, 1953). Based on the pediatric literature in the ensuing years, these reports appear to have had limited influence.

The 1960s – the decade of "the battered child"

A major turning point took place in 1962, when Kempe and his associates, in an influential article entitled "The Battered Child Syndrome" in a prestigious medical journal, drew attention to the problem (Kempe et al., 1962). This paper stimulated an outpouring of editorial concern in professional and lay media. It was the stimulus for the drafting by the Children's Bureau, the lead agency for children in the federal government, of a model child abuse reporting statute. A flurry of legislative activity ensued, and within 5 years all 50 states had promulgated child abuse reporting laws. Professionals responsible for children were mandated to report suspected abuse to public agencies, principally welfare departments, who in turn were required to ensure the safety of the children.

It is not coincidental that the new sensitivity to the needs of children occurred in a time of great public concern for the rights of disadvantaged citizens of the United States. This concern included a belief that government had a responsibility and a role to play in supporting those in need of help. Consequently, several major programs to benefit children were initiated: the regional centers for retarded children, Project Head Start, and Medicaid – a program offering health insurance to indigent adults and their children. Sensitivities were aroused to consider the rights, and abuse, of children.

Although published several years following Caffey's report, Kempe and his colleagues' article is seen as heralding the discovery of child abuse. The dramatic title of "The Battered Child Syndrome" held clear connotations. An etiological model of vicious aggression perpetrated by a psychologically disturbed caregiver upon a helpless child victim was suggested. It was the responsibility of physicians to recognize the syndrome, make the "diagnosis," and report the case to the child protection agency that would provide the necessary intervention. The suggested formulation successfully captured professional, media, and public attention, but led to certain problematic ramifications.

The perpetrator–victim model contributed toward, and reflected, a narrow view of etiology: helpless infants and children being maliciously battered by mentally ill or deviant adults. It would be approximately a decade later that serious mental illness would be shown to be as prevalent among abusive parents as in the general population (Steele, 1975; Wright, 1976; Gaines, Sandgrund, Green, and Power, 1978). This is, however, in need of reassessment using the clear diagnostic criteria laid out in *DSM-III* (see Cicchetti and Rizley, 1981). It appears likely that certain forms of abuse, such as sexual molestation or planned and severe maltreatment, are more likely correlated with parental psychopathology. The psychological difficulties of a caretaker by no means preclude a potential role of other contributory factors. Indeed, environmental factors can exert an important influence toward the development of the psychopathology.

It is interesting to speculate as to why the attribution of child abuse to parental psychopathology was so readily accepted as the major etiological factor. If such aberrant behavior as abusing a child is connected with mental illness, then those who are "normal" or healthy have little to fear. Although it now appears that the majority of people who maltreat children are not mentally ill, it can be seen that assigning a certain deviancy to such behavior serves a valuable protective function.

Another implication of the perpetrator–victim model is the focus on the violent transaction itself. With caregivers under the spotlight, attention has been diverted from other contributory factors and etiological theories. This has limited the understanding of child maltreatment and restricted the development of preventative and therapeutic interventions.

The perpetrator–victim model connotes intentionality of the maltreatment and, therefore, blame. This fosters a response that is likely to be more punitive than therapeutic as is evidenced in the recent report of the Attorney General's Task Force on Domestic Violence (National Institute of Justice, 1984). Although outcomes of the legal system's involvement remain to be studied, it seems that it is public outrage, rather than children's needs, that is being catered to. A substantial body of research exists that supports an ecological understanding of child maltreatment with a complex etiology of multiple interacting factors, in which "perpetrators" might be seen as only one piece of the puzzle (Belsky, 1980; Cicchetti and Rizley, 1981; Garbarino, 1977). To what extent have we resorted to blaming the victim (Ryan, 1977)? The perpetrator–victim model persists in current thinking, as reflected in recent laws passed by a number of states that include the involvement of law enforcement agencies and the court systems in managing child abuse cases (Hampton and Newberger, 1985; Helfer, Hoffmeister, and Schneider, 1978).

The distinction between "punitive" and "therapeutic" approaches is not as clear as advocates have argued. Psychotherapy, particularly when mandated by an agency in a position of authority, can be controlling, albeit subtly so, and perceived as punitive. In contrast, legal measures that lead to the protection of a child can be valuable and have a therapeutic effect. Appropriate interventions need to be tailored to individual cases, and a constructive integration of compassion and control appears optimal for most situations (Rosenfeld and Newberger, 1977).

The 1970s – a broadened conceptualization

In the 1970s, influenced by studies of child abuse that were stimulated by the public and professional activism of the 1960s, the laws mandating the reporting of child abuse were revised. In 1973 a new model child abuse reporting law was promulgated by the U.S. Children's Bureau, and Public Law 97–243 established the National Center on Child Abuse and Neglect. This statute broadened the definition of child abuse to include child neglect, emotional injury, parental deprivation of medical care, and factors injurious to a child's moral development. Almost all professionals with responsibilities for the care of children were mandated to report suspected child abuse cases. The subsequent expansion of state statutes resulted in an expected increase in reports of child abuse, but budgetary appropriations continued to lag far behind the necessary level of support. The federal government had played an important leadership role, but financial backing was minimal. Nevertheless, the 1970s witnessed the wide deployment of demonstration projects and treatment interventions. Studies of the foster care system demonstrated significant problems, (Fanshel and Schinn, 1978; Gruber, 1978), and new efforts were made to keep most maltreated children in their families wherever possible. Parents of abused children were seen as people who could be helped, and interventions centered around supporting them to better protect their children. *Helping the battered child and his family* edited by Kempe and Helfer (1972) illustrates the more humane approach of the time.

The broadening of the definition of child abuse, associated with the public awareness campaigns initiated both by the National Center and by the private National Committee for the Prevention of Child Abuse, facilitated the perspective that child abuse is not restricted to parents setting out to destroy their defenseless offspring. The states' broadened reporting laws held important implications for pediatricians, who now needed to diagnose and report a new array of conditions. Infants born drug addicted, newborns with features of fetal alcohol syndrome, children who were unimmunized or with health needs that were being neglected, deprived youngsters who were being psychologically abused at home, and infants with nonorganic failure to thrive were all within the newly defined realm of pediatric responsibility.

The development is consistent with the increasing focus within pediatrics on the so-called "new morbidity" (Haggerty, Goghmann, and Pless, 1975). This term embraces a range of psychosocial problems affecting children, such as drug addiction, behavioral difficulties, parental divorce or separation, teenage pregnancy, and child maltreatment. A Task Force on Pediatric Education and leaders in the profession declared the need for pediatricians to be responsive to these important problems confronting American children (American Academy of Pediatrics, 1978; Haggerty, 1985).

An underpinning of the broadened conceptualization of child maltreatment had been the development of the ecological theory of etiology. Child abuse was no longer seen as a discrete event but rather as a symptom of family distress. It made sense to more comprehensively examine contributory factors, and in addition, to consider other symptom manifestations under the rubric of abuse or neglect. These new dimensions added complexity to managing these problems and have warranted interdisciplinary collaboration of pediatricians with nursing, legal, social work, and mental health colleagues.

The 1980s – new forms of abuse

Sexual abuse has been uncovered as a major problem, with prevalence estimates ranging from 3 to 15 percent of boys and 12 to 38 percent of girls (Finkelhor, 1979; Kinsey, Pomeroy, Martin, and Gebhard, 1953; Russell, 1983). The last few years have seen a rapid increase in studies in this area and innovative efforts at prevention, including school programs and television public service announcements. Still, the knowledge base is extremely limited and much remains to be learned. A related concern has been the sexual abuse of children in day care settings, since several cases involving many children have received enormous media attention.

The federal government has in recent years proposed an active federal involvement in cases of multiply handicapped infants in newborn intensive care units. This followed a series of widely publicized lawsuits concerning infants born with various defects where physicians and families considered the prognosis to be hopeless. Treatment and, in some instances, fundamental life support, were withheld. The debate centered around the prognosis and quality of life with some viewing the outlook as sufficiently good to justify appropriate support and medical treatment. Denial of treatment was argued to be a form of child abuse. After a good deal of heated debate, the U.S. Department of Health and Human Services, the key medical associations, and citizen groups reached a compromise with guidelines for care. Although decisions are left for the most part to physicians and families, oversight is maintained by mandatory Infant Care Review Boards within hospitals. This provision was included in the 1984 Federal reauthorization of the National Center on Child Abuse and Neglect.

In summary, the number of reported cases of child abuse continues to rise. Resources to meet the identified needs remain woefully inadequate and professionals are called upon to be responsive despite a lack of training and preparation. Notwithstanding the progress of the last 25 years, the knowledge base is limited and many critical questions remain unanswered. Pediatrics is therefore confronted with an immense responsibility and needs to find new ways to be helpful to children and families.

Pediatric practice: conflicts and dilemmas

In this section, we will focus on a number of pragmatic and conceptual factors that impinge on current pediatric practice in the area of child maltreatment.

Pragmatic constraints

Involvement in cases of child abuse and neglect invariably demands a considerable time commitment from the pediatrician. Typically, physicians in a busy private practice allot 15–20 minutes for a regular "well-child check" and less time for "sick" visits. When a problem arises that calls for more time, the physician's schedule falls behind and patients are kept waiting.

There are few shortcuts in the assessment of possible maltreatment. An anxious child might require 15 minutes of reassurance before allowing the pediatrician to proceed with the examination. Aware of the immense ramifications that a report to a state agency might have, there is a need to cautiously evaluate the circumstances surrounding an injury, and how the family situation might have contributed to it. Beyond the initial assessment, a good deal of time can be consumed by the support and counseling of the family, collaborating with other professionals involved in the case, and possible court appearances.

Remuneration for medical care in child abuse cases is rarely commensurate with the time involved, providing a further disincentive for pediatricians to get involved. On the average, pediatricians earn less than any other group of physicians, and they depend upon seeing large numbers of children to support their income. Pediatricians are thus deterred from becoming involved in an area that many already deem peripheral to their work.

One possible solution is the training of pediatric specialists in abuse and neglect. Primary care physicians typically seek consultation from specialists for problems that they are not comfortable in handling. Identifying pediatricians or interdisciplinary clinics that are specialists in the assessment of child maltreatment could provide a valuable resource to physicians and others. Parents of maltreated children are frequently anxious that optimal medical consultation be obtained and that the nature of the injuries and likelihood of maltreatment be carefully evaluated. This is particularly so following alleged sexual abuse, when great anxiety and fears are experienced. In addition, child protection services and the juvenile courts require astute medical consultation to support their efforts. Not least, the children, under the circumstances, deserve optimal medical care. This arrangement has been successfully established in a number of states (Kremer, 1984).

Another pragmatic restraint confronting pediatricians is the relatively small amount of contact time they have with children and families. The actual time spent together is far less than with a school teacher or a visiting nurse, for example. Many physicians honestly question just how much they really know of what transpires in the homes of the children they take care of. Certainly, there are instances when the problems are flagrant and declare themselves overtly, but frequently the difficulties might not be at all obvious. This is not to minimize the potential opportunity for physicians to take an interest in the health related aspects of the lives of their patients and, in the context of a respectful and confidential relationship, to seek an understanding of the family situation. But it is humbling to acknowledge the limited insights gained from brief intermittent visits every 3, 6, or 12 months.

Biomedical focus

This had been alluded to earlier, where medicine has traditionally utilized a biomedical model with relatively scant attention to psychosocial factors in health and illness. The intern who exclaims: "What a fascinating case!" is no doubt referring to some rare, perhaps exotic, physical condition. Psychosocial problems rarely engender the same enthusiasm, and the treatment of organic disease represents the thrust of physician training.

It is only in recent years that a few medical schools have begun to teach students psychosocial aspects of medicine and that pediatric residents are being trained to manage these problems. Despite the attention given to the new morbidity in pediatrics, the psychosocial area of practice still occupies a lowly status in the priorities of pediatric training programs.

Without suitable training, it is understandable that pediatricians do not feel at ease and competent to grapple with problems such as child abuse and neglect. It might well seem preferable to confine one's practice to dealing with such problems as anemia, meningitis, or lead poisoning, which are well within the pediatrician's repertoire of skills.

There is, in addition, a more insidious consequence of the biomedical model. This stems from a linear theory of causality that is frequently invoked to explain disease processes. For example, an insufficient iron intake depletes the body stores and results in anemia. Although this model might be applicable to some problems, it is less useful in explaining child abuse and neglect. No single simple cause is explanatory, and understanding the symptom requires exploring multiple and interacting causal factors. A typical laceration or fracture seen in a busy emergency room generally evokes only a modest degree of interest. A cursory history might be obtained and the laceration sutured; the possibility of an injury being inflicted is frequently overlooked. (This is even more of a problem with adult women who are battered. All too often the physical injuries alone are taken care of and the patient discharged home.)

Professional bias

A 3-year-old with a fractured arm is more likely to be diagnosed and reported as having been abused if he or she is treated in a city hospital emergency room than in a private pediatrician's office. There are a number of reasons for the difference in diagnosis and reporting.

O'Toole, Turbett and Nalepka (1983) studied the responses of physicians (and others) to case vignettes of children with different injuries under varying circumstances. Each case vignette was held constant except for 3 descriptors that were experimentally manipulated: racial group, social class, and severity of the injury. Respondents were asked to diagnose "abuse" or "accident" for each vignette. Black children were more likely to be diagnosed as abused than white children when all other descriptors of the vignette were identical. Similar prejudicial judgments were made against families of lower social class and when the injury was more severe.

What is known about these factors? The incidence data based on *reported* cases do show a disproportionately high representation of minority and poor families (U.S. Department of Health and Human Services, 1984). To some extent this reflects a certain bias as to who gets diagnosed as abused and, once identified, reported (Hampton and Newberger, 1985). However, prejudice probably does not totally account for the disproportionate representation, and families in the lowest socioeconomic classes themselves reveal far more frequent violent behavior (Straus, Gelles, and Steinmetz, 1980). When the influence of social class is eliminated, no clear differences in child abuse between blacks and whites in the U.S. have been demonstrated.

Integration of the available data suggests that although discriminatory diagnoses are made against poor and minority families, there also does exist a greater degree of violent behavior in impoverished subcultures. It should be added that no study has demonstrated a correlation between the severity of an injury and the likelihood that it was inflicted.

Why do physicians (and others) have these prejudices? Faulty science is seen in the "woozle effect," where questionable research findings become "established facts" despite being based on an unsatisfactory methodology. A cyclical dynamic is set in motion. If more blacks are reported as abusive, this is then reflected in incidence data (of reported cases), and later can be misinterpreted as a "characteristic" of child abuse. A stereotype results, and blacks are more likely to be diagnosed and reported as abuse cases.

Another consideration is the emotional response of those who work with abused children. The bruised infant with several fractures evokes strong feelings of sadness and anger. For many, it is difficult to understand and accept how such violent behavior can be explained. For others it is frightening to acknowledge that indeed many of us have the *capacity* to be violent. How many parents who have experienced enormous frustration and anger towards their child have thought, "How close I came to hurting my child"? To avoid reconciling with this possibility, it might be easier to repress such a painful reality in the form of denial. In conjunction with this defense mechanism, violent behavior is attributed to those who are substantially different from oneself. For white middle class professionals, poor and minority groups fit this bill.

Confidentiality of the doctor–patient relationship

The respected confidentiality between physician and patient has facilitated the establishment of a trusting rapport, allowing patients to disclose their most private concerns to their physicians. Professional consultation is thus sought with the understanding that "it will go no further," and physicians have long respected this.

Pediatrics presents a somewhat complicated case. Although the health of the child is the primary responsibility, much of the care is necessarily implemented through the parents. Consequently, close relationships exist with both the child and the parents. A dilemma arises as to whether the primary affiliation is to the child or to the parents. Too often, problems of child abuse are couched in terms of the rights of parents versus those of children, and protection of the relationship with the parents can supersede intervention to safeguard the child. A more useful framework is to understand child abuse as a symptom of a family in distress, and we are therefore primarily concerned with the *rights of families.* In the majority of instances, children who have been abused or neglected will remain with their families or return to them after a temporary sojourn in foster care. The best interests of most children are inextricably bound together with the best interests of their families. Support and nurture of families should enable them to better protect and take care of their children. This constructive approach is not easy to implement today because, in order to obtain support services for a family, it is often first necessary to demonstrate that maltreatment has occurred.

The strength of the physician–family tie can wield significant influence on clinical management. This is especially the case in private practice settings where there is greater continuity of care – the child is seen by the same pediatrician over a period of time – compared with poor inner city populations using hospital clinics. When the subject of abuse arises, a report to a state protective agency is likely to be perceived by both the family and doctor as a breach of trust and confidentiality. That such a report is mandated by law and should lead to the delivery of much needed services to the family does not console the family, which is hurt by the stigma associated with such reports. In a conscious or unconscious effort to avoid antagonizing parents, pediatricians may not file a report. A valuable guiding principle for pediatricians should be that ensuring the safety of the child is their first responsibility, and since most children are best served by remaining in their families, a constructive approach to working *with* these families is called for.

Criminalization

In recent years there has been a trend toward greater criminalization of child abuse, with rapidly increasing involvement of law enforcement personnel and the judicial systems. For example, in Southern California the initial report is automatically filed with both the Department of Social Services and the Police Department. In Massachusetts, legislation passed in 1983 requires the Department of Social Services to report certain more serious categories of abuse to the District Attorney. Maryland State law requires a joint investigation of all cases by the Department of Social Services and the Police Department. Particularly in the area of sexual abuse, there is a consensus among most professionals that court authority is necessary at least to confront offenders and mandate therapy, if not to prosecute and punish them.

Quite precipitously, a social work approach of over 100 years duration has given way to a punitive "solution." Partly rooted in the frustration with the limited success of therapeutic interventions, and in the context of a generally conservative political climate, policemen, lawyers, and the courts have readily been embraced as resources needed to deal with the problem of child abuse. Considering their lack of education and training in this area, the inherently adversarial approaches and punitive philosophies of their disciplines, the implications for families and children are uncertain (Weiss and Berg, 1982).

Criminalization of child abuse further complicates the doctor–patient relationship. Now, perhaps, pediatricians are ethically bound to warn parents *in advance* that what is divulged to them might require the filing of a case report. This could involve the District Attorney, who then has the prerogative of whether or not to pursue criminal prosecution. It is feasible that this sequence of events could serve several deterrent functions: Families could be deterred from confiding in their physicians and other professionals; pediatricians might be deterred from becoming involved, especially if court appearances seem likely. On the other hand, it has been argued that when offenders are given the clear signal that abusive behavior is not tolerable and constitutes a crime, they can be deterred from such actions. The considerable effects of criminalization on all parties concerned have not been adequately studied, and evaluative research is critically needed.

Skepticism of social services

Many physicians and other professionals share a widely held belief that state social service agencies have not succeeded in helping a large proportion of the families reported to them (Morris, Johnson, and Clasen, 1985; Saulsbury and Campbell, 1985). State legislatures liberally expanded the definitions of reportable conditions, but failed to match this commitment with the appropriation of sufficient funds. Consequently, although large numbers of cases are being identified, resources for serving this population are seriously limited, and most child protection agencies have been overwhelmed. Lowly status, poor salaries, high case loads, limited supervision, and lack of office space and support staff are among the obstacles to quality professional work. Even the best intentions burn out under such circumstances (Daley, 1979).

There are, in addition, serious limitations to what social service agencies can realistically achieve. They rarely have the wherewithal to address underlying problems such as inadequate housing, unemployment, miserable poverty, and lack of community supports. Generally, they are constrained to applying "bandaids," when radical surgery is necessary. A number of critiques have assailed the whole system as less than a serious endeavor to improve the lives they are purporting to help; "a poor system for poor people" (Jenkins, 1974; Piven and Cloward, 1971).

Social service involvement can appear (and can be) more harmful than helpful, posing a difficult dilemma for physicians with their dictum: primum non nocere – first, do no harm. There is a danger, however, of physicians becoming nihilistic. The problems are complex, and the challenge is to seek new and better ways to enhance the lives of children and families. Partial solutions should not be cynically discarded while families are hurting, one such solution being an agency that competently offers a range of supportive services to families in need. Pediatricians can play a useful role in supporting this work by cooperating with the agency, offering consultation and training on health related matters, and advocating needed funding by state and federal governments.

Physician roles: present and potential

Central to the practice of pediatrics is the responsibility of overseeing the health of children – health being defined to include physical and mental health, growth, and development. As the new morbidity becomes an increasingly important part of pediatric practice, pediatricians have recognized the need to become competent in dealing with problems such as drug abuse, teenage pregnancy, and child abuse and neglect. This last section examines what role pediatricians are currently playing in the realm of child abuse, and to where this could lead in the future.

Despite the concerns many Americans have about the enormous cost of health care, physicians continue to command a good deal of respect and represent authority figures at all levels within our society. Because of the influence pediatricians wield with individual families and communities at large, they should be actively involved in issues that affect the well-being of children. There are many forms that this participation can take.

Screening and prevention

Early screening and detection of children at high risk for abuse and neglect is an important pediatric task. An example is the diagnosis of newborns who are born drug addicted or with fetal alcohol syndrome. Many states include this category as a reportable condition. It is especially during the infancy period that pediatricians might be the only professionals who have frequent contact with families, providing a good opportunity to assess how well a family is coping, the nature of their interactions and relationships, and whether the baby is being adequately nurtured and protected.

The astute and sensitive clinician is able to detect possible warning signals and, in addition, to actively seek an understanding of the parent's feelings and concerns. A depressed or angry mother, a father who refuses to come in for any of the appointments even though he is not employed, a severe diaper rash, or frustration expressed about the poor hygiene and lack of safety in a project apartment, are all indicators of certain difficulties that *might* reflect family conflict and violence.

There is a critical distinction between screening and diagnosis. None of the examples above per se constitute child abuse, nor can they be construed as causing child abuse. Rather, they reflect a high-risk situation that *could* involve family violence. A constraint on pediatric screening is the limited ability to predict maltreatment. The research literature primarily identifies risk factors that have been shown to correlate with, not to cause, child maltreatment. A few studies that followed high-risk families prospectively from the prenatal period identified relatively small numbers of cases of maltreatment and it was difficult to discern what it was about those families that explained their violent behavior (Egeland and Brunquell, 1979; Vietze, O'Connor, Hopkins, Sandler, and Altemeier, 1982). A number of research studies have been conducted to screen parents for potential maltreatment (Conger, 1981; Helfer, Hoffmeister, and Schneider, 1978; Milner, 1986). To date, none of these have been satisfactorily validated with sufficient sensitivity, specificity, and predictive value to be applied in clinical practice. Pediatricians thus do not have any definite measure for calculating high risk status; they need to rely upon their clinical intuition, experience, and those risk factors that research has correlated with maltreatment.

An important consideration is the goal of the screening measure. If the screening instrument is simply used to indicate whether further clarification is needed, there can be little damage. If it leads to supportive services for those in need, that would be laudatory. However, when simplistic diagnoses are rapidly made, or if harmful interventions ensue, this is an abuse of the screening measure, and is especially a problem for those who are falsely screened positive (Cicchetti and Aber, 1980).

Good pediatric practice would clarify the child's and family's strengths and difficulties, with help from colleagues in social work, mental health, and nursing. This assessment should identify specific needs and strengths and then lead to the implementation of appropriate services in a plan worked out with the family. Pediatricians typically play a supportive and counseling role, but if more intensive mental health intervention is indicated, a referral is generally made. Pediatricians also can be useful advocates to help ensure that needed services such as day care, an early intervention program, or a visiting nurse are implemented. Ideally, families should be supported to enable them to cope better with their difficulties and so be in a position to adequately nurture and protect their children.

Unfortunately, the resources in the United States for primary prevention are severely limited. All too frequently, services are only available "after the fact," once abuse or neglect have already occurred. For what purpose are efforts at primary prevention, if the needed resources to intervene effectively do not exist? An essential criterion of a screening test is that early detection of high-risk status yield some benefit to the patient or client. Detection alone is generally not helpful, and potentially harmful. The paucity of resources to help families provides a formidable challenge for the pediatrician to be as supportive as possible and to advocate the implementation of those services that are available.

Diagnosis and reporting

Pediatricians have an important role in the diagnosis of abuse and neglect and account for approximately 12 percent of reported cases nationwide (American Humane Association, 1985). Pediatricians are, in addition, frequently consulted to examine children to clarify allegations of abuse made from another source.

This medical evidence is extremely variable. At times there are physical findings such as bruises, a fracture, or failure to gain an appropriate amount of weight. In only a relatively small proportion of cases, however, the injuries are flagrantly the result of inflicted trauma. More typically, the medical data are quite ambiguous, necessitating a careful integration with the history and context of the injury together with an assessment of the family functioning and relationships. Given the possible ramifications of a child abuse report, it is critical that such a comprehensive evaluation be made to enable an educated formulation concerning the child's presenting signs and symptoms.

This more extensive assessment requires a considerable amount of time and might well go beyond the pediatrician's repertoire of skills. In many hospitals with pediatric departments, interdisciplinary groups including pediatricians, nurses, social workers, lawyers, and mental health professionals have been formed. This approach appears to be optimal to address the complexity of a good proportion of these cases, and also helps to alleviate the burden of responsibility from any one individual. Of course, there are cases where the issues are relatively straightforward, and the pediatrician alone can reasonably report the child to the appropriate child protection agency.

The pediatrician in a busy private practice is in a far more difficult situation with less access to colleagues in related disciplines. Consultation with staff at a nearby hospital or referral to a consultation interdisciplinary group such as those established in Florida might be the preferred route. In most parts of the country, pediatricians tackle the task alone, and their level of expertise varies greatly. One advantage of the private practitioner is the relationship and rapport established with a family over a period of time. This makes for a better understanding of the family's strengths and weaknesses, providing useful information to evaluate the presenting problem. This relationship can, however, complicate management in that the report might place in jeopardy the trust and rapport that have been established.

A sure diagnosis of abuse is not required by most state reporting laws. Rather, reports are mandated where a physician (or others), acting in good faith, has reasonable cause for concern that a child is being abused or neglected. Once a report is made, agency staff screen in those that will be investigated. Typically, reports made by physicians and other professionals are accepted for further investigation.

When a report is made in compliance with the law, the physician is immune from any liability. In contrast, should a report not be filed when there is reasonable indication to do so, the physician can be legally liable in the majority of states. In those states that have a penalty for not reporting, the intent is primarily to encourage professionals to comply with the reporting statute, although there have been a number of cases when a fine has been imposed.

Frustration with the modest success of child protection agencies has been raised in an earlier section. If limited help and possible harm are anticipated, physicians have a dilemma of whether or not to report. What are the alternatives? To do nothing, to ignore the situation, is not acceptable. To attempt to deal with the situation alone is clearly very difficult, and assumes considerable risk and responsibility. There does seem to be a compromise route.

The least detrimental and hopefully constructive approach might be for the physician to fulfill his or her legal obligation and file the report, but not to relinquish responsibility and involvement at that point. By staying involved, supporting the family, and helping to monitor the situation, the physician can play a valuable role after the report is made. This is a time when the pediatrician can strongly advocate on behalf of the child and family to help ensure that appropriate supportive services be implemented. There does exist the potential for pediatricians to considerably influence the subsequent course of events with regard to both social service and law enforcement agencies.

The public health perspective offers another interesting view. It has been suggested that one of the obstacles to high quality clinical management is the discrepancy between widely defined reporting laws and inadequate resources. The question raised is: Should the statutes be more restrictive so as to identify only the highest risk situations, thus targeting services where most needed? Lower risk families would then not be screened into the system, and this would allow the social service agencies to more competently address the needs of fewer clients.

The problem with this approach is that conditions already need to be quite desperate in order to obtain services. Little is being done in the way of primary prevention. By identifying families in trouble, at least a case is made to advocate for the supports they need. That is perhaps an idealistic view and certainly a long-term one, but it appears preferable to further tightening the criteria for receiving possible help. In addition, agencies do have a natural mechanism of adjusting their responses according to their available resources.

The role of the pediatrician as an advocate for the child and family is very important (Westman, 1979). Within the family, the pediatrician can convey to parents much that the infant or young child is unable to express. Frequently, parents are not able to understand a given behavior or appreciate why a child reacts in a particular way. By helping parents to understand and accept their child and to manage difficult behavior, the pediatrician might alleviate the frustration or anger a parent is feeling. In addition, by guiding child-rearing practices – offering alternatives to corporal punishment, for example – pediatricians can enhance the ability of families to support and protect their children. Thus, the pediatrician can be a powerful advocate for the child within his or her family.

This function can be extended. Pediatricians have been playing an important role by advocating the improvement of facilities for children in their communities. In cases of abuse and neglect, several therapeutic and monitoring agencies generally become involved, and here too the pediatrician can be a valuable ally of the child. In this sphere, the pediatrician is often in the position of advocating for the entire family, not only the child. This is not surprising because, as discussed earlier, in most situations the child's best interests are served by the better functioning of the family.

Despite these possibilities, physicians might still feel frustrated by their limited abilities to substantially improve the lives of children and families. This is especially the case in the many instances of abuse and neglect where there exist multiple major problems. Unemployment, inadequate housing, dangerous neighborhoods, drug abuse, parental history of child abuse, and paucity of community supports contribute to a situation that often seems beyond the realm of pediatric care. Efforts with individual families might seem like hopeless stop-gap measures against overwhelming circumstances.

It is therefore crucial that pediatricians be advocates for children and families at the local, state, and national levels. Their voice in calling for critical programs and policies to protect and enrich the lives of children is a valuable addition to the child advocacy groups. The battle to enhance the lives of children and families in our society is one that needs to be fought on many fronts. Treating an injured child, supporting a family so as to prevent further abuse, working for new community programs, enhancing the efforts of a child protection agency, testifying at a congressional hearing – all are valuable endeavors toward the central goal of pediatrics: the optimal health and welfare of all children.

References

American Academy of Pediatrics (1978). *Task force on pediatric education, final report.* Evanston, IL.

American Humane Association (1985). *Highlights of official child neglect and abuse reporting 1983.* Denver: American Humane Association.

Ariès, P. (1962). *Centuries of childhood.* New York: Random House.

Belsky, J. (1980). Child maltreatment: An ecological integration. *American Psychologist, 35,* 320–355.

Caffey, J. (1946). Multiple fractures in the long bones of infants suffering from chronic subdural hematoma. *American Journal of Radiology, 56,* 163–173.

Cicchetti, D., and Aber, J. L. (1980). Abused children – abusive parents: An overstated case? *Harvard Educational Review, 50,* 244–255.

Cicchetti, D., and Rizley, R. (1981). Developmental perspectives on the etiology, intergenerational transmission and sequelae of child maltreatment. *New Directions for Child Development, 11,* 32–59.

Conger, R. D. (1981). Assessment of dysfunctional family systems. In B. B. Lahey and A. E. Kazdin (Eds.), *Advances in clinical child psychology* (Vol. 4, pp. 199–242). New York: Plenum Press.

Daley, M. R. (1979). "Burnout": Smouldering problem in protective services. *Social Work, 24,* 375–379.

De Mause, L. (1984). The evolution of childhood. In L. De Mause (Ed.), *The history of childhood* (pp. 1–74). New York: Psychohistory Press.

Egeland, B., and Brunquell, D. (1979). An at-risk approach to the study of child abuse. *Journal of the American Academy of Child Psychiatry, 18,* 219–235.

Fanshel, D., and Schinn, E. B. (1978). *Children in foster care.* New York: Columbia University.

Finkelhor, D. (1979). *Sexually victimized children.* New York: Free Press.

Gaines, R., Sandgrund, A., Green, A. H., and Power, E. (1978). Etiological factors in child maltreatment: A multivariate study of abusing, neglecting and normal mothers. *Journal of Abnormal Psychology, 87,* 531–540.

Garbarino, J. (1977). The human ecology of child maltreatment: A conceptual model for research. *Journal of Marriage and the Family, 39,* 721–735.

Gruber, A. R. (1978). *Children in foster care.* New York: Human Services Press.

Haggerty, R. J. (1985). Reflection on "summer dreams" of better child health care. *American Academy of Pediatrics News, 1,* 8.

Haggerty, R. J., Goghmann, K. J., and Pless, I. B. (1975). *Child health and the community* (pp. 94–116). New York: John Wiley and Sons.

Hampton, R., and Newberger, E. H. (1985). Child abuse incidence and reporting by hospitals: Significance of severity, class and race. *American Journal of Public Health, 75,* 56–59.

Helfer, R. E., Hoffmeister, J. K., and Schneider, C. J. (1978). *MSPP: A manual for use of the Michigan Screening Profile of Parenting.* Boulder, CO: Express Press.

Jenkins, S. (1974). Child welfare as class system. In A. L. Schorr (Ed.), *Children and decent people* (pp. 3–23). New York: Basic Books.

Kempe, C. H., and Helfer, R. E. (1972). *Helping the battered child and his family.* Philadelphia: Lippincott.

Kempe, C. H., Silverman, F. N., Steele, B. F., Droegemueller, W., and Silver, H. K. (1962). The battered child syndrome. *Journal of the American Medical Association, 18* (1), 17–24.

Kinsey, A., Pomeroy, C. E., Martin, C. E., and Gebhard, P. H. (1953). *Sexual behavior in the human female.* Philadelphia: Saunders.

Kremer, A. (1984). *Community prioritization as a functional approach to child abuse prevention.* Paper presented at the Fifth International Conference on Child Abuse and Neglect, Montreal. September.

Lynch, M. A. (1985). Child abuse before Kempe: An historical literature review. *Child Abuse and Neglect, 9,* 7–15.

Maryland Law pertaining to the Department of Human Resources, Section 5–905.

Massachusetts General Laws, Chapter 288 of the Child Abuse Act of 1983, The District Attorney Reporting Bill.

Masson, J. M. (1984). *The assault on truth: Freud's suppression of the seduction theory.* New York: Farrar, Straus, and Giroux.

Milner, J. S. (1986). *The child abuse potential inventory: Manual.* Webster, NC: Psytec Corporation.

Morris, J. L., Johnson, C. F., and Clasen, M. (1985). To report or not to report: Physicians' attitudes toward discipline and child abuse. *American Journal of Diseases of Childhood, 139,* 194–197.

National Institute of Justice (1984). *Attorney general's task force on family violence.* Washington, DC: U.S. Governmental Printing Office.

O'Toole, R., Turbett, P., & Nalepka, C. (1983). Theories, professional knowledge and diagnosis of child abuse. In D. Finkelhor, R. J. Gelles, G. T. Hotaling, and M. A. Straus (Eds.), *The dark side of families: Current family violence research* (pp. 349–362). Beverly Hills, CA: Sage.

Pelton, L. H. (1978). Child abuse and neglect: The myth of classlessness. *American Journal of Orthopsychiatry, 48,* 608–617.

Piven, F. F., and Cloward, R. A. (1971). *Regulating the poor: The functions of public welfare.* New York: Random House.

Public Law 98–457, Child abuse amendments of 1984.

Rosenfeld, A. A., and Newberger, E. H. (1977). Compassion versus control. *Journal of the American Medical Association, 237,* 2086–2088.

Russell, D. (1983). The incidence and prevalence of intrafamilial and extrafamilial sexual abuse of female children. *Child Abuse and Neglect, 7,* 133–146.

Ryan, W. (1977). *Blaming the victim.* New York: Vintage Books.

Saulsbury, F. T., and Campbell, R. E. (1985). Evaluation of child abuse reporting by physicians. *American Journal of Diseases of Childhood, 139,* 393–395.

Silverman, F. N. (1953). The roentgen manifestation of unrecognized skeletal trauma in infants. *American Journal of Radiology, 69,* 413.

Steele, B. F. (1975). Working with abusive parents: A psychiatrist's view. *Children Today, 4,* 3.

Straus, M. A., and Gelles, R. J. (1986). Change in family violence from 1975 to 1985. *Journal of Marriage and the Family, 48,* 465.

Straus, M. A., Gelles, R. J., and Steinmetz, S. K. (1980). *Behind closed doors: Violence in the American family.* Garden City, NY: Doubleday.

Tucker, M. J. (1974). The child as beginning and end: Fifteenth and sixteenth century English childhood. In L. de Mause (Ed.), *The history of childhood.* New York: Harper and Row.

U. S. Department of Health and Human Services, National Center on Child Abuse and Neglect (1984). National study on child neglect and abuse reporting. Denver: American Humane Association.

Vietze, P., O'Connor, S., Hopkins, J. B., Sandler, H. M., and Altemeier, W. A. (1982). Prospective study of child maltreatment from a transactional perspective. In R. H. Starr, Jr. (Ed.), *Child abuse prediction: Policy implications* (pp. 135–156). Cambridge, MA: Ballinger.

Weiss, E. H., and Berg, R. F. (1982). Child victims of sexual assault: Impact of court procedures. *Journal of the American Academy of Child Psychiatry, 21* (5), 513–518.

Westman, J. C. (1979). *Child advocacy.* New York: Free Press.

Wright, L. (1976). The "sick but slick" syndrome as a personality component of parents of battered children. *Journal of Clinical Psychology, 32,* 41–45.

4   Sexual abuse of children: causes and consequences

Carol R. Hartman and Ann W. Burgess

Introduction

Mrs. G., in psychiatric treatment for over 12 years, vacillated between various states of integration and hospitalization. A referral for medical evaluation and a sigmoidoscopy for rectal bleeding connected a long-standing delusion that her brain was "rotten" with an early sexual trauma. Sections of therapy interviews illustrate how the event fragmented the ego and the memory recall of the event.

Memory 1   One time a long time ago – I don't even remember how long ago, when I was a lot younger, on Saturdays I used to have to take my two brothers and sister to the park. There was a man at the park and he did something to my rectum and he had to go to jail for it. I had to go to court. I was maybe about 10. . . . He made it bleed. Then I had to go to court and tell them. I remember what the man looked like, but I can't remember what he did. . . . He was an old man; he was a dirty man; he stunk; his clothes were dirty. I had on a bathing suit. It's such a bad thing. If it hadn't been bad, they wouldn't have sent him to jail and the policeman wouldn't have hit him. We were in the park. I must have told somebody. I think I was scared because I was bleeding.

Memory 2   I was just thinking that I could still feel it. . . . I always felt so dirty. I felt bad because they put him in jail for something I let him do.

Memory 3   I was in the park with my two little brothers and sister and we'd been swimming. And this man had his two grandchildren with him, and they were the same age as my brothers and they were all playing together. The man told me to go with him, that he had something to show me and I went with him in the bushes. There was a big, like a big heap of leaves, rotting leaves. And he said he wanted to show me something and he showed me himself, exposed himself to me and then he said he wanted to make me feel good. And I was all for that and then he did it to me. He held me down with his hand and he put his leg on my leg and he forced me to do it and he slapped me once and made me cry. He really frightened me. I thought he was going to kill me. . . . I just laid there. He got up and pulled his pants and said, "See, I didn't hurt you after all." Then he left. (Stoller, 1973)

Stoller's (1973) case history of an adult woman charged with attempted murder and with a history of childhood sexual trauma provides an opening for the major questions of this chapter: What causes sexual abuse of children, and what are the consequences of sexual abuse? This case is important for several reasons. First, the realization that many women institutionalized for mental illness have a childhood history of sexual abuse (Carmen, Rieker, and Mills, 1984). Second, the case demonstrates how the event is dissociated from conscious memory and is represented in a delusion focused on a rotting brain. Third, this case illustrates how an associated set of events (e.g., bleeding, impending intrusive examination by sigmoidoscopy, and fear of death) converge to surface the repressed memory.

The woman's preservation of these memories shows the impact of the interaction between child victim and adult abuser. This impact comes not only from the sexual assault itself, but also from the distortion of the act by the molester's disqualification of the child's perception and experience. The woman remembered the molester said he would make her feel good; then he hurt her. Her face was thrown into the leaves, and the smell of the dead leaves combined with the odor of the man became the delusion of her rotting brain. While there are many possible outcomes from unresolved childhood sexual abuse, the recovered memory details important aspects of the abusive interaction and its outcome. At first glance, the case appears to be a stereotypic stranger, dirty-old-man type. However, this child told of the abuse; the abuser was identified, apprehended, and convicted – a scenario that counters many of the myths, especially considering the time period – the 1930s. That the aftereffects were so profound (lifestyle dysfunction, psychotic thinking, and homicidal aggression), even with the disclosure, points to the need for intervention with victimization as well as respectful attention to trauma by therapists working with adults who have histories of childhood sexual abuse.

It is the thesis of this chapter that the sexual assault of a child, whether brief or over time, requires psychological, social, and cognitive adjustment by the child in order to survive. As illustrated in the case example, this adjustment, in turn, has an impact on the child's developing ego. Our own clinical work with children who have psychologically survived group and sex-ring assaults (Burgess, Hartman, McCausland, and Powers, 1984) supports the notion that dissociation plays a substantive role in the process of survival. We believe this dissociation results in a splitting and discontinuity in the child victim's further development of body, ego, affective continuity with self, and self-preservation and caring functions. Understanding the *causes* of child sexual abuse and the concomitant operations used by the victimizer to entice and control the child is critical to understanding the *consequences* of early sexual abuse on psychological and social development.

Clinical experience with child victims of sexual abuse as well as with adults who commit sexually abusive acts suggests that there is a specific link between early life victimization and subsequent adult behavior as a victimizer. Furthermore, clinical investigation of the impact of strategies used to control children who are being sexually abused suggests that victim survival during the event is dependent on the victim's own psychological strategies, which result in continued fragmentations and impairment of normal development and a tendency in some victims toward acceptance of sexually abusive behavior.

To explicate our premise that childhood sexual abuse requires adjustments that influence the child's subsequent development, this chapter reviews critical variables in the background and development of sexual offenders that have been found to be associated with sexually abusing behaviors and also the factors associated with postassault adjustment of child victims. Many of the studies cited for both offenders and victims present conflicting or inconclusive connections as to the importance of early sexual abuse in maladjustment and subsequent deviant behavior, including sexual abuse patterns as manifested by pedophiles and rapists. Literature in these areas is limited at this time; nevertheless, what does exist establishes that early sexual abuse does have a complex impact on the victim, dependent on the nature of the assault, and that sexually offending adults are characterized by a powerful sense of justification for their actions with little or no regard for their child victims. The literature suggests that offender violence and disregard for victims bears an association with patterns of victim maladjustment. This lends support to further investigation into the characteristics of maladjustment that might lead to offender activities.

Definitions of child sexual abuse

The definition of child sexual abuse used for this chapter is broad and in accordance with the 1981 definition of the National Center on Child Abuse and Neglect. *Child sexual abuse* is defined as follows:

Contact and interactions between a child and an adult when the child is being used for the sexual stimulation of the perpetrator or another person. Sexual abuse may also be committed by a person under the age of 18 when that person is either significantly older than the victim or when the perpetrator is in a position of power or control over another.

The term *sexual exploitation* may include situations in which the child is physically forced into sexual activities with an adult or is psychologically pressured into the activities, but either must include a commercial element, that is, an economic motive. Although generally used legally to mean a money exchange, in this chapter *exploitation* will be used to include social and psychological rewards for a child. This exploitation is most commonly seen through activities of pornography. As described in the 1984 Report of the Committee on Sexual Offenses Against Children and Youths of the Government of Canada, child pornography is a direct product of child sexual abuse and comes into existence through the exploitation of a young person's sexual vulnerability.

Sexual abuse of children is proscribed in all states. When sexual abuse occurs within a family unit, its social definition is *incest*. Sexual abuse by people outside the family (i.e., older children, more powerful children, adults, neighbors, caretakers, strangers, or family friends) is called *sexual molestation*. Legal charges vary from state to state, as do definitions of "child." For this chapter, *children* are young people under the age of 12, and *adolescents* range in age from 13 to 18. The *perpetrator* is generally so labeled if there is an age difference of at least five years between victim and abuser. The term *child molester* encompasses both the psychiatric term of *pedophile* and the clinical term of *incest offender*. Each of these two types of child molester may have similar as well as dissimilar characteristics.

Prevalence of child sexual abuse

With the current highly publicized accounts of sexual abuse of children, there is increased interest, both professional and public, in the area. It is difficult to estimate how widespread this problem is, as the incidence of child sexual abuse in the general population tends to be underreported. Statistics on child sexual abuse vary considerably. This is due to differences, primarily in victim age categories, among state reporting requirements and because children and family members are reluctant to report abuse due to both the dynamics of secrecy and pressure from the offender.

Nevertheless, several studies have reported incidence statistics. Russell's 1982 random survey (N = 930), which used 14 separate questions to probe for a variety of forms of child sexual abuse, found that 28% of 930 San Francisco women had been victimized before age 14 – 12% of that 28% had been victimized by a relative. When the age level was raised to 17 years, the figure rose to 38% (Russell, 1982). Finkelhor's 1979 survey of 796 college students found that 19% of females and 9% of males had experienced sexual abuse as children (Finkelhor, 1979). A 1980 mail survey of 1054 Texas driver's license holders reported a history of victimization of 3% for males and 12% for females (Kercher, 1983). Gordon and O'Keefe (1985) reported on a retrospective review of 502 randomly selected cases of family violence between the years 1880 and 1960. Fifty, or 10%, included incest. A survey of 521 Boston parents found that 6% of the males and 15% of the females had had an experience of sexual abuse before the age of 16 by a person at least 5 years older than themselves (Finkelhor, 1984).

Current statistics are fairly consistent from study to study in that 8–10% of child sexual abuse cases involve strangers as offenders; close to half (47%)

include family member offenders; and approximately 40% involve offenders who are acquaintances of the child. Statistics also show that victim breakdown, by gender, is changing. A decade ago the reporting incidence of victims was 97% female vs. 3% male (Burgess et al., 1978). Currently, agencies are reporting 80% female vs. 20% male victims (Conte, 1984).

By extrapolating from some of these incidence statistics, one can speculate as to the prevalence of child sexual abuse (Finkelhor, 1984). Using conservative estimates, even if no more than 10% of all girls and 2% of all boys were sexually abused (based on 60 million currently under the age of 18), roughly 210,000 new cases of sexual abuse would occur every year (Finkelhor, 1984). The best statistics find the number of new cases coming to professional attention each year to be 44,700 (National Incidence Study, 1981). Compared with the 210,000 speculated cases, this number illustrates how small a fraction of cases are being seen by professionals.

Causes of child sexual abuse – retrospective studies of deviant subpopulations

Even though there has been interest in recent years in determining the causes of sexual abuse, studies have been hindered significantly by this range of reporting problems. As a result, one approach to the initial exploration of the impact of early sexual abuse and its relationship to sexually abusive behavior patterns has been to investigate retrospectively the histories of deviant subpopulations. This type of approach, however, is associated with numerous methodological shortcomings. For instance, Browne and Finkelhor (1984) identify sampling problems and lack of control populations as reasons to exercise caution in concluding that child sexual abuse produces deviancy. Nevertheless, the prevalence of early childhood sexual abuse has been found in populations of juvenile delinquents (Reich and Gutierre, 1979), prostitutes (James and Meyerding, 1977; Silbert and Pines, 1981), and sex offenders (Groth, 1979; Seghorn, Boucher, and Prentky, in press). Conte (1985; see also Conte, Berliner, and Schurman, 1986) challenges several of the traditional clinical concepts applied to adults who have sexual interest in children on the basis of lack of empirical study or on the use of biased sample such as incarcerated offenders. For example, the typology of the fixated versus regressed child molester (Groth, Hobson, and Gary, 1982) was based on a prison population and suggests that discrete features exist in each group when in fact community-based therapists find that many offenders have combined features from both categories. In the typology of the incest versus the pedophilia offender – which is based on three core tenets: (1) incestuous fathers do not abuse outside the family, (2) incest is the sexual expression of nonsexual needs, and (3) every member of the family makes a psychological contribution to the development and maintenance of sexual abuse – there is increasing evidence that many incestuous fathers are in fact sexually acting outside of the home, that all sexuality contains sexual and nonsexual dimensions, and that stereotyped profiles of incest families do not hold up empirically (Conte, 1985; Conte et al., 1986).

Findings by Seghorn and colleagues of incarcerated offenders illustrate the abused–abuser cycle. This study found that

1. the incidence of sexual assault in childhood among child molesters was higher than the incidence of such abuse reported in the literature of both clinical and nonclinical sample groups,
2. the incidence of sexual assault in childhood among child molesters was more than twice that of the incidence among rapists,
3. rapists who were abused in childhood were three times more likely to have been victimized by a family member than were child molesters (three quarters of whom were victimized by strangers or casual acquaintances and who were more likely male abusers), and
4. when a sexual assault had occurred, among child molesters as well as rapists, it was associated with several other indices of familial turmoil and instability.

Classification of child abusers

Although the questions about the causes of sexual abuse of children do not yet have a definitive answer (Conte, 1984), attempts to address these questions have included efforts to develop child sexual abuse typology classification systems. These systems hypothesize that understanding *who* abuses children will elucidate the reasons *why* abuse occurs.

The results of an empirical study of classification efforts have revealed that people who molest or who are involved in incestuous relationships with children are a heterogeneous population (Knight, Rosenberg, and Schneider, 1985). This has contributed to dispelling myths about who child abusers are (i.e., old, demented men) and has focused clinicians and researchers on defining subpopulations (Fitch, 1962; Kopp, 1962; Gebhard, Gagnon, Pomeroy, and Christenson, 1965; McCaghy, 1967; Groth, 1978; Cohen, Garofalo, Boucher, and Seghorn, 1971). The salient offender characteristics have been derived from sociological studies, clinical studies, treatment outcome studies, ward behavior ratings, psychometric studies, projective tests, and personality inventory tests.

What has emerged from attempts to classify pedophiles and incest offenders is investigation of style of abuse obtained from offender self reports, criminal investigative reports, and victim reports. Critical factors in the style of sexual abuse are the degree of violence used (Finkelhor, 1984), the relationship of the victim to the offender (Panton, 1978), the age of the victim (Armentrout and Hauer, 1978), the age of the offender, and the level of education of the offender (Knight et al., 1985). Other criteria contributing to subgroupings when compared with sexual abuse style are: preoffense social and occupational adjustment, alcohol abuse, frequency of sexual abuse and other crimes, institutional behavior while incarcerated, and personality traits (Anderson, Kunce, and Rich, 1979).

Other studies seeking to classify child abusers have examined the physiological response of sex offenders, focusing on the relationship between sexual stimuli and violence stimuli and their respective arousal components. A number of studies report differences in penile responses between sex offenders with histories of forcible sexual assault and various control groups, including nonsexual offenders and offenders with histories of other unconventional sexual behavior, including pedophilia, exhibitionism, and homosexuality (Abel, 1976; Abel et al., 1977; Abel and Blanchard, 1974; Barbaree, Marshall, and Lanthier, 1979; Quinsey, Chaplin, and Varney, 1981). Study results support the theory that aggression and violence are linked with sexual abuse.

Knight et al. (1985) uses three major hierarchical levels for classifying offenders who sexually abuse children. The first level concerns the meaning of the aggression in the offense. This meaning is seen as a dichotomy between an assault whose aim is primarily sexual (i.e., instrumental aim) and an assault that is primarily aggressive and is accompanied by intent to hurt the child (i.e., expressive aim).

The second level concerns the manner in which the offender relates to the victim. This level breaks down into another dichotomy; relevant variables include sensitivity to the child's need, use of seduction, distortion of victim, emphasis on force or manipulation, and abuse of known or unknown victim.

The third level of the model concerns the offender's prior level of achieved interpersonal relationships, and dichotomized categories are assessed as to regressed or fixated parameters. Regressed indicates a higher level of achieved interpersonal relationships than fixated. This offender is more likely to have been married and have had age appropriate heterosexual relationships prior to regression, to have mastery in other areas, and to show regression as a decompensation. Fixated offenders, in comparison, have a low level of social competence except in relationships with children. These offenders distort the age of the victim and their offenses are often ego syntonic (Knight et al., 1985).

The model attempts to account for the variety of behavioral styles, both normative and deviant, manifested by sexual offenders of children. It does not, however, speak to the origins of these characteristics. Consequently, the question "Why a child?" remains unanswered. The model does underscore that children, by their nature of being children, are stimuli for adult emotions of sex and aggression, which are expressed regardless of consequences to either adult or child.

Research efforts are being made to bring together theoretical and empirical models. This combination would blend a hierarchical structuring of offender personality characteristics, behaviors, and symptoms with a quantitative and qualitative evaluation of overall offender social competency, sexual adequacy, and degree of importance of sex with children (Knight et al., 1985).

In Conte's (1985, see also Conte et al., 1986) review of studies of assessment areas for adults who use children sexually, the following were identified as important:

1. Measurement of sexual arousal through use of plythsmograph is essential to discriminate between various categories of sexual offenders (Abel, Becker, Murphy, and Flanagan, 1981; Avery-Clarke and Laws, 1984; Quinsey, Chaplin, and Carrigan, 1979).
2. Determination of the presence of sexual fantasies toward children is important due to its role in deviant sexuality (Abel and Blanchard, 1974). Wolf (1987) suggests that fantasies with children as sexual partners paired with sexual excitement through masturbation act as a disinhibitor or serve as cognitive rehearsals for sexual contact with children.
3. Determination of cognitive distortions or rationalizations that are common to adults who have sex with children. Abel, Becker, and Cunningham-Rathner (1984) identify seven distortions common to child molesters seen in their practice (A child who does not physically resist really wants sex. Having sex with a child is a good way to teach the child about sex. Children don't tell about sex with an adult because they really enjoy it. Some time in the future, our society will realize that sex with children is really all right. An adult who feels a child's genitals is not really being sexual with the child so no harm is really being done. When a child asks about sex it means that the child wants to see the adult's sex organ or have sex with the adult. A relationship with the child is enhanced by having sex with her or him).

The various research findings indicate that psychopathology, rather than being a direct, causal link with child sexual abuse, must be understood as a mediating variable to the abusive acts themselves. This means that offenders are most often distinguished by the outcomes they are seeking with children. These outcomes have been identified as power, control, sadistic pleasure, impulsive and explosive outlets, displaced anger, displaced and compensatory sexual aims, consequences of general amoral development, consequences of alcohol and drug abuse, and miscellaneous outcomes (such as sexual abuse secondary to organic mental impairment) (Knight et al., 1985).

Finkelhor's preconditions of sexual abuse of children

In addition to differentiating styles of sexual abuse in efforts to provide a context for understanding abuse, research also has been concentrated on the identification of the sources of abusive behavior patterns. A principally sociological view of the abuser has been proposed by Finkelhor (1984) and covers, broadly, preconditions that create a personal and social context for expressing sexually abusive behaviors. Of importance are personal motivations and other psychological and social conditions that allow for the overriding of inhibitions toward sexually abusive behaviors. This model underscores our basic clinical finding that psychological structures that emerge out of the experience of sexual abuse and attempts to survive it have a role in the development of aberrant sexual motivation and disinhibiting responses.

Stating the pressing need for new theory in the field of sexual abuse that takes into account the sociological dimensions of child abuse and clinicians' family systems approach to treating incest families, Finkelhor (1984) proposes a model called the Four Preconditions Model of Sexual Abuse. His review of the literature suggests that all factors relating to sexual abuse could be grouped as contributing to one of four offender preconditions that need to be met before sexual abuse can occur.

Precondition I: Motivation to sexually abuse. In Precondition I of the model, three components of a motivation to abuse a child sexually are stated to include emotional congruence (relating sexually to the child satisfies some important emotional need), sexual arousal (the child becomes the potential source of sexual gratification), and blockage (alternative sources of sexual gratification are not available or are less satisfying). These three components are not alone and in themselves preconditions; in many cases elements present from all three components account for the motivation.

The sources for this precondition, as well as for the other preconditions, can be explained on two levels: (1) the individual, or psychological level, and (2) the sociological level. Some of the individual explanations for the motivation to abuse sexually are arrested emotional development, need for power and control, unconscious reenactment of a childhood trauma, narcissistic identification with the self as a young child, presence of a childhood sexual experience that was traumatic or strongly conditioning, modeling of someone else's sexual interest in children, misattention to arousal cues, and biologic abnormality. Some of the sociological explanations include masculine requirements to be dominant and powerful in sexual relationships, child pornography, erotic portrayal of children in advertising, male tendency to sexualize emotional needs, and repressive normals about masturbation and extramarital sex.

Precondition II: Overcoming internal inhibitors. This precondition implies that the offender must overcome internal inhibitors in order to abuse a child sexually. Some of the individual explanations for overcoming internal inhibitors include alcohol, psychosis, impulse disorder, senility, and failure of incest inhibition in family dynamics. Some of the sociological explanations include social tolerance of sexual interest in children, weak criminal sanctions against offenders, ideology of patriarchal prerogatives for fathers, social tolerance of deviance committed while intoxicated, child pornography, and (adult) inability to identify with the needs of children.

Precondition III: Factors predisposing to overcoming external inhibitors. This precondition looks outside the offender to external social interactional factors. Most important in this area is the caretaking supervision a child receives. Although children can't always be in the presence of others, it is clear that the influence of third parties appears as a factor in creating a vulnerability to abuse. Some of the individual explanations include a mother who is absent, ill, not close to or protective of the child, or dominated or abused by the father; social isolation of the family; unusual opportunities to be alone with the child; lack of supervision of the child; and unusual sleeping or rooming conditions. Some of the sociological explanations include lack of social supports for the mother, barriers to women's equality, erosion of social networks, and loss of ideology of family sanctity.

Precondition IV: Factors predisposing to overcoming child's resistance. This precondition looks at the child's ability to resist abuse. Some of the individual explanations for this precondition include that the child is emotionally insecure or deprived, the child lacks knowledge about sexual abuse, a situation of unusual trust exists between child and offender, and coercion. Sociological explanations include unavailability of sex education for children and the social powerlessness of children.

Combined with the offender's abuse style, these preconditions are key to what is communicated to the abused child during the offense. Consequently, the ability to recover from this abuse tends to be correlated with the offender's abuse style (in particular, the degree of violence) as well as with various components of the preconditions (Burgess and Holmstrom, 1975; Finkelhor, 1979; Tufts study, 1984; Anderson et al., 1981; Russell, 1982). It is the impact of the abuser's message and the means by which that message is delivered that become important to the child's experience.

In summary, as our discussion of abusers illustrates, child sexual abuse has been explained both as a reaction by the offender to his own motivations and psychological needs and as a response to social structure. Additional research is needed to reconstruct the cognitive-behavioral impact of early victimization on belief patterns. Belief patterns are related to the social sensitivity of the offender, to cues that trigger assault of children, and to problems offenders have identifying with child victims. As the causes begin to be understood, the existence of this linkage becomes more visible.

Consequences of child sexual abuse

Studies reporting on the postassault adjustment of children contribute to our thesis regarding the child's employment of assault survival strategies and their role in subsequent cognitive–behavioral development. Manifestations in child victims of passivity and compliance, anger and aggression, betrayal and mistrust, and hypersexualized behavior are strongly linked to the sexual assault experience. In the preceding discussion of the causes of child sexual abuse we looked to the offenders for information. In addition, a range of behaviors and characteristics, including abandonment, discord, and victimization can be found in the life histories of child molesters (Conte, 1984, 1985; Conte et al., 1986). Also apparent from offender life histories are family lifestyles conducive to predatory behavior, alcohol and drug abuse, and criminality.

Despite the benevolence that many abusers claim to show children, the self-seeking interest of the abuser preempts the rights and individuality of the victim. The consistent attempts on the part of the offender to convince the child of the offender's rights over the child ultimately result in the dissociation of the victim from his or her sense of self and what is right for that self in order to survive the relationship with the offending adult.

Studies reporting on the consequences of sexual abuse of children can be categorized according to variables related to the offense, the offender, the victim's symptom stress response patterns, the disclosure phase, and parental and institutional reaction. It is important to keep in mind that drawbacks of these studies include dissimilarity of populations of abused children studied and the lack of control groups. In addition, the dissention of various studies within particular areas should temper conclusions drawn from these studies. However, these studies do serve as a guide to research on the consequences of child sexual abuse.

Offense variables

One approach to the investigation of the impact of childhood sexual abuse has been to evaluate adjustment of the victim to the meaning and use of force and aggression in the offense.

Level of aggression in offenses. Although there are studies cited in Browne and Finkelhor's 1984 review of the child sexual abuse literature that found no relationship between adjustment of the victim and offender use of violence, force, and aggression (Anderson et al., 1981) other studies have. Finkelhor (1979), Fromuth (1983), Russell (1984), and the Tufts study (1984) all make strong arguments showing that offender use of force, aggression, and violence is associated with increased trauma response in the child. Data from Burgess et al. (1984) further support the impact of force and violence in maladjustment, particularly when there is use of pornography in sex rings involving children. One speculation over reasons for the dissenting opinions has to do with varying definitions of force, violence, and aggression (i.e., signs of physical injury to child), and measurement of the outcome for child victims.

Duration and frequence of abuse. Although the association between trauma response and frequency of abuse is clinically sensible, it has not always been shown to be highly associated with later victim adjustment. The Tufts study (1984) and Finkelhor (1979) did not find a difference in adjustment according to the variable of duration. One study (Courtois, 1979) found the least amount of trauma with the longest duration of sexual contact. Russell's study (1984), however, found an association between abuser duration and victim adjustment among adult women who had been abused for more than five years. Tsai, Fieldman-Summers, and Edgar (1979), using the MMPI, found levels of victim personality dysfunction.

Offender variables

Relationship to the offender. Research has shown that although a perpetrator known to the child elicits in the victim a sense of betrayal as contrasted with the fear that accompanies abuse by a stranger, abuse by the father creates distress (Finkelhor, 1979; Groth, 1978; Russell, 1984). There is no consensus as to the level of distress, and whether or not this distress is greater when a stepfather is involved (Tufts study, 1984) or when the biologic father is the abuser (Groth, 1979). Clinicians looking at the issue of perceived participation have speculated that there is more trauma when the child sees her or himself actively participating in the sexual activity rather than avoiding or disclosing it.

Sexual activity

The negative impact of sexual activity (penetration, fellatio, anal intercourse) is supported by Russell's study (1984), in which women reflected on their childhood experiences. Other studies have found less severe responses to less invasive physical forms of sexual contact (Finkelhor, 1979). However, this variable is difficult to sort out as it perhaps interacts with other variables, such as the age of the child and characteristics of the assailant. In contrast, the Tufts study (1984) of incest victims found that children *not* sexually penetrated manifested more anxiety than those who reported penetration. Finkelhor (1979), in a self-report study of college students who had been molested as children, could find no differences between the group that reported penetration and the group that did not.

Age of onset of abuse. Research studies again reported mixed findings for this variable. The Tufts study has done the most rigorous investigation of the age of onset and its findings indicate increased symptoms in latency-age children. However, Finkelhor (1979) questions whether the evaluation of the children occurred during the latency period rather than at the time of onset of sexual abuse, his point being that the disturbance might reflect a developmental age rather than the abuse. Even if testing a latency-age victim reveals this child more upset or disturbed than victims of other ages, the disturbance may in fact still be related to the abuse and its earlier onset. The developmental demands of latency in terms of learning, relating, and impulse expression may reflect characterological difficulties that arose later in the victim's development (e.g., when negotiating intimacy or involved in parenting).

Age and gender of the offender. Several studies have been able to confirm assumptions about offender age and gender. The older the perpetrator is the greater the trauma for the victim; the victim trauma is also greater when the perpetrator is male (Finkelhor, 1979; Fromuth, 1983; Russell, 1983).

Primary stress response pattern variables

Many studies related to consequences of child sexual abuse document observed and expressed symptoms. These symptoms of primary stress response patterns appear to fall into three categories: primary or acute symptoms, secondary symptoms, and tertiary symptoms.

Acute symptoms of primary stress response patterns. Acute symptoms may be due to the disclosure process when the sexual activity is stopped and when the child must deal with the social meaning of abuse. That is, the child has to respond to other peoples' reaction to knowledge of the abuse. These symptoms may also be noted during early stages of abuse. Preliminary or acute signs and symptoms of sexual abuse in children can be detected by persons knowledgeable of the pattern. The symptoms may be physical, psychological, behavioral, and/or performance related.

A child's mediating force between self and the world is his or her body. Therefore, it is not surprising that acute symptoms of abuse manifest themselves primarily *physically* in such bodily signs as headaches, stomachaches, vomiting, appetite changes, genital complaints, urinary tract infections, and gynecological problems. *Psychologically* the child may be unable to concentrate, preoccupied with daydreams, depressed, less involved and interested in usual activities, anxious when around strangers, and generally more anxious or angry. Sleep disturbances and nightmares may also be present. *Behaviorally* children may be sexually oriented – masturbating openly; seductive in actions, language, or dress – or they may become clingy and withdrawn. School and social performance may decline; children may avoid school. Hyperactivity and the emergence of phobias and fears are often the most striking outcome of sexual abuse (Tufts study, 1984). Risktaking behaviors may increase following disclosure.

Symptoms of secondary stress response patterns. If the sexual abuse has continued for an extended time period, generally over several years, the child has made some adaptation to the abuse and developed a defensive armor, and thus later symptoms may differ from the acute symptoms. This difference appears more noted in children who adopt an avoidant pattern of response (Burgess et al., 1984).

Using existing measurement tools, sexually abused children are not necessarily distinguishable from normal populations. The Tufts study (1984) investigating incest victims compared victims to a normal control group and to a clinic group of children. This study found 17% of the sexually abused 4- to 6-year-olds meeting criteria for "clinically significant pathology" (Tufts study, 1984). Of the 7- to 13-year-old abused children, 40% were seriously disturbed. The adolescent victims were found to exhibit more neurotic-type symptoms. All these findings were higher than the normal control group, but only slightly less than the clinic population of children. Affective states of anger and hostility were found among 45% to 50% of abused children in the Tufts study. These findings were substantially higher than for either the normal control or the clinic group. The same outcome was true for the 4- to 6-year-olds and for 23% of the adolescents.

Shame, guilt, and depression as well as negative self-perceptions are some symptoms of secondary stress response patterns that have been reported in studies of the consequences of child sexual abuse. However, cross-comparison of empirical studies shows these findings do not always hold up. This may be a function of the measurement tools used and of the variety of populations studied, which suggests diversity in the populations studied. What accounts for this diversity is not evident.

Other studies have observed additional symptoms of secondary stress response patterns. Peters (1976) and Burgess et al. (1978) reported fear and avoidance of either the person who abused the child or people of the same sex as the abuser.

Long-term effects of child sexual abuse are examples of secondary stress response patterns. Study findings of these long-term effects can be summarized under three major headings: (1) emotional reactions and self-perceptions, (2) impact on interpersonal relating and sexuality, and (3) effects on social functioning (Browne and Finkelhor, 1984).

1. *Emotional reactions and self-perceptions:* The rate of depression among people in general is high. However, suicide attempts and self-mutilating behavior appear high among victims (Briere, 1984; Yorukoglu and Kemph,

1966; de Young, 1982; Carroll, Shaffer, and Abramanowitz, 1980) as do instances of hysterical seizures (Goodwin, Simms, and Bergman, 1979; Gross, 1979).

Fear, anxiety, isolation, and stigma are noted in follow-up studies (Herman, 1981; Courtois, 1979; Briere, 1984), whereas negative self-concept has been harder to confirm. Again, this is partially due to the methods by which investigators measured victim self-esteem. Although negative self-concepts were reported by Courtois (1979) and by Herman (1981), Fromuth (1983) found no relationship between negative self-esteem and childhood sexual assault.

2. *Impact on interpersonal relating and sexuality:* Herman (1981) studied adult women from incestuous families and reported victim rage toward mothers and less rage toward abusers. There appears to be a great deal of difficulty in women who have been abused in childhood in relating to both men and women. In addition, the women reported contempt for their mothers as well as for themselves (Herman, 1981; de Young, 1982).

Difficulty trusting others accompanied by reactions of fear, hostility, and a sense of betrayal are found in many follow-up victim reports (Courtois, 1979; Briere, 1984; Meiselman, 1979). Difficulty in parenting has been reported (Goodwin and DiVasto, 1979) and revictimization in later life has been found (Russell, 1984; Herman, 1981; de Young, 1982; Fromuth, 1983). Childhood sexual victimization has been associated with later abuse by husbands or other adult partners (Russell, 1984; Briere, 1984; Herman, 1981).

Sexual maladjustment has been found with incest victims (Meiselman, 1979; Herman, 1981; Finkelhor, 1979; Langmade, 1983). Becker, Skinner, Abel, and Traecy (1982) compared a group of rape victims (N = 22) and incest victims (N = 12) and found that the incest victims had significantly higher rates of primary and secondary nonorgasmia. McGuire and Wagner (1978) suggest that incest victims experience specific sexual dysfunctions, such as minimal arousal or disgust at nudity. Sexual dysfunction seems to be accompanied by flashbacks to the earlier sexual victimization and by a general sense of repugnance (Meiselman, 1979; de Young, 1982). Some empirical studies indicate that it is the victim who seeks therapy that reports the greatest amount of sexual dysfunction (Finkelhor, 1984) when compared to victims and controls who do not seek therapy.

3. *Effects on social functioning:* A connection has been made between sexual abuse and prostitution (James and Meyerding, 1977; Silbert and Pines, 1981), as well as between childhood sexual abuse and substance abuse (Briere, 1984; Herman, 1981). For example, Benward and Densen-Gerber (1975) found that 44 percent of a sample of drug addicted women had childhood histories of child sexual abuse. The major population on which follow-up data on long-term and short-term effects of childhood sexual abuse are based are females. Information on male children is less visible, although it

is becoming increasingly evident from studies of offenders that male childhood sexual abuse is more prevalent than presently reported (Burgess, Hazelwood, Rokous, Hartman, and Burgess, 1987).

Symptoms of tertiary stress. There is a third category of stress response patterns identified in the literature, in which acute and secondary symptoms are *not* observed. Instead, the victim assumes a position of identifying with the exploiter. This pattern is documented in studies reporting a high incidence of childhood sexual abuse in the life histories of molesters as well as in follow-up studies of child victims.

Disclosure variables

There are no firm findings concerning whether or not withholding information about being sexually abused is more traumatic than immediately disclosing the abuse. The social meaning of telling needs to be separated from the individual meaning of the abuse. That is, until the child discloses the sexual abuse, he or she only has to manage that information privately. When the abuse is disclosed, the child has to also manage the way other people react to the news. It is clear that there is a wide range in the manner in which family members, peers, and other authority persons will react to such news, all of which must be dealt with by the child in addition to the personal meaning of the abuse.

The Tufts study (1984) found that children who took the longest amount of time to tell had the least amount of reported trauma and hostility. However, the child's awareness of the social taboo against incest may be a factor in any increased distress (MacFarlane, 1978, MacFarlane and Bulkley, 1982). Again, this may be an interactive variable.

Parental and institutional reaction variables

Foley and Davis (1983) compiled from the literature a list of adaptive and maladaptive responses of families to sexual assaults. Families at risk for difficulties in resolving sexual assault include those with:

1. a high number of early preassault traumatic life events and poor early relationships (Brothers, Hilton, & Kunkes, 1982);
2. histories of emotional and psychiatric difficulties;
3. low levels of functioning in the nuclear and extended family;
4. histories of early sexual trauma (Burgess and Holmstrom, 1975; Nadelson et al., 1982);
5. expressed beliefs in rape myths;
6. pre-assault histories of chronic relationship difficulties, including disturbed communication patterns and lack of empathy for and understanding of family members' needs and concerns; and
7. social and sexual adjustment dysfunctions both pre- and postassault. (Foley and Davis, 1983)

In addition, MacFarlane (1982) reports on the impact to the child of unsupportive parents.

MacFarlane (1982) and Conte (1984) describe symptom-induced trauma, which is the result of insensitive handling of victims by professionals who lack both an understanding of the dynamics of sexual abuse and the skills to interact sensitively with victims. Additionally, trauma may be induced as the victim progresses through the various institutional systems and encounters the rules and regulations of these systems (Holmstrom and Burgess, 1979).

Psychodynamic impact of sexual abuse on children

The linking of childhood sexual abuse to subsequent problems is not a new idea. The field of psychiatry has a history of addressing this issue through various clinical observations. On one hand, a review of these papers illustrates psychiatry's early identification of the psychodynamic impact of child sexual abuse; on the other hand, the lack of follow-up response by clinicians illustrates their difficulty in believing the abuse actually occurred.

The magnitude of psychodynamic impact from childhood sexual trauma was presented by Freud in 1895. He stated that hysterical symptoms could be understood when traced to an early traumatic experience and the trauma was always related to the patient's sexual life. The trauma manifested itself when revived later – usually after puberty – as a memory.

However, Freud later reversed his belief and said that the sexual seductions his patients reported were not all reports of real events, but often fantasies created by the child (Freud, 1905). This reversal created a major shift in the priorities of psychological investigation. The external, realistic trauma was replaced in importance by infantile sexual wishes and fantasies. Clinicians, understanding the universality of those wishes and fantasies, began to focus attention on the person's reaction to them (Masson, 1985).

In 1932, Sandor Ferenczi presented a paper, "The Passions of Adults and Their Influence on the Sexual and Character Development of Children," at the Viennese Psychoanalytic Society on the occasion of Freud's seventy-fifth birthday. This paper presented Ferenczi's belief that childhood trauma had been unjustly neglected over the years and that factors were insufficiently explored, resulting in premature interpretations and explanations. Ferenczi noted that sexual trauma as the pathogenic factor could not be valued highly enough.

Ferenczi documented the following outcomes of early childhood trauma:

1. the introjection of the guilt feelings of the adult;
2. the undeveloped or perverted sexual life of the child;
3. the traumatic progression of a precocious maturity;
4. the terrorism of suffering.

In a later study of psychotic patients, Gleuck (1963) describes finding traumatic consequences of incestuous episodes from a clinical population of schizophrenic patients receiving electroshock treatments:

1. actual physical pain during the incestuous activity;
2. denial by the patient, either immediately after the event or on subsequent occasions, that the episode ever occurred;
3. accusation of the child by the parent, with the parent placing the responsibility for the episode on the child;
4. failure of the other parent to protect the child from the incestuous relationship. This may vary from a genuine ignorance of the situation (rarely), through a covert accpetance and pretended ignorance of the event, to an overt encouraging of the incestuous activity.

On the other side of the coin, there is literature that indicates that abused children have suffered no ill effects (Bender and Blau, 1937; Shane and Karpinski, 1942; Bender and Grugett, 1952; Lukianowicz, 1972). Conte (1984) suggests that the extent to which the reader of study results identifies negative effects or no effects may be a function of preexisting bias, citing Constantine's (1981) interpretation of the frequent outcome reported as "neutral" in the Bender and Grugett (1952) study. Conte's review of the same 15 case summaries stated that only two of the 15 patients had adjusted well at time of follow-up. Others had experienced long-term hospitalization or institutionalization, a successful suicide, and emotional and social isolation.

Utilization of literature on child sexual abuse

When examining studies on the consequences of child sexual abuse, one finds a wide range in the interpretations and uses of study results. Conte (1984) suggests that this variance can be attributed to several factors:

1. *Differential impact.* The question of why some victims appear to be affected more than others has been a troublesome one. There is considerable contradiction across studies measuring abuse variables (i.e., age, gender, use of force, duration, frequency). Conte suggests methodological problems in samples and instruments make it difficult to interpret the absence of significant findings.
2. *Substantive implications.* Two comprehensive reviews (Browne and Finkelhor, 1984; Mrazek and Mrazek, 1981) plus Conte's table of 25 studies (1984) illustrate some of the substantive findings to date about child sexual abuse effects. These effects are described in physical, behavioral, physiological, emotional, psychological, and interpersonal terms. The abuse characteristics strongly associated with negative effects appear to be presence of force in the abuse, longer duration of abuse, and older victim at last incident.
3. *Political contexts.* On one hand, Conte (1984) highlights the effects of politicizing the impact of the sexual abuse issue – that is, people who want to have sexual activity with children use the absence of ill effects as justification. On the other hand, clinicians aware of the negative effects may be pushed into stating "all children are harmed."

4. *Methodological issues.* Studies of the *effects* of sexual abuse have been criticized for being biased because of the use of special populations (prostitutes, drug addicts, college students, psychotherapy patients, or populations taken from court, probation departments, or child welfare). One response to such criticism is the use of comparison or control groups. Some recent studies have collected data from interesting comparison groups. For example, Becker et al. (1982) compared rape victims versus incest victims; Meiselman (1979) compared 58 incest victims in psychotherapy and 100 nonabused psychotherapy control patients. Briere (1984) compared walk-in patients with a history of child sexual abuse to a mental health clinic group of nonabused patients.

Other methodological issues are the timing of data collection and the reliability of memory of the abuse. Because victims appear to exhibit the effects of sexual victimization at various times, the absence of observable symptoms at one specific point in time does not mean that some effects will not appear in the future (Conte, 1984). Groth and colleagues (1979) noted memory difficulties in sex offenders asked about childhood sexual abuse. Many did not deny such an experience, but were not sure if something had happened.

Another methodological issue is *how* the effects of child sexual abuse are measured. Studies vary considerably in measurement strategies. Conte (1984) notes that recent studies have used one of three approaches to measurement: global self-reports of how affected the victim is, tallies of clinical problems, or standardized tests. In evaluating each approach, Conte notes that self-report of behavior is influenced by the balance of behavior, the degree of motivation the victim has to change the behavior, and whether there is a means to check the reliability of the self-report.

Measures of more global responses (for example, the question "How are you affected by the experience?") are also influenced by demand characteristics and reported bias. According to Conte, there is no methodological research examining psychometric properties and factors affecting victim reports of how they have been affected by sexual abuse.

There are also problems with tallies of clinical problems. For example, various stresses might have pressured an individual to report a problem. Victim behavior may not be seen as a problem (i.e., nightmares, masturbation). The causal nature of a problem may even be attributed to fantasy construction and internal drives as opposed to actual occurring events.

There are also validity problems in the use of readily available tests and instruments. Conte summarizes a 1984, carefully executed study by Seidner and Calhoun using several standardized instruments with undergraduates who had or had not been sexually victimized as children. Victims and nonvictims scored differently on several of the instrument scales. One of the findings (contrary to the authors' hypothesis) was that victims scored higher on the self-acceptance scale of the California Psychological Inventory. The authors note that this finding may be a function of the scale's tendency to measure self-reliance and independence. This suggests the sample group may have scored high as a function of victims having grown up distrusting others and therefore being more self-reliant. This same type of problem is apparent in the Tufts study (1984) of abused vs. nonabused child psychiatric patients and in Walker's (1979) study of abused women. The results are contrary to the suggested hypothesis of low self-concept and "appearance of normality."

Conte suggests researchers do conceptual work before instruments are used. Although well-known instruments have appeal to investigators and review panels, it is not at all clear that standardized measures will be useful in studying the effects of sexual abuse. Seidner and Calhoun (1984) caution that many dimensions of available instruments may not directly assess aspects of human functioning thought to be influenced by victimization.

Because recent studies have tended to describe victims and nonvictim comparison subjects in terms of specific problematic behaviors (e.g., Meiselman, 1979; Becker et al., 1982; Briere, 1984), Conte suggests researchers develop their instruments in order to avoid the difficulty encountered in using statistically generated factors, which are often highly abstract and not of direct utility in understanding the victims.

Conceptual framework for traumatic event processing of sexual abuse

This model was developed because of the lack of explicated or tested frameworks for understanding the linkage between child sexual victimization and level of adjustment. We are not aware of any related models and our confidence in this model comes from clinical and interview experiences with victims and victimizers. It also derives from victim data analysis originating from a case involving children who were all molested at the same age (five), for the same length of time (four months), and by the same adult abuser (Burgess, Hartman, Wolbert, and Grant, in press).

The conceptual framework has two major parts: (1) phases of sexual abuse and recovery, and (2) concepts for processing traumatic life events. The section of phases addresses the sequencing and time parameters involved in experiencing, disclosing, and recovering from sexual abuse. The concepts section addresses the event (the sexual victimization) and informational processing of the event, with subconcepts of encapsulation of the event, dissociation and splitting, and patterned responses of the individual (Hartman and Burgess, 1986).

The scheme of phases helps locate the child victim during particularly stressful time periods when there is demand for relieving not only the stress of the abuse but also the compounding stress generated by the child's social system. Following the assumption of stress and poststress response, we suggest concepts that contribute to a framework or model for assessing the populations of children, adolescents, and adults examined in this project.

Phase 1: Pretrauma – pre-abuse conditions

This is the period before the child is sexually abused. Environmental supports, stressors, quality of relationships with adults and siblings, personal organization, and ego development all give an indication of the child's strengths as well as vulnerabilities and risk factors for maladjustment.

These conditions can be described as falling into one of three categories. The first, early life history, includes quality of relationships with adults and siblings, early socialization experiences, and social resources. Preexisting beliefs and values are those pertinent to the abuse and to coping or patterns of adaptation. Level of life stress conditions may incorporate how stressful the child's life is in ways that may have an impact on the intensity of his or her reaction to the abuse.

Phase 2: Trauma encapsulation – processing the event

The event is the child sexual abuse, whether this abuse occurs only once or whether it continues to occur over time, and the disclosure of the abuse. It may include a wide range of behaviors within the context of the abuse including some of the following: dialogue and conversation regarding the victim's motivations, beliefs, and responses; the physical contact; the sexual contact; the use of force, orders, and threats (including threats to life); ploys used to guarantee secrecy and continuance of the sexual activity.

During the event phase, the child victim is forced to confront the details of the sexual abuse. Factors critical to this confrontation are the relationship of the assailant to the child; the degree of violence, threat, and intimidation used; the type of sexual and other physical acts; the child's age; the defenses and coping mechanisms used by the child throughout the assault period (including behavioral, cognitive, and psychological defenses); the patterns of inhibition and disinhibition demanded of the child for survival in response to the abuser's aggressive and erotic behaviors; the presence of multiple assailants; the use of pornography; the extent of distortion and bizarreness in the sexual activity; and the symptoms manifested by the child.

Phase 3: Disclosure – the process of revealing the event

The disclosure phase implies that outsiders now know of the sexual abuse. Was the disclosure voluntary or forced? How does the system respond to the child? This response includes physical examination, interviews about what happened, and contact with the criminal justice system, as well as family and extended social network reactions. What type of contact does the child have with the assailant? If the assailant is a family member, such as a parent or sibling, the impact of the social support system is important in how it shapes the victim's thoughts about himself or herself and the abuse experience. If the assailant is a stranger, has the stranger been apprehended? Is the offender released after a period of confinement? Does the offender attempt to threaten the child (which can occur in cases of group or sex ring involvement)? How many symptoms of stress manifest themselves? What are the characteristics of these symptoms and what are the stimuli that exacerbate their occurrence?

Phase 4: Post-trauma outcome – patterned responses to the event

This phase covers at least a two-year period following litigation, criminal investigation, and/or extended therapy. What life adjustments have been made? How much disruption has there been in pre-assault life activities? How are signs of aggression or avoidance handled by family or victim? How is sexualized behavior dealt with by family and victim? Has there been continuous goal-directed development in the child? To what extent does the family talk with the child about the abuse and about how is the child managing?

Informational processing of event: the mediating mechanism

In considering the victim's postabuse reactions, it is useful to think of cognitive–behavioral adjustment to a traumatic event as informational processing. Horowitz (1975) researched responses to stressful stimuli outside of the victim context. The intrusive imagery (flashbacks to sights, thoughts, sounds, feelings, and odors) is viewed as part of a general stress response. The presumption is that information is kept in active awareness until it can be placed in distant memory. That comes about when there is sufficient processing for the information to be stored. The event must be processed before it can be stored. Successful counseling facilitates this processing, allowing the victim to place the event in distant memory.

The premise of informational processing gives some clues to the intensity of defensive adjustment made by children who are assaulted over a prolonged period of time. Their initial distress is subdued by a level of cognitive operations that allows the abuse activities to be stored partially in past memory. It is merely speculation as to what the child goes through to do this, although the assumptions in the following discussion about dissociation provide some clues.

This information processing premise also suggests why disclosure is so upsetting to the child, as disclosure requires a breakdown of the defensive structures in order to retrieve or disclose the information. If disclosure comes from an outside source, the child may respond with distress and anger toward the outside person who reveals what is going on. The child's anger is defensive and protective of his or her adjustment to the long-term abuse.

Summarized from the literature review on child sexual abuse, the critical victim survivor responses highlight the following behaviors:

> visual reproductions of the event
> hypersensitivity to idiosyncratic stimuli
> uncontrollable thoughts regarding the event
> anxiety
> symbolic reenactment
> sleep disturbances
> dissociative states of consciousness
> conscious and unconscious reenactment of the event
> excessive passivity
> hypersexuality

The following concepts of encapsulation of the event, dissociation, splitting, ego fragmentation, and drive disharmony are used in our model, which shows how the traumatic event is processed and provides the conceptual link between the event experience and patterns of postabuse adjustment.

Encapsulation of the event. A growing body of literature supports the premise that sexual abuse of children is a traumatic event having personal repercussions over time (Browne and Finkelhor, 1984). Of particular importance to child sexual abuse is that often, after the first expression of acute symptoms are manifested by the child and no substantive response to the child's predicament follows, there is a quiescent period – still during the abuse phase – when the molestation, in many situations, continues. It is during this period of being "trapped" that the child must in some manner encapsulate the trauma of the abuse.

This encapsulation process has two components. First, silence about the abuse is demanded by the offender. Second, a defensive position is taken by the child to avoid discussion and any possible detection. This defensive silence encloses the sexual abuse that is ongoing; the informational processing of the ongoing event holds it in present memory.

This encapsulation process depletes the victims' psychic energy and thus disrupts the continuity of development of other areas of the children's psychological make-up. Of particular concern is its impact on the victims' sense of right and wrong, their sense of self, their arousal capacities and their inhibition capacities, their awareness or lack of awareness of body states, their sense of personal power, and their self-comforting, self-preserving, and protective behaviors. There is also concern for the reality-mediating strategies used by children to survive psychologically, cognitively, and (at times) physically.

Dissociation from event. One way to understand the impact of sexual abuse on the child's developing personality structure is to analyze the development of the ego and the mechanisms of its defense. Ego development is involved with individual coping and adaptation – processes highly relevant for understanding impairments and gains in individual maturation. One of this study's hypotheses is that the victim's motivation is affected by the abuse. Ego as used here denotes that part of the personality that perceives, experiences, judges, and controls behavior.

During the past several decades major contributors to writings on ego psychology have included Anna Freud (1981, 1983), Heinz Hartmann (1951), and Erik Erikson (1950), among other theorists. Anna Freud (1981, 1983), among others, has emphasized that in the battle for impulse control during normal ego development, developmental defects can take the place of regressive processes. This may be noted in an individual by a different rate of ego growth and a variance in the strength of the drives of sex and aggression. This state has the capacity to create internal disharmonies, which the individual resolves via compromise.

Anna Freud suggests that obsessive traits and uncontrollable impulsivity begin to develop if ego maturation is premature or if there is slower development of drives. This contrasts with uncontrollable impulsiveness that develops when ego development lags behind drive development or when, for constitutional reasons, ego strength is minimal and the given drive increases. These are important points regarding factors that impinge on the harmonious, simultaneous evolution of ego and drives. An imbalance in either one can create internal conflict.

Applying this theory to child sexual abuse, we believe the sexual abuse disrupts the evolution of equal development of drives and ego. That is, the drive component (sex and aggression) is being stimulated beyond ego development. Furthermore, the abuser accomplishes this disruption through intimidation and through distortion of reality and of the child's sense of right and wrong. In addition, the physical approaches enforce irregular patterns of inhibition and disinhibition, rather than the child's normal rhythmic response in usual drive development. To deal with this externally provoked disruption of internal harmony, the child must invoke a life-saving mechanism to survive psychologically. This mechanism is dissociation.

Dissociation from the sexual abuse appears to be a prime and immediate method used by children to survive sexual assault during the abuse phase.

Survival behaviors manifested by child victims during sexual assault include complying, negotiating, fighting, experiencing amnesia, crying, freezing in terror, and actively pretending to be somewhere or someone else. We define dissociation as a general process in which the mind fragments psychic integrity in the service of survival. In other words, the child victim diverts mental attention away from the abuse. Dissociation is a normal reaction to an emotionally loaded situation.

In order to understand dissociation, we need to discuss the role of ego and self-preservation. Self-preservation is vital to dissociation. Such self-preservation is an ego task, and external events that threaten people psychologically as well as physically call for this ego function. Because of extensive research, we understand this phenomenon clearly with adult victims of rape, combat, concentration camps, and hostage situations. However, less clear is the ego's role in child sexual abuse, where the variable of violence is culturally defined. Conte (1984) suggests that our culturally bound definition of violence is too narrow and sexually biased in favor of men by not taking into account the psychological violence and force men use against women and children. Every time an adult sexually abuses a child, coercion, manipulation, force, and violence are involved. To regard people who abuse children as nonviolent, argues Conte, is to fail to see them as their victims see them – as big and powerful.

Although no research exists regarding self-preservation and ego development in situations of child sexual abuse, we add this component to our model as an underlying assumption. In areas other than child sexual abuse, theorists have contributed to our understanding of the role of the ego in self-preservation. Hartmann's (1951) belief about the central role of the ego in relation to survival provides a basis for understanding the victim's capacity for self-care and self-protection.

Other contributors to the connection between ego and self-preservation include Glover (1933), Lowenstein (1949), Zetzel (1949), Rochlin (1965), and Mahler (1968). Kohut (1971) touches on the implications for self-preservation in the development of ego, especially in personality styles. The relationship between self-care and self-regulation is addressed by Sifneos, Apfel-Savitz, and Frankl (1977); victim studies by Krystal and Raskin (1970) and Krystal (1977) discuss developmental disturbances and traumatic regressed states in substance abusers, concentration camp survivors, and sufferers of psychosomatic illness. These studies relate to ego survival during various levels of experience and provide directions for inquiry for our project.

Khantzian and Mack (1982) examine self-preservation and self-care in drug abusers and summarize key points regarding these functions. They observe self-care to be a complex phenomenon involving multiple affective and cognitive processes, component functions, mechanisms of defense, and ego functions. The self-care function becomes internalized, primarily through the behaviors of the caretakers of the child. Their study (Khantzian and Mack, 1982) suggests that self-care capacities are closely associated with positive self-esteem and that a developing child needs to internalize the conviction, before self-care can begin, that he or she has value and is worth protecting. The need for protection by the child during sexual victimization suggests a comparison to the Khantzian and Mack study in that an adult forces a sexual act on a child; no adult protects the child, and the child is unable to protect him- or herself.

Splitting. Dissociation has the capacity to invoke the psychic mechanism of *splitting* (Benner and Joscelyne, 1984; Fagan and McMahon, 1984). The repeated nature of child sexual abuse further burdens the child's psychic structure, and thus the dissociation expands to the phenomenon of splitting, which is defined as a conflict between the demand of the instinct and the command of reality. The conflict persists as the center-point of a split in the ego; the rift never heals but, instead, increases with time (Freud, 1938). Two indicators that splitting has occurred for the child victim are ego fragmentation and drive disharmony.

Ego fragmentation can be observed through the victim's cognitions, self-representation, and body state. There is a split in trust in adult protection; a disruption of body-comforting states as well as of self-care, self-preservation, and protective functions; splits occur with amnesic states for bodily responses as well as ego states for competency. The victim may also exhibit a diffuse sense of right and wrong; a misplaced loyalty; a justification of violence, pain, or intimidation; and/or a self-depreciatory pattern (i.e., "I'm to blame," "I'm no good; that is why this is happening," "I deserve this because I have feelings," "I'm responsible for what will happen to others in my family if I tell"). This may be accompanied by a distorted sense of causality or a distorted sense of value of self, of others, or of personal rights.

Drive disharmony, or the split in drive function (sexual and aggressive drives) is noted through disharmonious levels of stimulation and inhibition. That is, drive disharmony is evidenced through confused body integrity (arousal stimulation), through disruption in an evenly patterned expression of sexuality (symptoms include hypersexuality and repeated sexual rubbing of body), and through sexualized relationships.

Patterned responses to event

The child adjusts to the sexual abuse through the use of defense mechanisms and certain behavior patterns. Four such precurser patterns that have been noted in children (Burgess et al., 1984) are presented below. These patterns may not necessarily be discrete, although whether or not and the extent to which they overlap are not known.

In the *integrated pattern,* the child has mastered the anxiety about the abuse. When asked about the event the child neither avoids nor encourages discussion but is able to talk of the event with reasonable objectivity. The child believes the adult was not only wrong but was responsible for initiating the behavior. Criminal prosecution of the adult is viewed positively. The child has a future orientation, reestablishes friendships with a new peer group, and shows evidence of making age-appropriate adjustments with peers, family, and school.

In the *avoidant pattern* the child's anxiety about the abuse remains sealed off, either consciously or unconsciously. When asked about the event, the child denies it, refuses to recognize it occurred, and may not be able to give a clear picture of it. The child often has a stoic demeanor and actively avoids discussion; he or she is afraid of the offender and tends to be oriented to the present. When not under stress, the child manages life as if nothing has happened.

Stress and a breakdown of avoidance patterns may bring forth such symptoms as depression and self-destructive behavior. Relationships with peers may be terminated, family relationships may be strained, school difficulties may persist, and minor antisocial acts may surface. This child does not have a sense of right and wrong, and believes other children are not exploited. The child refuses to talk about the event. Unconsciously the child feels responsible and "bad" and feels that he or she has injured both self and family.

In the *symptomatic pattern,* acute symptoms become chronic. The symptoms may be related to the event, or they may be a compound reaction to continued victimization or other traumatic events. There may be a cumulative reaction to additional stressful events, such as separation of the parents or death of a family member. The child's anxiety over being powerless is increased, and the child is unable to master and exert control over this anxiety.

When asked about the event, child victims in this pattern become quite anxious. They feel guilty and blame themselves – not the adult offender – for participating in the activity. These children are not in control of thoughts about the event; the event is still operant and conscious. Family relationships are often unstable, peer relationships may not be reestablished, and the victims are not successful in socializing with children of the same age and may associate with younger children. They may drop out of school, continue sexually explicit behaviors, and be victimized again. They believe they should have known better and they should have told their parents. In addition, they are oriented to the past and may be hopeless about the future, believing it impossible to make up for what happened.

In the pattern of *identification with the abuser,* the child has introjected some characteristics of the anxiety caused by the abuse and has assimilated the anxiety by impersonating the aggressor. The child transforms himself or herself from the person threatened into the person who makes the threat.

The child masters anxiety by exploiting others and by adopting an antisocial position toward peers, schools, and family.

In talking about the event, the child who identifies with the abuser minimizes the exploitation, resents the interference of the authorities, and feels there is "much ado about nothing." The child maintains emotional, social, and economic ties with the offender and feels sorry or angry that the adult was exposed. This child has difficulties with authorities, especially in school. Use of drugs and alcohol, which is often part of the sexual abuse, continues and increases. There is a shift in the child's belief system that supports the antisocial behavior.

There is another less well described pattern that is more visible in adolescent and adult populations. It is in the *psychotic pattern* that the most profound symptoms are noted. The individual is unable to distinguish reality; the ego boundaries are significantly blurred. Primary symptoms may herald the secondary (psychotic) symptoms, such as loose associations prior to the shattering of cognitive, emotional, and physiological integration of the victim. There is marked restricted ego development, and the traumatic event is split off and buried in delusional symptoms and material. There is splitting noted in interpersonal relationships, regressive behavior, and primitive, fixed, sexualized thinking patterns. The individual may exhibit a pattern similar to the case cited in the beginning of the chapter.

Framework utilization

Our conceptual framework for examining traumatic event processing in sexual abuse victims is an initial model approach to this topic. Nevertheless, it is important to keep in mind limitations associated with its use. First, using this model does not allow *direct* observation of the victim's cognitive processes. We are neither present at the time of the events nor are there adequate measurements for direct measuring of cognitive processes. Direct measurement is therefore impossible.

Second, the interval between victimization and development of complete response patterns allows other variables – such as time, life stresses, and events – to intervene. Research using this model cannot control for these intervening factors.

Third, the psychodynamic concepts of ego fragmentation and drive disharmony are abstract phenomena. Thus, they are subject to the above limitations imposed by intervening factors.

Summary

The material on child sexual abuse is presented separately for two major reasons: (1) it is a predominantly secret underreported phenomena and (2) there are political and emotional positions taken that exceed the resistance to the acknowledgment of physical abuse of children. As with physical abuse, the incidence of sexual abuse often occurs within the context of a trusted relationship. That perpetrators are usually male challenges the safety of the family as the primary social unit. Compounding the issue is the fact that "mental illness" does not explain this breach of social conduct. Rather, we find rationalizations justifying the acts or blaming the child for the "seduction." The fact that the child is often not believed is curious and raises a question: How is it possible for people to invoke the child's claim as a lie while thinking it impossible for an adult to so behave with a child? The paradox is that, if it is so hard to believe that an adult would "do such a thing" to a child, how is it then possible to believe that a child would know about sexual acts without the influence of an older person?

It is this singular shared information with regard to sex that pits the child against the assailant. Unlike physical abuse with physical signs and symptoms, disclosure by the child or another child is often the basis of initially identifying child sexual abuse. It is essential for professionals to identify the salient characteristics of children who are sexually abused that separate them from children who are not sexually abused. If the incidence continues to be underreported, it suggests that children suffer without our knowledge and without our understanding of the full range of its impact.

References

Abel, G. G. (1976). Assessment of sexual deviation in the male. In M. Herson and A. S. Bellack (Eds.), *Behavioral Assessment: A Practical Handbook.* New York: Pergamon Press.

Abel, G. G., Barlow, D., Blanchard, and Guild, D. (1977). The components of rapists' sexual arousal. *Archives of General Psychiatry. 34,* 895–908.

Abel, G. G., and Blanchard, E. B. (1974). The role of fantasy in the treatment of sexual deviation. *Archives of General Psychiatry, 30,* 467–474.

Abel, G. G., Becker, J. V., and Cunningham-Rathner, J. (1984). Complications, consent, and cognitions in sex between children and adults. *International J. Law and Psychiatry 7,* 89–103.

Abel, G. G., Becker, J. V., Murphy, W. D., and Flanagan, B. (1981). Identifying dangerous child molesters. In R. B. Stuart (Ed.), *Violent Behavior: Social Learning Approaches to Prediction, Management and Treatment.* New York: Brunner/Mazel.

Anderson, S. C., Bach, C. M., and Griffith, S. (1981). Psychosocial sequelae in intrafamilial victims of sexual assault and abuse. Paper presented at the Third International Conference on Child Abuse and Neglect, Amsterdam, The Netherlands.

Anderson, W. P., Kunce, J. T., and Rich, B. (1979). Sex offenders: Three personality types. *Journal of Clinical Psychology, 34,* 671–676.

Armentrout, J. A., and Hauer, A. L. (1978). MMPI's of rapists of children, and non-rapist sex offenders. *Journal of Clinical Psychology, 34,* 330–332.

Avery-Clark, C. A. and Laws, D. A. (1984). Differential erection response patterns of sexual child abusers to stimuli describing activities with children. *Behavior Therapy, 15:* 71–83.

Barbaree, H. E., Marshall, W. L., and Lanthier, R. D. (1979). Deviant sexual arousal in rapists. *Behavioral Research Therapy, 17,* 215–222.

Becker, J. V., Skinner, L. J., Abel, G. G., and Traecy, E. C. (1982). Incidence and types of sexual dysfunctions in rape and incest victims. *J. Sex and Marital Therapy, 8,* 65–74.

Bender, L., and Blau, A. (1937). The reaction of children to sexual relations with adults. *Am. J. Orthopsychiatry, 7,* 500–518.

Bender, L., and Grugett, A. E. (1952). A follow-up report on children who had atypical sexual experience. *Am. J. Orthopsychiatry, 7,* 500–518.

Benner, D. G., and Joscelyne, B. (1984). Multiple personality as a borderline disorder. *J. Nervous and Mental Disease, 172,* 98–104.

Benward, J., and Densen-Gerber, J. Incest as a causative factor in anti-social behavior: An exploratory study. *Contemporary Drug Problems,* (in press) *4:* 323–340.

Blumer, H. (1971). Social problems as collective behavior. *Social Problems, 18,* 298.

Briere, J. (1984). The effects of childhood sexual abuse on later psychological functioning: Defining a "post-sexual-abuse syndrome." Paper presented at the Third National Conference on Sexual Victimization of Children, Washington, DC.

Brothers, D., Hilton, I., and Kunkes, C. (1982). Trust disturbances among victims of rape and incest. *Journal of Adolescent Health Care, 3,* 150.

Browne, A., and Finkelhor, D. (1984). The impact of child sexual abuse. Unpublished paper, University of New Hampshire.

Browning, D. H., and Boatman, B. (1977). Incest: Children at risk. *Am. J. Psychiatry, 134* (1), 69–72.

Burgess, A. W. (Ed.) (1984). *Child Pornography and Sex Rings.* Lexington, MA: D. C. Heath Co.

Burgess, A. W., Hartman, C. R., McCausland, M. P., and Powers, P. (1984). Response patterns in children and adolescents exploited through sex rings and pornography. *Am. J. Psychiatry 141* (5), 656–662.

Burgess, A. W., Hartman, C. R., and McCormack, A. (1987). Abused to abuser: Antecedents to socially deviant behaviors. *Am. J. Psychiatry, 144,* 1431–1436.

Burgess, A. W., Hartman, C. G., Wolbert, W. A., and Grant, C. A. (in press). Child molestation: Assessing impact in multiple victims. *Archives of Psychiatric Nursing, 1,* 33–39.

Burgess, A. W., Hazelwood, R. R., Rokous, F. E., Hartman, C. R., and Burgess, A. G. (1987). Serial rapists and their victims: Reenactment and repetition (prepublication draft from study supported by Department of Justice, Office of Juvenile Justice and Delinquency Prevention, no. 84–JN–K010).

Burgess, A. W., and Holmstrom, L. L. (1975). Sexual trauma in children and adolescents: Sex, pressure and secrecy. *Nursing Clinics of North America, 10,* 551–563.

Burgess, A. W., and Holmstrom, L. L. (1979). *Rape: Crisis and Recovery.* Englewood Cliffs: Brady.

Burgess, A. W., Holmstrom, L. L., Groth, A. N., and Sgroi, S. M. (1978). *Sexual Assault of Children and Adolescents.* Lexington, MA: D. C. Heath Co.

Carmen, E. H., Rieker, P. P., and Mills, T. (1984). Victims of violence and psychiatric illness. *Am. J. Psychiatry, 141,* 378–83.

Carroll, J. L., and Fuller, G. B. (1971). An MMPI comparison of three groups of criminals. *Journal of Clinical Psychology, 27,* 240–242.

Carroll, J. L., Schaffer, C., and Abramanowitz, S. (1980). Family experiences of self-mutilating patients. *Am. J. Psychiatry, 137,* 852–853.

Cohen, M. L., Garofalo, R., Boucher, R., and Seghorn, T. (1971). The psychology of rapists. *Seminars in Psychiatry, 3,* 307–327.

Constantine, L. L. (1981). The effects of early sexual experience. In L. L. Constantine and F. Martinson (Eds.), *Children and Sex: New Findings, New Perspectives.* Boston: Little, Brown.

Conte, J. R. (1984). Progress in treating the sexual abuse of children. *Social Work,* 258–263.

Conte, J. (1985). The effects of sexual abuse on children: A critique and suggestions for future research. *Victimology: An International Journal, 10,* 110–130.

Conte, J. Berliner, I., and Schurman, J. (1986). The impact of sexual abuse on children: Final report. Available from the authors at the University of Chicago, 969 East 60th Street, Chicago, IL, 60637.

Courtois, C. (1979). The incest experience and its aftermath. *Victimology: An International Journal, 4,* 337–347.

de Young, M. (1982). *The Sexual Victimization of Children.* Jefferson, NC: McFarland & Company.

Erikson, E. H. (1950). *Childhood and Society* New York: Norton.

Fagan, J., and McMahon, P. P. (1984). Incipient multiple personality in children. *J. Nervous and Mental Disease, 172,* 26–36.

Ferenczi, S. (1949). Confusion of tongues between adult and the child. *Int. J. Psychoanalysis 30,* 227–229.

Finkelhor, D. (1979). *Sexually Victimized Children.* New York: Free Press.

Finkelhor, D. (1984). *Child Sexual Abuse: New Theories and Research.* New York: Free Press.

Fitch, J. H. (1962). Men convicted of sexual offenses against children: A descriptive follow-up study. *British J. of Criminology 3,* 18–37.

Foley, T. S., and Davis, M. A. (1983). *Rape: Nursing Care of the Victim.* St. Louis: Mosby.

Freud, A. (1981). The concept of developmental lines. *Psychoanalytic Study of the Child, 36,* 129–136.

Freud, A. (1983). Problems of pathogenesis. In *The Psychoanalytic Study of the Child,* ed. A. J. Solnit, R. S. Eissler, and P. B. Neubauer. New Haven: Yale University Press, pp. 383–388.

Freud, S. (1886). The etiology of hysteria. First published in the *Wiener klinische Rundschau,* 1886, Nr. 22 to 26. Amplification of a lecture delivered at the Society of Psychiatry and Neurology in Vienna, May 2, 1886. Trans. Cecil M. Baines and published in 1959 in *The Collected Papers of Sigmund Freud,* Vol. 1. New York: Basic Books.

Freud, S. (1905). My views on the part played by sexuality in the aetiology of the neuroses. In Joan Riviere (Trans.), *Sigmund Freud, Collected Papers* (Vol 1, 272–286). New York: Basic Books, 1957.

Freud, S. (1938). Splitting of the ego in the defensive process. First published posthumously *Int. J. Psychoanalysis Imago, 25* (1940). Translation, reprinted from *Int. J. Psychoanalysis, 22* (1941), 65, by James Strachey.

Freund, K. (1967). Erotic preference in pedophilia. *Behavior Research and Therapy, 5,* 339–348.

Fromuth, M. E. (1983). The long term psychological impact of childhood sexual abuse. Unpublished doctoral dissertation, Auburn University, Auburn, AL.

Garbarino, J., and Plantz, M. C. (1984). *Child maltreatment and juvenile delinquency: What are the links?* Unpublished manuscript, Pennsylvania State University.

Gebbard, P. H., Gagnon, J. H., Pomeroy, W. B., and Christenson, C. V. (1965). *Sex Offenders: An Analysis of Types.* New York: Harper & Row.

Gleuck, B. C. (1954). Psychodynamic patterns in sex offenders. *Psychiatric Quarterly, 28,* 1.

Gleuck, B. C. (1956). Final Report, Research Project for the Study and Treatment of Persons Convicted of Crimes Involving Sexual Aberrations, June 1952 to June 1955. New York: State Department of Hygiene.

Gleuck, B. C. (1963). Early sexual experiences in schizophrenia. In H. Biegal (Ed.), *Advances in Sex Research.* New York: Harper & Row.

Glover, E. (1933). The relation of perversion-formation to the development of reality sense. *Int. J. Psychoanalysis 14,* 486–504.

Goodwin, J., and DiVasto, P. (1979). Mother–daughter incest. *Child Abuse and Neglect, 3,* 953–957.

Goodwin, J., Simms, M., and Bergman, R. (1979). Hysterical seizures: A sequel to incest. *Am. J. Orthopsychiatry, 49,* 698–703.

Gordon, L., and O'Keefe, P. (1985). The "normality" of incest. In *Rape and Sexual Assault,* ed. A. W. Burgess, New York: Garland Publishing, 70–82.

Gross, M. (1979). Incestuous rape: A cause for hysterical seizures. *Am. J. Orthopsychiatry, 49,* 698–703.

Groth, A. N. (1978). Patterns of sexual assault against children and adolescents. In A. W. Burgess, A. N. Groth, L. L. Holmstrom, and S. M. Sgroi, *Sexual Assault of Children and Adolescents.* Lexington, MA: Lexington Books.

Groth, A. N. (1979). Sexual trauma in the life histories of rapists and child molesters. *Victimology, 4,* 6–10.

Groth, A. N., Hobson, W. F., and Gary, T. S. (1982). The child molester: Clinical observations. *J. Social Work and Human Sexuality, 1* (1), 129–144.

Hartmann, H. (1939). *Ego Psychology and Adaptation.* New York: International Universities Press.

Hartmann, H. (1951). *Ego Psychology and the Problem of Adaptation.* New York: International Universities Press, 1951.

Hartman, C. R., and Burgess, A. W. (1986). Child sexual abuse: Generic roots of the victim experience. *J. Psychotherapy and the Family, 2* (2), 83–92.

Hartmann, C. R., and Burgess, A. W. (in press). Information processing of a trauma: A case application of a model. *Journal of Interpersonal Violence, 4.* In press.

Hempel, C. G. (1965). *Aspects of Scientific Explanation.* New York: Free Press.

Herman, J. A. (1981). *Father–Daughter Incest.* Cambridge: Harvard University Press.

Herman, J. (1983). Recognition and treatment of incestuous families. *International Journal of Family Therapy, 5* (2), 81–92.

Herman, J., and Hirschman, L. (1981). Families at risk for father–daughter incest. *Am. J. Psychiatry, 138,* 967–970.

Holmstrom, L. L., and Burgess, A. W. (1979). *The Victim of Rape: Institutional Reactions.* New York: Wiley.

Horowitz, M. (1975). *Stress Response Syndromes.* New York: Jason Aronson.

James, J., and Meyerding, J. (1977). Early sexual experiences and prostitution. *Am. J. Psychiatry, 134,* 1381–1385.

Karpman, B. (1954). *The Sexual Offender and His Offenses, Etiology, Pathology, Psychodynamics and Treatment.* New York: Julian.

Kercher, G., and McShane, M. (1983). The prevalence of child sexual abuse victimization in an adult sample of Texas residents. Mimeographed manuscript. Sam Houston State University, Huntsville, TX.

Khantzian, E. J., and Mack, J. E. (1983). Self-preservation and self-care. In A. J. Solnit, R. S. Eissler, and P. B. Neubauer (Eds.), *The Psychoanalytic Study of the Child.* New York: International Universities Press.

Knight, R. A., Rosenberg, R., and Schneider, B. (1985). Classification of sexual offenders: Perspectives, methods and validation. In *Rape and Sexual Assault.* New York: Garland Publishing, 222–293.

Kohut, H. (1971). *The Analysis of Self.* New York: International Universities Press.

Kopp, S. B. (1962). The character structure of sex offenders. *Am. J. Psychotherapy, 16,* 64–70.

Krystal, H. (1977). Self representation and the capacity for self-care. *Annals of Psychoanalysis, 6,* 209–246.

Krystal, H., and Raskin, H. A. (1970). *Drug Dependence.* Detroit: Wayne State University Press.

Langmade, C. J. (1983). The impact of pre- and postpubertal onset of incest experiences in adult women as measured by sex anxiety, sex guilt, sexual satisfaction and sexual behavior. Universtiy Microfilms International, 3592.

Lanning, K. V., and Burgess, A. W. (1984). Child pornography and sex ring crimes, *FBI Bulletin, 53* (1), 10–16.

Lowenstein, R. M. (1949). The vital or somatic instinct. *Int. J. Psychoanalysis 21,* 377–400.

Lukianowicz, N. (1972). Incest: Paternal incest, *Int. J. Psychoanalysis, 120,* 301–318.

MacFarlane, K. (1978). Sexual abuse of children. In J. R. Chapman and M. Gates (Eds.), *The Victimization of Women,* Vol. 3 of Sage Yearbooks in Women's Police Studies. Beverly Hills, CA: Sage.

MacFarlane, K., and Bulkley, J. (1982). Treating child sexual abuse: An overview of current program models. In J. Conte and D. Shore (Eds.), *Social Work and Child Sexual Abuse.* Hawthorne, NY.

Mahler, M. S. (1968). *On Human Symbiosis and the Vicissitudes of Individuation.* New York: International Universities Press.

Maisch, H. (1972). *Incest.* New York: Stein & Day.

Masson, J. M. (1984). *The Assault on Truth: Freud's Suppression of the Seduction Theory.* New York: Farrar, Straus & Giroux.

Masson, J. M. (ed.) (1985). *The Complete Letters of Sigmund Freud to Wilhelm Fliess, 1887–1904.* Cambridge: Harvard University Press.

McCaghy, C. H. (1967). Child molesters: A study of their careers as deviants. In M. B. Clinnard and R. Quinney (Eds.), *Criminal Behavior Systems: A Typology.* New York: Holt, Rinehart & Winston.

McGuire, L., and Wagner, N. (1978). Sexual dysfunction in women who were molested as children: One response pattern and suggestions for treatment. *J. Sex and Marital Therapy, 4,* 11–15.

Meiselman, K. (1979). *Incest: A Psychiatric Study of Causes and Effects with Treatment Recommendations.* San Francisco: Jossey-Bass.

Mrazek, P., and Mrazek, D. (1981). The effects of child abuse: Methodological considerations. In P. Mrazek and C. H. Kempe (Eds.), *Sexually Abused Children and Their Families.* London: Pergamon Press.

Nadelson, C., Notman, M. T., and Jackson H. (1982). A follow-up study of rape victims. *Am. J. Psychiatry, 139,* 1266–1270.

National Study of the Incidence and Severity of Child Abuse and Neglect: Technical Report Number 1. Ed. K. Bergdorf and J. Edmonds. Washington, DC: DHHS Publ. No. (OHDS) 81–30326.

Panton, J. H. (1978). Personality differences appearing between rapists of adults, rapists of children, and non-violent sexual molesters of female children. *Research Communications in Psychology, Psychiatry and Behavior, 3,* 385–393.

Peters, J. J. (1976). Children who are victims of sexual assault and the psychology of offenders. *Am. J. Psychotherapy, 30,* 398–421.

Quinsey, V. L., Chaplin, T. C., and Carrigan, W. F. (1979). Sexual preferences among incestuous and non-incestuous child molesters. *Behavior Therapy 10,* 231–219.

Quinsey, V. L., Chaplin, T. C., and Varney, G. (1981). A comparison of rapists' and non-sex offenders' sexual preferences for mutually consenting sex, rape, and physical abuse of women. *Behavioral Assessment, 3,* 127–135.

Quinsey, V. L., Steinman, C. M., Bergersen, S. G., and Holmes, T. F. (1975). Penile circumference, skin conductance, and ranking response of child molesters and "normals" to sexual and non-sexual visual stimuli. *Behavior Therapy, 6,* 213–219.

Reich, J. W., and Gutierre, S. E. (1979). Escape/aggression incidence in sexually abused juvenile delinquents. *Criminal Justice and Behavior, 6,* 239–243.

Ressler, R., Douglas, J., Depue, R. (1984). Criminal profiling research on homicide. In A. W. Burgess (Ed.), *Rape and Sexual Assault.* New York: Garland.

Russell, D. (1982). *Rape in Marriage.* New York: Macmillan.

Russell, D. (1983). The incidence and prevalence of intrafamilial and extrafamilial sexual abuse of female children. *Child Abuse and Neglect: The International Journal,* 133–146.

Russell, D. (1984). *Rape, Incest and Sexual Exploitation.* Los Angeles: Sage.

Rochlin, G. (1965). *Griefs and Discontents.* Boston: Little, Brown.

Rosenfeld, A. A. (1979). The clinical management of incest and sexual abuse of children, *J. Am. Med. Assoc., 242,* 1761–1764.

Seghorn, T. K., Boucher, R. J., and Prentky, R. A. (in press). Childhood sexual abuse in the lives of sexually aggressive offenders. *J. Am. Acad. of Child Psychiatry.*

Seidner, A. L., and Calhoun, K. S. (1984). Childhood sexual abuse: Factors related to differential adult adjustment. Paper presented at the Second National Conference for Family Violence Researchers. Durham, New Hampshire.

Shane, P., and Karpinski, E. (1942). Effects of incest on the participants. *Am. J. Orthopsychiatry, 12,* 666–673.

Sifneos, P., Apfel-Savitz, R., and Frankl, F. (1977). The phenomenon of "alexethymia." *Psychother. Psychosom., 28,* 47–57.

Sgroi, S. M. (1981). *Handbook of Clinical Intervention in Child Sexual Abuse.* Lexington, MA: D. C. Heath.

Silbert, M. H., and Pines, A. M. (1981). Sexual child abuse as an antecedent to prostitution. *Child Abuse and Neglect, 5,* 407–411.

Skinner, H. A. (1981). Toward the integration of classification theory and methods. *J. Abnormal Psychology, 90,* 68–87.

Stoller, R. (1973). *Splitting: A Case of Female Masculinity.* New York: Delta Books.

Swanson, D. (1968). Adult sexual abuse of children. *Diseases of the Nervous System 29* (19), 677–683.

Swift, C. (1985). The prevention of rape. In A. W. Burgess (Ed.), *Rape and Sexual Assault.* New York: Garland Publishing, 415.

Tsai, M., Feldman-Summers, S., and Edgar, M. (1979). Childhood molestation: Variables related to differential impact of psychosexual functioning in adult women. *J. Abnormal Psychology, 88,* 407–417.

Tufts–New England Medical Center Study (1984). Final Report to the Department of Juvenile Justice and Delinquency Prevention. Sexual Abuse Treatment Project at Tufts. New England Medical Center, Boston, MA.

Walker, L. (1979). *The Battered Woman.* New York: Harper & Row.

Woodling, B., and Kossoris, P. (1981). Sexual misuse: Rape, molestation and incest. *Pediatric Clinical of North America, 28,* 481–499.

Wolf, S. C., Conte, J. R., and Engle-Menig, M. (1987). Community treatment of adults who have sex with children. In L. E. A. Walker (Ed.), *Handbook on Sexual Abuse of Children: Assessment and Treatment Issues.* New York: Springer Publishers.

Yorukoglu, A., and Kemph, J. (1969). Children not severely damaged by incest with a parent. *J. Am. Acad. of Child Psychiatry, 8,* 111–124.

Zetzel, E. R. (1949). Anxiety and the capacity to bear it. *Int. J. Psychoanalysis, 30,* 1–12.

5   The intergenerational transmission of child abuse

Joan Kaufman and Edward Zigler

Introduction

The belief that abuse is transmitted intergenerationally is widely acclaimed in the child abuse literature and popular press alike. Numerous professional reviews (i.e., Friedrich and Wheeler, 1982; Spinetta and Rigler, 1972) and newspaper articles have been published promulgating this idea. Although this belief is extensively held, and there are many media reports that suggest that 99 percent of all maltreated children become abusers themselves, there is a paucity of empirical evidence to support this claim.

Current research indicates that unqualified acceptance of the intergenerational hypothesis is unwarranted (see Kaufman and Zigler, 1987, for a review of the literature). Being maltreated as a child puts one at risk for becoming abusive, but the path between these two points is far from direct or inevitable.

In this chapter, several issues associated with the intergenerational hypothesis are addressed. In the first section, a sample of empirical studies are reviewed and an estimate of the true rate of transmission derived. Next, two mechanisms proposed to explain transmission, when it does occur, are discussed. In the third section, mediating factors shown to affect the likelihood of abuse being transmitted are outlined, and the complex relationships among these factors highlighted. The possibility of using information about child rearing experiences to predict whether or not parents are apt to become abusive is explored in the last section of this chapter.

The intergenerational hypothesis

There are many papers cited in support of the intergenerational hypothesis that make no more than assertions of its validity without providing any substantive evidence (Bleiberg, 1965; Blue, 1965; Corbett, 1964; Harper, 1963; Kempe, 1973; Wasserman, 1967). Until recently, three types of data sources were used to investigate the intergenerational hypothesis: case study materials, clinical interviews, and agency records. The value of most of these studies is diminished, however, because of a number of methodological problems, including: (1) the use of small, nonrepresentative samples without comparison subjects, which limits the generalizability and interpretability of research findings; (2) the use of observers who were not blind to parents' maltreatment status, which increases the likelihood of biased reporting; and (3) the failure to develop formal criteria for the terms "history of abuse" and "current abuse," which obfuscates the meaning of investigators' conclusions.

In this section four studies are detailed to evaluate the validity of the intergenerational hypothesis and derive an estimate of the true rate of transmission. Since the likelihood of the intergenerational hypothesis being confirmed is affected by the criteria utilized to substantiate transmission claims, the parameters of the intergenerational hypothesis are first delimited.

Defining the intergenerational hypothesis

The intergenerational hypothesis states that maltreated children are likely to become abusive parents. In this chapter, evidence of transmission is restricted to incidents of physical abuse, sexual abuse, and/or extreme neglect that occur in successive generations. The hypothesis is considered substantiated regardless of which form of maltreatment is experienced in subsequent generations, because the intervention implications of these three forms of maltreatment are quite similar. As this definition of transmission is consistent with most lay people's and professionals' conceptualization of transmission, the conclusions presented in this chapter are not likely to be misinterpreted and inappropriately applied within the mental health and judiciary systems.

The criteria for transmission used by the investigators of the studies reviewed in this section vary greatly. A number of the other basic elements of these studies differ as well, including the subjects studied (identified abusers versus high risk populations versus nationally representative samples), definitions of "history of abuse" and "current abuse" used, experimental design employed (retrospective versus prospective), and type of data sources tapped to substantiate claims of past and current abuse. The methodology and results of the four studies are now detailed to illustrate how variations in the research designs affected the transmission rates obtained by different investigators. An estimate of the true rate of transmission is then derived.

Studies cited in support of the intergenerational hypothesis

The study by Steele and Pollock (1968) is one of the most widely cited reports, despite the authors' cautionary note at the onset of their paper stating that their "study group of parents was not to be thought of as useful statistical proof of any concepts" (p. 90). The subjects of this study were 60 child abusing parents who were participating in a psychological treatment program. Most parents were referred to the study by hospital personnel after their children were treated for nonaccidental injuries. Information about the parents' background and current functioning was collected through psychiatric diagnostic and therapeutic interviews. The authors reported that the abusing parents in their study recreated the pattern of rearing they experienced with their own children, "without exception." But they also stated that a number of parents reported "never having had a hand laid on them," which leaves one uncertain about what is meant by "rearing experiences" being "recreated" (p. 97).

Steele and Pollock later expanded on this point and stated that, "all [the parents in their study] had experienced . . . a sense of intense, pervasive, continuous demands from their parents" (p. 97). This definition is rather removed from what is usually implied by the intergenerational hypothesis, and it is not particularly useful to law providers or service workers needing to make clinical decisions in individual cases. In addition, without an appropriate comparison group it is impossible to determine if these experiences are unique to abusive parents, or simply true of most adults receiving psychological services. The number of adults who were subjected to similar demands in childhood who neither abuse their children nor receive psychological services cannot be determined from the findings of this study. Although this study was clearly valuable in generating hypotheses about the possible relationship between being abused and becoming abusive, it simply cannot be considered conclusive evidence in support of the intergenerational hypothesis.

Over the past five years, standardized self-report measures (e.g., written questionnaires, structured interviews) have become the primary data source of most studies investigating the intergenerational question. Studies using these types of measures are far more methodologically sound than studies that used case study materials, clinical interviews, and/or agency records. In these studies, the terms "history of abuse" and "current abuse" were consistently defined, comparison groups were always employed, and multiple etiological factors were always assessed. Measures of stress, social isolation, and child characteristics were often included, representing a shift from the focus of earlier investigations that concentrated solely on detecting pathology in the parents who abused their children.

In all studies that used self-report instruments as their primary data source, consistent differences emerged between abusers and comparison subjects on measures assessing the variable "history of abuse" (Altemeier, O'Connor, Vietze, Sandler, and Sherrod, 1984; Conger, Burgess, and Barrett, 1979; Egeland and Jacobvitz, 1984; Gaines, Sandgrund, Green, and Power, 1978; Herrenkohl, Herrenkohl, and Toedtler, 1983; Hunter and Kilstrom, 1979; Quinton, Rutter, and Liddle, 1984; Smith and Hanson, 1975; Spinetta, 1978; Straus, 1979). There was, however, considerable overlap between the two groups reported. This implies that, although a history of abuse is more common among parents who maltreat their children, many parents who do not report abusive childhood experiences become abusers and a sizable number of parents who were maltreated as children do not.

The rate of intergenerational transmission reported by different investigators that used self-report questionnaires ranges from 18 percent to 70 percent. Three studies are detailed here to illustrate how variation in research designs produced such discrepant figures. The findings of these studies are then integrated to derive an estimate of the most accurate transmission rate.

The first study was conducted by Hunter and Kilstrom (1979), who interviewed 282 parents of newborns admitted to a regional intensive care nursery for premature infants. Information about the parents' childhood, mothers' pregnancy, child's health, and families' social networks were obtained through a semistructured interview. A history of abuse was defined to include incidents of neglect as well as physical abuse. Current abuse was determined by searching the state central registry for confirmed reports of abuse or neglect when the children were 1 year old. At the time of the initial interview, 49 parents reported a childhood history of abuse or neglect. At follow-up, 10 babies in the study were identified as maltreated. Nine of these infants had parents with a history of abuse or neglect; however, 40 parents with comparable childhood histories were not detected as maltreaters. Since only 9 of the 49 parents who initially reported childhood abuse were identified as maltreaters, the rate of intergenerational transmission reported in this investigation was 18 percent.

This study pointedly illustrates how variations in the subjects (identified abusers versus high-risk sample) and experimental design (retrospective versus prospective) affect the outcome of research findings. If this study had been conducted retrospectively with only the parents who were identified as maltreaters, the link between a history of abuse and subsequent child abuse would have appeared deceptively strong, since 9 out of 10 of the abusive parents reported a history of abuse (90 percent). By employing a prospective research design, Hunter and Kilstrom demonstrated that the majority of parents who had been abused did not maltreat their children (82 percent).

The parents in this study who broke the cycle of abuse differed from those parents who did not in that they had more extensive social supports, physically healthier babies, and fewer ambivalent feelings about their child's birth. In addition, the parents who broke the cycle were more openly angry about their earlier abuse and better able to give detailed accounts of those experiences. They were also less likely to have been abused by both their parents, and more apt to have reported a supportive relationship with one of their parents when growing up.

The generalizability of Hunter and Kilstrom's study, however, is restricted because of the nonrepresentative nature of their sample (parents of ill infants), the limitations associated with the data source used to detect current incidents of abuse (agency records), and the fact that follow-up did not extend beyond one year. Despite these caveats, this study clearly demonstrates the superiority of prospective research designs and highlights the need to interpret retrospective studies with caution.

The second study was conducted by Egeland and Jacobvitz (1984) who used a semistructured interview to collect information about the childhood histories and current disciplinary practices of 160 high-risk, low-income, predominantly single-parent mothers. Each mother had at least one child between four to five years of age. In addition, measures of stress, isolation, and child characteristics were also obtained. In this study, a history of abuse was restricted to incidents of severe physical punishment, including being thrown against a wall, hit repeatedly with an object, or intentionally burned. Current abusers were subdivided into three categories: a "physical abuse" group who used severe physical punishment tactics, a "borderline abuse" group who administered daily or weekly spankings that did not cause bruises or caused red marks that disappeared, and an "other" group that included women whose children were being cared for by someone else. (Reasons for the out-of-home care were not specified.) The authors reported an intergenerational transmission rate of 70% for mothers with a history of severe physical abuse. This percentage, however, included mothers who physically abused their children (34%), mothers who fell into the borderline abuse category (30%), and mothers whose children were being reared away from the home (6%).

The findings of this study are confounded by the high-risk nature of Egeland and Jacobvitz's sample. The influence of a history of abuse upon subsequent parenting cannot be separated from the effects of poverty, stress, and social isolation. The results of this study actually reflect the interaction of multiple determinants on the etiology of abuse (e.g., history of abuse, poverty, stress, isolation), and not the influence of a single determinant (e.g., history of abuse). It is important to keep in mind the simultaneous effects of these different variables when interpreting the findings of this study. Unless the independent effects of these variables are tested empirically, it is impossible to determine their separate influences on subsequent parenting.

The broad definition of "current abuse" used also affected the results. In general, the broader the definitional criteria employed, the greater the apparent link between a history of abuse and current abuse. As noted, Egeland and Jacobvitz included the borderline abuse category in their computation of the rate of intergenerational transmission. They found that 30% of the mothers who reported a history of abuse fell into this category, but an even larger percentage of mothers who reported emotionally supportive child-hoods were categorized as borderline abusers (39%). Given the failure of the borderline abuse category to differentiate these two groups, the validity of this category, and the conclusion that aberrant childhood histories "caused" the borderline parenting, is questionable. In fact, a national survey of disciplinary practices reported that 97% of all children in the United States have been physically punished (Straus, 1983). It appears the borderline abuse group's parenting is more reflective of a cultural norm than a parenting deviation. Although on a continuum of parenting, the behaviors associated with the borderline abuse group are not optimal, they can best be understood in light of cultural (e.g., acceptance of corporal punishment as a legitimate means of discipline) and environmental determinants (e.g., stress, isolation), and not developmental factors (e.g., history of abuse).

Egeland and Jacobvitz also reported a number of factors that differentiated the repeaters from the nonrepeaters in their study. They found that nonrepeaters were more likely to have one parent or foster parent who provided support and love during childhood, to be currently involved in a relationship with an emotionally supportive spouse or boyfriend, and to report fewer current stressful life events. They also showed a greater awareness of their history of being abused and were consciously resolved not to repeat the pattern of abuse with their own children. These factors are highly similar to those reported by Hunter and Kilstrom (1979).

Although the 70% transmission rate reported by Egeland and Jacobvitz is most likely an overestimation for the aforementioned reasons, this study provides a valuable contribution to understanding the interrelationships among the many determinants of abuse. Because the effects of a history of abuse upon subsequent parenting often cannot be determined without considering the effects of poverty, stress, and social isolation, this study highlights the importance of assessing multiple factors and giving careful thought to the choice of comparison groups used in investigations of this kind.

The last self-report study was conducted by Straus (1979), who interviewed a nationally representative sample of 1,146 two-parent families with a child between the ages of 3 and 17. Straus obtained an estimate of 18 percent for the rate of intergenerational transmission of abuse, which is probably somewhat low for the following reasons: The definition of a history of abuse included only experiences of physical punishment or abuse that occurred during adolescence, an age when physical punishment is least likely to occur (Straus, Gelles, and Steinmetz, 1980); numerous individuals who were mistreated when they were younger but not as teenagers were undoubtedly omitted from the history of abuse category by this criterion. In addition, the exclusion of single parents and parents of children in the 0–3 age range is problematic, as these two groups are at greater risk for abuse than two-parent families with older children. Despite these problems, this study demonstrates that the link between being maltreated and becoming abusive is far from inevitable.

The findings of the different investigations reviewed are not easily integrated because of their methodological variations. Nonetheless, we feel the best estimate of the rate of intergenerational transmission of abuse is 30% ± 5%. For the reasons discussed previously, we believe the estimates obtained by Hunter and Kilstrom (1979) and Straus (1979) are somewhat low. Although we questioned the validity of the borderline abuse category used by Egeland and Jacobvitz (1984), we relied heavily on their finding that only 34 percent of the severely abused mothers in their study physically abused their children. Because they employed a high-risk sample, it is reasonable to assume that when a more representative population is surveyed, less than one-third of all individuals who were abused or extremely neglected will be found to maltreat their own children in either of these ways.

In the past, uncritical acceptance of the intergenerational hypothesis has caused undue anxiety in many victims of abuse, led to biased responses by mental health workers, and influenced the outcome of court decisions, even in routine divorce child custody cases. In one such case that was brought to the attention of the second author, a judge refused a mother custody rights because it was discovered during the trial that the mother had been abused as a child. Despite the fact that much of the evidence supported the children's placement with their mother, the judge concluded that the mother was an unfit guardian, since everyone "knows" abused children become abusive parents.

As stated elsewhere, "the time has come for the intergenerational myth to be placed aside" (Kaufman and Zigler, in press). The association between abuse in childhood and poor parenting is far from complete – the majority of parents who were abused do not maltreat their children. Although a 30% ± 5% transmission rate is scarcely inconsequential, it is a long cry from the 99 percent figure promulgated in the popular press. Undoubtedly, a history of abuse is a considerable risk factor associated with the etiology of child maltreatment, but the pathway to abusive parenting is far from inevitable or direct.

The value of using information about early abusive experiences to predict subsequent parenting difficulties is the subject of the last section of this chapter: First, a brief discussion of the mechanisms proposed to explain transmission when it does occur, then an analysis of the mediating factors that affect the likelihood of abuse being transmitted from one generation to the next.

Mechanisms of transmission

Investigators from divergent schools of psychological thought have proposed different mechanisms to explain why some parents who were abused
repeat the pattern and others do not. Two hypothesized mechanisms
advanced by social learning and attachment theorists are briefly outlined in
this section. Both of these views approach the problem of transmission from
a psychological perspective, but a sociological analysis is equally plausible.
Advocates of the sociological view believe that when parents and children
share a common cultural milieu with norms that support abusive behavior,
transmission is likely to occur (Zigler, 1983). Because a sociological perspective, however, relies in part on psychological mechanisms, the following
discussion of transmission mechanisms is restricted to this level, rather than
a sociological analysis.

Using a social learning perspective Feshbach (1974), Hertzberger (1983),
and others (Burgess and Youngblade, in press; Gelles and Straus, 1979)
hypothesized that abusive parenting behaviors are transmitted by teaching
children that aggression is appropriate. Children learn this by observing
abusive behavior and developing a set of rules that support it. This increases
the likelihood that they will repeat the pattern of behavior with their own
offspring. Hertzberger speculated that abused children are most likely to
form rules supporting abusive behavior if the parent's action is seen as normative, if the abuse is accompanied by rationalizing verbalizations, and if
the abuse occurs during discipline following an actual wrongdoing.
Although the validity of this perspective has not been tested in its entirety,
Hertzberger and Tennen (1982) found some support for this hypothesis
when they asked college students to judge the abusive treatment of children
described in case histories. They found that students who had been physically abused regarded the treatment received by the children in the stories
as more appropriate than students who had not been abused. Furthermore,
when students were given a description of a child's moderately provocative
behavior along with a description of the parent's abuse, the child was judged
by the students to be more responsible for the parental discipline, and the
disciplinary act was rated as less severe.

In contrast to the social learning perspective, attachment theorists are more
psychoanalytic in their approach to the intergenerational question. They
consider representational schemata of past attachment figures primary in
determining the nature of future relationships (Bowlby, 1973, 1980; Sroufe
and Fleeson, 1986). These representational models are produced through
interactions with significant others from birth through adolescence. The
likelihood that abusive patterns of behavior will be passed from one generation to the next is presumed to increase when early negative experiences

are not remembered and integrated, and coherent working models of relationships are not formed (Bowlby, 1980).

To test this hypothesis, Main and Goldwyn (1984) interviewed 30 women about their relationships with their mothers and observed them interacting with their children in the Ainsworth Strange Situation (Ainsworth and Wittig, 1969), a research paradigm designed to assess mother–child attachment. They found that women who remembered their mothers as rejecting were more likely to reject their own children than women who reported supportive child rearing experiences. Women who were rejected as children were also more likely to have incoherent recollections of childhood experiences. If coherent accounts of rejecting experiences were formed, however, mothers were not likely to reject their children.

The study by Main and Goldwyn (1984) provides some preliminary support for the hypothesis that mental representations of past relationships mediate the transmission of abuse. Because no alternative hypotheses were investigated, however, and the factors responsible for the more coherent memories in the one group of women not identified, one must consider the possibility that other variables contributed to the observed differences in parenting. For example, although Hunter and Kilstrom (1979) and Egeland and Jacobvitz (1984) reported that mothers who had coherent recollections of their early abusive experiences were less likely to repeat the pattern with their children, these investigators also identified numerous other factors (e.g., quality of marital relationship, number of stressful life events) that differentiated the repeaters from the nonrepeaters.

The two hypotheses outlined above raise many questions. For example, from a social learning perspective, what sort of experiences are necessary to change rules that support abusive behavior? From the vantage point of attachment theorists, is the establishment of coherent childhood recollections a prerequisite for the creation of future positive relationships, or can positive experiences affect the solidification of representational models? More generally, what is the relationship between representational models and the existence of rules that support abusive behavior? Understanding the relationships between these mechanisms will have implications for understanding the etiology of abuse, as well as the etiology of many other forms of psychopathology. Unfortunately, further research is required to understand the individual mechanisms and their interrelationships.

Mediating variables

The literature reviewed highlighted a number of factors that differentiate repeaters from nonrepeaters. Further exploration of these variables, together with variables that have been shown to increase the likelihood of abuse, is essential to determine the conditions under which the transmission of abuse is most likely to occur. In this section, a framework for organizing these factors is presented, and the complexity of the relationships among the associated variables is highlighted.

Organizing child abuse risk factors

Belsky (1980), in extending a model presented by Garbarino (1977), proposed the most comprehensive model of abuse to date. He integrated Bronfenbrenner's (1977, 1979) conceptualization of the contexts in which development occurs and Tinbergen's (1951) analysis of ontogenetic development, and organized the factors associated with the etiology of abuse into a framework comprised of four ecological levels: the ontogenetic, microsystem, exosystem, and macrosystem. On the ontogenetic level he included characteristics of parents who mistreat their children, such as a history of abuse or low self-esteem. On the microsystem level he discussed aspects of the family environment that increase the likelihood of abuse occurring, such as a poor marital relationship or a child with behavior problems. On the exosystem level he included work and social factors, such as unemployment and isolation; and on the macrosystem level he depicted cultural determinants, such as our society's acceptance of corporal punishment as a legitimate form of discipline.

The studies reviewed in the last section highlighted the importance of both compensatory and risk factors in understanding the transmission of abuse. Consequently, together with Cicchetti and Rizley (1981), we believe a complete conceptualization of the factors associated with the etiology of abuse should include both risk and compensatory factors. Risk factors increase the likelihood of abuse occurring (e.g., history of abuse, poverty), compensatory factors decrease the likelihood of abuse occurring (e.g., being involved in a relationship with a supportive spouse). Although compensatory factors are implied in Belsky's model, their explicit delineation will be useful to both clinicians and researchers. Table 5.1 includes a number of compensatory and risk factors that have been organized utilizing Belsky's ecological framework. Many of these factors were derived from the work of Cicchetti and Rizley (1981).

As can be seen from the table, the factors that have been shown to mediate the transmission of abuse can be organized using the ecological system. Having a high IQ, an awareness of early abusive experiences, resolve not to repeat the abuse, and a history of a positive attachment relationship with one caregiver, are some ontogenetic compensatory factors (Egeland and Jacobvitz, 1984; Hunter and Kilstrom, 1979). Microsystem level compensatory factors include having physically healthy children (Hunter and Kilstrom, 1979; Smith and Hanson, 1975) and a supportive spouse (Egeland and Jacobvitz, 1984; Herrenkohl et al., 1983; Hunter and Kilstrom, 1979; Quinton, Rutter, and Liddle, 1984). Good social supports (Hunter and Kil-

Table 5.1. *Determinants of abuse: Compensatory and risk factors*

	Ontogenetic level	Microsystem level	Exosystem level	Macrosystem level
Compensatory Factors	High IQ Awareness of past abuse History of a positive relationship with one parent Special talents Physical attractiveness Good interpersonal skills	Healthy children Supportive spouse Economic security/ savings in the bank	Good social supports Few stressful events Strong, supportive religious affiliation Positive school experiences and peer relations as a child Therapeutic interventions	Culture that promotes a sense of shared responsibility in caring for the community's children Culture opposed to violence Economic prosperity
Risk Factors	History of abuse Low self esteem Low IQ Poor interpersonal skills	Marital discord Children with behavior problems Premature or unhealthy children Single parent Poverty	Unemployment Isolation; poor social supports Poor peer relations as a child	Cultural acceptance of corporal punishment View of children as possessions Economic depression

strom, 1979) and few stressful life events (Egeland and Jacobvitz, 1984) are important exosystem factors. Other compensatory factors identified through clinical and/or research experience include having special talents (Cicchetti and Rizley, 1981), economic security (Straus, 1979), a strong, supportive religious affiliation (Helfer, 1984), positive school experiences (Rutter and Quinton, 1984), and/or good peer relations (Freud and Dann, 1951). Therapeutic interventions are also capable of producing compensatory effects (Egeland and Jacobvitz, 1984). It is not enough to merely identify and conceptually organize these factors, however. The key to predicting the likelihood that any one individual will become abusive is understanding the relative importance of each of these factors.

Understanding the relationships among the factors

Belsky (1984) has asserted that the factors on the ontogenetic level are most important in determining parenting behavior. He believes this because, although marital relations, for example, have been shown to contribute to the etiology of abuse, as the quality of the marital relation is influenced by personality and developmental characteristics, its influence can be traced back to the ontogenetic level.

In a recent study of the parenting of women raised in institutions because their parents could not cope with child rearing responsibilities, the effect of a history of abuse on subsequent parenting was demonstrated as Belsky predicted (Quinton et al., 1984). Women who were raised in institutions were more likely to marry deviant, unsupportive spouses; and women in these marriages tended to be less adequate parents. The ability of the spousal relationship to ameliorate the impact of institutional rearing was evidenced as well, however. The authors reported that when marital support was available, poor parenting was rare and occurred in only 3 percent of all cases, irrespective of childhood rearing experiences.

As the Quinton et al. (1984) study illustrates, the compensatory and risk factors outlined in Table 5.1 are capable of producing bidirectional effects. Early experiences can influence the quality of the spousal relationship, and good marital relations can ameliorate the effects of childhood adversities. However, because the direction of the effect of a given factor is not specific, the prediction of its impact is problematic.

The relationships among the variables associated with the etiology and transmission of abuse are complicated further. For example, in addition to being nonspecific, the effect of each stressor is also variable. Differences in the configuration of the remaining compensatory and risk factors and variations in the causes of the stressor affect the impact of the stressor. For example, the effect of unemployment due to characterological (individualistic) reasons will be different than the effect of unemployment caused by a sociological reason (e.g., economic depression). In addition, the impact of the unemployment caused by individualistic or socioeconomic causes will differentially affect individuals depending on the availability of the other compensatory and risk factors (e.g., personality characteristics, savings in the bank, social supports; Elder, Caspi, and Nguyen, in press). Given the changing value of each risk factor in differing contexts and the possibility of bidirectional effects, it is extremely difficult to determine the likelihood that any individual parent will become abusive.

There is one other phenomenon that further diminishes the likelihood of accurately predicting which parents are most likely to confirm the intergenerational hypothesis – luck, "the roulette wheel of life's chances" (Rutter, 1984; p. 53). The notion that chance constitutes one of the major influences on people's lives was demonstrated by Jencks and his colleagues (1972) and has been elaborated upon elsewhere (Bandura, 1982; Rutter, 1984). The following case study illustrates the importance of chance experiences in determining life circumstances and subsequent parenting.

Elizabeth's parents were both alcoholics. She was physically and sexually abused by her father, and grossly neglected by her mother. At ten, shortly after her mother abandoned the family, Elizabeth was placed in a foster home.

Elizabeth changed foster placements five times before she came of age – once because she was sexually abused by her foster-care father.

Despite these adversities, Elizabeth had a lot going for her. She was pretty, had good social skills, and was well liked by her peers. She was also quite intelligent and managed to graduate high school on schedule, in spite of the multiple moves that resulted from changes in her foster-care placements.

All these assets helped Elizabeth, but it is probably the following chance experience that aided her most.

When Elizabeth was fourteen she was permanently injured in a car accident. The injury was not the least bit debilitating, but she received $8,000 in an insurance settlement.

After high school, Elizabeth used this money to earn a degree in computer programming. She then got a job with excellent medical benefits. Shortly thereafter she got pregnant out of wedlock. Her employee medical plan, however, guaranteed her a six month maternity leave with 70% pay.

A year later Elizabeth was married. She, her husband, and her two year old son are all doing well. Elizabeth is still haunted by many painful memories which therapeutic interventions have helped her deal with, but she has the resolve and resources to see that her son has a better life.

Elizabeth was endowed with many assets, but luck played an important part in shaping her life. It is ironic that a seemingly negative chance experience (i.e., a car accident) had such a positive effect on Elizabeth's life; but without the insurance settlement that resulted from the accident, she would never have been able to receive training as a computer programmer. Without that training, it is unlikely that Elizabeth would have been employed by a company with such an excellent medical plan, as 60 percent of all working women have absolutely no maternity leave benefits. Without these instances of good fortune, the likelihood of Elizabeth experiencing difficulties in parenting would have been significantly increased.

Breaking the cycle of abuse is not an easy endeavor; it takes work. With some luck and positive relations, however, most victims of abuse appear to overcome the dire prediction of the intergenerational hypothesis. The complexity of the relations among the variables that affect the likelihood of transmission occurring undermine efforts to predict which individuals are most likely to repeat the pattern of abuse in subsequent generations. These problems, however, are further compounded by several probabilistic considerations. In the next section, issues associated with child abuse prediction are explored.

Child abuse prediction

It has been argued that to prevent child abuse, we must be able to predict its occurrence (Helfer and Kempe, 1976). To facilitate prediction, screening instruments were developed to assess factors implicated in the etiology of abuse by a number of retrospective studies (see Starr, 1982, for a review of the literature). Reports suggesting that maltreaters were themselves abused as children were given special attention in the construction of most screening techniques. In fact, the aim of prediction efforts has been described as the identification of "high-risk parents . . . who themselves had unfortunate childhood experiences" (Helfer, 1976, p. 363).

Currently there are three major screening methods used to predict individuals' likelihood to abuse their children: written questionnaires (e.g., Milner, 1986; Schneider, Helfer, and Pollock, 1972); standardized interviews (e.g., Altemeier et al., 1984); and direct parent–child observations (e.g., Gray, Cutler, Dean, and Kempe, 1977). In this section the utility of one predictive questionnaire, the Family Stress Checklist (Schneider et al., 1972), is discussed to illustrate the statistical improbability of devising sensitive screening devices (see also Cicchetti and Aber, 1980, for a discussion of this issue). The success rate of this instrument is consistent with the best rates reported in the literature (see Schneider, Helfer, and Hoffmeister, 1982, for a review). We chose to discuss this instrument because it assesses risk factors at multiple ecological levels and is most compatible with the risk-factor model of abuse outlined in the previous section. Although the Family Stress Checklist and other available screening methods have not been used to predict which individuals are apt to confirm the intergenerational hypothesis, the utility of employing these instruments for such purposes is discussed hypothetically at the conclusion of this section. First, a few probability concepts are discussed. (See Meehl and Rosen, 1973, for an extensive discussion of the clinical applications of probability principles.)

Probability concepts

A predictive instrument's performance is evaluated in terms of two measures: its sensitivity and its specificity (Daniel, Newberger, Reed, and Kotelchuck, 1978). In the case of predicting child abusers, sensitivity refers to the probability that future child abusers will be accurately detected; and specificity refers to the probability that nonabusers will be correctly identified. These two probabilities are also referred to as valid positives and valid negatives (Meehl and Rosen, 1973). Associated with these probabilities are two types of errors: false positives and false negatives. A nonabusive parent labelled abusive by a screening device is an example of a false positive prediction; and an abusive parent that misses detection and is labelled nonabusive is an example of a false negative prediction. The magnitude of these two types of errors must be considered against the prevalence rate – or base rate – of abuse, as a 5% error rate that applies to 95% of the population (e.g., percent of parents who do not abuse their children) will result in a greater number of misclassifications than a 5% error rate that applies to only 5% of the population. These principles are presently applied.

Table 5.2. *Prenatal predictions of abuse and follow-up classifications*

		Actual abuser	
		Yes	No
	Yes	20 valid positive	18 false positive
Predicted abuser	No	5 false negative	152 valid negative

Source: Adapted from Murphy, S., Orkow, B., and Nicola, R. (1985). Prenatal prediction of child abuse and neglect: A prospective study. *Child Abuse and Neglect, 9,* 225–235.

Evaluation of the Family Stress Checklist

Murphy, Orkow, and Nicola (1985) administered the Family Stress Checklist to 587 lower income mothers during their third trimester of pregnancy. The checklist produces scores for the following ten categories: history of abuse; stress; isolation and/or depression; provocative and/or difficult child; unwanted child; unrealistic expectations of child behavior; harsh punishment practices; suspected parenting difficulties in past; record of violent temper outbursts; and criminal or mental illness record. Possible scores range from 0 to 100. The greatest proportion of mothers scored between 5–25 points (61%); mothers scoring over 40 points (7%) were considered "at-risk" for abusing or neglecting their children. When the children were 1 to 2 years old, the children's medical charts were examined for evidence of abuse and/or neglect.

At follow-up, 20 of the 38 children whose mothers scored 40 or above were identified as abused or neglected. Two of the 100 children whose mothers scored between 0–10, and three of the 57 children whose mothers scored between 25–35 were identified as abused or neglected. These figures were then used to compute sensitivity and specificity rates. The proportion of children who were correctly and incorrectly identified by the screening technique are shown in Table 5.2. The authors computed an 80% sensitivity rate, as 20 of the 25 abused children were correctly identified by the screen (i.e., $20/25 \times 100\% = 80\%$); and a 90% specificity figure, as 152 of the 170 nonabused children were accurately predicted (i.e., $152/170 \times 100\% = 90\%$). These figures suggest that 20% of actual abusers and 10% of nonabusers were misclassified. These error rates are now considered in relation

Table 5.3. *Proportion of parents accurately labelled abuser by the screening interview assuming a 5% base rate of abuse*

Sensitivity rate*	Specificity rate**	Proportion of parents accurately labelled abuser
.80	.90	.30
.95	.95	.50

*The proportion of actual abusers correctly identified.
**The proportion of actual non-abusers correctly identified.

to the base rate figure of abuse reported in this study to determine the proportion of parents who were mislabelled as abusers.

Murphy et al. (1985) reported a 5% prevalence rate of abuse, but there are many different base rate figures reported in the literature. Depending on the definition of abuse used and data sources tapped to obtain base rates of abuse, estimated prevalence rates range from 1% (Light, 1973) to 14% (Straus, 1979). Since the 5% incidence rate reported by Murphy et al. (1985) is comparable to the rate most often reported in the literature (see Parke & Collmer, 1975, for a review), this figure is used in all subsequent analyses.

Bayes' Theorem was used to calculate the proportion of parents who were accurately labelled by the Family Stress Checklist in its present form, and the proportion of parents who could be accurately identified if the sensitivity and specificity rates were increased to 95%. These figures are reported in the first and second rows of Table 5.3.

Bayes' Theorem derives screening accuracy estimates from information about the rate of abuse and the number of valid and false positive predictions. Utilizing the 5% abuse rate to determine the screening accuracy of the Family Stress Questionnaire, according to Bayes' Theorem only 30% of parents who were labelled abusive were accurately identified. This figure was computed as follows (for illustrative purposes, a sample of 100 parents is employed in the example. Utilizing a 5% abuse rate implies that 5 parents in 100 are actual abusers; 95 are nonabusers): The 90% specificity figure reported by Murphy et al. (1985) assumes that approximately 10 parents in 100 would be erroneously labelled abusers (i.e., 95 nonabusers $\times$ .10 error rate = 9.5 nonabusers labelled abusers). The 80% sensitivity rate suggests that four of the five real abusive parents would be correctly identified (i.e., 5 abusers $\times$ .80 sensitivity rate = 4 abusers labelled abusers). In total then, of the fourteen parents labelled abusive, only four (30%) would have been labelled correctly. If sensitivity and specificity ratings could be increased to 95%, utilizing the 5% prevalence rate, misclassifications would still be as high as 50%.

Because the 5% abuse rate implies that 95 out of every 100 parents will not become abusers, accuracy could be assured 95% of the time by always predicting that parents will not abuse their children. This hit rate is considerably higher than any rate achieved with existing screening methods. In order for a screening device to be considered efficient, it must increase the number of correct predictions that are possible using the base rates alone. As the application of Bayes' Theorem illustrated, and as has been noted elsewhere (Meehl and Rosen, 1973), when the base rate of a given phenomenon deviates greatly from a 50 percent split (as in the case of child abuse), use of a screening instrument with moderate validity will cause an increase in the number of erroneous predictions. It appears that it is simply not statistically feasible to accurately predict a low base rate phenomenon like child abuse, even when screening devices assess multiple etiological factors and sensitivity and specificity ratings are increased to 95%.

Using screening devices to predict individuals likely to confirm the intergenerational hypothesis

The feasibility of using screening devices to predict future abusers is limited by the low base rate of abuse. The base rate for abuse among individuals with a history of abuse (30% ± 5%), however, is approximately six times higher than the base rate for abuse in the general population (5%). Using Bayes' Theorem, the magnitude of expected errors in labelling "abusers" within this group is considerably less than they are when screening techniques are applied more universally, suggesting that it may be feasible to employ screening techniques to identify individuals likely to confirm the intergenerational hypothesis. Given the complexity of the relations among the factors that affect the likelihood of abuse being transmitted across generations, however, the probability of making accurate predictions in individual cases is still severely hampered. Standardized screening procedures are not likely to properly evaluate the effects of chance events, or sufficiently explore the simultaneous effects of various compensatory and risk factors to assure accurate predictions.

Because the issue of misclassification is not merely an abstract, statistical question (Daniel et al., 1978), the infeasibility of devising sufficiently sensitive measures and the cost of mislabelling parents as potential abusers must be weighed seriously. "Child abuser" is an extremely value-laden and derogatory term. The stigma of being called a "potential abuser," and the stress it causes parents, may put children at greater risk than before the prediction of abuse was cast (Solnit, 1980). Being labelled a potential abuser, in fact, may create a self-fulfilling prophecy (Gelles, 1982).

In addition, mistakes in labelling abusive families will not be random.

Certain social groups (e.g., minorities, single-parent families, and low income families) will be more vulnerable than others to false accusations (Gelles, 1982; Solnit, 1980). The threat to personal liberty and the family's integrity caused by these biases in error prediction is quite substantial (Uviller, 1980).

Furthermore, unless services are available to offset the negative consequences of labelling and improve the prognosis of identified families, screening is not warranted (Cicchetti and Aber, 1980; Hobbs, 1974). Because adequate resources have not been supplied to meet the needs of all the reported abuse cases that have flooded government agencies since the mandated reporting laws were passed in the early 1970s (Solnit, 1980), it is unlikely that sufficient services can be provided to justify the screening procedures. Given the realistic constraints of social service funding and many of the other considerations noted, a prediction approach to prevention is simply not viable. Whether this approach is applied globally, or only to specific targeted groups (i.e., parents who were abused as children), the costs associated with prediction errors far exceed the potential benefits of using screening procedures to identify individuals likely to abuse their children.

Consequently, we believe that efforts at predicting individual cases of child abuse should be abandoned. While it is feasible to predict high-risk communities and changes in the national prevalence rates of abuse based on fluctuations in the economy (Zigler, 1976), accurate prediction of individual cases is not possible. In contrast to a prediction approach to prevention, in agreement with Solnit (1980), we advocate the implementation of voluntary services to ameliorate the conditions that promote abuse. Possible services include neighborhood health care, home visitor services, parent education programs, social service guidance, employment counseling, day care facilities, and hot line supports for parents in crisis. A full discussion of prevention strategies is beyond the scope of this chapter, but we advocate interventions aimed at multiple ecological levels that are targeted towards high-risk communities, and not high-risk individuals. (For further discussion of prevention strategies, see Garbarino and Stockman, 1980; Olson, this volume; and Ross and Zigler, 1980.)

Conclusions

Our review has demonstrated that the link between being maltreated and becoming abusive is far from inevitable. The time has come for researchers to cease to ask: "Do abused children become abusive parents?" and ask instead: "Under what conditions is the transmission of abuse most likely to occur?" In future studies, to untangle the complex relationships among the factors that affect the transmission of abuse, it will be important to systematically explore the affect of numerous compensatory and risk factors using statistical procedures that are sensitive to both main and interaction effects (i.e., linear logistic modeling). Once the relative importance of these factors is better understood, more effective intervention programs can be designed and implemented.

In the past, uncritical acceptance of the intergenerational hypothesis has had many negative consequences. It has impeded progress in understanding the etiology of abuse, and led to misguided judicial and social policy interventions. Despite the long held popularity of this belief, the fact is that the majority of abused children do not become abusive parents. Until this fact is promulgated by professionals and lay people alike with the same enthusiasm the intergenerational myth enjoyed, innocent victims of abuse will continue to be unjustly stigmatized.

References

Ainsworth, M., and Wittig, B. (1969). Attachment and exploratory behavior of one-year-olds in a strange situation. In B. Foss (ed.), *Determinants of Infant Behavior* (Vol. 4). London: Methuen.

Altemeier, W., O'Connor, S., Vietze, P., Sandler, H., and Sherrod, K. (1984). Prediction of child abuse: A prospective study of feasibility. *Child Abuse and Neglect, 8,* 393–400.

Bandura, A. (1982). A psychology of chance encounters and life paths. *American Psychologist, 37,* 747–755.

Belsky, J. (1980). Child maltreatment: An ecological integration. *American Psychologist, 35,* 320–335.

Belsky, J. (1984). The determinants of parenting: A process model. *Child Development, 55,* 83–96.

Bleiberg, N. (1965). The neglected child and the child health conference. *New York State Journal of Medicine, 65,* 1880–1885.

Blue, M. (1965). The battered child syndrome from a social work viewpoint. *Canadian Journal of Public Health, 56,* 197–198.

Bowlby, J. (1973). *Attachment and Loss. Vol. 2: Separation.* New York: Basic Books.

Bowlby, J. (1980). *Attachment and Loss. Vol. 3: Loss.* New York: Basic Books.

Bronfenbrenner, U. (1977). Toward an experimental ecology of human development. *American Psychologist, 32,* 513–531.

Bronfenbrenner, U. (1979). *The Ecology of Human Development.* Cambridge, MA: Harvard University Press.

Burgess, R., and Youngblade, L. (in press). The intergenerational transmission of abusive parental practices: A social interactional analysis. In R. Gelles, G. Hotaling, D. Finkelhor, and M. Straus (Eds.), *New Directions in Family Violence Research.* New York: Sage.

Cicchetti, D., and Aber, L. A. (1980). Abused children–abusive parents: An overstated case? *Harvard Educational Review, 50,* 244–255.

Cicchetti, D., and Rizley, R. (1981). Developmental perspectives on the etiology, intergenerational transmission, and sequelae of child maltreatment. *New Directions for Child Maltreatment, 11,* 31–55.

Conger, R., Burgess, R., and Barrett, C. (1979). Child abuse related to life change and perceptions of illness: Some preliminary findings. *Family Coordinator, 58,* 73–77.

Corbett, J. (1964). A psychiatrist reviews the battered child syndrome and mandatory reporting legislation. *North-West Medicine, 63,* 920–922.

Daniel, J., Newberger, E., Reed, R., and Kotelchuck, M. (1978). Child abuse screening: Implications of the limited predictive power of abuse discriminants from a controlled family study of pediatric social illness. *Child Abuse and Neglect, 2,* 247–259.

Egeland, B., and Jacobvitz, D. (1984). Intergenerational continuity of parental abuse: Causes and consequences. Paper presented at the Conference on Biosocial Perspectives in Abuse and Neglect, York, Maine.

Elder, G., Caspi, A., and Nguyen, T. (in press). Resourceful and vulnerable children: Family influences in stressful times. In R. Silbereisen and K. Eyterth (Eds.), *Development in Context: Integrative Perspectives on Youth Development.*

Feshbach, S. (1974). The development and regulation of aggression: Some research gaps and a proposed cognitive analysis. In J. De Wit and W. Hartup (Eds.), *Determinants and Origins of Aggressive Behavior.* Mouton, Paris.

Friedrich, W., and Wheeler, K. (1982). The abusing parent revisited: A decade of psychological research. *The Journal of Nervous and Mental Disease, 170,* 577–587.

Freud, A., and Dann, S. (1951). An experiment in group upbringing. *Psychoanalytic Study of the Child, 6,* 127–168.

Gaines, R., Sandgrund, A., Green, A., and Power, E. (1978). Etiological factors in child maltreatment: A multivariate study of abusing, neglecting, and normal mothers. *Journal of Abnormal Psychology, 87,* 531–540.

Garbarino, J. (1977). The human ecology of child maltreatment: A conceptual model for research. *Journal of Marriage and the Family, 39,* 721–736.

Garbarino, J., and Stockman, S. (1980). *Protecting Children from Abuse and Neglect.* San Francisco: Jossey-Bass.

Gelles, R. (1982). Problems in defining and labelling child abuse. In R. Starr (Ed.), *Child Abuse Prediction: Policy Implications.* Cambridge: Ballinger Publishing Company.

Gelles, R., and Straus, M. (1979). Determinants of violence in the family: Toward a theoretical integration. In W. Burr, R. Hill, F. Nye, and I. Reiss (Eds.), *Contemporary Theories about the Family.* Free Press, New York.

Gray, J., Cutler, C., Dean, J., and Kempe, H. (1977). Prediction and prevention of child abuse and neglect. *Child Abuse and Neglect, 1,* 45–55.

Harper, F. (1963). The physician, the battered child, and the law. *Pediatrics, 31,* 899–902.

Helfer, R. (1976). Basic issues concerning prediction. In R. Helfer and C. H. Kempe (Eds.), *Child Abuse and Neglect: The Family and the Community.* Cambridge, MA: Ballinger Publishing Company.

Helfer, R. (1984). The epidemiology of child abuse and neglect. *Pediatric Annals, 13,* 747–751.

Helfer, R., and Kempe, C. H. (1976). *Child Abuse and Neglect: The Family and the Community.* Cambridge: Ballinger Publishing Company.

Herrenkohl, E., Herrenkohl, R., and Toedtler, L. (1983). Perspectives on the intergenerational transmission of abuse. In D. Finkelhor, R. Gelles, G. Hotaling, and M. Straus (Eds.), *The Darkside of Families: Current Family Violence Research.* Beverly Hills, CA: Sage.

Hertzberger, S. (1983). Social cognition and the transmission of abuse. In D. Finkelhor, R. Gelles, G. Hotaling, and M. Straus (Eds.), *The Darkside of Families: Current Family Violence Research.* Beverly Hills, CA: Sage.

Hertzberger, S., and Tennen, H. (1982). The social definition of child abuse. Paper presented at the Annual Meeting of the American Psychological Association, Washington, D.C.

Hobbs, N. (1974). *The Futures of Children: Categories, Labels, and their Consequences.* Nashville: Vanderbilt University Press.

Hunter, R., and Kilstrom, N. (1979). Breaking the cycle in abusive families. *American Journal of Psychiatry, 136,* 1320–1322.

Jencks, C., Smith, M., Acland, H., Bane, M., Cohen, D., Gentis, H., Heyns, B., and Michelson, S. (1972). *Inequality: A Reassessment of the Effect of Family and Schooling in America.* New York: Basic Books.

Journal News. *Rockland Review and Extra.* Rockland County, NY, June 26, 1986.

Kaufman, J., and Zigler, E. (1987). Do abused children become abusive parents? *American Journal of Orthopsychiatry, 57,* 186–192.

Kempe, C. (1973). A practical approach to the protection of the abused child and rehabilitation of the abusing parent. *Pediatrics, 51,* 804–812.

Light, R. (1973). Abused and neglected children in America: A study of alternative policies. *Harvard Educational Review, 43,* 556–598.

Meehl, P., and Rosen, A. (1973). Antecedent probability and the efficiency of psychometric signs, patterns, or cutting scores. In P. Meehl (Ed.), *Psychodiagnosis: Selected Papers.*

Main, M., and Goldwyn, R. (1984). Predicting rejection of her infant from mother's representation of her own experiences: A preliminary report. *International Journal of Child Abuse and Neglect, 8,* 203–207.

Milner, J. S. (1986). *The Child Abuse Potential Inventory: Manual* (2nd. Ed.). Webster, NC: Psytec.

Murphy, S., Orkow, B., and Nicola, R. (1985). Prenatal prediction of child abuse and neglect: A prospective study. *Child Abuse and Neglect, 9,* 225–235.

Parke, R., and Collmer, C. (1975). Child abuse: An interdisciplinary review. In E. M. Hetherington (Ed.), *Review of Child Development Research* (Vol. 5). Chicago: Chicago University Press.

Quinton, D., Rutter, M., and Liddle, C. (1984). Institutional rearing, parental difficulties and marital support. *Psychological Medicine, 14,* 107–124.

Ross, C. J., and Zigler, E. (1980). An agenda for action. In G. Gerbner, C. Ross, E. Zigler (Eds.), *Child Abuse: An agenda for action.* New York: Oxford University Press.

Rutter, M. (1984). Continuities and discontinuities in socioemotional development: Empirical and conceptual perspectives. In R. Emde and R. Harmon (Eds.), *Continuities and Discontinuities in Development.* New York: Plenum Press.

Rutter, M., and Quinton, D. (1984). Long-term follow-up of women institutionalized in childhood: Factors promoting good function in adult life. *British Journal of Developmental Psychology, 2,* 191–204.

Schneider, C. (1982). In R. Starr (Ed.), *Child Abuse Prediction: Policy Implications.* Cambridge: Ballinger Publishing Company.

Schneider, C., Helfer, R., and Pollock, C. (1972). The predictive questionnaire: A preliminary report. In C. H. Kempe and R. Helfer (Eds.), *Helping the Battered Child and His Family.* Philadelphia: Lippincott.

Schneider, C., Hoffmeister, J., and Helfer, R. (1982). A predictive screening questionnaire for potential problems in mother–child interaction. In R. Helfer and C. H. Kempe (Eds.), *Child Abuse and Neglect: The Family and the Community.* Cambridge, MA: Ballinger Publishing Company.

Smith, S., and Hanson, R. (1975). Interpersonal relationships and child-rearing practices in 214 parents of battered children. *British Journal of Psychiatry, 127,* 513–525.

Solnit, A. (1980). Too much reporting and too little services: Roots and prevention of child abuse. In G. Gerbner, C. Ross, and E. Zigler (Eds.), *Child Abuse: An Agenda for Action.* New York: Oxford University Press.

Spinetta, J. (1978). Parental personality factors in child abuse. *Journal of Consulting and Clinical Psychology, 46,* 1409–1414.

Spinetta, J., and Rigler, D. (1972). The child-abusing parent: A psychological review. *Psychological Bulletin, 77,* 296–304.

Sroufe, L. A., and Fleeson, J. (1986). Attachment and the construction of relationships. In W. Hartup and Z. Rubin (Eds.), *Relationships and Development,* New York: Cambridge University Press.

Starr, R. (1982). *Child Abuse Prediction: Policy Implications.* Cambridge, MA: Ballinger Publishing Company.

Steele, B., and Pollock, C. (1968). A psychiatric study of parents who abuse infants and small children. In R. Helfer and C. Kempe (Eds.), *The Battered Child Syndrome.* Chicago: University of Chicago Press.

Straus, M. (1979). Family patterns and child abuse in a nationally representative sample. *International Journal of Child Abuse and Neglect, 3,* 23–225.

Straus, M. (1983). Ordinary violence, child abuse, and wife beating: What do they have in common? In D. Finkelhor, R. Gelles, G. Hotaling, and M. Straus (Eds.), *The Darkside of Families: Current Family Violence Research.* Beverly Hills, CA: Sage.

Straus, M., Gelles, R., and Steinmetz, S. (1980). *Behind Closed Doors: Violence in the American Family.* Garden City, NJ: Anchor/Doubleday.

Tinbergen, N. (1951). *The Study of Instinct.* London: Oxford University Press.

Uviller, R. (1980). Save them from their saviors: The constitutional rights of the family. In G. Gerbner, C. Ross, and E. Zigler (Eds.), *Child Abuse: An Agenda for Action.* New York: Oxford University Press.

Wasserman, S. (1967). The abused parent of the abused child. *Children, 14,* 175–179.

Zigler, E. (1976). Controlling child abuse in America: An effort doomed to failure. In D. Adamovics (Ed.), *Proceedings of the First National Conference on Child Abuse and Neglect.* Washington, DC: Department of Health, Education, and Welfare.

Zigler, E. (1983). Child Abuse. Speech presented at the "Building Bridges" Conference sponsored by the Illinois Department of Children and Family Services, Chicago.

Part II

Parental and contextual influences on maltreatment

6   Lessons from child abuse: the determinants of parenting

Jay Belsky and Joan Vondra

The determinants of parenting: a process model

By tradition, students of socialization have directed their primary energies toward understanding processes whereby parents' child rearing strategies and behaviors shape and influence their offsprings' development. Whereas great effort has been expended studying the characteristics and consequences of parenting, much less attention has been devoted to studying why parents parent the way they do – beyond, of course, social-class and cross-cultural comparisons (e.g., Hess and Shipman, 1965; Lewis and Wilson, 1972; Whiting and Whiting, 1975), and investigations examining the effect of the child on parenting behavior (e.g., Bell, 1968; Lewis and Rosenblum, 1974). This is not to say, however, that no data have been collected on this topic beyond the general areas of inquiry just outlined. In point of fact, it is suprising to learn that, despite the *relative* neglect of the study of the determinants of parenting, a large quantity of empirical information is available that addresses this general issue.

It is unfortunately the case that much of the research relevant to this area of concern remains unintegrated and underutilized. One reason for this is that many of the research findings pertinent to the study of parental determinants are found in a diverse set of studies that have little to do with each other beyond some secondary result or focus that speaks to this issue. But probably the major reason studies pertinent to the determinants of parenting remain unrelated is, in part, the general absence of conceptual models capable of integrating the disparate findings in the literature into a coherent

Work on this chapter was supported by grants from the National Science Foundation (No. SES–8108886), the National Institute of Child Health and Human Development (No. R01HD15496–01A1), the Division of Maternal and Child Health of the Public Health Service (No. MC–R–424067–02–0), the March of Dimes Birth Defects Foundation (Social and Behavior Science Branch, No. 12–64), and the National Institute of Mental Health (R01MH39741–01).

whole. It is the basic premise of this chapter that research on and interest in child abuse – a concern of applied science – has much to contribute toward an empirical synthesis with regard to the determinants of individual differences in parenting – a concern of basic science.

In asking questions about the etiology of child abuse and neglect, clinicians and research scientists alike have been inquiring into the determinants of parental functioning – or, more precisely, parental dysfunction. In the course of this chapter we shall (1) consider those sources of influence that have been implicated by research on dysfunctional parenting (i.e., child abuse) as playing a causal role in the maltreatment process; (2) summarize data gathered on nonabusive samples consistent with general hypotheses raised by child abuse researchers regarding the determinants of parenting; and, (3) on the basis of these analyses, provide support for a multicausal model of the determinants of parental functioning emphasizing the role played by social forces both within and beyond individual parents and the families in which they function. This model is informed by a systems approach with an emphasis upon interrelated components and processes whereby certain stresses upon parenting are buffered by other supports. In sum, our goal is to show that concern for the etiology of child maltreatment has much to say to an important, but long neglected, issue in the study of socialization – namely, the causes of individual differences in parenting.

The etiology of child abuse

By tradition, three general perspectives have been employed to account for the etiology of child maltreatment; these can be referred to as the psychiatric or psychological model, the sociological model, and the effect-of-the-child-on-the-caregiver model (Belsky, 1978a; Parke and Collmer, 1975). By far the account of child maltreatment most widely subscribed to by the lay public falls within the psychiatric model, which focuses exclusive attention on the individual abusive parent. Essentially, the psychiatric model emphasizes the role that the parent plays, because it is the parent who is the direct perpetrator of mistreatment. Probably the most compelling evidence that implicates psychological factors in the etiology of child mistreatment, and thereby focuses attention on the psychiatric make-up of the individual abuser, derives from reports linking parents' own childrearing histories with subsequent parenting (e.g., Altemeier, O'Connor, Vietze, Sandler, and Sherrod, 1982; Sherrod, O'Connor, Altemeier, and Vietze, 1986; Spinetta and Rigler, 1972).

A radical sociological critique of the psychiatric model argues that the psychiatric perspective "blames the victim" (Belsky, 1978a). That is, it fails to recognize that social conditions create stresses that undermine family functioning and cultural values and practices that encourage societal violence and the corporal punishment of children, which are primarily responsible for child maltreatment (Gelles, 1973, 1975; Gil, 1971; Light, 1973). Some of the most compelling evidence in support of this model derives from studies linking unemployment, labor market shrinkage, and social isolation with child abuse and/or neglect (Garbarino, 1976, 1977; Gelles, 1975; Light, 1973; Steinberg, Catalano, and Dooley, 1981; for a review, see Siegal, 1982). According to this viewpoint, parents must be considered the victims of these social forces. The basic premise of the sociological model of child abuse is that in a society in which violence is rampant and frequently encouraged as a strategy for settling human relations disputes; in which children are regarded as property of their parents; and in which beliefs like "spare the rod and spoil the child" are promulgated, the fact that parent–child conflict eventuates in child abuse should not be surprising. In essence, the cultural soil is regarded as fertile when it comes to fostering the mistreatment of children.

Implicit in both psychiatric and sociological models of child abuse is the assumption that parent–child relations are unidirectional, with only parents exercising influence in this subsystem of family relations. The effect-of-child-on-caregiver model challenges this basic assumption and underscores the role the child's own behavior plays in determining the course of parent–child relations. Evidence to suggest that children might be responsible for the mistreatment they experience comes from reports that a single child within a family is typically the recipient of abuse (Kadushin and Martin, 1981); that mistreated children exhibit deviations in social interaction and general functioning prior to their reported abuse (Starr, Dietrich, Fischhoff, Ceresnie, and Zweier, 1984); and that prematurity and low birthweight characterize the perinatal histories of a disproportionate number of abused children (Fontana, 1971; Klein and Stern, 1971; Martin, Conway, Breezley, and Kempe, 1974).

Ecological integration. It has become apparent that a model narrow in scope, whether emphasizing the personality and developmental history of abusive parents, the social stresses that abusive families experience and the social context in which they function, or the role the children play in eliciting their own mistreatment, must inevitably fail in its attempt to account for the multifaceted processes at work in child abuse. In response to the widely recognized need to integrate these distinct approaches to the etiology of child maltreatment, Belsky (1980) offered an ecological synthesis of these clearly complementary approaches using a modified version of Bronfenbrenner's (1977) ecological framework. Belsky's review of past research highlighted the components of each prior model:

While abusing parents enter the microsystem of the family with developmental histories that may predispose them to treat children in an abusive or neglectful manner (ontogenic development), stress-promoting forces both within the immediate family (the microsystem) and beyond it (the exosystem) increase the likelihood that parent-child conflict will occur. The fact that a parent's response to such conflict and stress takes the form of child maltreatment is seen to be a consequence both of the parent's own experience as a child (ontogenic development) and of the values and child-rearing practices that characterize the society or subculture in which the individual, family, and community are embedded [the macrosystem]. (Belsky, 1980, p. 33)

The determinants of parenting

Available theory and research on the etiology of child abuse and neglect draw attention to three general sources of influence upon parental functioning: (1) the parents' ontogenic origins and personal psychological resources (psychiatric model/ontogenic development), (2) the child's characteristics of individuality (effect-of-child-on-caregiver model/microsystem) and (3) contextual sources of stress and support (sociological model/exo- and macrosystems). It still remains to be determined, however, whether processes identified as exerting an influence in extreme cases (i.e., child abuse) also function in the normal range of parental behavior. It is noteworthy that researchers and theorists often conceptualize child maltreatment as a "quality of care" issue, a qualitative extreme along a broader continuum of caregiving. From this perspective, sensitive parenting, inconsistent or unresponsive caregiving, and child maltreatment simply represent different points or segments along the same caregiving continuum. Such a position, however, has little bearing on the issue of common determinants. It is possible that the most prominent influences on high-quality parenting are quite distinct from those contributing to maltreatment. It is more likely, however, that the same factors operate across the entire continuum of parenting but vary according to whether they function as an asset or a handicap.

The critical question, then, which this chapter raises, concerns whether or not there exists a continuum of *influence;* that is, whether the determinants of parenting highlighted by child abuse research also play a role in influencing parenting that falls within the range of normal functioning. To facilitate this analysis, discussion is organized around the three general sources of influence delineated in the preceding paragraph. As already noted, the principal goal of this chapter is to draw upon this analysis, itself based upon the study of dysfunctional parenting, in order to substantiate a general model of the determinants of parental functioning.

The model to be explicated in the course of reviewing relevant data is presented in schematic form in Figure 6.1. As can be seen from the diagram, the model presumes that parenting is directly influenced by forces emanating from within the individual parent (personality), within the individual child (child characteristics of individuality), and from the broader social context in which the parent–child relationship is embedded – specifically,

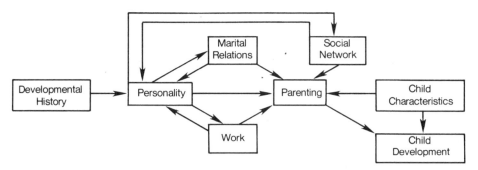

Figure 6.1. The determinants of parenting: a process model. (Reprinted with the permission of the Society for Research in Child Development.)

the marital relations, social networks, and occupational experiences of parents. Further, the model assumes that parents' developmental histories, marital relations, social networks, and jobs influence their individual personalities and general psychological well-being and, thereby, parental functioning and, in turn, child development. By reviewing research pertinent to each of these lines of argument, support for three general conclusions regarding the determinants of parenting will be provided: First, that parenting is multiply determined; second, that, with respect to their influence on parenting, the characteristics of the parent, of the child, and of the social context are *not* equally influential in supporting or undermining growth-promoting parenting; and finally, that developmental history and personality shape parenting indirectly by first influencing the broader context in which parent–child relations exist (i.e., marital relations, social networks, occupational experience).

In its emphasis on the multiple determinants of parenting, our model resembles the framework Cicchetti and Rizley (1981) have proposed to understand the etiology of maltreatment. According to their framework, parenting outcomes are determined by the relative balance of potentiating (risk) factors and compensating factors experienced by a given family. Child maltreatment occurs only when risk factors – whether transient or chronic – outweigh any compensatory influences that are operating. Common to both models, then, is a recognition of the multiple pathways by which individual (parental personality attributes or child characteristics), historical (parental developmental history), and social (marital satisfaction an social network support), as well as circumstantial factors (poverty, job dissatisfaction, ignorance about child development) combine to shape parental functioning. Neither is a "main effects" model; abusive or neglectful parenting is the consequence of an interaction between parental stresses and supports. In arguing for each element cited in our model, however, we will rely heavily

on research that considers only main effects, for it is rare to find studies that
examine interactive influences. Only after we have reviewed data supporting each individual domain of influence will we proceed to consider research
that examines combinations of factors, the most persuasive evidence for our
respective models.

The parents' contribution

Research on child maltreatment indicates that parenting, like most dimensions of human functioning, may be influenced by enduring characteristics
of the individual – characteristics that are, at least in part, a product of one's
developmental history. To obtain a better sense of just how developmental
history and personality influence parenting, it is useful to consider briefly
the kind of parenting that appears to promote optimal child functioning and
to speculate on the type of personality most likely to provide such developmental care.

In the infancy period, detailed observational studies reveal that cognitive–motivational competence and healthy socioemotional development
are promoted by attentive, warm, stimulating, responsive, and nonrestrictive caregiving (e.g., Clarke-Stewart, 1973; Stayton, Hogan, and Ainsworth,
1971; Yarrow, Rubenstein, and Pedersen, 1975). During the preschool years
the work of Baumrind (1967, 1971) demonstrates that it is high levels of
nurturance and control that foster the ability to engage peers and adults in
a friendly and cooperative manner, as well as the capacity to be instru-
mentally resourceful and achievement-striving. As children grow older,
parental use of induction or reasoning, consistent discipline, and expression
of warmth have been found to relate positively to self-esteem, internalized
controls, prosocial orientation, and intellectual achievement during
the school-age years (e.g., Coopersmith, 1967; Hoffman, 1970; McCall,
1974).

Consideration of these findings and others suggests that, across childhood,
parenting that is *sensitively* attuned to children's capabilities and to the
developmental tasks they face promotes a variety of highly valued developmental outcomes, including emotional security, behavioral independence, social competence, and intellectual achievement (Belsky, Lerner, and
Spanier, 1984). In infancy this sensitivity translates into being able to read
babies' often-subtle cues and repsond appropriately to their needs in reasonably brief periods of time (Ainsworth, Blehar, Waters, and Wall, 1978;
Lamb and Easterbrooks, 1980). In childhood, sensitivity means continuing
the warmth and affection provided in the early years, but increasing the
demands for age-appropriate behavior. Parents must be willing and able to
direct children's behavior and activities without squelching their developing
independence and industry. Ultimately, the sensitive and thus competent
parent must be willing to wean the child from this overt control to permit

the testing of personal limits through the exercise of internalized rules and regulations. Indeed, by the time the child reaches adolescence, the competent parent has set the stage so that the child has the psychological building blocks to encounter successfully the transition from childhood to adolescence.

What kind of person should be able to provide such developmentally flexible and growth-promoting care? The sensitive individual, one might argue, is able to decenter and appraise the perspective of others accurately, is able to empathize with them and, in addition, is able to adopt a nurturant orientation. Without the capacity to escape the egocentrism of one's own psychological state and the ability to nurture others, it is difficult to imagine how a parent could recognize, much less respond to, immediate and long-term developmental needs of children on a daily basis. Indeed, only by possessing the skills outlined above is it likely that an individual faced with the very real demands and challenges that parenting presents would not abdicate responsibility (as in neglectful and permissive rearing) or rely on absolute power (as in child abuse or authoritarian rearing). Moreover, to function in this way, the individual will likely need to experience a sense of control over his/her own life and destiny, as well as feel that his/her own psychological needs are being met. Because the essence of parenting, especially in the childhood years, involves "giving," it seems reasonable that parents most able to do this in a sensitive, competence-inducing manner, will be mature, psychologically healthy adults. Having advanced this hypothesis, we now turn attention to evidence bearing upon the relationship between personality and psychological resources of parents and the quality of care they provide.

Personality. The literature linking personality and parenting is not nearly as rich nor as extensive as one might expect. Nevertheless, the limited data that are available can be marshalled to provide some support for the notion that psychological maturity and competent parenting covary with each other. We purposefully employ the statistical term "covary" here to underscore the fact that those studies that will be cited do not demonstrate a cause–effect relationship between personality and parenting, since virtually all studies of this topic are correlational and fail to consider competing explanations (like: parenting shapes personality).

In general, psychological maturity is presumed to be an accomplishment of young adulthood that requires, as a prerequisite, the establishment of a stable identity, or sense of self. In Erikson's (1950) epigenetic framework, in fact, the stage of generativity follows both the establishment of identity and intimacy. On the basis of such theorizing, it is plausible that age may serve as a marker for maturity and be positively related to parental competence. There are two sets of data that speak to the issue and, indeed, provide some support for this hypothesis. The first set of investigations treat age as a continuous variable and evaluate the interrelation of mother's age and her parenting. The second set of studies treat age as a categorical variable and involve comparisons of the caregiving attitudes and behavior of teenage and older women.

With respect to the first set of investigations, a group of researchers in Seattle found that primiparous mothers interact with four-month-old infants in a more positively affectionate, stimulating, and sensitive manner the older they are (Ragozin, Basham, Crnic, Greenberg, and Robinson, 1982). Consistent with these results are data from a Boston study indicating that older mothers show greater adaptation to the mothering role and display more reciprocity when interacting with their 2-month-olds (Grossman Eichler, and Winickoff, 1980). Feldman and Nash (1982), in their work at Stanford, have also observed that older women are more skilled at maintaining longer interactive sequences with their 6-month-olds, and Wandersman and Unger (1983) have reported that even within a sample of teenage mothers, age positively covaries with the amount of stimulating and responsive care mothers provide to their babies.

Comparisons of teenage and older mothers are generally consistent with the findings just summarized. Not only is there evidence that such young mothers express less desirable childrearing attitudes and have less realistic expectations for infant development than do older mothers (Epstein, 1979; Field, Widmayer, Stringer, and Ignatoff, 1980; Seth and Khanna, 1978) but, from a more behavioral standpoint, it has been observed that they also tend to be less responsive to their newborns (Jones, Green, and Krauss, 1980) and to engage infants in less verbal interaction (Osofsky and Osofsky, 1970). Indeed, Levine, Coll, and Oh (1984) have reported that, when observed in face-to-face interaction and in teaching tasks with their eight-month-olds, adolescent mothers display less positive affection, talk less, and demonstrate activities less often than do older mothers. The fact that comparable age-related differences were discerned in ego development scores derived from a sentence completion task suggests that the parental functioning of younger and older women is directly related to their psychological maturity.

Ego development was also the focus of inquiry in an investigation of the verbal interaction between psychiatrically hospitalized and normal adolescents and *their* parents. Hauser, Powers, Noam, and Jacobson (1984) found an interesting pattern of contemporaneous relationships suggestive of a sequence whereby parental ego development influences the quality of parental verbal interaction with the adolescents which, in turn, facilitates or impedes adolescent ego development. Ego development in both parents and adolescents was consistently related to the amount of "enabling" versus "constraining" remarks contributed to family discussions, determining the extent to which discussion was conducive to idea exchange and elaboration, important on a conceptual basis for fostering further ego development.

Thus, a direct link between ego development and verbal parenting behavior was discerned, in this case between parents and their adolescents.

More detailed evidence in support of the proposition that psychological maturity and parenting are linked can be found in studies that measure disposition and state characteristics of the parent and relate these personal psychological resources directly to indices of parental functioning. Work of this kind tends also to fall in one of two camps – research focusing upon multivariate indices of psychological functioning presumed to reflect broad constructs like psychological maturity and well-being and research focusing upon particular psychological constructs like self-esteem, irritability, locus of control and the like.

Brunquell, Crichton, and Egeland (1981) implemented a multivariate approach in studying some 267 economically disadvantaged families from the Minneapolis/St. Paul area. Those mothers who proved to be abusive or neglectful during their children's first few years displayed, prenatally and at three-months postpartum, a configuration of personality attributes indicating that they were less psychologically complex and less personally integrated than mothers who did not mistreat their offspring. More specifically, these mothers received less optimal scores on summary scales comprised of several specific personality and attitudinal assessments, including anxiety, locus of control, aggression, succorance, suspicion, and defendence. Indeed, these inadequate caregivers lacked understanding of the complexity of a parent–child relationship, reacted negatively to pregnancy, were more aggressive and suspicious, and described themselves negatively.

In another investigation that also included some abusive families, Conger and his colleagues (Conger, McCarty, Yang, Lahey, and Kropp, 1984) assessed psychological well-being with the nonphysical health items of the Cornell Medical Index, which tapped depression, anxiety, and irritability. When these items were composited to create a measure of emotional well-being, it was observed that those mothers of preschool and school-age children showing the most emotional distress displayed less positive and more negative affect when engaged in structured interactive activities with their offspring.

Data linking parenting with global constructs of psychological maturity and psychological complexity are not confined to mothers alone. In Heath's (1976) longitudinal study of 60 professional men, scores on standardized personality assessments like the MMPI and Rorschach consistently predicted paternal competence. Such competence was defined as emotional and affectional involvement and time spent playing with offspring, and was discerned in men who displayed more personality integration, less depression and anxiety, and who were more independent and stable.

In his extensive program of research on the developmental effects of the Great Depression, Elder (1974) provides a good deal of data with relevance to the model we are presenting, particularly in regard to the contribution of personality to parental functioning. Elder, Caspi, and Downey (1986) have recently examined patterns of marriage, parenting, and child functioning across four generations in an effort to illuminate continuities in development within and between lifespans. Using data from the original participants of the Berkeley Growth Study, Elder and his colleagues were able to link personality to parenting and then to child development in a cycle that spanned several generations. They discovered that growing up in a home in which parents' personalities could be described as unstable and in which parental care could be depicted as controlling, hostile, and lacking in affection led to the development of unstable personalities in these children as adults. This personal instability on the part of Berkeley parents, derived as it seemed to be from poor developmental experiences in their families of origin, was itself predictive of tension in their own marriages. Marital tension, in the fact of another generation of personal instability, contributed to extreme and arbitrary discipline for the third generation of Berkeley children. And finally, exposure to such care resulted in the development of behavior problems in this third generation of children that were predictive of undercontrolled behavior in adulthood. Thus, parenting difficulties, apparently originating from personality problems, seemed to leave a legacy of personal adjustment problems that were passed down through parenting from one generation to the next, testimony indeed for the hypothesized role that personality plays as a determinant of parenting and, thus, an indirect influence on child development.

Confirmation of this pathway of influence is also evident in Engfer and Schneewind's (1982) cross-sectional study of the causes and consequences of harsh parental punishment. Relying upon self-report data provided by parents and children (8–14 years of age) from some 570 representative German families, these investigators sought to test, using path analytic techniques, Gelles's theoretical model of the etiology of child abuse. Results revealed, consistent with our own thinking, that, in the case of both mothers and fathers, unfavorable socialization experiences in parents' own childhoods were reliably related to parental personality problems of irritability and nervous tension as well as family conflict (i.e., marital conflict). These personality problems, through their effect on parental anger proneness and helplessness, along with family conflict and a difficult, problem child, each contributed to the prediction of harsh parental punishment (especially in the case of mothers). Such childrearing was itself related to a "conduct disordered" personality on the part of the child, to perceived rejection and, thereby, to feelings of anxiety and helplessness by the child.

In this German study, as well as in the Berkeley work, we find evidence to support our model of the determinants of parenting. More specifically, there is evidence in their theoretically guided, multivariate inquiries that positive developmental experiences foster healthy personality development and, thereby, positive family functioning, particularly marital and parent–child relations. Through this process, child development is promoted.

Narrower, more specific psychological constructs tend to show the same patterns of association with assessments of parental functioning. For example, Elder, Liker, and Cross (1984) found, in another analysis of the families that lived through the depression, that the father's irritability was an important predictor of the arbitrariness of his behavior, which was itself linked to problematical social behavior on the part of offspring. On a more positive note, both Cowan and Cowan (1983a) and Gamble and Belsky (1984) have reported that self-esteem is positively related to parental functioning. In the former study, fathers with higher self-esteem were observed to be more involved with their infants, and in the latter it was observed that working mothers of preschoolers provided more stimulating, responsive, and positively affectionate care when they felt good about themselves and had active (as opposed to avoidant) coping styles. Consistent with these data are those presented by Farber and Egeland (1980) indicating that mothers who are more tense and irritable and have lower self-esteem display less interest in their newborns, are less effective in soothing their babies, and are less able to maintain synchronous exchanges.

In addition to maintaining a reasonably positive sense of self and an ability to decenter so as to assume the perspective of others, the mature, healthy personality is also expected to appraise situations accurately in terms of his or her ability to exert control over the environment. Except under unusual circumstances (in circumstances beyond individual control), such an individual should operate from an internal locus of control, recognizing the influence that his/her own actions have upon the world. Given that psychological maturity and parental competence are linked within the model being formulated, one would expect locus of control to be associated with growth-promoting parenting as well. Support for this prediction can be found in studies of the infancy and the preschool period. Schaeffer, Bauman, Siegel, Hosking, and Sanders (1980) reported, for example, that an internal (as opposed to external) locus of control (assessed prenatally) forecasted high levels of observed maternal stimulation and interaction when infants were 4 and 12 months of age in their sample of 321 medically indigent women. Consistent with these results are findings of Mondell and Tyler (1981) who discerned positive associations between a composite personal resource measure consisting of three subscales (locus of control, interpersonal trust, and coping style) and supportive parenting behavior displayed during a structured laboratory teaching task.

How is it that psychological maturity in general or particular personality attributes like self-esteem, locus of control, and psychological complexity lead to nurturant, sensitive parenting? One possible mechanism might involve attributions parents make about their children; and one set of attributions that would seem especially important involves the intentionality ascribed to child behavior. Consider, for instance, the differential behavioral consequences of assuming that a child disobeys because she or he does not comprehend a rule or request versus because she or he is simply "out to get" the parent. Another potentially influential attribution involves assumptions made about a child's disposition. Is the child perceived as a generally sweet, loving individual, or as a "bad sort"? The likelihood that such differential attributions can be tied directly to individual differences in parental personality seems great.

But is there any evidence that attributional processes like those detailed above affect parenting? Probably as a result of the behavioral emphasis in most research and the disfavor into which attitudinal studies of parenting have fallen, there is little evidence that speaks to this issue of cognitive processes mediating parental responses to child functioning (Parke, 1978). Nevertheless, clinical analyses of the personalities of child abusing parents do provide additional support for the role of attributional processes in shaping parenting (Rosenberg and Reppucci, 1982). A common observation is that parents who mistreat their children interpret developmentally appropriate behavior as willful disobedience or intentional behavior when child activities clash with parental needs and desires (Helfer, McKinney, and Kempe, 1976; Pollock and Steele, 1972). Additionally, mistreating parents appear to appraise their offsprings' dispositions globally through such negative terms as stubborn, unloving, or spoiled (Steele, 1970). In view of the fact that scientists who study child development disagree frequently on exactly what compels children to act the way they do, it should not be surprising that, in the face of uncertainty, interpretations and, consequently, attributions, may be as much a function of the parent's personality as of the child's behavior.

Psychological disturbances. Up through this point our review has focused upon investigations linking personality with parenting that relied upon populations of nonpsychologically disturbed individuals. Evidence that is potentially more compelling in its demonstration of the influence of personal psychological attributes on parental functioning can be found in investigations of psychologically disturbed adults. Baldwin, Cole, and Baldwin (1982) have recently reported an extensive investigation examining the relationship between parental psychopathology and parenting. Although this cross-sectional study of 145 families with 4-, 7-, or 10-year-olds does not permit comparison of family functioning to households with nondisturbed parents, it does provide information on relating child functioning, as well as family functioning, to parental personality. Observations revealed that families with a parent suffering from a psychotic and/or affective disorder were less active, had a lower proportion of patient-initiated interactions, and exhibited less warmth when engaged in a laboratory free play situation than families of nonpsychotics. Moreover, only these impaired dimensions of parenting were subsequently related to the child's school functioning. For example, children with an active and warm relationship with their fathers were rated by peers as more bright and less dull, and by teachers as being more cognitively and motivationally competent. When neither parent–child relationship could be classified as active and warm, children were less compliant and more intrusive. On the basis of these data, Baldwin et al. (1982) conclude that the patient's illness influences the likelihood of active and warm interactions that are well balanced in terms of adult and child initiations, which in turn affects the competence the child displays in school.

Studies focusing specifically upon schizophrenia also reveal the influence of psychological disturbances upon parental functioning. Although the limited data available on the topic suggest that mothers with a history of schizophrenia do not differ from controls in the amount of time they spend with their infants or the adequacy of the biological care they provide, investigations of the affective aspects of maternal behavior do highlight differences between normal and disturbed mothers (Walker and Emory, 1983). Ragins, Schachter, Elmer, Preisman, Bowes, and Harway (1975), for example, rated quality of caregiving during the first year of life and found that schizophrenic mothers provided less environmental stability and nurturance when compared to normal control mothers. Consistent with these results are those of Sameroff and his colleagues (Sameroff, Barocas, and Seifer, 1984) who found that schizophrenic and neurotic-depressed mothers were significantly less spontaneous and proximal with their 4-month-old infants than were nondisturbed mothers – important to note here is that severity and chronicity of mother's illness, across diagnostic groups, were negatively related to the quality of maternal care.

The disturbance in parental psychological functioning that has received the most attention from investigators interested in the personality–parenting link is depression (Fabian and Donahue, 1956; Pollitt, 1965). One of the most extensive and informative studies of the parenting and developmental consequences of depression is provided by Weissman and her colleagues (Orraschel, Weissman, and Kidd, 1980; Weissman and Paykel, 1974). Relying upon self-reports from semistructured interviews with 40 depressed and 40 nondisturbed, mostly middle- and low-income mothers, these investigators concluded that depressed parents provide a disruptive, hostile, rejecting home environment which, not surprisingly, undermines child functioning. This conclusion was based upon the fact that depressed mothers reported being only moderately involved in their children's lives, having difficulty communicating with them, and experiencing considerable friction in parent–child relations. It is of interest from a developmental perspective that parental pathology, although evident across all stages of the family life cycle, was most pronounced in the postpartum, infancy, and early adolescent periods. Depressed mothers of infants, for example, were either overconcerned, helpless, and guilty, or directly hostile. But even during the school-age years, mothers' low self esteem and hopelessness impaired their ability to be positive models or to be responsive to requests for help at meals, when dressing, or with homework. From their own reports, disorganization and chaos were the frequent results as mothers withdrew from all aspects of home management. The children appeared to respond to such noninvolvement with hyperactivity and excessive sibling rivalry (possibly for whatever limited attention mother provided); some even began to display acute symptoms of agitated depression themselves.

However, Patterson's (1980) recent observation that mothers of aggressive, out-of-control sons are "victims," bearing the brunt of coercive behavior and developing feelings of depression and low self-esteem, raises the possibility that depression may be a consequence as much as it it a cause of behavioral problems in children. In all likelihood, a reciprocal process of influence is at work, so it may be empirically futile to attempt to disentangle cause from consequence once such a vicious cycle has been established.

Findings consistent with Weissman's data have been reported recently by Colletta (1983), who interviewed 75 urban adolescent parents. Teenage mothers who were depressed were more often dissatisfied with their maternal role and displayed little understanding of the developmental needs of their children. Possibly as a consequence, these depressed parents appeared hostile, indifferent, and rejecting of their children on a self-report measure tapping parental acceptance–rejection. These results highlighting the poor maternal care depressed women provide are also consistent with recent data showing that depressed mothers of disabled infants are less emotionally and verbally responsive to their offspring (Affleck, Allen, McGrade, and McQueeney, 1982).

The research summarized provides evidence for the general notion that an individual's personality can function to support or undermine his or her parenting ability. If our principal concern is the determinants of parenting, we need to ask, in the face of such an observation, about the developmental origins of personality as they pertain to childrearing. There can be little doubt that an individual's mental health is in large measure determined by the immediate stresses to which one is exposed and the supports available to him or her. The role of just such contextual forces will be considered as determinants of parental functioning in a subsequent section. For now, our attentions focus on the developmental histories of parents under the assumption that earlier experiences, particularly in the family, shape the personality that subsequently contributes to parenting.

Developmental history. Three distinct sets of data illuminate the relationship between developmental history and parenting. Literature on child abuse furnishes the first set by underscoring an association between the experience of mistreatment in one's own childhood and mistreatment of one's children. Because this relationship has been mentioned earlier and discussed elsewhere (Belsky, 1978a, 1980; Parke and Collmer, 1975), little else will be said regarding it. The second set of data linking developmental history and parenting derives from the study of depression (e.g., Heinecke, 1970; Langner and Michael, 1963), and the third from studies of individual differences in father involvement.

Empirical work already reviewed indicates that depression contributes to difficulties in parenting. Of particular interest here is evidence that early developmental history and susceptibility to depression are correlated, making plausible the postulated process of influence from developmental history to personality, and finally to parental functioning and, thereby, child development. As part of an investigation concerned specifically with the social origins of depression, Brown and Harris (1978) conducted clinical interviews, psychological testing, and case-record reviews on some 114 randomly sampled clinic patients and 95 neighborhood controls. Separation from mother prior to the age of 11 emerged as one important feature distinguishing female patients (47 percent) from controls (17 percent), though only those individuals who had lost a mother *and* experienced a severely stressful life event or major difficulty actually became depressed.

The potential implications of such early experiences for parenting are suggested specifically by several studies revealing a direct association between early separation from parent(s) and subsequent parental dysfunction. For example, Frommer and O'Shea (1973a) found, in the course of clinical work at a day center for disturbed preschool children, that an unduly high proportion of the mothers whose children were disturbed, or who themselves reported difficulties in mothering, also reported a history of separation from one or both of their parents in childhood. In a second investigation replicating this general finding from the first study, Frommer and O'Shea (1973b) observed further that mothers reporting parenting difficulties, and who had experienced parental separation in their own childhoods, were likely to be suffering from depression.

Having observed that early separation may be related to depression as well as to mothering, the results of still another English study are especially intriguing, particularly with respect to the model being developed. Hall, Pawlby, and Wolkind (1979) found, in their observational research on 68 primiparous working-class women, that not only was experience in a family of origin disrupted by parental death, separation, or divorce associated with lower levels of mother–infant interaction but, possibly as a consequence of receiving less social stimulation, that children of such mothers displayed less linguistic competence when tested at 27 months. When these several studies concerned with the origins of depression and the consequences of separation are jointly considered, there certainly appears to be a basis for concluding that, at least under certain stressful conditions, developmental history influences psychological well-being, which in turn affects parental functioning and, as a result, child development. Evidence in support of such a causal sequence is furnished by Crook, Raskin, and Eliot (1981), who compared the parenting reported retrospectively by 714 hospitalized depressed patients with that of 387 matched normals. Using self-reports and ratings of interview data from other family members, Crook et al. discovered that the parents of depressed patients were more likely to be described as rejecting of their children and to have controlled them through psychologically harmful techniques (e.g., derogation, manipulation through guilt or anxiety, etc.). Because depression undermines parenting and one's own experiences during childhood forecast depression, there is justification on the basis of data such as these for our argument that the parenting experienced during childhood shapes personality, which, in turn, shapes an individual's future parental functioning.

The final set of data to be considered regarding the relationship between developmental history and parenting pertain to the functioning of men as parents. Several investigators have found that a father's involvement in parenting is positively related to the involvement exhibited by his own father (Reuter and Biller, 1973). In one study of the antecedents of paternal involvement in Israel, for example, Sagi (1982) reported that highly involved fathers of preschoolers recalled having fathers who were highly involved with them. Similarly, Manion (1977) observed that fathers who were particularly active in their infants' child care described their own fathers as very nurturant. At first glance, these findings suggest that fathers model the behavior of their own fathers. But other data, indicating that unsatisfactory childhood experiences (Gersick, 1979; Mendes, 1976) and insufficient paternal involvement during childhood (De Frain, 1979; Eiduson and Alexander, 1978) are correlated with *high* levels of parental interest and involvement on the part of fathers, raise questions about the accuracy of this simple observational learning interpretation.

One would expect fathers who are warm, nurturant, and involved to be modelled because their sons are more likely to identify strongly with them. In contrast, it seems likely that a noninvolved father would generate a weak identification in the son, reducing the likelihood that he will be modelled, but perhaps initiating a compensatory process that later prompts the son to parent in a manner expressly opposite that of his own father. In any case, understanding of the process by which one's childhood experience of fathering is linked to one's own fathering seems to require consideration of personality development, especially in regard to processes of identification and role modelling. In other words, we find implicit support, once again, for a pathway of influence from developmental history to personality, to parenting.

Conclusion: specification of process. The evidence considered broadly indicates that developmental history influences parenting. If this is indeed the case, it is very possibly because experience shapes personality. Analysis of such a hypothesis demands simultaneous consideration of developmental history, personality, and parenting if understanding of the individual parent's contribution to parenting is to be achieved. Progress at this point requires not only demonstrations of relationships between early experience and parental functioning, but conceptions of why such relations should obtain.

The problems that arise from failing to address this important issue of process are quite evident in the child abuse literature. Does mistreatment during childhood eventuate in dysfunctional parenting because parenting behavior is modelled involuntarily or because personality development is disrupted? Because treatment programs are based upon etiological theories, the failure to address questions such as this are of practical as well as scientific concern (Belsky, 1978b). Acceptance of the modelling hypothesis would lead one to believe that behavior modification should prove effective in remediating child abuse. In contrast, a more psychodynamic explanation, emphasizing personality development, would suggest that the behavioristic approach would merely address the symptom, not the underlying problem, and thus do little to remediate mistreatment over the long term.

The issue of process must also be considered in efforts to link parental personality to child development. When connections between personality and child development are made without measuring parenting, one is left to presume a genetic process of influence. Although such sources of influence should not be discounted, the contention advanced here is that parenting, as shaped by personality and developmental history, serves to transmit much of the parental influence on children. Indeed, a conclusion that can be drawn at this point is that, in general, supportive developmental experiences give rise to a mature healthy personality that is then capable of providing sensitive parental care which, in turn, promotes optimal child development. Rohner's empirically based argument on the origins of dysfunctional parenting provides support for this causal sequence. As a result of his cross-cultural research on the universal effects of parental acceptance–rejection, he was led to conclude that

rejected children everywhere tend more than accepted children to be: hostile, aggressive, passive aggressive, or to have problems in the management of hostility and aggression; to be dependent or "defensively independent," depending on the degree

of rejecton; to have an impaired sense of self-esteem and self-adequacy; to be emotionally unstable; emotionally unresponsive and to have a negative world view. We
expect each of these personality dispositions to result from rejection for the following
reasons. First, all of us tend to view ourselves as we imagine "significant others" view
us, and if our parents as the most significant of "others" rejected us as children, we
are likely to define ourselves as unworthy of love, and therefore as unworthy and
inadequate human beings. In this way we develop a sense of overall negative self-
evaluation, including feelings of negative self-esteem and negative self-adequacy.
(Rohner and Rohner, 1980, p. 192)

Adults who were rejected as children tend to have strong need for affection, but they are unable to return it because they have become more or less
emotionally insulated from, unresponsive to, or highly suspicious of potentially close interpersonal relations (Kempe and Kempe, 1978). Any of these
adults who become parents are therefore much more likely to reject their
own children than parents who were accepted as children (Rohner and Rohner, 1980, p. 194).

The child's contribution

It is now widely recognized that what transpires in the parent–child relationship is determined not only by the parent, but by the child as well. We
speak, therefore, in terms of bidirectional influences and of the effect of the
child on the caregiver (Bell, 1968; Lewis and Rosenblum, 1974). During the
past 15 to 20 years, an abundance of evidence has been amassed documenting the manner in which child characteristics influence caregiver
behavior. For illustrative purposes, we consider here two sets of data, that
bearing on the effects of prematurity and that of child temperament.

There is much about the infant born at or before 37 weeks gestational age
or less than 5½ pounds that leads to differences in the way such children are
treated and, indeed, may explain why they are disproportionally at-risk for
child maltreatment (Belsky, 1980; Parke and Collmer, 1975). In the opening
weeks of life premature infants are less alert, harder to quiet if distressed,
and weaker than full-term infants and, probably as a consequence, their
mothers tend to be less stimulating, spending less time in close face-to-face
encounters, and smiling, touching, and talking to them less often than mothers of full-term infants (Goldberg, 1978). Beyond the newborn period, at
least through the first six months of life, premature babies tend to be more
lethargic and less responsive than full-terms and, probably as a result, their
mothers tend to be more active in interacting with them (Beckwith and
Cohen, 1978; Brown and Bakeman, 1977; DiVitto and Goldberg, 1979;
Field, 1977). Such heightened activity is likely to stress the premature baby,
as it seems that they have a narrower band of arousal in which to function
(Field, 1982). The fact that it is very easy to overstimulate them by doing
too much, and very easy to understimulate them by doing too little, makes

it more difficult for parents of such babies to engage them in synchronous interaction.

In many respects, we might think of the premature infant as having a more difficult temperament or behavioral disposition. And although the evidence concerning the effects of difficult temperament in the population of nonrisk children is mixed (Bates, 1980), select evidence does exist certainly in support of the notion that difficult temperament can undermine parental functioning. Campbell (1979) reported, for example, that when mothers rated their infants as having difficult temperaments at 3 months, they interacted with them less and were less responsive to their cries at 3 and 8 months, in comparison to a set of matched controls. Similarly, Milliones (1978) discerned a significant negative association between mothers' perceptions of difficultness and outreach workers' rating of maternal responsiveness when infants averaged 11 months of age. Kelly (1976) reported that mothers of more difficult 4-month-olds tended to respond negatively to negative infant emotions. Interestingly, a follow-up analysis of these same mother–infant dyads at 12 months indicated that mothers of these difficult infants more often avoided social interaction with them than did other mothers (Sameroff, 1977).

The effect of a difficult temperament upon parenting appears to extend beyond the first year of life. In a short-term longitudinal study, Maccoby, Snow, and Jacklin (1984) discovered that mothers who regarded their sons as difficult at 1 year of age engaged in less effort in teaching them when the boys were 18 months. Studying a group of 24-month-olds, Bates (1980) found that there was more conflict between mothers and toddlers rated as difficult, with mothers displaying more power assertion, including frequent use of controlling actions, frequent repetition of prohibitions and warnings, and more frequent removal of objects from their children. Consistent with these data are the results of a recent cross-sectional study indicating that mothers' reports of their 3- and 4-year-olds' temperaments accounted for almost 50 percent of the variance in independent evaluations of the growth-promoting nature of the home environment, with mothers of more difficult preschoolers providing less stimulating, affectionate, and responsive care (Gamble & Belsky, 1984). In considering data such as these, and when thinking about the effect of the child on the caregiver, it is important to keep in mind that the older the child, the more likely it is that the very care parents have provided in the past influences what comes to be labeled as child temperament. Evidence of child effects, then, may be construed as evidence of parental effects, with caregiver influencing child who, in turn, influences caregiver.

It must also be recognized that the influence children have on the actual care they receive from their parents may be indirect and mediated by the effect of the child on the parents' psychological resources. There are several sets of data that provide support for this contention. In one recent study, for example, Sirignano and Lachman (1984) found that parents, especially fathers, of infants described as difficult experience a decline in their sense of personal efficacy across the transition to parenthood, whereas parents whose infants were characterized as easy actually experience a positive change in feelings of control. Consistent with these findings are data from a study of much older children indicating that mothers of 3- to 7-year-olds whose children are difficult suffer from emotional distress (Conger et al., 1984).

Personality assessments of parents of retarded and emotionally disturbed children provide insight into what some of the psychological consequences of a lowered sense of control and a heightened sense of emotional distress might be and thus go a long way toward accounting for the less growth-promoting care which difficult children appear to elicit. In work by Erickson (1968, 1969) and by Miller and Keirn (1978), MMPI profiles of parents of atypical children revealed problems in impulse control, accompanied by aggressive feelings. Work by Cummings and his colleagues indicated that mothers of retarded children display greater depressive and dysphoric affect (Cummings, Bayley, and Rie, 1966), whereas fathers display depression and low self-esteem, and undergo personality changes resembling a pattern of neuroticlike constriction (Cummings, 1976). These data suggest, then, that children do not simply affect the way in which mothers and fathers care for them but also their parents' psychological state and well-being.

Contextual sources of stress and support

Although both parent and child contributions to differences in parenting have been addressed here, an ecological perspective on this topic requires consideration of the *context* of parent–child relations as well. For this purpose one may turn to the abundant evidence that highlights the generally beneficial impact of social support on both psychological and physical health. Some data indicate, for instance, that supports of all kinds, formal or informal, enable individuals to cope with stress and thereby both lessen the risk of ill health and facilitate a more optimal recovery from illness (Caplan, 1974; Cassell, 1974; Cobb, 1976; Mitchell and Trickett, 1980; Powell, 1979). In terms of psychological functioning, Pearlin and Johnson (1977) report that women who reside in neighborhoods for an extended period, have really close friends, and belong to voluntary associations are less likely than those without such social bonds to suffer from depression.

Of particular significance to the topic of this discussion is research chronicling a relationship between support and general well-being in the case of parents. Nuckolls, Cassell, and Kaplan (1972) report, for example, that the availability of social support buffers women experiencing stress occasioned by many life changes from complications of pregnancy, labor, and delivery.

Working with adolescent mothers, Colletta finds total social support to be the single strongest predictor of self-reported emotional stress (Colletta and Gregg, 1981), as well as a significant correlate of depression, in that mothers receiving high levels of emotional support, material aid, and overall assistance tend to report the lowest depressive symptomatology (Colletta, 1983; Lee and Colletta, 1983).

Not only does overall support positively influence psychological well-being in general and the mental health of parents in particular but, possibly as a consequence, it is also related to parenting itself. Feiring and her colleagues (Feiring, Fox, Jaskir, and Lewis, 1985) found significant relationships between the number of people low-income mothers reported as providing them with goods and services and three measures of maternal behavior during a 15-minute laboratory observation with their infant. Mothers citing a greater number of friends or relatives who provided such assistance spent more time in close proximity to and playing with their 3-month-olds and less time at a distance from them during the observation session. Open-ended interviews by Colletta (1979) with three groups of mothers with preschoolers (low- and middle-income single parents, middle-income married mothers) revealed that total support (provided by friends, relatives, and spouse) was negatively associated with maternal restrictiveness and punitiveness. In fact, she was led to conclude, on the basis of her data, that "mothers receiving the least amount of total support tended to have more household rules and to use more authoritarian punishment techniques" (p. 843). Similar results were reported in Lee and Colletta's (1983) study of teenage mothers, in which it was found that mothers who were highly satisfied with their total support were more affectionate with their 1- to 3-year-olds, showing their love by comforting, cuddling, playing with, and praising their offspring, whereas mothers who were unsatisfied with their support tended to be hostile, rejecting, and indifferent toward their children. Consistent with these findings are results of a study indicating that the social support available to mothers of 3-year-olds who had required intensive care as neonates predicted the extent to which they were stimulating in their parenting (Pascoe, Loda, Jeffries, and Earp, 1981).

What is especially intriguing about these data is that it is just these kinds of parenting that research has linked to child competence (e.g., attentiveness, responsiveness) and incompetence (e.g., authoritarian rearing). On the basis of these findings, then, there seems good reason to suppose that social support not only plays an influential, but still largely unexplored role in the development and maintenance of competent parenting (Cochran and Brassard,1979; Unger and Powell, 1980) but, in consequence, also indirectly affects child functioning.

The fact that parenting appears to be positively associated with social support should not be surprising. As noted already, support and general well-being have been linked repeatedly. And if one conceptualizes growth-promoting parenting as a dimension of mental health, then the link between parenting and support may be but one way in which the more general support–well-being relationship manifests itself. But even after highlighting such general associations, we need to consider the sources of stress and support in parents' lives. It is to this issue that we now turn.

Sources of support/stress

The work on child abuse highlights three distinct sources of stress and support that are likely to promote or undermine parental competence: the marital relationship, social networks, and employment. We consider each of these in turn.

The marital relationship. Belsky (1981) has argued that consideration of the father's role in child development necessitates consideration of the marital relationship, since the addition of the father to the more commonly studied mother–child dyad does more than create an additional parent–child relationship; it creates a family system comprised of husband–wife as well as mother–child and father–child relationships. And although the evidence to date is not sufficient to document his claim that the marital relationship serves as the principal support system for parents, the effect of spousal relations on parenting has been suggested by studies of quite different developmental periods (Belsky, Lerner, and Spanier, 1984).

Much of the evidence for marital effects comes from non-process-oriented investigations linking marital functioning and child development directly. During the infancy and toddler periods, for example, Honzik (1967) reported that marital adjustment predicted daughters', but not sons', mental test performance from 21 months through the school-age years; and Bronson (1966), working with the same data set from the Berkeley Growth Study, found that poor marital adjustment, marital hostility, and indifference were all predictive of reactive/explosive, as opposed to placid/controlled, styles of emotional expression during the elementary school-age years. More recently, Goldberg (1982) and Soloman (1982) discerned positive associations between marital quality and the quality of infant–parent attachment; parents of infants who displayed avoidance and resistance toward their parents reported less marital adjustment and emotional sharing between spouses.

At older ages, the principal finding has been that conflicted, disharmonious marriages and antisocial, aggressive, or otherwise problematical child behavior covary with each other (e.g., Gibson, 1969; Johnson and Lobitz, 1974; Kimmel and Van der Veen, 1974; Nye, 1957; O'Leary and Emery, 1983; for review see Emery, 1982). Although a modelling process might account for such direct associations between marital relations and child functioning, one can reason, consistent with the line of argument we are developing, that all-too-*in*frequently studied parenting practices are likely to mediate such seemingly direct effects. The evidence reviewed below provides support for this contention.

It has been suggested that during the infancy years the influence of fathers on child functioning may be primarily indirect, that is, mediated by the wife in her capacity as mother (Lewis and Weinraub, 1976; Parke, 1978; Pedersen, Yarrow, Anderson, and Cain, 1978). Several studies have begun to illuminate these types of indirect effects (Moss, 1974; Switzky, Vietze, and Switzky, 1979). In an investigation of family relations during the infant's first month of life, Pedersen (1975,1982; Pedersen, Anderson, and Cain, 1977) found that tension and conflict between husband and wife (as reported by fathers) was strongly and negatively correlated with independent observational evaluations of maternal feeding competence. These data are consistent with those of Belsky and Volling (in press), indicating that high levels of marital conflict and low levels of father involvement also tend to occur early in infancy. Returning to the Pedersen study, it is also worth noting that, in contrast to the negative effect of tension and conflict, the husband's esteem for his wife as a mother (i.e., direct emotional support) was positively related to feeding skill. Price (1977) reported data remarkably consistent with Pedersen's observations linking marital support and maternal feeding ability. On the basis of her investigation of changes in mother–infant reciprocity across the first month of the baby's life, she was led to conclude, in fact, "that the mother's ability to enjoy her infant, and regard it with affection may be in part a function of the quality of her relationshp with her husband" (p. 7).

Further evidence of these conclusions is available from still other studies of parent–infant relations (Cowan and Cowan, 1983b; Dickie, Schuurmans, and Schang, 1980; Donovan, Leavitt, and Balling, 1975; Feiring and Taylor, n.d.; Wandersman and Unger, 1983). Belsky (1979) observed that in families marked by frequent marital communication about the baby, fathers were highly involved with their 15-month-olds, both when alone with them and while in their wives' presence. More recently, he and his colleagues found that at 1, 3, and 9 months of age, high levels of fathering and marital interaction covary positively with each other (Belsky, Gilstrap, and Rovine, 1984; Belsky and Volling, in press). Consistent with these results are findings reported by a group of Stanford University researchers indicating that marital quality was one of the most powerful predictors of fathering observed in free and structured laboratory play situations (Feldman, Nash, and Aschenbrenner, 1983). Also consistent are the findings of Gibaud-Wallston and Wandersman (1978) indicating that fathers who feel support from their wives have a high sense of parental competence regardless of the temperamental difficulty of their infants. The recently reported results of Goldberg and Easterbrooks (1984) also underscore the positive influence of marital relations on parenting. In this cross-sectional study of families with 20-month-olds, it was found that mothers with higher marital adjustment expressed warmer attitudes toward their offspring, encouraged independence in their toddlers, and experienced less aggravation in caring for their children. Fathers, too, who were satisfied with their marriages were less aggravated by parenting and were more emotionally supportive of their children when observed in a laboratory playroom.

Investigations linking marital relations and parenting during the preschool years are generally consistent with those just summarized that focus upon the parent–infant relationship. In fact, two classic studies foreshadow Hetherington, Cox, and Cox's (1977) divorce research demonstrating that it is primarily when ex-spouses continue to bicker after separation that parenting and, ultimately, child functioning are undermined. In one, Bandura and Walters (1959) observed that mothers inclined to nag and scold their sons felt less warmth and affection toward their husbands. Since comparable findings were absent in the case of daughters, the possibility must be entertained that mothers were projecting their hostile feelings toward their husbands on the other males with whom they had a presumably close relationship. Complementing these findings are data from a study by Sears, Maccoby, and Levin (1957) indicating that mothers' professed esteem for their husbands is systematically related to the praise they direct at their preschool children. More recently, Gamble and Belsky (1984) found that working mothers who were satisfied with their marriages provided more responsive, stimulating, and positively affectionate care to their laterborn 3- and 4-year-olds. Since it is just the kind of parenting observed in these investigations that predicts less than optimal or competent child functioning, there are once again grounds for inferring a marriage-to-parenting-to-child development process of influence (Belsky, 1981; Crouter, Belsky, and Spanier, 1984).

During the school-age and adolescent years, high interspousal hostility has been linked to the frequent use of punishment and the infrequent use of induction or reasoning as a disciplinary strategy (Dielman, Barton, and Cattell, 1977). Johnson and Lobitz (1974) report, for example, consistent negative relationships between marital satisfaction and the level of observed negativeness to children in their study of 31 boys, aged 2 to 12 years, who had been referred for behavioral counseling. Further, Kemper and Reichler (1976a) found that undergraduates who reported a satisfying spousal relationship between their parents also reported receiving more rewards and less intense and frequent punishment. The reason for this, Olweus's (1980) recent work on the development of aggression indicates, is that the quality of the emotional relationship between spouses influences mothers' negativism toward their adolescent sons, which itself leads to aggressive, antisocial behavior.

On a more positive note, and with respect to fathering, Heath (1976) observed that paternal competence is predicted by marital happiness and the ability to communicate with one's spouse. The benefits of such marital harmony are evident in a current study of 6- to 11-year-old boys raised in reconstituted families comprising a stepfather and biological mother. These boys were found to be more socially competent than agemates reared in families comprising both biological parents (Santrock, Warshak, Lindbergh, and Meadows, 1982). This surprising result, further inquiry revealed, coincided with the more competent parenting displayed by the stepfathers. Most important to us here, though, was the observation that these more competent stepfathers, with more socially skilled stepsons, reported less marital conflict than did the biological fathers whose parenting and sons' functioning appeared less competent.

In sum, the data reviewed in this section strongly suggest that to understand parenting and its influence upon child development, attention must be accorded the marital relationship (Belsky,1981). Indeed, the possibility must also be entertained that marital relations do not so much influence parenting directly as they do indirectly – by influencing the general psychological well-being of individuals, and only thereby the skills they exercise in the parenting role. Gamble and Belsky (1984) provide support for an indirect pathway by demonstrating that when a composite index of mother's psychological well-being is controlled statistically, the reliable relationship between marital satisfaction and supportive parenting is significantly attenuated. More indirect support for a marriage-to-personality-to-parenting process comes from several studies documenting relationships between marital quality and parents' psychological well-being. In two such studies, Brown and Harris (1978) and Zur-Spiro and Longfellow (1981) each discerned an association between the presence of a supportive husband or boyfriend and lower frequency of depression, which we have observed already to be related to parenting. Carveth and Gottlieb (1979) reported that only contact with husband (not with friends and relatives) predicted perceived stress among 99 primiparous and multiparous middle-class mothers of young infants. Johnson and Lobitz (1974) found that scale ratings of depression, schizophrenia, and social introversion were significantly and negatively related to marital adjustment in their sample of 31 families referred for behavioral counseling as a result of child behavior problems. Finally, in an investigation of the adaptive effect of participation in parenting groups during the transition to parenthood, Wandersman, Wandersman, and Kahn (1980) found that maternal sense of fullness in life, sense of energy, and sense of relaxation were all positively related to marital cohesion. (See also Wandersman and Unger, 1983, for similar findings with a sample of adolescent mothers.) Considered together, these investigations provide support for the hypothesis that marital relations enhance or undermine general psychological well-being, which contributes to parental competence.

Social network. If the marital relationship is the principal support system of parents, as Belsky (1981) suggests, it is likely that the interpersonal relations between parents and their friends, relatives, and neighbors – the significant others in their lives – function as the next most important system of support. In many households, particularly those in which a spouse is not present or the marital relationship is in conflict, the social network may well function as the primary system of support.

It is clear that the availability of significant others and the support received from them exert a beneficial impact on parent–child relations (Aug and Bright, 1970; Feiring and Taylor, n.d.; Hetherington, Cox, and Cox, 1977; Kessen, Fein, Clarke-Stewart, and Starr, 1975; McLanahan, Wedemeyer, and Adelberg, 1981; Toms-Olson, 1981). During the infancy period, Powell (1980) discovered that the qualities of mothering predictive of child competence during the preschool years, namely verbal and emotional responsivity, are more characteristic of mothers who have weekly or more frequent contact with friends. Similarly, Crnic, Greenberg, Ragozin, and Robinson (1983) in their study of the parents of preterm and term infants, found that, although assistance from friends does not relate to observed behavior per se, more positive maternal attitudes toward parenting are evident among mothers who have more friends and who receive greater support from those that they do have. Fathers, too, seem to be influenced by contact with their social networks; Feldman et al. (1983) reported, for example, that a man's positive relationshp with his own mother is predictive of high levels of playfulness in interacting with his infant, and that a positive relationship with both parents is related to high levels of paternal involvement in the provision of basic care.

The last set of evidence to be considered that links social network contact and support with parenting during infancy comes from an experimental study designed to reduce the stress associated with bearing a high-risk infant. Minde and his colleagues observed that parents of premature infants who participated in a self-help group seemed to cope more effectively with their premature infants (Minde, Shosenberg, Marton, Thompson, Ripley, and Burns, 1980). More specifically, during the time the babies were still in the hospital, experimental mothers visited their infants and touched, talked to, and looked at them significantly more often than did a control group of mothers; they also expressed more confidence in their caregiving. At three months after discharge, those mothers who had the opportunity to share their feelings and experiences with other parents in the same stressful situation continued to display more involvement (during feedings) and were more concerned about their infants' development than mothers who were randomly excluded from this supportive intervention. Moreover, at one year the experimental mothers provided their infants more freedom and stimulation and judged their babies' competencies more accurately relative to their biological abilities and – possibly as a consequence – had infants who displayed more social and exploratory behavior in playing, food sharing, and self-feeding.

Turning to the preschool years, Abernethy (1973) found the presence of a tightly-knit social network to be positively associated with parents' sense of competence in the caregiving role, defined in terms of the mother's recognition of the malleability of her children, an appreciation of individual differences, and knowledge of how childrearing practices need to be adjusted to match the child's developmental capabilities. The results of Pascoe et al.'s (1981) investigation of mothers of 3-year-olds and of Colletta's (1981) study of teenage mothers indicate that supportive contact with friends, neighbors, and relatives may enhance more than just the parental self-concept. In the former, social network contact and supportiveness correlated positively with the physical and temporal organization of the child's world and with mothers' avoidance of punishment and restriction; in the latter, adolescent parents having a close family that could be counted on for help were more likely to display affectionate behavior toward their own young children and were less likely to be hostile, indifferent, rejecting, and/or dissatisfied with the maternal role. Consistent with these findings are results reported by Weinraub and Wolf (1983) showing that in single-parent households satisfaction with parenting support was related to higher levels of observed mother–child communication and nurturance, whereas in two-parent homes satisfaction with emotional support, parenting support, and help with child care predicted high levels of communication and nurturance. Finally, Jennings, Stagg, and Connors (1985) found that mothers' satisfaction with the emotional support received from network members predicted both the amount of praise (more) and level of control (less) used during structured teaching tasks at home with their 4- and 5-year-olds. Potential developmental consequences for the child of such supportive social networks are revealed in Hess, Shipman, Brophy, and Bear's (1968) analyses of mother–child interaction in structured teaching situations. Mothers who were well integrated in social networks were not only more likely to engage their preschoolers in goal-oriented tasks (like model building and block sorting) than were their network-isolated counterparts, but the children of the presumably better-supported mothers performed more competently in these structured task situations and in preschool as well.

Although social isolation, identified as a risk condition in the child abuse literature (Garbarino, 1977), may be associated with less supportive parenting, it would be inappropriate to conclude, on the basis of the above findings, that more social network contact is always advantageous. Contact that would normally function supportively may become stressful if taken to an extreme (French, Rodgers, and Cobb, 1974). Indirect evidence of such a diminishing-returns effect can be found in Minturn and Lambert's (1964) cross-cultural study of parenting in six cultures. These investigators observed maternal warmth to be inversely related to the number of adult kin with young children that lived in close proximity to the mother. Strikingly similar results were also reported in two of the studies cited above. In the first case, high levels of social network contact by single parent mothers was associated with low levels of maternal nurturance (Weinraub and Wolf, 1983), and in the second, closer proximity to and more frequent contact with network members was related to less praise and more control by mothers in a structured teaching task (Jennings et al., 1985). When considered in conjunction with the results cited above, these data suggest the existence of some optimal, but as yet unspecified, degree of contact and support which, when surpassed or unrealized, serves to undermine rather than enhance parenting. Indeed, what is probably most beneficial is what French, Rodgers, and Cobb (1974) refer to as a goodness of fit, representing the match between support desired and support received.

In the case of social network support, just as in the case of the marital relationship, one must speculate on the possible mediating role played by the parents' own psychological well-being. That is, social networks may serve to enhance the personal psychological functioning of the parent and, by these means, promote effective parenting behavior and practices. In this regard, Cochran and Brassard (1979) hypothesized that the support social networks provide can enhance self-esteem and, as a consequence, increase the patience and sensitivity individuals exercise in the parenting role. Some data presented by Colletta, Lee, and Gregg (n.d.) and by Lee and Colletta (1983) tend to substantiate this hypothesis by showing that, in the case of teenage mothers, the support provided by indivdiuals (but not by formal community services) decreases the stress and enhances the self-esteem and coping style of these high-risk mothers. Similarly, Aug and Bright (1970) found positive attitudes toward self to be characteristic of out-of-wedlock mothers who enjoyed the support of family members and relatives. Belle's (1981) investigation of other low-income mothers also confirms this pattern. She discovered that the more instrumental assistance women had available in the form of routine childcare assistance, the less depressive symptomology they reported, and the more sense of control and mastery they experienced in their lives. Presumably, these are the kinds of personal psychological resources that increase the patience an individual can exercise in the parenting role, thereby enhancing sensitivity to the child's individual needs as well as overall parental competence.

Work. The third and final contextual source of stress/support on parenting considered here is suggested by research that links unemployment and labor market shrinkage with child maltreatment (Light, 1973; Steinberg, Catalano, and Dooley, 1981). It is not only investigations of child abuse, however, that highlight the deleterious consequences of unemployment with respect to parent–child relations (Bronfenbrenner and Crouter, 1983a). Over four decades ago, Komarovsky's (1940) detailed interview study of intact families with fathers on relief revealed that, especially in households with adolescent children, paternal authority declined with unemployment. Elder's (1974) investigation of children during the Great Depression documented similar consequences but, in doing so, was able to illustrate how the experience of adversity could actually benefit adolescent offspring – especially sons – when families realigned themselves adaptively to cope with their circumstances. More recent analyses of children growing up in the Great Depression, however, continue to underscore the negative impact of unemployment and underemployment, as indexed by income loss, on men's parenting. In several recent papers, Elder and his colleagues have found that income loss increased the arbitrariness and punitiveness of the father's behavior while decreasing the supportiveness of his parenting (Elder, Liker, and Cross, 1984; Elder, Nguyen, and Caspi, 1985). In view of the work discussed earlier, it is not surprising to learn that such effects of the absence of work on men also took a toll on children's development.

Beyond the study of unemployment, the greatest source of information pertinent to the impact of work on parenting is found in the literature on maternal employment.[1] Even though a sizeable proportion of studies fail to document any such effects (e.g., Cohen, 1978; Hock, 1980; Schubert, Bradley-Johnson, and Nuttal, 1980), several others do suggest that the mother's employment status influences both the quantity and quality of her own and her spouse's parenting behavior. Quite a few investigations indicate, for example, that maternal employment creates strain in the father–son relationshp in lower income families (Douvan, 1963; Gold and Andres, 1978; Kappel and Lambert, 1972; McCord, McCord, and Thurber, 1963; Propper, 1972). This may be due to the fact that in such households the mother's entry into the work force is regarded as an indication of the inadequacy of father as provider (Bronfenbrenner and Crouter, 1983a; Hoffman, 1979). A number of studies also demonstrate that parental expectations of children are greater when both parents are employed outside the home, particularly with respect to those aspects of home and self-maintenance for which children are held responsible (Douvan, 1963; Johnson, 1969; Propper, 1972; Walker, 1970). Other studies record positive developmental outcomes as a consequence of such demands (Elder, 1974; Johnson, 1969; Woods, 1972).

There is also some evidence that paternal involvement is altered by mother's work. Gold and Andres (1980) found, for example, in their study of 10-year-olds, that fathers report greater involvement when their wives are employed. These findings are consistent with results from diary and survey studies conducted in this country (Pleck, 1981; Robinson, 1977) and from an investigation conducted in Australia (Russell, 1981). Important to note, though, are the results of an investigation by Bloom-Feshbach (1981), which indicate that, at least in the case of 7- to 14-month-old infants, women's employment increases men's instrumental, but not their affective–expressive, involvement with their offspring.

In contrast to these investigations documenting a "positive" impact of wives' work on fathering, Pedersen, Cain, Zaslow, and Anderson (1983) found that working mothers tend to "crowd out" fathers, leaving them less opportunity to interact with their infant offspring during the evening. But these data are themselves somewhat inconsistent with the results of a survey by Hill and Stafford (1978) revealing that maternal employment has no effect on the time middle-class mothers spend with their preschoolers, but is related to lower levels of involvement among lower-class families. Further discrepancies are evident in Stuckey, McGhee, and Bell's (1982) lab-based observational investigation of mother–father–preschooler triads; these researchers found maternal employment to be related to increased parental attention to daughters but decreased attention to sons. Obviously, a variety of factors may account for such inconsistency in the literature, including the age of child studied, research methodology, and the failure to distinguish child gender or family social class.

Above and beyond such points of confusion, a major limitation of all the studies cited here attempting to document the effect of maternal employment on parenting is their undifferentiated classification of employment (Bronfenbrenner and Crouter, 1983b; Crouter, Belsky, and Spanier, 1984). Research on maternal attitudes toward work establishes clearly the need to consider maternal employment as more than simply a "social address" if an understanding of *how* it affects parenting and thereby child development is to be achieved. Not only is there evidence that mothers who are dissatisfied with their employment status have offspring whose development is less optimal than those whose mothers are more satisfied with their work situation (Farel, 1980; Hock, 1978, 1980; Hoffman, 1961; Yarrow, Scott, DeLeeuw, and Heinig, 1962), but several studies suggest that parenting itself is compromised under such stressful conditions. In their previously mentioned investigation of 40 preschool family triads, Stuckey and her colleagues (1982) found that "parental negative affect was exhibited more frequently by parents with attitudes toward dual roles for women that did not match the employment status of the mother in their family" (p. 643). Similarly, Hoffman (1963) found that the working mothers who liked their work displayed more affection and used less severe discipline with their children, whereas Yarrow et al. (1962) reported that mothers dissatisfied with their employment status expressed more problems in childrearing.

It is of interest to learn that although maternal employment has been treated, for the most part, as an undifferentiated phenomenon, this is much less the case in research on paternal employment and its effects on family functioning. The earliest work of this kind was reported by Miller and Swanson (1958), who found that the wives of men from bureaucratic organizations (characterized by secure work conditions, regular hours, stabilized wages) described their parenting as more permissive, and as placing greater emphasis on the development of interpersonal skills and the importance of getting along with others, than that of women whose husbands' jobs were entrepreneurial in nature (characterized by greater initiative, competitiveness, risk taking, and insecurity regarding the future). These latter mothers valued individual achievement and achievement striving, were not as indulgent, and placed less importance on interpersonal relationships in rearing their children. In conjunction with Candell and Weinstein's (1969) replication study, using a Japanese sample of mothers of infants, these data provide clear support for Aberle and Naegele's (1952) hypothesis that value-orientations in the husband's work situation are operationalized in childrearing attitudes and behavior (Bronfenbrenner and Crouter, 1983a).

Additional support for this claim is to be found in Kohn's (1963) research demonstrating "that working-class men, whose jobs typically require compliance to authority, tend to hold values that stress obedience and conformity in their children" and to favor physical punishment (Bronfenbrenner and Crouter, 1983b, p. 23). Middle-class fathers, whose jobs require self-direction and independence, instead value the latter attributes in their children (see also Mortimer and Kumka, 1982). Pursuing this line of inquiry, Mortimer's (1974, 1976) work suggests that it is fathers' parenting that prompts some sons to select the same occupation as their fathers. Specifically, warmth in the father–son relationship mediates the extent to which sons are biased toward their father's work when choosing their own occupations.

In addition to self-direction, work absorption, work stress, and satisfaction, other dimensions of employment have been linked to parenting. In his longitudinal study of men in professional jobs, Heath (1976) found the characteristics Kanter (1978) referred to as "work absorption" related to paternal inadequacy. Specifically, the more time and energy fathers devoted to their occupations, the more irritable and impatient they were with their children, as indicated by both husbands' and wives' reports (see also Clarke and Gecas, 1971; Moen, 1982; Pleck, Staines, and Long, 1978). Cowan and Cowan (1983b) and McHale and Huston (1984) have also reported, in their longitudinal studies of families rearing firstborn infants, that time on the job is related to low levels of father involvement.

Whereas work absorption seems to undermine parental behavior, job satisfaction seems to exert the opposite effect. Kemper and Reichler (1976b)
and McKinley (1964) demonstrated that a father's job satisfaction is
inversely related to the severity of punishment he dispenses and his reliance
upon reasoning as a disciplinary strategy. Belsky and Volling (in press),
studying fathers of infants, found that high levels of job satisfaction were
related to high levels of father involvement when infants were 1 and 3
months old.

As was postulated in prior discussion of marital relations and social networks, it is quite conceivable that many of these work–parenting associations are actually mediated by effects that employment and work conditions
have upon personality and general psychological well-being. Komarovsky
(1940) showed over 40 years ago that unemployment caused men to become
moody, irritable, and depressed (see also Liker and Elder, 1983). More
recently, Miller, Schooler, Kohn, and Miller's (1979) interviews with more
than 500 women revealed that specific conditions of work, including closeness of supervision, routinization of job, and the substantive complexity of
tasks performed "are related to effective intellectual functioning and an
open, flexible orientation to others, while those that constrain opportunities
for self direction or subject the worker to pressures or uncertainties are
related to ineffective functioning, unfavorable self conceptions, and a rigid
social orientation" (p. 91). These latter personal styles could hardly be considered encouraging portents of sensitive, growth-promoting parenting
practices.

Further evidence that work has an impact on general psychological functioning is derived from Kohn's program of research. Kohn and Schooler's
(1973, 1978) initial examinaiton of the complexity of skills required at work,
the autonomy that is granted on the job, and the absence of routinization,
revealed that such job characteristics facilitate intellectual flexibility which,
in turn, feeds back to affect work. Since then, these scholars have extended
their model of employment effects to other components of personality in a
study of more than 3,000 men representative of most male civilian occupations in the United States (Kohn and Schooler, 1982). Highly sophisticated causal modelling analyses demonstrated that occupational self-direction leads to the internalization of this kind of orientation. Men who are
self-directed in their work were less likely to become authoritarian and fatal-
istic and more likely to become self-confident and to develop personally
responsible standards of morality. Job conditions that instead generate feelings of distress are lack of job protection, dirty work, close supervision, and
a low position in the supervisory hierarchy. In sum, the data provide support for Kohn's learning-generalization hypothesis, which stipulates that lessons learned on the job generalize to the world beyond, including the parental role.

The potential implications for parental functioning of such effects of work on personality are even more apparent in Piotrkowski's (1979) small, but intensive, study of 13 working- and middle-class families. Case analysis indicated that "work experience is brought into the family via the worker-parent's emotional state, which in turn determines in part the person's avail-ability to family members, particularly children" (Bronfenbrenner and Crouter, 1983a, p. 28). Specifically, when workers are stressed and upset at work due to role conflict and overload, boredom, and underutilization of skills, they come home fatigued, irritable, and worried; they attempt to cre-ate "personal space" between themselves and other family members, thus blocking out their wives and their children. When children do not maintain this distance, fathers become angry and irritable. However, when fathers feel satisfied and challenged on their jobs, "positive carryover" occurs, with the worker actively initiating family contact and with parent–child and spousal interactions characterized by interest, concern, closeness, and warmth. Note how consistent this perspective is with Heath's (1976) study linking energy invested in the job and irritability and impatience with children.

Conclusion: relative importance of contextual sources of stress/ support

Throughout the preceding discussion of the roles that marriage, social net-works, and work assume in supporting or undermining growth-promoting parental functioning, only the consequences of variation within any single sphere of influence have been considered. What remains to be addressed is the *relative* contribution made by each of these three contextual dimensions. We remain of the opinion that the marital relationship is the first-order sup-port system, with inherent potential for exerting the most positive or nega-tive effect on parental functioning. This seems reasonable if only because emotional investment is routinely greater in the marriage, as is time spent in this relationship.

Several studies have been reported recently that address this issue of the *relative* importance of marital support versus certain other kinds of support. In Colletta's (1981) investigation of 50 adolescent mothers, the emotional assistance received from family of origin (i.e., social network) was found to be the most predictive of maternal attitudes and affectionate behavior, and that support received from boyfriend or spouse was next in order of impor-tance, followed finally by friendship support. In another investigation, com-prised of 105 mothers and their full-term and pre-term 4-month-olds, "inti-mate support [from the spouse] proved to have the most general positive effects, although community and friendship support appear[ed] valuable to maternal attitudes as well" (Crnic, Greenberg, Ragozin, Robinson, and Bas-ham, 1983, p. 14). The fact that the availability of, and mothers' satisfaction with, spouse support turned out to be the most significant predictors of the mother's positive attitude toward parenting and of the affect she displayed in face-to-face interaction, led Crnic et al. to express strong agreement with "Belsky's (1981) notion that a positive marital relationship is a major support of competent parenting" (p. 14). Moreover, their discovery that empirical relations between all types of maternal social support and infant functioning became insignificant once the mother's observed behavior was statistically controlled provided the basis for the conclusion that support exerts a primarily indirect effect on the child. Consistent with our own thinking, the hypothesis was also advanced by Crnic et al. that with age, the possibility of direct influences probably increases.

The results of the Crnic et al. investigation are generally consistent with two other recent studies in showing that, at least in comparison to social network support, quality of marital relations is the stronger predictor of parenting. In one such investigation, Wandersman and Unger (1983) focused on the care that primiparous teenage mothers provide their high-risk infants; in another, Gamble and Belsky (1984) focused on the care that working mothers provide their preschoolers.

Under certain conditions marriage probably plays a less influential role than that chronicled in the investigations cited above. Under circumstances such as single parenthood and teenage parenthood, social networks may well serve as the principal source of support, as Colletta's (1981) data indicate. The same may be true for traditional blue-collar marriages, in which husband and wife roles typically serve more instrumental than intimate functions, and in which neither friendship nor romance (and thus emotional support) are the principal reasons for the relationship. Young and Willmott's (1957) description of social network ties in East London, particularly those of mothers to their families of origin, clearly suggests that this is the case.

If we add occupation to our causal model of parenting, we must remain unclear about its relative influence at this time. In the Gamble and Belsky (1984) investigation, however, marital quality was a stronger predictor of mothering than employment strain. The greater the status a work role has in one's hierarchy of identities, the more influence it probably exerts. The job absorption that Kanter (1978) discussed and Heath (1976) chronicled as undermining the father's patience, for example, will function principally when work is conceptualized as a career, and when achievement is an important source of motivation. Obviously, both mothers and fathers are susceptible to this influence.

Unfortunately, both our assumption of the primacy of marital relations as a source of support/stress and our inclination to emphasize social networks as second in importance must remain speculative propositions. The only completed study to date looking at all three determinants is Gamble and Belsky's (1984), and a single investigation is never sufficient evidence for determining the validity of a model or its components. Until more work is carried out, then, on the multiple determinants of parenting, strong conclusions cannot be advanced. A clear imperative for future research is highlighted by this lacuna.

Parenting: a buffered system

This analysis of the determinants of parental functioning, informed as it is by concern for the etiology of child mistreatment, suggests that parental functioning is influenced by a variety of forces, with its three major determinants being the personality/psychological well-being of the parent, the characteristics of the child, and contextual sources of stress and support. Because parental competence is multiply determined, it stands to reason that the parenting system is buffered against threats to its integrity that derive from weaknesses in any single source. Evidence to this effect can be found in several recent studies by Elder and his colleagues that involve analyses of data gathered on children who grew up during the Great Depression. In one such analysis it was found that unemployment or underemployment, through the income loss it occasioned, undermined the father's parenting principally when marital relations were poor *prior* to the economic insult the family experienced (Elder, Liker, and Cross, 1984). In another analysis, income loss, precipitated by loss of work, was found to increase fathers' punitive behavior toward daughters, principally when these girls were unattractive (Elder, Nguyen, and Caspi, 1985). What we see in these instances, then, is that both positive child characteristics (attractiveness) and healthy marital relations can buffer the parenting system from threats to its integrity that come from the world of work.

The interaction effects just illustrated, of stresses that occur in the context of certain supports – or occur in the context of further hardship – are precisely the sort of dynamic relations captured both in our model of the determinants of parenting and in Cicchetti and Rizley's (1981) model of risk factors, mentioned at the outset of this chapter. In each case, maltreatment is conceived as the outcome of accumulated risk factors accompanied by a deficiency in support or compensatory factors. In their framework, Cicchetti and Rizley make an additional distinction among factors in terms of the duration of their effect. "Vulnerability factors" represent the sort of chronic risk characteristics or conditions we could describe as deficits within our developmental history (childhood experiences of cold, rejecting parenting), child characteristics (a congenital handicap), or personality categories (low self-esteem, psychological disturbance), for example. More transient "challengers" are short-term circumstantial stresses that could, for instance, belong in the category of marriage (a marital argument, death of or divorce from one's spouse) or work (a rough day on the job), as well as characteristics of the child (another virus, a cranky morning, a poor report card). Similarly, supportive factors may be enduring or short-lived. When we note a caring, affectionate spouse (marriage), and active and cohesive neighborhood (social network), or bright, adaptable child (child characteristics), we are identifying long-range "protective factors." Even potentially short-term "buffers" such as a raise in pay or some money in the bank account (work) or the child care assistance of a relative or friend (social network) figure in the maltreatment equation. Clearly, then, these two models share a common perspective, although each adopts its own focus: One looks at the locus of effect (our model of the determinants of parenting), the other is concerned with the quality and duration of effect (the Cicchetti and Rizley model). And this perspective is an emphasis on interactions, the total pattern of stresses and supports that enhance or undermine competent parenting.

At this point let us explore in more detail the nature of these hypothesized interactions. We just described data reported by Elder and his colleagues that demonstrate a potential buffering effect of child characteristics and marital relations when the work situation represents a stress on parenting. This buffering property can be expressed in the form of several general propositions: The undermining effect of a difficult child on parental functioning will be lessened when the parent has an abundance of personal psychological resources. Conversely, an easy-to-rear child can compensate for limited personal resources on the part of the parent in maintaining parental effectiveness. In analogous fashion, an abundance of personal resources can compensate for the absence of social network support, whereas an abundance of such support can reduce the threat to successful parenting that derives from limited parental psychological resources. Finally, the easy-to-rear child may preclude the need for extensive social support, whereas an abundance of support may ameliorate the stress usually encountered when rearing a problematic child.

The preceding hypotheses all describe relationships between pairs of the major determinants of parenting when one contributor is at risk (i.e., does not function to promote parental effectiveness). When two of three determinants of parenting are at risk, it is proposed that parental functioning is most protected when the personal resource subsystem still functions to promote sensitive involvement and least protected when only the subsystem of child characteristics fulfills this function. What this implies, of course, is that if something goes wrong in the parenting system, optimal functioning (defined in terms of producing competent offspring) will occur when the personal resources of the parents are the only determinants that remain intact.

Evidence in support of the claim that risk characteristics in the child are relatively easy to overcome can be found in the literature on high-risk and difficult infants. Premature birth does not compromise subsequent development when rearing takes place in middle-class homes, where both personal resources and support systems are likely to function effectively (Sameroff and Chandler, 1975). Moreover, although studies of the effects of difficult infant temperament on maternal behavior show mixed results, the strongest support for the hypothesis that maternal perceptions of difficultness are concurrently associated with negative aspects of the mother–child relationship comes from samples that seem a priori at risk for relationship problems (Bates, 1980). Thus, unless the subsystems of support or personal resources are at risk, as they are more likely to be in impoverished homes, we do not find problematic parental functioning in the face of difficult child characteristics.

In support of this conclusion are the results of studies by Vincent, Cook, Brady, Harris, and Messerly (1979; Cook, 1979) and by Gibaud-Wallston and Wandersman (1978) on the interactive influence of infant characteristics and on contextual support provided by the marital relationship. In the former case, disorganized infant functioning predicted nonsynchronous patterns of mother–infant and father–infant interaction *only* when marriages were evaluated as low in satisfaction. In the latter case, it was reported that mothers of difficult babies had a poor sense of parental competence unless they experienced support from people around them, particularly their husbands. Parental competence appears to be undermined by stress-generating child attributes, then, principally when contextual support systems fail to buffer the parent–child relationship.

At present, no studies are available that test the claim that personal resources have the greatest potential for buffering the parenting system, as no studies have examined simultaneously all the determinants identified in a single research effort. There are several investigations, however, that have simultaneously examined personal resources and one or another contextual sources of stress and support, and these prove instructive. In one recent study of adolescent and adult women, Levine et al. (1984) observed, using multiple regression procedures, that the mother's level of ego development was a stronger predictor of her positive affect and responsiveness while interacting with her infant in a face-to-face situation than was an index of social support in child care. Important to note, however, is the fact that child care support proved to be a better predictor of the mother's teaching activity in a structured teaching task than the ego development index used to assess her psychological maturity.

In another recent investigation – this one of German mothers and their newborn infants – Engfer (1984) related personality, marriage, and temperamental assessments to nurses' and doctors' evaluations of maternal sensitivity to their babies' needs. The evidence clearly indicated that both indices of personality (e.g., depression, composure) and marriage (e.g., conflict, communication) were stronger predictors than were indices of infant temperament (e.g., soothability, fussiness). Although the personality measures tended to be somewhat stronger predictors than the marital indicators, there was sufficient overlap to prevent one from drawing strong conclusions.

In two other studies examining both the psychological characteristics of the mother and evaluations of her marriage, findings emerged that actually run counter to the proposition advanced above regarding the primacy of parental characteristics. In his analysis of the determinants of coping behavior of mothers of handicapped children, Friedrich (1979) found that even though the mothers' psychological well-being was a reliable predictor of maternal coping, as was a measure of social support, marital satisfaction emerged from the regression analysis as the best of 19 predictors examined. In their study of the determinants of parenting, Belsky, Hertzog, and Rovine (1986) also found that marriage indicators were stronger structural equation predictors of observed mothering at nine months than were indicators of maternal personality. It must be noted, however, that in this latter study – and possibly in the Friedrich investigation as well – marital functioning and personality were significantly and positively correlated; such multicollinearity among predictor variables poses interpretive difficulties when it comes to drawing conclusions about the most important source of influence on parental functioning.

Despite the interpretive restrictions imposed and the few, contradictory findings just reviewed, we believe our hypothesis regarding the primacy of parental characteristics remains tenable because personal psychological resources are themselves likely to be instrumental in determining the quality of support one receives (see Figure 6.1). Consider, for example, the very real possibility that individual psychological characteristics affect not only the selection of a mate, but the quality of the relationshp that marital partners establish. Indeed, this may explain why personality indices and measures of marital quality are often found to covary positively with each other. Because it is also conceivable, at least according to our process model (see Figure 6.1), that developmental history shapes personal psychological well-being, marital influences upon parenting may themselves be traced back to developmental history through personality characteristics. Indeed, upon finding that dependency (as measured by the MMPI) is greater among women who lost their mothers before age ten, Birtchnell (1975) speculated that the effects of such early experiences upon personality may predispose women to poor marriages, as they might be willing to settle for the first man professing to care for them.

With respect to social network, there is suggestive evidence that personal resources do indeed influence the support one receives, which, we have seen, can affect parental functioning. Both Colletta (1981) and Kleiner and Parker (reported in Pattison, Llams, and Hurd, 1979) found low self-esteem associated with impoverished social networks. That this potential effect of personality on social networks, and thereby on parenting, can be traced back to developmental history is suggested by Colletta's (1981) study; she found that the extent to which teenage mothers were oriented toward social networks was related to familial socialization regarding doing things for oneself rather than asking for help. Developmental experience is also likely to affect one's ability to gather social network support through the social skills it fosters, in addition to the attitudes toward help-seeking it imparts. Thus, although the temptation certainly exists to explain social network impoverishment and personal dysfunction (parental or otherwise) in terms of the effect of social network support on psychological well-being, the possibility must be entertained that it is personal psychological inadequacies that generate network impoverishment and thereby undermine parental competence (Belsky, 1980).

Finally, work stresses must also be recognized as being, at least potentially, of the parents' own making and, conceivably, derivative of one's life-course history. In this regard, Kohn and Schooler's (1982) work that documents the reciprocal influence of job and personality, although not addressing the influence of developmental history, clearly demonstrates that personality can shape occupation, which influences parenting.

It should be evident, then, that we regard personal psychological resources as the most influential determinants of parenting not simply for their direct effect on parental functioning, but also because of the role they undoubtedly play in recruiting contextual support. By assigning them so central a role in our model, the very keystone of the design, we draw both our model and the ensuing discussion into the realm of developmental psychopathology. When the outcome is a qualitative extreme on the order of child maltreatment, the psychologically-based model we propose to explain its etiology is one of the development of psychopathology. Indeed, we see this area of inquiry – the determinants of parenting – as a vital expansion of the field, for what more critical aspect of adult functioning can we consider than the demanding, long-term commitment of raising children?

Conclusion

In his writings on the ecology of human development, Bronfenbrenner (1977, p. 77) is fond of quoting Goethe ("What is the most difficult of all? That which seems to you the easiest, to see with one's eyes what is lying before them") and Walter Fenno Dearborn, a graduate school mentor ("If you want to understand something, try to change it"). When these statements are juxtaposed, they illustrate quite effectively the general reason why dysfunction can illuminate normal functioning and, specifically, how the study of the etiology of child abuse can inform an analysis of the determinants of parenting.

In the routine ebb and flow of life it is often difficult to discern normal processes. Any dysfunction, by creating a perturbation in this flow, reveals elements and/or relationships that might otherwise go unnoticed. The determinants of parental functioning are considered to be one such set of relatively unnoticed events and processes. The significance of parental dysfunction – in the form of child maltreatment – is its power to reveal mechanisms of influence, at least in the pathological range, governing parental behavior. Because parenting is not readily manipulated, it is difficult to implement the strategy promulgated by Bronfenbrenner's mentor for the study of socialization. But here is found an illuminating example of the "natural experiment," in that the concern of applied scientists for the etiology of child abuse instructs inquiry into more basic scientific issues. If one regards child maltreatment as a departure from normal parenting practices, then the study of child abuse, representing "changes" in parenting, serves not only to enhance understanding of the socialization process but, in so doing, reveals that which is hardest to see because it lies right in front of our eyes – the determinants of individual differences in parenting, a topic that, despite this lengthy review, has received insufficient attention in the long history of socialization research.

Note

1. This section of the paper draws heavily from Bronfenbrenner and Crouter's (1983b) excellent analysis of work and family, which itself relied greatly upon past reviews of the maternal employment literature.

References

Aberle, D. F., and Naegele, K. D. Middle-class fathers' occupational role and attitudes toward children. *American Journal of Orthopsychiatry*, 1952, *22*, 366–378.
Abernethy, V. D. Social network and response to the maternal role. *International Journal of Sociology of the Family*, 1973, *3*, 86–92.
Affleck, G., Allen, D., McGrade, B. J., & McQueeney, M. Home environments of developmentally disabled infants as a function of parent and infant characteristics. *American Journal of Mental Deficiency*, 1982, *86*, 445–452.
Affleck, G., Allen, D., McGrade, B. J., and McQueeney, M. Maternal and child characteristics associated with mothers' perceptions of their high risk/developmental delayed infants. *The Journal of Genetic Psychology*, 1983, *142*, 171–180.
Ainsworth, M., Blehar, M., Waters, E., and Wall, S. (1978). *Patterns of attachment.* Hillsdale, N.J.: Erlbaum.
Altemeier, W. A., O'Connor, S., Vietze, P. M., Sandler, H. M., & Sherrod, K. B. Antecedents of child abuse. *Journal of Pediatrics*, 1982, *100*, 823–829.
Aug, R. G., & Bright, T. P. A study of wed and unwed motherhood in adolescents and young adults. *Journal of the American Academy of Child Psychiatry*, 1970, *9*, 577–592.
Baldwin, A. L., Cole, R. E., and Baldwin, C. T. Parent pathology, family interaction, and the competence of the child in school. *Monographs of the Society for Research in Child Development*, Serial No. 197, 1982.

Bandura, A., and Walters, R. *Adolescent aggression*. New York: Ronald Press, 1959.

Bates, J. The concept of difficult temperament. *Merrill-Palmer Quarterly*, 1980, *26*, 299–319.

Baumrind, D. Child care practices anteceding three patterns of preschool behavior. *Genetic Psychology Monographs*, 1967, *75*, 43–88.

Baumrind, D. Current patterns of parental authority. *Developmental Psychology Monographs*, 1971, *4* (1).

Beckwith, L., and Cohen, S. E. Preterm birth: Hazardous obstetrical and postnatal events as related to caregiver-infant behavior. *Infant Behavior and Development*, 1978, *1*, 403–412.

Bell, R. Q. A reinterpretation of the direction of effects in studies of socialization. *Psychological Review*, 1968, *75*, 81–95.

Belle, D. E. *The social network as a source of both stress and support to low-income mothers.* Paper presented at the biennial meeting of the Society for Research in Child Development, Boston, Mass., April, 1981.

Belsky, J. Three theoretical models of child abuse: A critical review. *International Journal of Child Abuse and Neglect*, 1978 (a), *2*, 37–49.

Belsky, J. A theoretical analysis of child abuse remediation strategies. *Journal of Clinical Child Psychology*, 1978 (b), *7*, 113–117.

Belsky, J. Child maltreatment: An ecological integration. *American Psychologist*, 1980, *35*, 320–335.

Belsky, J. Early human experience: A family perspective. *Developmental Psychology*, 1981, *17*, 3–23.

Belsky, J., Gilstrap, B., and Rovine, M. The Pennsylvania Infant and Family Development project I: Stability and change in mother-infant and father-infant interaction in a family setting: 1-to-3-to-9 months. *Child Development*, 1984, *55*, 692–705.

Belsky, J., Hertzog, C., and Rovine, M. (1986) Causal analysis of the determinants of parenting. In M. Lamb, A. Brown, and B. Rogoff (Eds.), *Advances in developmental psychology* (Vol. 4, pp. 153–202). Hillsdale, N.J.: Erlbaum.

Belsky, J. (1979). The interrelation of parental and spousal behavior during infancy in traditional nuclear families: an exploratory analysis. *Journal of Marriage and the Family, 41,* 749–755.

Belsky, J., Lerner, R., and Spanier, G. *The child in the family*. Reading, MA: Addison-Wesley, 1984.

Belsky, J., and Volling, B. Mothering, fathering, and marital interaction in the family triad during early infancy: Exploring family systems processes. In F. A. Pedersen and P. Berman (Eds.), *Men's transitions to parenthood: Longitudinal studies of early family experience* (pp. 37–63). Hillsdale, N.J.: Erlbaum, 1987.

Birtchnell, J. The personality characteristics of early bereaved psychiatric patients. *Social Psychiatry*, 1975, *10*, 97–103.

Bloom-Feshbach, J. Historical perspectives on the father's role. In M. E. Lamb (Ed.), *The role of the father in child development*, 2nd edition. New York: Wiley, 1981.

Bronfenbrenner, U. Toward an experimental ecology of human development. *American Psychologist*, 1977, *52*, 513–531.

Bronfenbrenner, U., and Crouter, A. C. The evolution of environmental models in developmental research. In P. Mussen (Ed.), *The handbook of child psychology*. New York: Wiley, 1983 (a).

Bronfenbrenner, U., and Crouter, A. C. Work and family through time and space. In C. Hayes and S. Kamerman (Eds.), *Families that work: Children in a changing world*. Washington, DC: National Academy of Sciences, 1983 (b).

Bronson, W. Early antecedents of emotional expressiveness and reactivity control. *Child Development*, 1966, *37*, 793–810.

Brown, G. W., and Harris, T. *Social origins of depression: A study of psychiatric disorder in women.* New York: Free Press, 1978.

Brown, J., and Bakeman, R. *Antecedents of emotional involvement in mothers of premature and full-term infants.* Paper presented at the biennial meeting of the Society for Research in Child Development, New Orleans, March, 1977.

Brunnquell, D., Crichton, L., and Egeland, B. Maternal personality and attitude in disturbances of child-rearing. *Journal of Orthopsychiatry*, 1981, *51*, 680–691.

Campbell, S. Mother–infant interaction as a function of maternal ratings of temperament. *Child Psychiatry and Human Development*, 1979, *10*, 67–76.

Candell, W., and Weinstein, H. Maternal care and infant behavior in Japan and America. *Psychiatry*, 1969, *12*, 32–43.

Caplan, G. *Support systems and community mental health.* New York: Behavioral Publications, 1974.

Carveth, W. B., and Gottlieb, B. H. The measurement of social support and its relation to stress. *Canadian Journal of Behavioral Science*, 1979, *11*, 179–188.

Cassell, J. Psychosocial processes and "stress": Theoretical formulation. *International Journal of Health Services*, 1974, *4*, 471–482.

Cicchetti, D., and Rizley, R. Developmental perspectives on the etiology, intergenerational transmission and sequelae of child maltreatment. *New Directions for Child Development*, 1981, *11*, 31–56.

Clarke, R., and Gecas, V. *The employed father in America: A role comparison analysis.* Paper presented at the annual meeting of the Pacific Sociological Association, 1971.

Clarke-Stewart, K. A. Interactions between mothers and their young children: Characteristics and consequences. *Monographs of the Society for Research in Child Development*, 1973, *38*(6–7, Serial No. 153).

Cobb, S. Social support as a moderator of life stress. *Psychosomatic Medicine*, 1976, *38*, 300–314.

Cochran, M., and Brassard, J. Child development and personal social networks. *Child Development*, 1979, *50*, 601–616.

Cohen, S. E. Maternal employment and mother-child interaction. *Merrill-Palmer Quarterly*, 1978, *24*, 189–197.

Colletta, N. D. Support systems after divorce: Incidence and impact. *Journal of Marriage and the Family*, 1979, *41*, 837–846.

Colletta, N. D. *The influence of support systems on the maternal behavior of young mothers.* Paper presented at the biennial meeting of the Society for Research in Child Development, Boston, Mass., April, 1981.

Colletta, N. D. At risk for depression: A study of young mothers. *Journal of Genetic Psychology*, 1983, *142*, 301–310.

Colletta, N. D., and Gregg, C. H. Adolescent mothers' vulnerability to stress. *The Journal of Nervous and Mental Disease*, 1981, *169*, 50–54.

Colletta, N. D., Lee, D., and Gregg, C. H. *The impact of support for adolescent mothers.* Unpublished manuscript, n.d.

Conger, R., McCarty, J., Yang, R., Lahey, B., and Kropp, J. Perception of child, childrearing values, and emotional distress as mediating links between environmental stressors and observed maternal behavior. *Child Development*, 1984, *55*, 2234–2247.

Cook, N. I. *An analysis of marital and infant factors in evolving family relations.* Paper presented at the biennial meeting of the Society for Research in Child Development, San Francisco, Calif., March, 1979.

Coopersmith, S. *The antecedents of self-esteem.* San Francisco: W. H. Freeman, 1967.

Cowan, C. P., and Cowan, P. A. *Men's involvement in the family: Implications for family well-being.* Paper presented at the annual meeting of the American Psychological Association, August, 1983 (a).

Cowan, P. A., and Cowan, C. P. *Quality of couple relationships and parenting stress in beginning families.* Paper presented at the biennial meeting of the Society for Research in Child Development, Detroit, April, 1983 (b).

Crnic, K. A., Greenberg, M. T., Ragozin, A. S., Robinson, N. M., and Basham, R. Effects of stress and social support on mothers and premature and full-term infants. *Child Development*, 1983, *54*, 209–217.

Crook, T., Raskin, A., and Eliot, J. Parent-child relationships and adult depression. *Child Development*, 1981, *52*, 950–957.

Crouter, A., Belsky, J., and Spanier, G. The family context of child development. In G. Whitehurst (Ed.), *Annals of child development,* Vol. 1. Greenwich, CT: JAI Press, 1984, 201–238.

Cummings, S. T. The impact of the child's deficiency on the father: A study of fathers of mentally retarded and of chronically ill children. *American Journal of Orthopsychiatry,* 1976, *46,* 246–255.

Cummings, S. T., Bayley, H., and Rie, H. Effects of the child's deficiency on the mother: A study of mothers of mentally retarded, chronically ill, and neurotic children. *American Journal of Orthopsychiatry,* 1966, *36,* 595–608.

De Frain, J. Androgynous parents tell who they are and what they need. *The Family Coordinator,* 1979, *28,* 237–243.

Dickie, J., Schuurmans, S., and Schang, B. *Mothers, fathers, and infants: What makes the triad work.* Paper presented at the annual meeting of the American Psychological Association, Montreal, September, 1980.

Dielman, T., Barton, K., and Cattell, R. Relationships among family attitudes and childrearing practices. *Journal of Genetic Psychology,* 1977, *130,* 105–112.

DiVitto, B., and Goldberg, S. The development of early parent-infant interaction as a function of newborn medical status. In T. Field, A. Sostek, S. Goldberg, and H. H. Shuman (Eds.), *Infants born at risk.* Holliswood, NY: Spectrum, 1979.

Donovan, W. L., Leavitt, L. A., and Balling, J. D. *Physiological correlates of mother–infant interaction.* Paper presented at the biennial meeting of the Society for Research in Child Development, Denver, CO, 1975.

Douvan, E. Employment and the adolescent. In F. I. Nye and L. W. Hoffman (Eds.), *The employed mother in America.* Chicago: Rand McNally, 1963.

Eiduson, B. T., and Alexander, J. W. The role of children in alternative family styles. *Journal of Social Issues,* 1978, *34,* 149–167.

Elder, G. H., Jr. *Children of the Great Depression.* Chicago: University of Chicago Press, 1974.

Elder, G. H., Jr., Caspi, A., and Downey, G. Problem behavior and family relationships: Life course and intergenerational themes. In A. Sorensen, F. Weinert, and L. Sherrod (Eds.), *Human development: Interdisciplinary perspectives* (pp. 293–340). Hillsdale, NJ: Erlbaum, 1986.

Elder, G. H., Jr., Liker, J. K., and Cross, C. E. Parent–child behavior in the Great Depression: Life course and intergenerational influences. In P. B. Baltes and O. G. Brim (Eds.), *Lifespan development and behavior,* Vol. 6. New York: Academic Press, 1984.

Elder, G. H., Jr., Nguyen, T. V., and Caspi, A. Linking family hardship to children's lives. *Child Development,* 1985, *56,* 361–375.

Emery, R. E. Interparental conflict and the children of discord and divorce. *Psychological Bulletin,* 1982, *92,* 310–330.

Engfer, A. *Early problems in mother–child interaction.* Paper presented at the European Study Group on Child Abuse and Neglect, David Solomans House, Tunbridge Wells, June, 1984.

Engfer, A., and Schneewind, K. *Causes and consequences of harsh parental punishment: An empirical investigation in a representative sample of 570 German families.* Paper presented at the third International Congress on Child Abuse and Neglect, Amsterdam, April, 1981.

Engfer, A., and Schneewind, K. Causes and consequences of harsh parental punishment. *Child Abuse and Neglect,* 1982, *6,* 129–139.

Epstein, A. S. *Pregnant teenagers' knowledge of infant development.* Paper presented at the biennial meeting of the Society for Research in Child Development, San Francisco, March, 1979.

Erickson, M. T. MMPI comparisons between parents of young emotionally disturbed and organically retarded children. *Journal of Consulting and Clinical Psychology,* 1968, *32,* 701–706.

Erickson, M. T. MMPI profiles of parents of young retarded children. *American Journal of Mental Deficiency,* 1969, *73,* 728–732.

Erikson, E. *Childhood and society.* New York: Norton, 1950.

Fabian, A. A., and Donohue, J. F. Maternal depression: A challenging child guidance problem. *American Journal of Orthopsychiatry*, 1956, *26*, 400–405.

Farber, A., and Egeland, B. *Maternal, neonatal and mother–infant antecedents of attachment in urban poor.* Paper presented at the Annual Meeting of the American Psychological Association, Montreal, September, 1980.

Farel, A. N. Effects of preferred maternal roles, maternal employment, and sociographic status on school adjustment and competence. *Child Development*, 1980, *50*, 1179–1186.

Feiring, C., Fox, H., Jaskir, J., and Lewis, M. *The relationship between social support, infant risk status, and mother–infant interaction.* Unpublished manuscript, Rutgers Medical School, 1985.

Feiring, C., and Taylor, J. *The influence of the infant and secondary parent on maternal behavior: Toward a social systems view of infant attachment.* Unpublished manuscript, University of Pittsburgh, n.d.

Feldman, S. S., and Nash, S. C. *Prediction of mothering behavior from pregnancy.* Unpublished manuscript, Stanford University, 1982.

Feldman, S. S., Nash, S. C., and Aschenbrenner, B. Antecedents of fathering. *Child Development*, 1983, *54*, 1628–1636.

Field, T. M. Maternal stimulation during infant feeding. *Developmental Psychology*, 1977, *13*, 539–540.

Field, T. M. Infants born at risk: Early compensatory experiences. In L. Bond and J. Joffee (Eds.), *Facilitating infant and early childhood development.* Hanover, NH: University Press of New England, 1982.

Field, T. M., Widmayer, S. M., Stringer, S., and Ignatoff, E. Teenage, lower-class, black mothers and their preterm infants: An intervention and developmental follow-up. *Child Development*, 1980, *51*, 426–436.

Fontana, V. *The maltreated child.* Springfield: Thomas, 1971.

French, J., Rodgers, W., and Cobb, S. Adjustment as person–environment fit. In G. Cochlo, D. Hamberg, and J. Adams (Eds.), *Coping and adaptation.* New York: Basic Books, 1974.

Friedrich, W. N. Predictors of the coping behavior of mothers of handicapped children. *Journal of Consulting and Clinical Psychology*, 1979, *47*, 1140–1141.

Frommer, E., and O'Shea, G. Antenatal identification of women liable to have problems in managing their infants. *British Journal of Psychiatry*, 1973 (a), *123*, 149–156.

Frommer, E., and O'Shea, G. The importance of childhood experiences in relation to problems of marriage and family building. *British Journal of Psychiatry*, 1973 (b), *123*, 157–160.

Gamble, W., and Belsky, J. *Stressors, support, and maternal personal resources as determinants of mothering: A comparison of three models.* Unpublished manuscript, The Pennsylvania State University, University Park, PA, 1984.

Garbarino, J. A preliminary study of some ecological correlates of child abuse: The impact of socioeconomic stress on mothers. *Child Development*, 1976, *47*, 178–185.

Garbarino, J. The price of privacy in the social dynamics of child abuse. *Child Welfare*, 1977, *56*, 565–575.

Gelles, R. Child abuse as psychopathology: A sociological critique and reformulation. *American Journal of Orthopsychiatry*, 1973, *43*, 611–621.

Gelles, R. The social construction of child abuse. *American Journal of Psychiatry*, 1975, *132*, 363–371.

Gersick, K. E. Fathers by choice: Divorced men who receive custody of their children. In A. Levinger and O. C. Moles (Eds.), *Divorce and Separation.* New York: Basic Books, 1979.

Gibaud-Wallston, and Wandersman, L. P. *Development and utility of the parenting sense of competence scale.* Paper presented at the annual meeting of the American Psychological Association, Toronto, 1978.

Gibson, H. Early delinquency in relation to broken homes. *Journal of Abnormal Psychology*, 1969, *74*, 33–41.

Gil, D. Violence against children. *Journal of Marriage and the Family*, 1971, *33*, 639.

Gold, D., and Andres, D. Developmental comparisons between 10-year-old children with employed and nonemployed mothers. *Child Development,* 1978, *49,* 75–84.

Gold, D., and Andres, D. Maternal employment and development of 10-year-old Canadian Francophone children. *Canadian Journal of Behavioral Science,* 1980, *12,* 233–240.

Goldberg, S. Prematurity: Effects on parent–infant interaction. *Journal of Pediatric Psychology,* 1978, *3* (3), 137–144.

Goldberg, W. A. *Marital quality and child–mother, child–father attachments.* Paper presented at the International Conference on Infant Studies, Austin, TX, March, 1982.

Goldberg, W. A., and Easterbrooks, M. A. The role of marital quality in toddler development. *Developmental Psychology,* 1984, *20,* 504–514.

Grossman, F., Eichler, L., and Winickoff, S. *Pregnancy, birth, and parenthood: Adaptations of mothers, fathers, and infants.* San Francisco: Jossey-Bass, 1980.

Hall, F., Pawlby, S., and Wolkind, S. Early life experience and later mothering behavior: A study of mothers and their 20 week old babies. In D. Schaffer and J. Dunn (Eds.), *The first year of life.* New York: Wiley, 1979.

Hauser, S. T., Powers, S. I., Noam, G. G., and Jacobson, A. M. Familial contexts of adolescent ego development. *Child Development,* 1984, *55,* 195–213.

Heath, D. H. Competent fathers: Their personality and marriages. *Human Development,* 1976, *19,* 26–39.

Heinecke, C. M. *Parental deprivation in early childhood: A predisposition to later depression?* Presented at the symposium on Separation and Depression: Clinical and Research Reports. Annual meeting of the American Association for the Advancement of Science, Chicago, Dec. 26–30, 1970.

Helfer, R. E. McKinney, J., and Kempe, R. Arresting or freezing the developmental process. In R. E. Helfer and C. H. Kempe (Eds.), *Child abuse and neglect: The family and the community.* Cambridge, MA: Ballinger 1976, 55–73.

Hess, R., & Shipman, V. Early experience and the socialization of cognitive modes in children. *Child Development,* 1965, *36,* 869–886.

Hess, R. D., Shipman, V. C., Brophy, J. E., & Bear, B. M. *The cognitive environments of urban preschool children.* Graduate School of Education, University of Chicago, 1968.

Hetherington, E., Cox, M., and Cox, R. The aftermath of divorce. In J. Stevens and M. Mathews (Eds.), *Mother-child, father-child relations.* Washington, DC: National Association for the Education of Young Children, 1977.

Hill, C. R., and Stafford, F. P. *Parental care of children: Time diary estimates of quantity, predictability, and variety.* Unpublished manuscript, Institute of Social Research, University of Michigan, 1978.

Hock, E. Working and nonworking mothers with infants: Perceptions of their careers, their infant's needs, and satisfaction with mothering. *Developmental Psychology,* 1978, *14,* 37–43.

Hock, E. Working and nonworking mothers and their infants: A comparative study of maternal caregiving characteristics and infant social behavior. *Merrill-Palmer Quarterly of Behavior and Development,* 1980, *26,* 79–101.

Hoffman, L. W. Mothers' enjoyment of work and its effects on the child. *Child Development,* 1961, *32,* 187–197.

Hoffman, L. W. Mother's enjoyment of work and effects on the child. In F. I. Nye and L. W. Hoffman (Eds.), *The employed mother in America.* Chicago: Rand McNally, 1963.

Hoffman, L. W. Changes in family roles, socialization, and sex differences. *American Psychologist,* 1979, *32,* 644–657.

Hoffman, M. L. Moral development. In P. H. Mussen (Ed.), *Carmichael's manual of child psychology,* Vol. 2. New York: Wiley, 1970.

Honzik, M. Environmental correlates of mental growth: Prediction from a family setting at 21 months. *Child Development,* 1967, *38,* 337–364.

Jennings, K. D., Stagg, V., and Connors, R. *Social support and mothers' interactions with their preschool children.* Paper presented at the biennial meeting of the Society for Research in Child Development, Toronto, April, 1985.

Johnson, C. L. *Leadership patterns in working and nonworking mother middle-class families.* Unpublished doctoral dissertation, University of Kansas, 1969 (University Microfilms 69–11).

Johnson, S., and Lobitz, G. The personal and marital adjustment of parents as related to observed child deviance and parenting behaviors. *Journal of Abnormal Child Psychology,* 1974, *2,* 193–207.

Jones, F. A., Green, V., and Krauss, D. R. Maternal responsiveness of primiparous mothers during the postpartum period: Age differences. *Pediatrics,* 1980, *65,* 579–583.

Kadushin, A., and Martin, J. *Child abuse: An interactional event.* New York: Columbia University Press, 1981.

Kanter, R. Families, family processes, and economic life: Toward a systematic analysis of social historical research. In J. Demos and S. Boocock (Eds.), *Turning points: Historical and sociological essays on the family.* Chicago: University of Chicago Press, 1978.

Kappel, B. E., and Lambert, R. D. *Self worth among the children of working mothers.* Unpublished manuscript, University of Waterloo, Ontario, 1972.

Kelly, P. The relation of infant's temperament and mother's psychopathology to interactions in early infancy. In K. F. Riegel and J. A. Meacham (Eds.), *The developing individual in a changing world,* Vol. 11. Chicago: Aldine, 1976.

Kempe, H., and Kempe, R. *Child abuse.* Cambridge, MA: Harvard University Press, 1978.

Kemper, T., and Reichler, M. Marital satisfaction and conjugal power as determinants of intensity and frequency of rewards and punishments administered by parents. *Journal of Genetic Psychology,* 1976 (a), *129,* 221–234.

Kemper, T., and Reichler, M. Fathers work integration and frequencies of rewards and punishments administered by fathers and mothers to adolescent sons and daughters. *Journal of Genetic Psychology,* 1976 (b), *129,* 207–219.

Kessen, W., Fein, G., Clarke-Stewart, A., and Starr, S. *Variations in home-based infant education.* Final report to the Office of Child Development, Grant #OCD–CB–98, August, 1975.

Kimmel, D., and Van der Veen, F. Factors of marital adjustment in Locke's Marital Adjustment Test. *Journal of Marriage and the Family,* 1974, *36,* 57–63.

Klein, M., and Stern, L. Low birthweight and the battered child syndrome. *American Journal of Diseases of Childhood,* 1971, *122,* 15–18.

Kohn, M. L. Social class and parent–child relationships: An interpretation. *American Journal of Sociology,* 1963, *68,* 471–480.

Kohn, M. L., and Schooler, C. Occupational experience and psychological functioning: An assessment of reciprocal effects. *American Sociological Review,* 1973, *38,* 97–118.

Kohn, M. L., and Schooler, C. The reciprocal effects of the substantive complexity of work and intellectual flexibility: A longitudinal assessment. *American Journal of Sociology,* 1978, *84,* 24–52.

Kohn, M. L., & Schooler, C. Job conditions and personality: A longitudinal assessment of their reciprocal effects. *American Journal of Sociology,* 1982, *87,* 1257–1286.

Komarovsky, M. *The unemployed man and his family.* New York: Dryden Press, 1940.

Lamb, M., and Easterbrooks, M. Individual differences in parental sensitivity. In M. Lamb and L. Sherrod (Eds.), *Infant social cognition.* Hillsdale, N.J.: Erlbaum, 1980.

Langner, T. S., and Michael, S. T. *Life stress and mental health.* London: Collier-Macmillan, 1963.

Lee, D. M., and Colletta, N. D. *Family support for adolescent mothers: The positive and negative impact.* Paper presented at the biennial meeting of the Society for Research in Child Development, Detroit, April, 1983.

Levine, L., Coll, C., and Oh, W. *Determinants of mother–infant interaction in adolescent mothers.* Paper presented at the International Conference on Infant Studies, New York, April, 1984.

Lewis, M., and Rosenblum, L. (Eds.), *The effect of the infant on its caregiver.* New York: Wiley, 1974.

Lewis, M., and Weinraub, M. The father's role in the infant's social network. In M. E. Lamb (Ed.), *The role of the father in child development*. New York: Wiley, 1976.

Lewis, M., and Wilson, C. D. Infant development in lower-class American families. *Human Development*, 1972, *15*, 112–127.

Light, R. Abused and neglected children in America: A study of alternative policies. *Harvard Educational Review*, 1973, *43*, 556–598.

Liker, J. K., and Elder, G. H., Jr. Economic hardship and marital relations in the 1930s. *American Sociological Review*, 1983, *48*, 343–359.

Maccoby, E. E., Snow, M. E., and Jacklin, C. N. Children's dispositions and mother–child interaction at 12 and 18 months: A short-term longitudinal study. *Developmental Psychology*, 1984, *20*, 459–472.

Manion, J. A study of fathers and infant caretaking. *Birth and the Family Journal*, 1977, *4*, 174–179.

Martin, H., Conway, E., Breezley, P., and Kempe, H. C. The development of abused children, Part I: A review of the literature. *Advances in Pediatrics*, 1974, *21*, 43.

McCall, R. B. Exploratory manipulation and play in the human infant. *Monographs of the Society for Research in Child Development*, 1974, *39* (No. 155).

McCord, J., McCord, W., and Thurber, E. Effects of maternal employment on lower-class boys. *Journal of Abnormal and Social Psychology*, 1963, *67*, 177–182.

McHale, S. M., and Huston, T. L. Men and women as parents: Sex role orientations, employment, and parental roles with infants. *Child Development*, 1984, *55*, 1349–1361.

McKinley, D. *Social class and family life*. New York: Free Press, 1964.

McLanahan, S., Wedemeyer, N., and Adelberg, T. Network structure, social support, and psychological well-being in the single-parent family. *Journal of Marriage and the Family*, 1981, *43*, 601–612.

Mendes, H. Single fatherhood. *Social Work*, 1976, *21*, 308–312.

Miller, D. R., and Swanson, G. E. *The changing American parent: A study in the Detroit area*. New York: John Wiley and Sons, 1958.

Miller, J., Schooler, C., Kohn, M. L., and Miller, K. A. Women and work: The psychological effects of occupational conditions. *American Journal of Sociology*, 1979, *85*, 66–94.

Miller, W. H., and Keirn, W. C. Personality measurement in parents of retarded and emotionally disturbed children: A replication. *Journal of Clinical Psychology*, 1978, *34*, 686–690.

Milliones, J. Relationship between perceived child temperament and maternal behavior. *Child Development*, 1978, *49*, 1255–1257.

Minde, K., Shosenberg, N. E., Marton, P., Thompson, J., Ripley, J., and Burns, S. Self-help groups in a premature nursery – a controlled evaluation. *The Journal of Pediatrics*, 1980, *96*, 933–940.

Minturn, L., and Lambert, W. W. *Mothers of six cultures: Antecedents of childrearing*. New York: Wiley, 1964.

Mitchell, R., and Trickett, E. Task force report: Social networks as mediators of social support. *Community Mental Health Journal*, 1980, *16*, 27–44.

Moen, P. The two-provider family: Problems and potentials. In M. Lamb (Ed.), *Nontraditional families: Parenting and child development*. Hillsdale, NJ: Erlbaum, 1982.

Mondell, S., and Tyler, F. Parental competence and styles of problem solving/play behavior with children. *Developmental Psychology*, 1981, *17*, 73–78.

Mortimer, J. T. Patterns of intergenerational occupational movements: A smallest-space analysis. *American Journal of Sociology*, 1974, *79*, 1278–1299.

Mortimer, J. T. Social class, work, and the family: Some implications of the father's career for familial relationships and son's career decisions. *Journal of Marriage and the Family*, 1976, *38*, 241–256.

Mortimer, J. T., and Kumka, D. A further examination of the "Occupational Linkage Hypothesis." *The Sociological Quarterly*, 1982, *23*, 3–16.

Moss, H. A. *Communication in mother–infant interaction*. Reprinted from: *Nonverbal communication*. Edited by L. Krames, P. Pliner, and T. Alloway, Plenum Press, 1974.

Nuckolls, C. G., Cassel, J., and Kaplan, B. H. Psychological assets, life crises and the prognosis of pregnancy. *American Journal of Epidemiology*, 1972, *95*, 431–441.

Nye, I. Child adjustment in broken and in unhappy unbroken homes. *Marriage and Family Living*, 1957, *19*, 356–361.

O'Leary, K., and Emery, R. Marital discord and child behavior problems. In M. Levine and P. Satz (Eds.), *Developmental variations and dysfunction*. New York: Academic Press, 1983.

Olweus, D. Familial and temperamental determinants of aggressive behavior in adolescent boys: A causal analysis. *Developmental Psychology*, 1980, *16*, 644–660.

Orraschel, H., Weissman, M. M., and Kidd, K. K. Children and depression: The children of depressed parents; the childhood of depressed patients; depression in children. *Journal of Affective Disorders*, 1980, *2* (1), 1–16.

Osofsky, J. J., and Osofsky, J. D. Adolescents as mothers. *American Journal of Orthopsychiatry*, 1970, *40*, 825.

Parke, R. D. Parent–infant interaction: Progress, paradigms and problems. In G. P. Sackett (Ed.), *Observing behavior, Vol. 1: Theory and applications in mental retardation*. Baltimore: University Park Press, 1978.

Parke, R., and Collmer, C. Child abuse: An interdisciplinary review. In E. M. Hetherington (Ed.), *Review of child development research* (Vol. 5). Chicago: University of Chicago Press, 1975.

Pascoe, J. M., Loda, F. A., Jeffries, V., and Earp, J. A. The association between mother's social support and provision of stimulation to their children. *Developmental and Behavioral Pediatrics*, 1981, *2*, 15–19.

Patterson, G. Mothers: The unacknowledged victims. *Monograph of the Society for Research in Child Development*. Serial No. 186, 1980.

Pattison, E. M., Llamas, R., and Hurd, G. Social network mediation of anxiety. *Psychiatric Annals*, 1979, *9*, 56–67.

Pearlin, L., and Johnson, T. Marital status, life-strains, and depression. *American Sociological Review*, 1977, *42*, 704–715.

Pedersen, F. *Mother, father and infant as an interactive system.* Paper presented at the annual convention of the American Psychological Association, Chicago, September, 1975.

Pedersen, F. Mother, father and infant as an interactive system. In J. Belsky (Ed.), *In the beginning: Readings on infancy*. New York: Columbia University Press, 1982.

Pedersen, F. Anderson, B., and Cain, R. *An approach to understanding linkages between the parent–infant and spouse relationships.* Paper presented at the biennial meeting of the Society for Research in Child Development, New Orleans, March, 1977.

Pedersen, F., Cain, R., Zaslow, M., and Anderson, B. Variation in infant experience associated with alternative family roles. In L. M. Laosa and I. E. Sigel (Eds.), *Families as learning environments for children*. New York: Plenum, 1983.

Pedersen, F., Yarrow, L., Anderson, B., and Cain, R. Conceptualization of father influences in the infancy period. In M. Lewis and L. Rosenblum (Eds.), *The social network of the developing infant*. New York: Plenum, 1978.

Piotrkowski, C. S. *Work and the family system: A naturalistic study of working-class and lower-middle class families*. New York: The Free Press, 1979.

Pleck, J. H. *Wives' employment, role demands and adjustment: Final report*. Unpublished manuscript, Wellesley College Center for Research on Women, 1981.

Pleck, J. H., Staines, G. L., and Long, L. *Work and family life*. Final reports on Work-Family Interference and Worker's Formal Childcare Arrangements, from the 1977 Quality of Employment Survey. Unpublished manuscript, Wellesley College, 1978.

Pollitt, J. *Depression and its treatment*. London: Heinemann, 1965.

Pollock, C., and Steele, B. A therapeutic approach to the parents. In C. H. Kempe and R. E. Helfer (Eds.), *Helping the battered child and his family*. Philadelphia: J. B. Lippincot Co., 1972, 3–21.

Powell, D. R. Family–environment relations and early childrearing: The role of social networks and neighborhoods. *Journal of Research and Development in Education*, 1979, *13*, 1–11.

Powell, D. R. Personal social networks as a focus for primary prevention of child maltreatment. *Infant Mental Health Journal,* 1980, *1,* 232–239.

Price, G. *Factors influencing reciprocity in early mother–infant interaction.* Paper presented at the biennial meeting of the Society for Research in Child Development, New Orleans, March, 1977.

Propper, A. M. The relationship of maternal employment to adolescent roles, activities, and parental relationships. *Journal of Marriage and the Family,* 1972, *34,* 417–421.

Ragins, N., Schachter, J., Elmer, E., Preisman, R., Bowes, A., and Harway, V. Infants and children at risk for schizophrenia. *Journal of Child Psychiatry,* 1975, *14,* 150–177.

Ragozin, A. S., Basham, R. B., Crnic, K. A., Greenberg, M. T., and Robinson, N. M. Effects of maternal age on parenting role. *Developmental Psychology,* 1982, *18*(4), 627–634.

Reuter, M. W., and Biller, H. B. Perceived paternal nurturance-availability and personality adjustment among college males. *Journal of Consulting and Clinical Psychology,* 1973, *40,* 339–342.

Robinson, J. P. *How Americans use time.* New York: Praeger, 1977.

Rohner, R., and Rohner, E. Antecedents and consequences of parental rejection: A theory of emotional abuse. *Child Abuse and Neglect,* 1980, *4,* 189–198.

Rosenberg, M., and Reppucci, N. *Abusive mothers: Perceptions of their own and their children's behavior.* Unpublished manuscript, University of Virginia, 1982.

Russell, G. Shared-caregiving families: An Australian study. In M. E. Lamb (Ed.), *Nontraditional families.* Hillsdale, NJ: Erlbaum, 1981.

Sagi, A. Antecedents and consequences of various degrees of paternal involvement in child-rearing: The Israeli Project. In M. E. Lamb (Ed.), *Nontraditional families: Parenting and child development.* Hillsdale, NJ: Erlbaum 1982.

Sameroff, A. Concepts of humanity in primary prevention. In G. Albee and J. Jaffe (Eds.), *Primary prevention of psychopathology,* Vol. 1. Hanover, NH: University Press of New England, 1977.

Sameroff, A. J., Barocas, R., and Seifer, R. The early development of children born to mentally-ill women. In N. F. Watt, E. J. Anthony, L. C. Wynne, and J. Rolf (Eds.), *Children at risk for schizophrenia: A longitudinal perspective.* New York: Cambridge University Press, 1984.

Sameroff, A., and Chandler, M. J. Reproductive risk and the continuum of caretaking casualty. In F. D. Horowitz (Ed.), *Review of child development research* (Vol. 4), Chicago: University of Chicago Press, 1975.

Santrock, J. W., Warshak, R., Lindbergh, C., and Meadows, L. Children's and parent's observed social behavior in stepfather families. *Child Development,* 1982, *53,* 472–480.

Schaefer, E., Bauman, K., Siegel, E., Hosking, J., and Sanders, M. *Mother–infant interaction: Factor analyses, stability and demographic and psychological correlates.* Unpublished manuscript, University of North Carolina, Chapel Hill, 1980.

Schubert, J. B., Bradley-Johnson, S., and Nuttal, J. Mother–infant communication and maternal employment. *Child Development,* 1980, *51,* 246–249.

Sears, R., Maccoby, E., and Levin, H. *Patterns of child rearing.* Evanston, Ill.: Row, Peterson, 1957.

Seth, M., and Khanna, M. Childrearing attitudes of the mothers as a function of age. *Child Psychiatry Quarterly,* 1978, *11,* 6–9.

Sherrod, K., O'Connor, S., Altemeier, W. A., and Vietze, P. Toward a semispecific, multidimensional, threshold model of maltreatment. In D. Drotar (Ed.), *New directions in research and practice on failure to thrive.* New York: Plenum, 1986.

Siegal, M. Economic deprivation and the quality of parent-child relations. In his *Fairness in children.* New York: Academic Press, 1982.

Sirignano, S., and Lachman, M. Personality change during the transition to parenthood: The role of perceived temperament. *Developmental Psychology, 21,* 1985, 558–567.

Soloman, J. *Marital intimacy and parent-infant relationships.* Unpublished doctoral dissertation, University of California, Berkeley, 1982.

Spinetta, J., and Rigler, D. The child abusing parent: A psychological review. *Psychological Bulletin*, 1972, *77*, 296–304.

Starr, R. H., Dietrich, K. N., Fischhoff, J., Ceresnie, S., and Zweier, D. The contribution of handicapping conditions to child abuse. *Topics in Early Childhood Special Education*, 1984, *4*, 55–69.

Stayton, D., Hogan, R., and Ainsworth, M. Infant obedience and maternal behavior: The origins of socialization reconsidered. *Child Development*, 1971, *42*, 1057–1069.

Steele, B. F. Parental abuse of infants and small children. In E. J. Anthony and T. Benedek (Eds.), *Parenthood, its psychology and psychopathology*, 1970, 449–477.

Steinberg, L., Catalano, R., and Dooley, D. Economic antecedents of child abuse and neglect. *Child Development*, 1981, *52*, 975–985.

Stuckey, M., McGhee, P., and Bell, N. Parent–child interaction: The influence of maternal employment. *Developmental Psychology*, 1982, *18*, 635–644.

Switzky, L. T., Vietze, P., and Switzky, H. N. Attitudinal and demographic predictors of breast-feeding and bottle-feeding behavior by mothers of six-week-old infants. *Psychological Reports*, 1979, *45*, 3–14.

Toms-Olson, J. The impact of housework on childcare in the home. *Family Relations*, 1981, *30*, 75–81.

Unger, D., and Powell, D. *Supporting families under stress: The role of social networks*. Unpublished manuscript, Merrill-Palmer Institute, Detroit, MI, 1980.

Vincent, P., Cook, N., Brady, C., Harris, G., and Messerly, L. *Learning to be a family: Struggle of the emergent triad*. Symposium presented at the biennial meeting of the Society for Research in Child Development, San Francisco, March, 1979.

Walker, E., and Emory, E. Infants at risk for psychopathology: Offspring of schizophrenic parents. *Child Development*, 1983, *54*, 1269–1285.

Walker, K. E. How much help for working mothers? The children's role. *Human Ecology Forum*, 1970, *1*, 13–15.

Wandersman, L., and Unger, D. G. *Interaction of infant difficulty and social support in adolescent mothers*. Paper presented at the biennial meeting of the Society for Research in Child Development, Detroit, Michigan, April, 1983.

Wandersman, L., Wandersman, A., and Kahn, S. Social support in the transition to parenthood. *Journal of Community Psychology*, 1980, *8*, 332–342.

Weinraub, M., and Wolf, B. M. Effects of stress and social supports on mother–child interactions in single- and two-parent families. *Child Development*, 1983, *54*, 1297–1311.

Weissman, M. M., and Paykel, E. S. *The depressed woman: A study of social relations*. Chicago: University of Chicago Press, 1974.

Whiting, B., and Whiting, J. *Children of six cultures*. Cambridge: Harvard University Press, 1975.

Woods, M. B. The unsupervised child of the working mother. *Developmental Psychology*, 1972, *6*, 14–25.

Yarrow, L., Rubenstein, J., and Pedersen, F. *Infant and environment*. New York: Wiley, 1975.

Yarrow, M. R., Scott, P., DeLeeuw, L., and Heinig, C. Childrearing in families of working and nonworking mothers. *Sociometry*, 1962, *25*, 122–140.

Young, M., and Willmott, P. *Family and kinship in East London*. London: Penguin, 1957.

Zur-Spiro, S., & Longfellow, C. *Support from fathers: Implications for the well-being of mothers and their children*. Paper presented at the biennial meeting of the Society for Research in Child Development, Boston, April, 1981.

7 The antecedents of maltreatment: results of the Mother–Child Interaction Research Project

Robert Pianta, Byron Egeland,
and Martha Farrell Erickson

Introduction

Interest in the antecedents of child maltreatment has been present in a wide variety of disciplines for many years. Psychologists, particularly developmental psychologists, express interest in the extent to which this knowledge contributes to an understanding of the parenting process and developmental psychopathology (Maccoby and Martin, 1983). Professionals in applied fields such as medicine, social work, education, and clinical psychology depend upon research on the antecedents of child maltreatment in order to construct prediction, prevention, and intervention efforts in their work with individuals and families as well as in communities and social policy efforts. Despite the advances made in research and theory in child maltreatment over the past thirty years, only recently have there been attempts to develop integrated theoretical models of such a complex phenomenon (Cicchetti and Rizley, 1981). These efforts to produce empirically derived theories of the etiology of child maltreatment have been hindered by a number of central issues.

These major issues are discussed at various points in this chapter and in others in this volume. It is important to realize that each of the disciplines contributing to maltreatment research must in some way address these issues. They include reliance on retrospective research designs, use of conceptual models that postulate isolated or single causes for maltreatment, and the lack of a heuristically generated theoretical foundation based on previous empirical findings (Belsky, 1980; Cicchetti and Aber, 1980; Cicchetti and Rizley, 1981; Egeland and Brunnquell, 1979). This chapter presents a

This research was supported by a grant from the Maternal and Child Health Service to the Department of Health, Education, and Welfare (MC–R–270416–01–0). This research is currently supported by a grant from the Office of Special Education, Department of Education, Washington, D.C. (G008300029) and the Wm. T. Grant Foundation, New York City.

summary of the results of research conducted on the antecedents of child maltreatment by the Mother–Child Interaction Research Project at the University of Minnesota, which was specifically designed to address these issues. As will be described in further detail in a later section, this is a prospective, longitudinal research program that has employed a multivariate measurement strategy to examine the antecedents and consequences of child maltreatment in a sample of mothers selected for being "at risk" for poor parenting. As such, the Mother–Child Project represents a unique opportunity to examine the complex etiology of child maltreatment.

This chapter consists of four major sections. First, a brief review of the literature on the antecedents of child maltreatment is presented in order to create a context in which to present and discuss the empirical findings of the Mother–Child Project. Next the project is described in detail, with special emphasis on the extent to which its research strategy addresses the issues noted earlier. Empirical findings on the antecedents of child maltreatment in the Mother–Child Project high-risk sample are then presented, and in a final section these results are discussed with specific emphasis on the development of an integrated theoretical framework for understanding the antecedents of child maltreatment.

Etiological factors in child maltreatment

In addition to the major issues in the literature noted above, studies on the antecedents of child maltreatment present other problematic issues that contribute to difficulty in reviewing this literature. First, as noted by other reviewers (Cicchetti and Rizley, 1981), there has been inconsistency across studies in the definition of maltreatment; some focus on legal definitions, whereas others have used psychological or medical definitions to frame their inquiry. Heterogeneity in definition, although perhaps useful for some applied purposes, makes it difficult to establish consistent linkages between cause and effect that can then be replicated (Aber and Zigler, 1981). The possible existence of subtypes of maltreatment within superficially similar groups of victims and perpetrators further confounds the task of integrating this literature.

The child maltreatment literature has also been biased toward research on just one type of maltreatment – physical abuse. Physical and emotional neglect or other forms of psychological maltreatment have not been regularly researched. As a result, the literature available for a review of antecedent factors is largely imbalanced toward studies on the antecedents of physical abuse. This review will of necessity reflect these issues of definitional inconsistency and bias toward physical abuse.

Parental characteristics

The majority of investigations of the antecedents of child maltreatment have focused on the role of parental characteristics in causing physical abuse (Wolfe, 1985). Historically, these investigations have derived from the "psychiatric" model of maltreatment, whereby physical abuse is viewed as the result of emotional illness in a parent (Gelles, 1973; Wooley and Evans, 1955). The literature that has followed from this model has attempted to demonstrate that physically maltreating parents can be characterized by cognitive factors, personality traits or attitudes that distinguish them from nonmaltreating controls. This conceptual model has placed relatively little emphasis on the roles of environmental stressors or child characteristics (Wolfe, 1985). For example, differences between abusive and nonabusive parents have been reported on a vast number of descriptors and symptoms such as anger, rigidity, immaturity, impulsivity, overall adjustment, and depression (summarized by Wolfe, 1985).

Studies consistently demonstrating a pattern of specific personality characteristics or traits in physically abusing parents have been lacking and generally have not been replicated (Parke and Collmer, 1975; Wolfe, 1985), mostly due to the great disparity across samples of parents, the different ways investigators have operationalized the same characteristics, and the extent to which there is overlap in the wide variety of personality traits and characteristics that can be measured. However, recent reviews suggest that the abusive parent is enmeshed within a multiproblem family with deficits and liabilities that encompass a wide range of dysfunction (Belsky, 1980; Wolfe, 1985). This progress marks a shift in emphasis from the psychiatric model, which viewed abuse as the result of static traits, to a focus on more interactive processes, of which the parent is a critical component.

Recently, investigators have turned to examining parental characteristics that are more directly tied to mothers' thoughts and feelings about caretaking rather than measuring static personality traits, such as aggression, which at best may have only a hypothetical link to caretaking skills. (Brunnquell, Crichton, and Egeland, 1981; Newberger, 1980; Newberger and Cook, 1983; Sameroff and Feil, 1984). These studies have begun to demonstrate rather consistently that one characteristic differentiating maltreating from adequate caretakers is their lack of understanding of the complexity of social relationships, especially caretaking, and their feelings about meeting the needs of another person. Again, there has been a movement away from measuring static traitlike characteristics toward examining the affective and cognitive aspects of the caretaker–child relationship within a conceptual model that is more process oriented.

There is recent evidence suggesting that maltreating parents share a common misunderstanding with regard to the nature of childrearing and their relationship with the child whom they maltreat (Newberger, 1980; Newberger and Cook, 1983; Sameroff and Feil, 1984). Independent studies by Sameroff and Newberger and colleagues have isolated similar sets of social cognitive factors associated with maltreating parents. Sameroff and Feil (1984) describe four stages of parents' conceptualizing about childrearing (symbiotic, categorical, compensating, and perspectivistic), which vary by the extent to which the parent is able to interpret the behavior of their children in the increasingly broad and complex contexts of the child's motivations and intentions. The stages vary from being embedded in here and now action to separating the behavior of their children from the life circumstances in which they were raised. Similarly, Newberger and Cook (1983) report on four levels of parents' conceptualizing about childrearing that represent increasingly comprehensive perspectives from which the parent–child relationship is viewed. Each level successively expands the reasoning perspective of the preceding level. This hierarchical organization is reflected in the labels of egoistic (self orientation), conventional (norms orientation), individualistic (child orientation), and analytic (systems orientation). Both sets of investigators have conceptually linked these social cognitive processes to child maltreatment through the ability of the parents to interpret their own needs and desires vis-à-vis the child's behavior within the context of the parent–child relationship. Thus the parent that provides good quality care is able to take the child's perspective and understand the child's behavior in terms of the context or situation and the developmental level of the child. The empirical validation of these a priori theoretical linkages between parental social-cognitive processes and quality of care is a major step forward for research on the parental determinants of child maltreatment.

The work of Sameroff and Feil and Newberger suggests that parental social-cognitive and affective processes that are directly tied to mothers' perceptions of their relationships with their children and caretaking behaviors may be more useful than static personality traits in empirically predicting who in the general population will maltreat their children and in understanding the roots of maltreatment cases found in clinical practice. The importance of social-cognitive processes tied to relationships fits well with the need to consider the maltreating parent within a developmental framework. Aber and Zigler (1981) suggest that in order to truly understand the parental determinants of maltreatment, researchers and clinicians alike must consider the developmental level of the maltreating parent, including their own history of parenting, struggles with dependency and autonomy, cognitive stages, and internal models of relationships.

The developmental perspective adds clarity to hypotheses regarding why these broad psychological processes are such powerful predictors of quality of care. One reason may be the extent to which they reflect the caretakers' own unresolved conflict with respect to the developmental issues of nurturance and dependency. Women who have not resolved interpersonal issues of trust, dependency, and autonomy are likely to be considerably stressed when faced with the demands of a highly dependent child. With respect to meeting the needs of a child, these women will have difficulty viewing the child's behavior from the perspective of an independent, mature adult. They may also find themselves seeking to meet their own emotional needs in the context of the parent–child relationship and may experience hostility toward the child when those needs are not met. This explanation is also congruent with many of the factors that place women in a group at high risk for maltreatment. For example, parents who are young, who have a history of being maltreated as a child, or who are currently in maltreating relationships are all considered to be at risk for poor parenting (Straus, 1983).

These considerations fit well with Wolfe's (1985) conclusion that parents' vulnerability to environmental and child-induced stress are major determinants of their treatment of a child. Wolfe's emphasis on the interaction between parental vulnerability, environmental stress, and child behavior is representative of the recent process-oriented conceptual models of child maltreatment and also reflects a multifactor causal model. Wolfe provides a framework within which a variety of parental characteristics can contribute to vulnerability. The application of the developmental perspective to a multifactor model of the antecedents of maltreatment as well as a focus on broad social-cognitive processes involving parents' perceptions of relationships is likely to make a significant contribution to theoretical advances in the future.

Child characteristics

Much has been written, studied, and speculated upon concerning the possibility that the behavior of children may contribute to their own maltreatment. This possibility has been referred to as the main effects model of child characteristics as a cause of maltreatment (Cicchetti and Rizley, 1981). Just as the section on parental characteristics emphasized a complex, interactive, multivariate model of etiology, this section summarizes literature that refutes the child main effects model and argues in favor of the process-oriented multivariate model.

The child main effects model has rested upon two independent foundations. The first is Bell's (1968) paper, which calls for the reinterpretation of correlational evidence in socialization studies so that effects are seen as bidirectional, that is, that children's influences upon parents are represented in correlational evidence. The second support for child effects in maltreatment is the literature that cites the relationship between maltreatment and child features such as prematurity, handicaps, and facial features (Belsky, 1980; McCabe, 1984). The assumption underlying the child main effects literature and the studies on prematurity is that some children, because they may be difficult to care for and nonrewarding for parents, elicit maltreatment from parents who, with otherwise normal children, would not maltreat. This is an assumption which is not often made explicit in studies purporting to validate the child effects position.

Integrating the child effects position with much of what has been written recently concerning the bidirectionality of effects (Maccoby and Martin, 1983), and studies of the parenting of children with developmental delays and difficulties (Brachfield, Goldberg, and Sloman, 1980; Crnic, Greenberg, Ragozin, Robinson, and Basham, 1983; Sameroff and Chandler, 1975) suggests that there is little evidence to substantiate it in its full form. Maccoby and Martin, in their extensive review of studies of the socialization process, have outlined the process of parenting in developmental progression as the child ages from birth to the early adolescent years. Their conclusion concerning the child effects position is that, by and large, the child's effects upon parents are short-term and short-lived. That is, at a molecular level, within a particular bout or sequence of behavior the child is an active elicitor of parental responses that may differ with respect to the child's behavior. However, there is little evidence to suggest that the infant or young child *actively* contributes to the overall quality of parenting it receives or to the quality of the relationship it has with its mother and father over a long period of time. The distinction here is that child effects are likely to be present in cross-sectional or sequential episodes of parent–child interaction (Patterson, 1983); however, they do not appear to account for the variability in caretaking outcomes over time.

This is not to deny the fact that some children are difficult to parent and unrewarding or that within isolated bouts of interaction the child's behavior may elicit parental reactions that could be considered maltreating. Several studies have documented, through parental report and observation, that there are wide individual differences in children's social behavior, arousal levels, and sleep and feeding states (Thomas and Chess, 1977). Child characteristics such as irritability, fussiness, and dependency have been associated with physical abuse (Gil, 1970), and others have suggested that the unenjoyable and unrewarding-to-care-for child is likely to be a victim of maltreatment (Gelles, 1973; Parke and Collmer, 1975). In one sample of physically abused children there was an increased proportion of hyperactive or mentally retarded children (Terr, 1970), and Kempe (1971) has noted the risk for physical abuse associated with adoption and prematurity. In addition, Patterson's research (Patterson, 1983) has established reciprocal linkages between aggressive boys' behavior and the quality of parental responses.

Conversely, reviews of the literature on the consequences of raising children with "risk" characteristics overwhelmingly suggest that these characteristics alone are not enough to infer that the child will have later difficulties or will be the victim of maltreatment (Brachfield et al, 1980; Sameroff and Chandler, 1975). These reviews and observational studies are in agreement in noting the power of parental responsiveness and the caretaking milieu in overcoming early developmental difficulties as well as the inability to predict that these children will be maltreated simply on the basis of their own characteristics or behavior. Also, despite the evidence linking child behavior with adult responses to that behavior, these studies have not established that the quality of adult responses can be categorized as maltreating.

It is important to note that many of these studies are retrospective – using already identified victims of maltreatment – making it impossible to separate the effects of the child's hyperactivity or unrewardingness from the possibility that poor parenting has resulted in a child with these characteristics. The inability to separate child characteristics from quality of parenting is a fundamental problem with this literature. Many of these studies neglect the possibility that early infant problems may not be the cause of maltreatment, but instead might be a result of a breakdown in the caretaking process that may have started during pregnancy. Also, the use of retrospective designs and measures of infant temperament that are not predictive of infant behavior make many of these studies highly suspect from a variety of validity criteria (Vaughn, Deinard, and Egeland, 1980).

From a developmental viewpoint, the child is an active part in the socialization process to the extent that he or she presents parents with a set of cues for responsiveness and sensitivity as well as a set of demands upon time and resources, both personal and financial. Complicating the picture for parents is the fact that these demands change over time. Adults can be considered to be "ready" to parent at any given point in time to the extent that they are capable of being sensitive and responsive to the appropriate cues and possess adequate stores of personal and financial resources. To the extent that the child with extreme individual differences is placed in a family that may not be "ready" to parent, characteristics of that child may exacerbate an already difficult situation. This child may become the victim of maltreatment, not because of its own behavior, but because the child places added burdens upon an already stressed or incapable family system, resulting in a breakdown in the processes of good parenting. For example, parents who have yet to resolve their feelings about their own upbringing, who are involved in dysfunctional interpersonal relationships, or who are experiencing environmental stress such as unemployment may also find it difficult to meet the needs of any child, especially one who presents challenges for caretakers. It is also possible that children with substantially deviant behavioral or temperamental characteristics might place extreme stress on otherwise competent caretakers who may engage in maltreating behavior. The important point is that child, parental, and environmental characteristics may be important for determining whether maltreatment will occur (Maccoby and Martin, 1983).

This point is consistent with the "risk factor" model presented by Cicchetti and Rizley (1981). The main premise of the model is to point out that antecedents of maltreatment can only be understood from a multifactorial perspective, whereby the multiple influences of a variety of risk and protective factors are considered simultaneously. As applied to the child effects position, this model would emphasize the importance of risk and protective factors due to both parent and child characteristics as well as environmental stressors in attempting to account for the development of maltreatment. From this perspective the main effects model of child characteristics as a cause of maltreatment is not tenable.

Having discussed the extent to which both members of the parent–child dyad may influence the development of maltreating parenting styles, and alluding to the importance of environmental factors, it is important to discuss more fully the role of the environment as an antecedent to child maltreatment. The following section addresses this task.

Characteristics of the environment

Characteristics of the psychosocial environments of families engaging in child maltreatment have been repeatedly implicated as possible causes of the maltreatment (Belsky, 1980). Specific factors such as family violence, unemployment, a lack of social support, and household poverty and disorganization have been noted as possible determinants (Belsky, 1980; Straus, 1983; Tonge, James, and Hillam, 1975).

In their examination of family violence in America, Straus, Gelles, and Steinmitz (1980) and Straus (1983) have noted the powerful relationship between violence in the marital relationship and child maltreatment. Straus has recently reported that high rates of ordinary violence in families, such as the use of physical punishment, is a factor that predicts rates of more extreme violence such as physical abuse. In this paper Straus also notes that wives who experience violence in their marital relationships tend to be more violent toward their children; the more extreme the violence they experience themselves, the greater is their tendency to physically abuse their children.

Marital violence and the associated parenting also appears to be one important determinant of maltreatment in the next generation. Boys who have witnessed physical spouse abuse are prone to physically abuse their own spouses and children when they become husbands and fathers (Rosenbaum and O'Leary, 1981). Straus (1983) demonstrated that this relationship also holds for both boys and girls who experience ordinary violence as a child. Straus concludes that ordinary violence and the more extreme forms of violence, such as spouse abuse, are culturally sanctioned forms of problem solving learned by wives, children, and siblings and practiced in the family context. A different theoretical perspective suggests these children may have difficulty developing internal working models for human relationships based on expressions of warmth, sensitivity, affection, and trust (Bowlby, 1980). The extent to which these internal working models are validated when the children become adults (Sroufe and Fleeson, 1986) may also account for some cases of intergenerational continuity in maltreatment. A more specific discussion of intergenerational continuity in maltreatment will be presented in a later section of this chapter.

Parental unemployment is another factor in the psychosocial environment that has been associated with physical abuse of children and spouses (Galdston, 1965; Gelles, 1973; Gil, 1970; Light, 1973; Steinmitz and Straus, 1974). Although loss of self-esteem, economic hardship, and frustration have been speculated to be the reasons for this association, few studies have directly addressed the actual process by which unemployment is linked with maltreatment. In addition, maternal unemployment, occurring when single mothers are unable to be employed, has been associated with material deprivation and physical abuse of and neglect of children (Horowitz and Wolcock, 1981). The fact that studies have been unable to isolate a single process by which unemployment affects caretaking suggests that unemployment is a general stressor that involves many areas of family life. Therefore, it is likely that its effect on caretaking will be due to differences in family and individual coping styles.

One environmental factor noted as both a risk factor and a means of buffering the family system against the negative effects of conditions such as unemployment is the quality of relationships in the family social network (Garbarino, 1982). For example, Garbarino and Sherman (1980) have demonstrated that when neighborhoods are equated on such characteristics as SES, race, income, and education, there was a significantly greater amount of child maltreatment in the area identified as "at risk" on the basis of residents' reports. Distinguishing characteristics of the at risk neighborhood were the lack of supervision for children, the lack of a network for alternative child care for working mothers, and a general lack of helpfulness among neighbors. However, the presence of community resource centers and availability of social service agencies appeared to distinguish the "healthy" neighborhoods in this study.

The most salient difference between the two types of neighborhoods, however, was the availability of networks of neighbors who performed specific, concrete tasks for parents (mostly single mothers), tasks directed at reducing economic stresses and personal burdens. For example, the single, working mother who was struggling to earn a living and provide care for her children received relief from neighbors who took care of her children after school or were able to do food shopping and provide transportation (Belle, 1982).

Other investigators have also noted the prevalence of single mothers in maltreating families (Horowitz and Wolcock, 1981). Mothers involved in coercive relationships with their sons often report significant experiences of isolation and are also likely to be single mothers, and this isolation appears to be causally linked to bouts of aggression and hostility between parent and child (Wahler, Leske, and Rogers, 1980). Belle (1982) has emphasized the stresses of single parenting as a drain on the emotional and financial resources of the woman.

The importance of social support networks is underscored in the single parent literature and has been demonstrated in the literature on parenting difficult children and in studies that have addressed the prevention of maltreatment (Garbarino, 1982; Crnic, Greenberg, Ragozin, Robinson, and Basham, 1983). The social support literature indicates that the emotional resources of the caregiver, although obviously taxed by parenting a young child or infant, need to be replenished in some way if the parent–child dyad is to function within developmentally appropriate constraints. Lack of intimate emotional support may be a factor that increases the likelihood of maltreatment when it is severe or if it occurs within a constellation of other exacerbating factors such as physical violence or poverty. The role in determining maltreatment of a variety of the psychosocial factors noted above is especially emphasized in a study by Tonge, James, and Hillam.

In a sample of poverty households in England, Tonge, James, and Hillam (1975) noted that the majority of the children were neglected physically and emotionally and at least half of the marriages were marked by lack of support and discord in the form of aggressive and physically abusive husbands. The majority of these mothers handled discipline in an inconsistent and highly punitive manner with their children, were unprotective of their children, and did not supervise them when in dangerous situations. Tonge et al. note that this sample was characterized by a disorder of lifestyle, where the parents were often poorly educated, unemployed, and themselves had come from highly disorganized, disordered homes. The constellation of the characteristics of poverty, poor education, authoritarian child rearing, insularity, maternal depression, and paternal alcohol abuse and unemployment was present within these families for generations.

Extreme disorganization and insularity were noteworthy characteristics of the homes studied by Tonge et al. The family context was marked by constant crisis and chaos. For many families daily events were highly unpredictable and there was little organization or structure to family life. For example, meals were unplanned, children roamed the city unsupervised, and there was a lack of daily routines surrounding parental employment, going to school, or family activities. Within this atmosphere, children had few means of developing self control and often this lack precipitated struggles with parents that ended with violence. These families also tended to consistently neglect the physical and emotional needs of the children.

Although this study is not meant to characterize all maltreating families, it portrays a picture of the extent to which environmental factors are linked within the family system to domestic violence and several forms of child maltreatment. The importance of this study to understanding the antecedents of child maltreatment lies in its emphasis on the linkages among these factors and the manner in which each particular antecedent may create the context for other risk conditions that ultimately produce the more visible outcome of physical abuse and neglect of children. Once again, it is useful to conceptualize these multiple antecedents using the type of risk factor model noted by Cicchetti and Rizley (1981) with respect to intergenerational continuity and applied earlier in this chapter in the discussion of parent and child effects.

The selection of an appropriate integrative model for research on the antecedents of child maltreatment

As alluded to earlier, there are a number of issues that have plagued research on the antecedents of child maltreatment. Generally, maltreatment research has employed a single-cause research model that has relied on examining differences in a particular domain – parental, child, or environmental – between maltreatment and control groups as opposed to multivariate research incorporating measures from each of these domains. Methodological problems also plague much single cause research. These issues are discussed in this section, with the intention of deriving what could be a more appropriate integrative model for research and theory.

Single cause research: methodology and models. The methodology employed by studies of the antecedents of child maltreatment is a critical factor in evaluating the importance of a particular "cause." The majority of studies demonstrating relationships between maltreatment and antecedent factors have used retrospective designs (Belsky, 1980; Cicchetti and Aber, 1980; Cicchetti and Rizley, 1981; Egeland and Brunnquell, 1979). That is, a group of maltreatment victims or maltreating parents has been identified after the fact and investigators have looked backward in time, within this group, to examine relationships between present maltreatment and past child or parent characteristics. Such an approach suffers from what Garmezy (1977a) calls the "etiological error," whereby looking backward in time will always produce a "cause." From a developmental perspective, these studies fail to enlighten our knowledge about the processes underlying maltreatment and, at an applied level, they fail to produce efficient prediction.

For this reason we emphasize the value of prospective studies of maltreatment and studies of at risk populations (Garmezy, 1977b). In this type of research, groups of parents and their children are identified on the basis of broad risk factors related to nonoptimal parenting – for example, low income populations. These families are then enrolled in longitudinal studies that trace the development of the parent–child relationship and the child outcomes. Heuristically, the factors identified through single-cause retrospective research are useful as broad indicators of risk, although they are not viewed as necessary or sufficient in a causal sense. In prospective research it is possible to examine the antecedents of maltreatment in predictive fashion and to identify those characteristics that enhance the development of nonoptimal caretaking, those that maintain it, and those that appear to discriminate at risk groups that do not maltreat from those who do.

Another flaw in research using a single cause model has been the failure to consider the error involved in using single causes in prediction. For example, it has been hypothesized that lack of an appropriate mother–infant "bond" in the immediate postpartum period may be a reason why mothers engage in subsequent maltreatment (Fanaroff, Kennell, and Klaus, 1972; Klaus and Kennel, 1970, 1976). However, for the great majority of children reared in the United States in the last several decades, separation from mothers in the immediate postpartum period was routine. If the bonding hypothesis were true, one would expect rates of child maltreatment to approach the base rate of maternal–infant separation, which is clearly not the case. This example highlights the consequences of failing to examine the results of using single causes to predict rates or cases of child maltreatment, whereby the linkages among hypothesized causal agents and possible moderator variables, as well as the effects of base rate on prediction, are ignored. The overall result of this single cause research is a literature that purports to identify causes, but is inefficient when used for predictive purposes.

Theoretical attempts to address the causes of child maltreatment have relied on this type of single cause research, and models have been proposed that attempt to include many of the antecedents identified by it (Gelles, 1973). The resulting theories have been important to developing an understanding that child maltreatment is a multidimensional and multidetermined phenomenon, yet they have less adequately addressed questions regarding which, if any, antecedents are most critical in predicting maltreatment in the general population or in understanding why particular parents maltreat their children. As has been noted elsewhere, researchers must begin to focus their efforts toward developing a more process-oriented theory of maltreatment if these questions are to be answered (Cicchetti and Rizley, 1981).

In the previous section we emphasized that poverty, unemployment, poor and crowded living conditions, social isolation, and marital conflict all stress caretakers in ways that may influence the quality of caretaking (Egeland, Cicchetti, and Taraldson, 1976). However, it is true that not all caretakers exposed to these stressors maltreat their children and not all maltreated children have a particular pattern of stressors in common. In addition, we have noted the existence of particular patterns of social-cognitive processes in some samples of maltreating parents. The numerous factors that apparently distinguish samples of maltreating and control groups in single cause studies present a dilemma for researchers seeking to identify a causal pattern among the antecedents of maltreatment and for the practitioner searching for targets of prevention and intervention efforts. Rather than being faced with a linear model of single causes, conceptualizations of maltreatment now acknowledge the multidimensionality of the phenomenon (Maccoby and Martin, 1983), including a complex network of causal agents linked together in cycles of potentiating, buffering, and reciprocal effects (Cicchetti and Rizley, 1981).

Multivariate models. Faced with this more complex conceptualization of the antecedents of maltreatment, it has been a temptation to embark upon multivariate model building based on single cause research. The resulting models of maltreatment attempt to incorporate many possible antecedents and effects in one comprehensive structure often resembling a flow chart (Gelles, 1973). A major problem with these models is that they are often pictorial reviews of the single cause literature, depicting the results of studies that are quite heterogeneous with respect to definitions of maltreatment, samples, and measurements. Given this methodological and conceptual heterogeneity, it becomes difficult to draw valid inferences regarding either causal processes in any particular population or with respect to the relative strength of any specific causal agent.

Integrative multivariate models. This criticism of some multivariate models of maltreatment highlights a distinction between multivariate models based upon single cause research and comprehensive, integrative models based upon multivariate research. The second type of model, as opposed to the first, has its roots in the identification of multiple antecedents within the same research program or study. Given relatively narrow definitions of maltreatment and its different forms (Aber and Zigler, 1981) and a prospective methodology, these integrative models have the potential to enlighten our understanding of the causes of maltreatment. Many of the research programs described in this volume are representative of this second type of model building.

The model proposed by Cicchetti and Rizley (1981) to account for intergenerational transmission of maltreatment is a specific example of a model that may be tested and refined using multivariate research. Within that model it is proposed that a number of risk and protective factors influence the family in such a way as to account for intergenerational continuity or discontinuity in maltreatment. The time trajectory and relative severity of these factors also affect the parameters of caretaking in such a way as to be influential in causing maltreatment in the second generation. As has been implied in earlier sections of this chapter, this model may also be useful in accounting for the influence of a number of antecedent factors of all forms of maltreatment, not just intergenerational types.

The task of integration is a large and important one in the field of child maltreatment if theoretical and social policy needs are to be addressed (Aber and Zigler, 1981). Integration may involve the development of research paradigms or models of maltreatment, such as the one described above (Cicchetti and Rizley, 1981), that provide researchers and clinicians with an overall framework within which to conceptualize and test hypotheses regarding antecedents of maltreatment in a variety of research and clinical populations. For example, questions regarding the interaction between the risk factors of poverty and single parenthood with the protective factor of social support may be conceptualized and tested within the Cicchetti and Rizley type of framework through some type of short-term longitudinal risk research.

However, another aspect of integration exists that has been less adequately developed in the field of child maltreatment. This is the identification of specific factors that capture the integrated effects of the multiple antecedents of maltreatment identified in any specific population or sample. This second integrative task is focused more directly on identifying the causal processes that explain maltreatment within any one specific case and across a variety of cases. For example, given that we may know that in some populations social support of a particular type may buffer the effects of poverty and single parenthood, what are the social and psychological processes that explain this finding? Related to this is the question: Given a particular constellation of stressors and supports in one family and a related but different pattern in another, what processes account for differences between the families in quality of care?

Starting with the premise that all cases of maltreatment have in common the existence of a relationship between caretaker and child in which the caretaker is "obligated" to meet the physical and emotional needs of the child (Maccoby and Martin, 1983), a starting point in the search for integrative factors may be the parental psychological processes that guide their caretaking behaviors and may also be affected by child behaviors and psychosocial factors. In this chapter we have proposed that parents' understanding and feelings about caretaking as well as their own personal emotional state are central determinants of the quality of care they give children.

We emphasize that it is highly likely that the psychological characteristics of maltreating caregivers are intertwined in mutually causal relationships with child characteristics, external stressors to which they are currently exposed, and their own developmental history. Addressing the second aspect of the task of integration noted above, it is possible to consider that the psychological characteristics of maltreating caregivers may be more central to the process of maltreatment than factors such as psychosocial stressors. The broad social-cognitive processes discussed in an earlier section represent the current state of the parents' own developmental journey (Aber and Zigler, 1891) and may be representative of the internal working model of self and relationships (Bowlby, 1980) that parents use to interpret and filter the environmental input of caretaking demands, children's characteristics, and behavior and environmental stressors.

In earlier sections we reviewed studies linking parental, child, and environmental variables to child maltreatment. In evaluating this research we used as a criterion the extent to which hypothesized causal agents fit within a conceptual model that is developmentally and process oriented. This review process has derived several conclusions with regard to research and theory on the antecedents of child maltreatment.

In an integrative, multivariate model for research on the antecedents of child maltreatment, consideration is given to the interaction, over time, of the three domains of antecedents discussed previously: parent, child, and environmental characteristics. This model differs from other multivariate etiological models by emphasizing the central role of parental psychological characteristics as the primary agent through which child or environmental factors influence caretaking. These parental factors may be broad psychological processes of a social cognitive nature that are linked to parents' feelings about caretaking (Newberger and Cook, 1983, Sameroff and Feil, 1984) and their internal working models of self and relationships (Bowlby, 1980). This model suggests that, although certain features of children may be important for understanding why maltreatment may occur in isolated instances, research that emphasizes the importance of child characteristics is not likely to further our understanding of the causes of maltreatment without making reference to factors influencing parents' interpretation of these characteristics. Environmental factors linked with maltreatment play a critical role in the integrative multivariate model. The complex network of buffering and exacerbating relationships that may exist within any family's social network is seen as a major determinant of a family's level of vulnerability to maltreatment, primarily due to influences upon parental psychological processes and resources.

Validation of this type of integrative model requires prospective, longitudinal multivariate research that adheres to a multifactor, process-oriented view of maltreatment. We maintain that in order for integrative models of child maltreatment to be developed there is a need for multivariate research to address the roles of parental characteristics, developmental history, and environmental stress and support in predicting maltreatment. The Mother–Child Interaction Research Project, as mentioned earlier, has been specifically designed to address these needs. The following sections will present a summary of research conducted by the Mother–Child Project on the antecedents of child maltreatment and a discussion of the extent to which this research contributes to an integrated understanding of etiology.

The Mother–Child Interaction Research Project: a brief overview

The Mother–Child Interaction Research Project at the University of Minnesota has been specifically designed to address the need for developing an integrative model of the antecedents of child maltreatment (Egeland and Deinard, 1975–1978; Egeland, Deinard, and Sroufe, 1978–1983, 1983–1987). This research is a prospective, longitudinal study of 267 primiparous women and their children, who at the time of enrollment in the study were considered to be "at risk" for maltreatment due to economic disadvantage. In order to increase the probability of finding a greater than average incidence of poor quality caretaking and developmental problems and disorders, subjects were selected as economically disadvantaged on the basis of receiving their prenatal care through public assistance clinics. Many of the risk factors presented earlier were present in the sample. For example, the mothers were young – mean age at the time of birth of their child was 20.5 (range 12 to 37); 62% were single; 40% had not completed high school; and 86% of the pregnancies were unplanned. As a group these were and are multiproblem families living in chaotic and disruptive environments. Since the early stages of the research project several mothers have moved on to live very stable lives without economic hardship. At this point in time, although the project sample retains much of its at risk status, there is also a great deal of variability in child and family outcomes.

Detailed and comprehensive multiple assessments of child and parental competence began at birth and have continued at regularly scheduled intervals through the early school years. Extensive data has also been collected on characteristics of the children, parents, child–parent interaction, and the environment, including life circumstances, stress, and support. These assessments have allowed us to account for adaptive as well as maladaptive outcomes at each developmental period through the early school years, a process that has enabled us to isolate some of the factors that appear to account for continuities and discontinuities in development. Table 7.1 provides a description of the measures used in the analyses presented in this chapter and in the Erickson, Egeland, and Pianta chapter, this volume.

Table 7.1. *List of measures: Mother-Child Interaction Project*

Information obtained during last trimester		
Measure	Variable measured	Developed by
Shipley Hartford Vocabulary Test	Intelligence	Shipley and Hartford (1946)

Personality Research form
  Aggression
  Defendence
  Impulsivity
  Succorance
	Personality characteristics	Jackson (1967)

IPAT Anxiety scale questionnaire	Anxiety	Cattell and Scheier (1963)
Inventory of beliefs	Locus of control	Rotter (1966)
Neonatal perception inventory	Mother's expectations	Broussard and Hartner (1971)

Maternal Attitude Scale:
Questionnaire for mothers
  Appropriate versus inappropriate control of child's aggression
  Encouragement versus discouragement of reciprocity
  Acceptance versus denial of emotional complexity in child care
	Mother's attitude toward developing mother–child relationship	Cohler, Weiss, and Grunebaum (1970)

Pregnancy Research Questionnaire
  Fear for self
  Desire for pregnancy
  Dependency
  Fear for baby
  Maternal feelings
  Irritability and tension
	Mother's feelings regarding pregnancy	Schaefer and Manheimer (1960)

Knowledge of child care and expectations of child development questionnaire	Mother's knowledge	Staff
Interview of mother	General information, social support, family background	Staff
Information obtained at birth		
Nurses' ratings of newborn	Infant temperament and characteristics	Staff
Brazelton Behavioral and Neurological Assessment Scale	Psychological and physiological characteristics of newborn	Brazelton (1973)
First days questionnaire	General information	Staff

Table 7.1 *(cont.)*

Information obtained at three months[a]		
Measure	Variable measured	Developed by
Life Stress Scale	Amount of environmental stress on mother	Cochrane and Robertson (1973); Staff
Enjoyment of baby scale	Mother's feelings regarding infant	Staff
Carey Infant Temperament Scale	Infant temperament	Carey (1970)
Three-month observation and rating:	Observation of mother–infant interaction	Staff
Waiting room rating scale		Staff
Doctor's rating scale		Ainsworth (1969);
Observation of feeding situation in home		Staff

Information obtained at six months		
Observation of feeding and play in home	Observation of mother–infant interaction	Ainsworth (1969); Staff

Information obtained at nine months		
Bayley Scale of Infant Development	Infant's mental and motor development	Bayley (1969)
Mother's expectations of child's ability	Mother's expectation of child's performance on Bayley	Staff
Observation of mother and infant during Bayley	Mother–Infant interaction	Staff

Information obtained at 12 months		
Strange Situation	Security of attachment	Ainsworth and Wittig (1969)
Interview of mother	General information including involvement with Child Protection Services	Staff
Habituation task	Attentional development of child	Staff
Life Stress Scale	Amount of environmental stress on mother	Cochrane and Robertson (1973); Staff
Prohibition of forbidden objects	Ratings of mother's style of discipline	Staff

Throughout first year		
Childcare rating scale	Ratings of quality of care during home observation	Staff

220

Table 7.1 *(cont.)*

Tests given at 18 months		
Measure	Variable measured	Developed by
Strange Situation	Security of attachment	Ainsworth and Wittig (1969)
Interview of mother	General information regarding social support, involvement with Child Protection	Staff

Information obtained at 24 months		
Tool Using and Problem Solving Laboratory Observation Procedure	Seven point ratings of child dependency, frustration, noncompliance, persistence, coping, enthusiasm, anger, maternal assistance, and support	Matas, Arend, and Sroufe (1978)
Child development scale	Mother's knowledge of child development norms	Staff
Childcare practices	Mother's knowledge of childcare practices	Staff
Acquiring childcare information	Where mother acquires information	Staff
Interview	Mother's knowledge of children and childcare practices, quality of emotional support, referral to Child Protection Services	Staff
Childcare rating scale	Quality of childcare observed in home	Staff

Information obtained at 30 months		
Life Events Inventory	Stressful life events	Cochrane and Robertson (1973); Staff
Source of information questionnaire	Source of knowledge about child rearing	Staff
Caldwell HOME Inventory, home observation	Social, emotional, and cognitive stimulation, quality of the home environment	Caldwell, Heider, and Kaplan (1966)
Interview of mother	General information, life circumstances, quality of emotional support, referral to Child Protection Services	Staff

221

Table 7.1 *(cont.)*

Information obtained at 42 months		
Measure	Variable measured	Developed by
Life Event Inventory	Stressful life events	Cochrane and Robertson (1973); Staff
Interview of mother	Involvement with Child Protection, social agencies, childcare practices, quality of emotional support	Staff
Barrier box laboratory procedure	Seven point ratings of Child Dependency, self-esteem, ego control, apathy, flexibility, creativity, agency, hyperactivity, positive and negative affect	Staff
Teaching task laboratory procedure	Mother var: supportive, respect for autonomy, struct., hostility, qual. of inst., confidence. Child var: persistence, enthusiasm, negativity, exp. in session, reliance on mother, affect for mother, avoidance of mother	Staff
Information obtained at 48 months		
Life Event Inventory	Stressful life events	Cochrane and Robertson (1973); Staff
Profile of Moods	Mother's affective mood	McNair, Lorr, and Droppleman (1971)
CES–D Scale	Maternal depression	Radloff (1977)
Symptom checklist	Child behavior problems	Staff
Wechsler Adult Intelligence Scale	Maternal intelligence	Wechsler (1955)
IPAT Anxiety Scale	Maternal anxiety	Cattell and Scheier (1963)
Interview of mother	General information, relationship status, quality of emotional support, mother's experience of maltreatment as a child, referral of mother to Child Protection Services	Staff

Table 7.1 *(cont.)*

Information obtained at 54 months		
Measure	Variable measured	Developed by
Mother interview	General information, life circumstances, maternal childrearing history, quality of emotional support, referral to Child Protection Services	Staff
Life Event Scale	Stressful life events	Cochrane and Robertson (1973); Staff

Information obtained at 64 months		
Mother interview	Family and work status, feelings about present life situation and child, social life, quality of emotional support, referral to Child Protective Services	Staff
Childcare rating scale	Quality of child care observed in home	Staff
Life Event Scale	Stressful life events	Cochrane and Robertson (1973); Staff
16 PF	Maternal personality	Cattell (1967)
Wechsler Preschool and Primary Scale of Intelligence	Child intelligence	Wechsler (1967)

Definitions of maltreatment

As noted by other investigators (Aber and Zigler, 1981; Cicchetti and Aber, 1980; Cicchetti and Rizley, 1981), definitional issues account for a great deal of the variance in the results of empirical studies of child maltreatment. The lack of precise, developmentally based definitions has impeded the progress toward an understanding of the processes by which child maltreatment develops.

Our conceptualization of maltreatment has been based upon what we consider to be the parameters of caretaking outcomes that enhance the optimal development of the child. It has been a consistent finding in the parenting literature that predictable, available, sensitive, and responsive caretaking within a structured and organized home environment enhances the development of children (Maccoby and Martin, 1983). Therefore, the way we have defined maltreatment concerns the extent to which parents qualitatively or quantitatively deviate from that pattern. The forms of maltreatment we have identified using this framework have ranged from a global identification of inadequate care to the more specific subtypes of physical abuse, physical neglect, psychological unavailability, and sexual abuse. What follows is a brief description of the maltreatment groups we have periodically formed on the basis of information collected between birth and age 6. In all cases of physical or sexual abuse and in many cases of the other types of maltreatment the children were known to county child protection agencies and some type of intervention was present. Information on families' involvement with child protection services was provided by mothers and cross checked with county files.

Maltreatment groups at one year. When the children were approximately 1 year old we made an assessment of global maltreatment without identifying specific subtypes. At each visit to the mothers' homes (3, 6, 9, and 12 months) a Child Care Rating Scale (Egeland and Brunquell, 1979) was administered. This involved ratings of evidence of violence in the household, poor physical care, unsanitary conditions, and neglect. On the basis of these direct observations, subjects were assigned to an inadequate care group by conferenced judgment of interviewers and project staff. Within the total sample, 32 mothers were identified as seriously maltreating their infant during the first year of the child's life (inadequate care group). Some examples of signs leading to a classification of maltreatment were untreated wounds, no place for the child to sleep, leaving the child without supervision, and exposure to hazards. All of the mothers in the maltreatment group were identified using the observational Child Care Rating Scale and all of the interviewers who had contact with the families agreed upon this classification. In support of this categorization, 11 of these cases had been previously detected by independent child protection referrals and no child protection cases were missed by our procedure. Again, information on families' involvement with child protection was provided by mothers in the course of obtaining interview data and periodically cross-checked with county files.

A control group of 33 adequate mothers (excellent care group) was identified on the basis of observation in the home by trained testers. These women, from the same high-risk sample, met the physical and emotional needs of their children in a competent manner. They responded to their infants' cues in a sensitive and predictable fashion, interacted in a cooperative way with their children, and encouraged growth and development.

The results from comparing these groups lends credence to considering the role of maternal characteristics in maltreatment (Brunnquell, Crichton, and Egeland, 1981; Egeland and Brunnquell, 1979). In general, mothers in the abusive group were younger, less educated, and less prepared for pregnancy and they differed on a wide variety of personality and attitude measures (Egeland and Brunnquell, 1979). However, a particularly salient variable that discriminated the good from maltreating caretakers was a measure of "psychological complexity" (Cohler, Weiss, and Greenbaum, 1970) that tapped the mother's understanding of and relationship with the infant.

Specifically, by combining baby variables, mothers' psychological characteristics, and mother–infant interaction variables, a correct classification rate of 85 percent was obtained (Egeland and Brunnquell, 1979). The variables, in order of importance, were: quality of mothers' feeding behavior and mothers' level of affective responsiveness observed at 3 months in a feeding situation, babies' orienting behavior as measured by the Brazelton Neonatal Assessment Scale at 7 days postpartum, babies' social behavior observed in the 3-month feeding situation, and the measure of mothers' "psychological complexity." The remainder of the variables in the multiple discriminate function analysis did not add to the prediction of group membership. The global ratings of mothers in the feeding situation and the comprehensive measure of "psychological complexity" were each highly predictive of the quality of care received by children in a high-risk sample.

The role of environmental stress was also addressed in examining these groups. In distinguishing the inadequate care and excellent care groups, it was found that even though maltreating mothers experienced more stressful events than controls, there were a number of maltreating families that experienced a relatively small number of stressful events. Similarly, many of the families providing adequate care were experiencing large amounts of stress (Egeland, Breitenbucher, and Rosenberg, 1980). The investigators examined what distinguished the mother with a high life events score who did not mistreat her child from one with a similar score who did maltreat. It was not the number or type of stressors that appeared to distinguish the groups. Instead, the maltreating mothers were characterized prenatally by their relatively high level of anxiety, aggression, dependence, and defensiveness as well as being less aware of the difficulties and demands of parenting. These high-stressed mothers who maltreated their children appeared to cope with stress in an angry and ineffective fashion. The stressful life events appeared to permeate every aspect of their lives and were not isolated to specific situations. These results suggest that the maltreating mothers may have been predisposed to react more vulnerably to psychosocial stressors in a manner that led them to maltreat their children. In terms of the integrative model, it was the interaction between the psychological characteristics of vulnerable, at risk mothers and exposure to environmental stressors that predicted maltreatment at 1 year.

Maltreatment groups at two years. A wide variety of data was collected on children and families in the child's second year of life. This included extensive interviewing of mothers, observations in homes using the Child Care Rating Scale, and a laboratory assessment of mother–child interaction during play and semistructured tasks. In addition, as before, the maternal interview included information regarding involvement with county child protective services. Each set of data provided us with an opportunity to make judgments regarding the quality of care received by the children. Using all available data, a team of project staff members conferenced and classified subjects into one or more of several maltreatment categories. Despite the subjective nature of identifying maltreating mothers, there was nearly perfect agreement among staff members.

This process identified four groups of women from the original sample of 267 mothers who were maltreating their children at 2 years of age: physically abusive ($n = 24$), hostile/verbally abusive ($n = 19$), psychologically unavailable ($n = 19$), and neglectful ($n = 24$). As is often the case in maltreatment classifications using specific categories (Cicchetti and Rizley, 1981; Gersten, Coster, Scheider-Rosen, Carlson, and Cicchetti, 1986) there were some women who fit more than one classification. Altogether there were 44 women who fit at least one category of maltreatment. The specific breakdown of overlapping cases, with number of corresponding subjects in parentheses, was as follows: psychologically unavailable and neglectful (2), psychologically unavailable and physically abusive (1), physically abusive and neglectful (1), neglectful and verbally abusive (0), physically and verbally abusive (4), psychologically unavailable and verbally abusive (1), psychologically unavailable, physically abusive, and neglectful (4), psychologically unavailable and verbally and physically abusive (3), verbally and physically abusive and neglectful (4), and there were three cases who met the descriptions of all four of the maltreatment types. All overlap cases were mothers who clearly fit the criteria for each group in which they were placed despite our efforts to make the groups as mutually exclusive as possible. It is unfortunate – from a classification perspective – that behavioral patterns that compose a function as complex as caretaking do not group themselves into neat, nonoverlapping categories. However, it is apparent from our observations of these mothers that it is not unlikely for children to experience more than one subtype of maltreatment at a given point in time.

Behaviors of the mothers in the physically abusive group ranged from frequent and intense spanking in disciplining their children to unprovoked angry outbursts resulting in severe injuries, such as cigarette burns. In many cases these were actually observed in the home or during laboratory tasks; in the other cases these behaviors were reported by mothers. In all instances the abuse was seen as physically damaging to the child. All of the women in this group were involved with child protection services as reported by the mothers and cross-checked with county files.

Mothers in the hostile/verbally abusive group chronically found fault with their children and criticized them in an extremely harsh fashion. This form of maltreatment involved constant berating and harassment of the child. For example, in an assessment of mother–child interaction during a problem-solving task at 24 months, children experiencing verbal abuse would be met with insults when they asked for assistance or would be told "you're so dumb." Other examples include more blatant hostility indicated by a very angry tone of voice or yelling at the child (e.g., "listen to me").

The mothers in the psychologically unavailable group were unresponsive to their children and in many cases passively rejected them. These mothers appeared detached and uninvolved with their children, interacting with them only when it appeared necessary. For example, in the problem-solving situation at 24 months, these mothers would ignore their child's cues for help and assistance, offer no encouragement to the child even if the child was failing to perform the task, and would appear comfortable even when the child was highly frustrated. These women took very few steps to protect their childrens' self esteem. In general, they were withdrawn, displayed flat affect and seemed depressed. There was no indication that these mothers derived any pleasure or satisfaction from their relationship with their children.

Mothers in the neglect group were irresponsible or incompetent in managing the day-to-day activities and care of their children. Their responses to interview procedures indicated that they failed to provide for the necessary health care of their children. Observation in the home indicated that they did not provide adequate physical care and did little to protect the children from dangers in the home. For several cases, the children were observed to have extremely poor hygiene and appeared malnourished. Although these mothers might have expressed interest in the well-being of their children, they lacked the skill, knowledge, or understanding to provide consistent, adequate care.

Finally, we identified a group of good caretakers to use as a control and comparison group ($n = 85$). These mothers were again identified by conferenced agreement among staff members using the criterion that they could not have been considered candidates for classification in any of the maltreatment groups. Therefore, they represent an average sample within the high-risk group and were not selected for excellent care. Generally, mothers in this group were characterized by responsive, sensitive caretaking; they managed to see to it that their children's needs for emotional and physical nurturance were met on a regular basis and there was no evidence whatsoever that any of their children suffered from any form of maltreatment. These good caretaking controls were selected from the same high-risk sample as the maltreatment groups and did not differ from them on the demographic characteristics of age or income level.

Our definition of maltreatment at 24 months, based upon developmentally appropriate caretaking parameters and not solely upon "casedness," identified 44 maltreating parents out of a sample of 267. This reflects a base rate for maltreatment in our high-risk sample of approximately 16 percent; in excess of the 5 percent cited nationwide (Gil, 1970) and confirmation of the risk status of the group. This increased prevalence of maltreatment within our sample may be explained by three possibilities. First, the sample was selected in order to increase the probability of maltreatment and therefore was intended to include a greater than base rate prevalence of maltreating mothers. Second, conceptualizing maltreatment in terms of the broad parameters of good parenting mentioned earlier increases the prevalence of identified maltreatment victims beyond the prevalence based upon overt physical or sexual insult, the common basis of identification. This results in a less stringent definition of maltreatment than the legal definition that is commonly used. Finally, our close association with these families over the years has enabled us to obtain information on quality of care that would not be possible to obtain in cross-sectional or retrospective studies.

These three possibilities – a high risk sample, use of a less than stringent definition of maltreatment, and close knowledge of families – all contribute to the high rate of maltreatment obtained in this sample. The difference in prevalence of maltreatment between the Mother–Child Project sample and other estimates suggests that studies of the antecedents of maltreatment that use county or state child protection records as their means of sample selection (i.e., a legal definition of maltreatment) may not be reflective of the factors associated with maltreatment in families who do not come to the attention of child protection agencies. In fact, most discussions of the prevalence of child maltreatment suggest that it is a more prevalent phenomenon than statistics indicate (Garbarino, 1982).

Continuity of maltreatment at one and two years. Continuity of maltreatment was determined by examining the overlap between the 1 year inadequate care group and the maltreatment groups formed at 2 years (collapsed to form a broad maltreatment group). Overall, 27 of the original 32 women in the Inadequate Care group remained in the study at 2 years. The five subjects who dropped out of the study between one and two years tended to be characterized by extremely chaotic households and parental psychopathology. Of the 27 subjects remaining in the study, 23 were classified in at least one of the maltreatment groups at 2 years, an overlap of 85 percent. Of the four subjects with a history of maltreatment at 1 year who were not classified in the maltreatment groups at 2 years, one child had been adopted out of the home, one had been placed with the grandmother as the primary caretaker, and two were being maltreated by their fathers. These last two were considered to be not maltreating at two years because it was the mothers who were identified as maltreating at 1 year.

Generally, this analysis suggests that inadequate care was consistent across the period measured and that there is a high rate of continuity within families for maltreatment of children. Further examination of the "discontinuous" subjects supports this conclusion in that the changes in caretaking arrangements appeared to be due to ongoing maltreatment and the fact that, despite two of the mothers no longer maltreating, the children were still being maltreated by fathers.

Maltreatment groups at six years. Recently a determination was made as to whether the children in the sample were receiving adequate caretaking at approximately 6 years of age based upon information collected concurrently and in the previous two years. As before, this information was obtained through a variety of data gathering procedures: observation of the home environment, anecdotal observation of mother–child interaction in the home, and maternal interview (see Table 7.1 for a list of data gathering procedures). We had the opportunity to interview the mothers in detail during the summers following kindergarten and first grade and to visit the children's homes. These interviews involved extensive questioning regarding child care practices, the mother's feelings about caretaking and her perceptions of her child. Classification of subjects as maltreating or not was made by conferenced agreement by projects staff and interviewers.

Once again, a developmental perspective guided our selection of nonoptimal styles of caretaking. As in previous years, we continued to be concerned with whether the child was being physically abused, as this constitutes a gross violation of interpersonal boundaries and reflects blatant insensitivity. We also continued to identify psychologically unavailable caretaking, as the uninvolvement and unresponsiveness of a caretaker constitutes a great risk to the child's continued emotional development through the early school years (Maccoby and Martin, 1983). The definitions of these groups remained the same as at 2 years, although the contexts of observing the signs and signals of these forms of maltreatment had changed.

The physical abuse group ($n = 16$) at 6 years continued to present a similar picture to the group identified at an earlier time period. For example, these mothers engaged in unprovoked violent outbursts, excessive physical punishment, and beatings of their children. The children in this group were identified on the basis of the mothers' admission of abusive parenting practices, observation of physically abusive behaviors in the home, or by additional cross-checking of child protection records.

The psychologically unavailable group ($n = 16$) also remains similar in characterization to the group identified at 2 years. These women often admitted that they did not like their children and would rather be left without them. Many of these mothers did not attempt to provide comfort to their children in distress and they openly did not enjoy interacting with them. These mothers often appeared depressed and listless and made no effort at emotionally engaging their children.

The third maltreatment group at 6 years was composed of neglecting mothers ($n = 17$), who were identified on the basis of the child's physical environment or needs for appropriate supervision. Neglected children were exposed to unsupervised, unstructured, and unorganized home environments. Mothers in this group left their young children unsupervised for long periods of time or in dangerous conditions, such as crossing busy city streets, and many of these children were required to take responsibility for feeding themselves. This group continued to be characterized by the physical neglect of the child, unhealthy and unsanitary living conditions, and continual household transitions.

At this assessment period we did not identify verbal abuse and hostility as a form of maltreatment as we had at 2 years. Our experience with this subtype of maltreatment at age 2 suggested that it was the most subjective classification and also had a high degree of overlap with the other maltreatment groups at 2 years, especially physical abuse. In addition, we had the opportunity to observe mother–child interaction in a standardized laboratory procedure at age 2 and did not have a similar type of standardized assessment available for the 6-year classification. For these reasons it was very difficult to gather a sample of verbal interaction between each mother and child pair in a relatively similar situation. The conceptual and methodological problems associated with verbal abuse forced us to drop this as a classification of maltreatment at 6 years.

Finally, we included a group of children who had been the victims of sexual abuse ($n = 11$). The age of the children at this point had made them more likely to be targets of sexual interaction with older relatives and peers as well as affording a greater probability of reporting the abuse when it occurred. This group was identified through mothers' reports of current and ongoing involvement with Child Protection Services and verified through cross-checking county files. Two of the children in this group were abused sexually by their mothers, five children had experienced direct physical (genital) sexual contact with an assortment of (male) family members, and four had experienced sexual contact with older (male) children. In each case the perpetrator of the sexual contact was at least in the teenage years. There were no children placed in this group due to what could be construed as reporting of routine sexual curiosity or play.

In addition to these maltreatment groups, we identified a control group of good caretakers similar to the one identified at 2 years. These caretakers were identified on the basis of the same sources of information used to identify the maltreatment groups. First, the 85 mothers classified in the control group at 2 years were used as a sample from which to choose mothers for the control group at 6 years. Any of the 85 mothers who – on the basis of the information for the 6-year classification – could be classified as questionably maltreating, were excluded from further consideration. The 65 mothers remaining from the 2-year control group were used as the 6-year control group.

As at 2 years, there was some overlap between groups. However, at this period it was less extensive. Maltreatment group overlap was as follows, with frequency in parentheses: psychologically unavailable and physical abuse (2), physical abuse and neglect (3), psychologically unavailable and sexual abuse (1), physical and sexual abuse (1), neglect and sexual abuse (1), and psychologically unavailable, physical abuse and sexual abuse (1).

Using these categories to describe maltreatment in our sample at six years resulted in identifying 47 cases as being members of at least one of the groups. Because our sample now numbers approximately 200, this reflects a prevalence of maltreatment approaching 25 percent in this sample. Once again, this exceeds expectations based upon national base rates; however, the justifications presented earlier still apply here. Our broader conceptualization of maltreatment, our intimate knowledge of these families, and the fact that they were selected as a high risk sample probably account for much of this increase in prevalence. Our selection of subjects for the physical and sexual abuse groups was validated by their having all been referred to county child protection as verified by our checking county files after the mothers' reports to us. In addition, several members of the neglect and psychologically unavailable groups were also involved with child protection.

Continuity of maltreatment from one to six years. As previously, we examined the extent to which women classified as maltreating at 1 year were also classified similarly at later time periods. This particular analysis of overlap spanned approximately five years. Our expectations were that continuity across this period would not be as high as the 85% reported earlier for the span from 1 to 2 years.

Of the 32 women classified as providing inadequate care at 1 year, 24 remained in the study at 6 years. Of the eight subjects who dropped from the study, two mothers were seriously mentally ill. One of the dropouts had moved out of state and refused to continue to participate after she had been brought to court on charges of killing her second child. Based on this information it would be reasonable to assume that these three mothers could be continuing to maltreat at 6 years; however, they were not members of the sample at that time and so were not classified.

Of the 24 mothers maltreating at 1 year who remained in the sample at 6 years, 17, or 71% were members of at least one of the maltreatment groups identified at 6 years. Of the seven subjects maltreating at 1 year who were not classified as maltreating at 6 years, one of the children was living with a grandmother, another was in the father's custody, and a third had been adopted. The 71% figure given as evidence of continuity in maltreatment is likely to be somewhat conservative given the information about the three subjects who were dropped from the study and the fact that the children who were no longer living with their mothers at 6 years were doing so at least partially as a result of their mothers' inability to care for them.

Relationship of maltreatment at two and six years. Examination of overlap between the same types of maltreatment across our 2- and 6-year groups indicates that there is much less continuity within subtypes of maltreatment than there is for a more general classification of maltreatment. For the neglect groups, 33% ($n = 8$) of the mothers classified as neglectful at 2 years were neglectful at 6 years. For the psychologically unavailable groups, 32% ($n = 6$) of the mothers classified as psychologically unavailable at 2 years remained in this classification at 6 years. Of the twenty-four mothers classified as physically abusive at 2 years, 21% ($n = 5$) were physically abusing their children at 6 years. These data suggest that neglectful and psychologically unavailable forms of caretaking may be more chronic conditions than physical abuse. However, these data are far from conclusive, largely due to the small sample sizes and moderate overlap among the groups at 24 months.

Considering the extent to which the mothers classified in the maltreatment groups at 2 years were still perpetuating some form of maltreatment at 6 years yields evidence of greater continuity than is suggested by the within-subtypes analysis described above. Of the 24 women classified as physically abusive at 2 years, 22 remained in the study at 6 years, one of the women who dropped out did so because of mental illness, the other was the woman brought on charges for killing her second child. Of the remaining 22 women (73%), 16 were classified in at least one of the maltreatment groups at 6 years. Two of the discontinuous subjects were in the custody of caretakers other than their mothers at 6 years.

Two women from the 2-year verbal abuse classification were dropped from the study by 6 years, leaving 17 of the women classified as verbally abusive at 2 years in the study at 6 years. One was the woman charged with the death of her second child, the other dropped out for unknown reasons. Twelve, or 70%, of these women were classified in at least one of the maltreatment groups at 6 years.

Four of the 24 women classified as neglectful at 2 years had dropped from the study at 6 years, leaving 20 in the study. One of the women dropped out for unknown reasons, two were mentally ill, and one was the woman charged with the death of her second child. Of these 20 women (65%), 13 were classified in at least one maltreatment group at 6 years. Four of the "discontinuous" caretakers continued to have some type of problem with caring for their children at 6 years; at best they were borderline caretakers but not able to be clearly classified as maltreating.

Finally, two subjects were dropped from the psychologically unavailable group in the period from 2 to 6 years, leaving 17. One dropped out for unknown reasons, the other was the woman charged with the death of her second child. Of these 17 women (71%), 12 were classified as maltreating in at least one form at 6 years. Again, at least three of the discontinuous group were not able to be clearly classified as maltreating at 6 years but continued to have problems in caretaking.

The evidence for continuity in maltreatment from the infancy and early preschool years to beginning school age is relatively strong. As noted earlier, 71% (17 out of 24) of the women classified as maltreating at 1 year who remained in the sample were still maltreating at 6 years. Of the women classified as maltreating at two years, 61% continued to maltreat at 6 years; however, 4 of these 44 women dropped from the sample, leaving a corrected continuity rate of 67%.

As noted in several of these cases, the reason for a classification of "no maltreatment" at 6 years was due to the child no longer living with the mother, a possible consequence of the earlier maltreatment. In addition, examination of the mothers who maltreated but were no longer classified as maltreating suggests that they were at best marginal caretakers, no longer so inadequate as to fit a maltreatment classification but by no means appropriate for inclusion with a group of adequate caretakers. For many women, their apparent improvement as caretakers, based on their own report and perceptions of interviewers who have known these mothers for years, was strongly influenced by the quality of their relationships with husbands or boyfriends. Changes in the quality of primary relationships appeared to have marked consequences for these mothers' caretaking ability, which remained highly variable and subject to fluctuation.

Having presented a description of our research project, we will now direct our attention to summarizing the results of our efforts to document the antecedents of maltreatment at 6 years of age. In addition, we will examine the factors associated with changes in quality of care and the extent to which mothers' own history of being maltreated as children might affect the manner in which they treat their own children.

Antecedent factors associated with child maltreatment in a disadvantaged sample

In this section, we will present a summary of data analyses conducted with the most recently formed maltreatment groups in order to address the following questions:

1. What antecedent factors distinguish the four types of maltreatment at 6 years of age from good caretaking outcomes at the same age?
2. Are there antecedent factors that distinguish among cases where parents

were maltreating their children at both 2 and 6 years and those where maltreatment occurred at either one or neither of those times?
3. Is there evidence that women who were abused as children are more likely to maltreat their own children, and are there factors that distinguish cases of intergenerational continuity from those in which mothers have been abused as children but do not maltreat their own children?

After presenting data addressing these questions, we will conclude this chapter with a brief discussion of the results.

Antecedents associated with different forms of maltreatment

In this section, we will summarize results concerning factors that distinguish between good caretaking and the different forms of maltreatment at 6 years. Several of the analyses presented compare maltreatment and control groups on factors measured prior to 6 years, and in some cases the dependent variables were measured concurrently with the maltreatment classification. Therefore, the word "antecedent" is used in a broad sense, not in a manner that infers causality. The analyses summarized in Table 7.2 consist of comparisons between each maltreatment group and a control group of good caretakers on variables of maternal personality and mood, life stress, experienced emotional support, and the quality of the home environment collected between 24 and 64 months.

As noted in Table 7.1, maternal personality was measured when the children were 64 months old using the 16PF (Cattell, 1967); maternal mood and personality were measured when the children were 4 years old using the Profile of Moods (POMS) (McNair, Lorr, and Droppleman, 1971), CES–D (Radloff, 1977), and the IPAT Anxiety scale (Cattell and Scheier, 1963). In addition, maternal intelligence was measured at 48 months with the WAIS (Wechsler, 1955). Life stress was measured at 30, 42, 48, 54, and 64 months using a version of Cochrane and Robertson's (1973) Life Events Inventory adapted by our staff for use with low income populations. Experienced emotional support was measured by rating mothers' responses to several interview questions regarding their close relationships. Finally, the quality of the home environment was measured at 30 months using the HOME (Caldwell, Heider, and Kaplan, 1966).

Within the cells of the table, letters are used to indicate the direction of significant differences, and highly significant differences ($p < .001$) are highlighted with an asterisk. Redundant comparisons have been omitted.

Not surprisingly, there are numerous highly significant differences between each of the maltreatment groups and the control group on many of the 2- to 6-year variables. Our interest in analyzing such a large number of comparisons is not to emphasize individual results but rather to examine the table for patterns of significant and nonsignificant findings across domains of variables or in the timing of differences.

Table 7.2. *Comparisons between controls and maltreatment groups on 24- to 64-month data*

Variables	Control group versus			
	Physical abuse	Neglect	Psychologically unavailable	Sexual abuse
Quality of emotional support:				
24 months	C>P*		C>U*	C>S*
30 months	C>P*	C>N	C>U*	C>S*
42 months	C>P*	C>N	C>U*	C−S*
48 months	C>P*	C>N	C>U*	C>S*
54 months	C>P	C>N		
54 months	C>P	C>N*		C>S*
Stressful life events:				
30 months	P>C	N>C	U>C*	S>C*
42 months	P>C	N>C	U>C	S>C
48 months				S>C
54 months	P>C	N>C	U>C	S>C
64 months	P>C			S>C
Home environment at 30 months:				
Responsivity	C>P*	C>N*	C>U*	C>S*
Avoidance of restrictions	C>P	C>N	C>U	
Organization		C>N		C>S
Provision of play materials	C>P	C>N*	C>U	C>S
Maternal involvement	C>P*	C>N	C>U	C>S
Opportunity for variety				
HOME total score	C>P*	C>N*	C>U*	C−S*
Maternal mood at 48 months				
Profile of moods:				
Tense	P>C	N>C	U>C	S>C*
Depressed	P>C		U>C	S>C
Angry	P>C		U>C	S>C
Vigorous				
Fatigued				
Confused	P>C		U>C	S>C*
Depression inventory: CES-D	C>P			
Maternal intelligence: WAIS	C>P	C>N*		
Maternal anxiety: IPAT	C>P			
*Maternal personality: 16PF**				
Impersonal–outgoing				
Concrete–abstract		N>C		
Unstable–mature	C>P	C>N	C>U*	C>S
Mild–aggressive				
Prudent–impulsive				
Breaks/follows rules				
Restrained–bold	P>C			
Realistic–unrealistic				

Table 7.2 *(cont.)*

Variables	Control group versus			
	Physical abuse	Neglect	Psychologically unavailable	Sexual abuse
Maternal personality: 16PF*				
Adaptable–skeptical		N>C	U>C	S>C
Careful–careless				
Natural–calculating				S>C
Secure–worrying	P>C			
Traditional–liberal	P>C			
Joining–self sufficient				
Careless–precise				
Tranquil–restless			U>C*	S>C

*Scales are bipolar dimensions; a low score is reflected by the first label, a high score by the second label.

There were consistent, ongoing differences between the maltreatment and control groups on the emotional support that the mother experienced from her husband/boyfriend, family members, and close friends. The physically abusive and psychologically unavailable mothers were easily distinguished by their insularity and lack of social support, as were homes in which the child was being sexually abused or neglected. Lack of social support and insularity appeared characteristic of all types of maltreatment.

The maltreatment groups were also distinguished from the good caretaking group by the mothers' experience of greater life stress for the assessments conducted over the 2- to 6-year period. The physical abuse, neglect, and psychologically unavailable groups experienced significantly greater amounts of life stress than the good caretaking groups at several points in time. The group of households where the children were being sexually abused was characterized by extreme amounts of stress at all assessment points.

Further analysis of the items on which the sexually abusing groups tended to score high suggests that these homes were marked by extreme disorganization and chaos: frequent moves, physical abuse of the mothers by husbands and boyfriends, maternal chemical abuse, extreme dependence by the mothers on husbands and boyfriends; in many cases the children were experiencing other forms of maltreatment. These mothers appeared to be living such jumbled and confused lives themselves that they were unable to take the steps necessary to ensure their childrens' sexual safety. There are two possible explanations for the association between excessive stress and sexual abuse. It is possible that the personal histories and interpersonal incompetence of these women led them to engage in relationships with men in which they and their children were victimized and that produced great stress. It is also possible that the general life stress experienced by these mothers taxed their coping and caretaking resources to the extent that they could no longer protect their children from the sexual advances of older males.

Given the differences between the maltreatment and control groups on stress and emotional support, it was not surprising to find the highly significant differences in the quality of the home environment at 30 months indicated in Table 7.2. All of the maltreatment groups were extremely different from the control group on home environment variables that appear to tap maternal interest in and knowledge about their child's development, such as responsivity, involvement and provision of appropriate play materials. The physically abusive, neglectful, and psychologically unavailable mothers also engaged in more restrictive caretaking practices. The households that were neglectful and in which there was sexual abuse also scored lower than the control group on the organization scale of the HOME. In addition, all of the maltreatment groups had significantly lower scores than the controls on the total HOME score, a measure of the global quality of the home environment.

The pattern of differences between the groups on maternal mood, personality, and ability variables is congruent with our earlier discussion of the importance of maternal characteristics as critical in distinguishing maltreatment and control families. The women in the physical abuse group at 6 years were more tense, depressed, angry, and confused than the control group on the Profile of Moods (POMS) and were also more depressed according to the CES–D, less intelligent and more anxious according to the IPAT. The women in the neglect group were more tense according to the POMS and less intelligent than the control group on the WAIS. Women in the psychologically unavailable group were more tense, depressed, angry, and confused than the controls according to the POMS. Finally, mothers of chidren who had been sexually abused were also more tense, depressed, angry, and confused according to the POMS.

When the children were 64 months, the 16PF (Cattell, 1967) was administered to the mothers. According to the maltreatment classifications done at 6 years, women in the physical abuse group were more emotionally unstable than the controls and tended to take more impulsive, bold actions, worried more, and endorsed more liberal views. Women in the 6-year neglect group showed more concrete thought patterns than the controls and were also more emotionally unstable and more skeptical of interpersonal relationships. The six-year psychologically unavailable group was also emotionally unstable, skeptical of interpersonal relationships, and restless when compared with the good caretakers. Finally, the mothers of children who had been sexually abused were more emotionally unstable, skeptical of interpersonal relationships, calculating, and restless when compared with the controls.

The pattern of differences between the control and maltreatment groups on personality and mood variables indicates that, collectively, these are experiencing marked emotional turmoil. The measures on which they differed from the control group suggest that these mothers felt threatened by interpersonal demands placed upon them and perhaps were unable to establish any type of intimate relationship in which mutual interdependency and trust are crucial to adaptive functioning.

The relative importance of maltreatment predictors. Throughout this chapter, we have referred to the importance of prospective studies in testing causal models of child maltreatment. We have cited a number of studies indicating differences between maltreatment groups and control groups on factors such as parental psychological characteristics, social support, and environmental stress. The data presented above are congruent with this pattern. Because it is of critical importance to establish models of maltreatment antecedents that have predictive validity (Cicchetti and Aber, 1980; Cicchetti and Rizley, 1981), we examined the extent to which several variables that appeared to consistently distinguish the maltreatment and control groups in the *t*-tests could be used to predict maltreatment group membership.

Due to the small size of our individual maltreatment groups at 6 years, we were unable to use discriminant function analysis to predict the specific groups. Instead, we chose to collapse the groups to form a general maltreatment group at 6 years and perform the discriminant function analysis to distinguish that group from the control group of good caretakers.

We chose seven variables to enter into the discriminant analysis: an index of total support formed by summing the ratings of experienced emotional support from 24 to 64 months, an index of total stress formed by summing the totals from the Life Events Scales from 24 to 64 months, an index of the overall quality of the home environment at 30 months (total score from the HOME), maternal IQ (WAIS), a factor score taken from a factor analysis of the Profile of Moods, CES–D and IPAT Anxiety Scale representing a negative maternal mood state, a measure of maternal emotional stability and maturity (the Stability Scale of the 16PF) and a measure of maternal interpersonal trust (the Suspiciousness Scale of the 16PF).

These variables were chosen for two reasons. First, they were representative of the factors that distinguished the maltreatment and control groups in the *t*-tests – namely, maternal psychological characteristics, stress, and support. Second, they generally distinguished *all* of the maltreatment groups from the control group and, as we had collapsed the maltreatment groups for this analysis, we were interested in using broad band predictors. The

Table 7.3. *Results of discriminant function analysis and classification analysis*

Discriminant function analysis	
Standardized function weights	
Maternal emotional stability[1]	.51
Home environment[2]	.50
Stress[3]	−.36
Support[4]	.34
Maternal IQ[5]	.27
Maternal negative mood factor[6]	.23
Maternal interpersonal trust[7]	−.04

Classification analysis			
		Predicted	
Actual group	*n*	Not maltreating	Maltreating
Not maltreating	38	33 (86.8%)	5 (13.2%)
Maltreating	20	5 (25.0%)	15 (75.0%)
	Percent correctly classified: 82.8		

1 16 PF Emotional and Stability Scale
2 Total score from HOME
3 Composite of Quality of Emotional Support rating at 24, 30, 42, 48, 54, and 64 months
4 Composite of Life Events Scale total score at 30, 42, 48, 54, and 64 months
5 WAIS
6 First factor from factor analysis of POMS, IPAT, CES-D
7 16 PF Skeptical Scale

discriminant function weights and results of the classification analysis are presented in Table 7.3.

The analysis indicates that the maternal psychological characteristic of emotional stability was the largest single contributor to distinguishing child maltreatment from good caretaking in our sample. The home environment also contributed highly to the discriminant function. This is not surprising because by definition the home environment of the subjects in the maltreatment groups was highly deviant and we expected it to make a large contribution to the discriminant function for that reason. Of secondary importance in discriminating the maltreatment and control groups were support and stress, followed by maternal IQ and negative mood state.

The discriminant function weights were used to perform a classification analysis in order to determine the "hit rate" that would be achieved if they were used for screening purposes. Overall, the discriminant function correctly predicted 83% of the total cases; 87% of the control group cases were correctly classified, as were 75% of the maltreatment group cases. The classification analysis misclassified 25% ($n = 5$) of the actually maltreating cases (false negatives) and 13.2% ($n = 5$) of the actually not maltreating cases (false positives).

It is unfortunate that we were unable to perform this type of analysis for the different forms of maltreatment. As it was, there were 38 control and 20 maltreatment subjects with complete data files on the variables used in the analysis, resulting in a subject to variable ratio that limits the reliability of the results. Cross-validation with a larger sample size would certainly be necessary before these results could be applied in any screening procedure. However, the main finding that maternal emotional stability was the most powerful discriminating variable has certain theoretical implications which will be discussed later.

Ongoing and periodic maltreatment

Another advantage of the prospective, longitudinal design of the Mother–Child Project is that it affords the opportunity to examine factors associated with continuity or deflection in a particular developmental path. This is especially important in the field of child maltreatment because there has been little investigation of whether the factors that have been implicated in the development of maltreatment in a previously nonmaltreating case are also those associated with ongoing maltreatment.

In order to classify ongoing and periodic maltreatment, we used the maltreatment groups identified at 2 and 6 years. Unfortunately, because group sizes were small for the specific maltreatment types (e.g., physical abuse) and there was considerable overlap among the 2-year maltreatment groups, we were forced to collapse the maltreatment groups and examine factors associated with continuity or discontinuity in maltreatment in general rather than for specific types. More specifically, we collapsed the psychologically unavailable, physical abuse and neglect groups at both 2 and 6 years to form general maltreatment groups at both of those time periods. Table 7.4 presents the groups we examined and the labels we used to distinguish them.

The "control" group (consistently nonmaltreating) involved all subjects in the sample who were not maltreating their children at 2 and 6 years. The late maltreating group did not maltreat their children at 2 years but were maltreating at 6, the early maltreating group maltreated at 2 and were not maltreating at 6, and the consistently maltreating group was maltreating at both ages. Because the group of parents who were not maltreating at either age consisted of such a large number of subjects, we randomly selected 30 of them for use in the comparisons.

We were interested in which, if any, factors would distinguish women who consistently maltreated their children from those who once maltreated and then stopped. Therefore, we conducted t-tests comparing the consis-

Table 7.4. *Frequency of ongoing or changing maltreatment group status*

		Maltreatment at six years		
		No	Yes	
		203	20	223
	No	Consistently nonmaltreating or dropped from sample	Late maltreating	
Maltreatment at two years				
		17	27	44
	Yes	Early maltreating	Consistently maltreating	
		220	47	267

tently maltreating and early maltreating groups on the measures of maternal characteristics and the psychosocial environment that were used as a basis for the comparisons between the maltreatment and control groups presented earlier.

It should be noted that the findings based upon these comparisons are highly tentative. The sample sizes are small and the groups are inherently unstable. It is quite possible that parents who were not classified as maltreating their child at age 2 but were maltreating at a later age may have been misclassified at one period. Possibly they were maltreating their child at age 2 and we were not aware of it. Classifying parents as maltreating their child is not an "either-or" issue. As noted earlier, in many instances parents who are no longer classified as maltreating their child are continuing to provide poor-quality care. There is a large gray area on the quality of caretaking continuum, and many of our parents who were assigned different classifications between the 2- and 6-year period may simply have moved from maltreating to this borderline area or vice versa.

In comparing the consistently maltreating and early maltreating groups, the only variables that differentiated these groups were maternal personality variables measured by the 16PF. At 6 years the women who were no longer maltreating were more outgoing and personable ($p = .037$), tended to be more mature and less reactive to their feelings ($p = .065$), and were more realistic and practical in problem solving ($p = .017$) than the continually maltreating mothers.

Interestingly, the groups did not differ on emotional support and life stress. We examined the means of these two groups relative to the consistently nonmaltreating group on the stress and emotional support measures, and both groups experienced more stress and less support at each assessment period between 2 and 6 years than the consistently nonmaltreating group. This comparison is revealing in that it suggests that in the presence of a lack of emotional support and high life stress, the psychological characteristics of the mothers differentiated ongoing maltreatment from that which stops.

We then systematically reviewed our interview data from 2 to 6 years to examine the extent to which any of the Early Maltreatment mothers had been involved in some type of intervention. Included on each interview at 24, 30, 42, 48, 54, and 64 months was a question regarding whether the mothers had sought help for any problems regarding childrearing or their own mental health and their feelings about the effectiveness of the intervention. Our interview data indicated that several of the women who were maltreating at 2 years and not maltreating at 6 years (early maltreatment group) were involved in treatment programs directed at changing their maltreating parenting styles, and nearly all of those women reported that they felt supported by their therapists. They specifically mentioned feeling accepted by their therapists, which gave them a feeling that the therapist was genuinely interested in their wellbeing. Some dealt specifically with issues concerning their own victimization in relationships, whether as a child or as an adult. These responses suggest that therapy may have played a role in helping these women gain insight into their own roles in being victimized in relationships and to help them address their own emotional needs. Other interview responses suggested the importance of educating mothers about their children's needs and providing concrete instructions about how to meet these needs.

Apparently, a combination of education and available support was critical for these mothers' feelings and knowledge about themselves and their relationships. The 16PF traits that distinguished the early maltreating and consistently maltreating groups are cognitive (i.e., more realistic in problem solving) and social (more outgoing, less reactive in emotional stimuli) variables that may tap their perceptions and feelings about close interpersonal relationships. These perceptions and feelings about relationships have distinguished maltreatment and control groups in other studies (Newberger and Newberger, 1982; Sameroff and Feil, 1984). The changes these women reported undergoing as a function of therapy tend to support the perception that mothers' internal models of relationships (Bowlby, 1980) play a very important role in the development, maintenance, and suspension of maltreating parenting practices.

Given what appeared to be an association between mothers' internal models of relationships and maltreatment, we examined whether factors in the developmental histories of maltreating women could point toward their current problems in intimate relationships and thus help account for the importance of many of the maternal characteristics we have reported. For this reason we examined the extent to which women in the 2- and 6-year groups had, as children, been maltreated by their own parents.

Intergenerational continuity of maltreatment

During interviews conducted when the children were 48 and 54 months we asked the mothers a series of questions about their childhood, including whether or not they had been raised by a relative or placed in a foster home. They were asked how they were disciplined and whether or not they were beaten, physically abused, sexually molested, or neglected. On the basis of their responses, the mothers were divided into groups consisting of those who had been maltreated or not maltreated. The maltreated group included women who experienced physical or sexual abuse or neglect as children.

For each type of maltreatment, a group of mothers was identified who had clearly and consistently experienced that form of inadequate care (Egeland, Jacobvitz, and Papatola, 1984). There were 47 women who were physically abused as children. In the case of sexual abuse by an older relative during childhood, there were 13 women who had experienced physical sexual contact as children. Finally, 9 women had experienced pervasive or extreme neglect of basic physical needs during their childhood.

To obtain information on the intergenerational continuity of maltreatment, Egeland, Jacobvitz, and Papatola (1984) examined the extent to which mothers who had experienced abuse as children were classified as maltreating their children at 2 years of age. As part of this chapter, we extended these analyses to examine intergenerational continuity using the maltreatment groups at 6 years.

Of the 47 women who were physically abused as children, 70% were maltreating their children at 2 years. Of the physically abused mothers, 16 were physically abusive, 14 were questionable caretakers, and 3 had other caretaking problems resulting in foster placement. At 6 years, 28 or 60% of the women who were physically abused as children were maltreating their own children, 8 were physically abusive, 8 were neglectful, 6 were psychologically unavailable, and in 6 of their homes children were being sexually abused. It is clear that being physically abused as a child constitutes a significant risk factor for the quality of parenting that that individual will provide when she becomes a parent – although there is also considerable evidence that intergenerational continuity is by no means complete (i.e., present in 100% of the cases), and it is true that there is not a type-to-type correspondence for transmission of physical abuse. In addition, our data suggest that there is a decrease in intergenerational continuity over time such that there appears to be a greater chance of a maltreated woman to maltreat her toddler-age child than there is for her to maltreat her school-age child.

The cross-generational association between a mother having been sexually abused by her parents and her maltreatment of her own children is also high. As children, 13 of our mothers were sexually abused. Of these, 12 were maltreating their children at 2 years: 6 were clear cut physical abuse cases, 2 had other caretaking problems, and 4 were in the questionable physical abuse group. Only one mother who had a history of being sexually abused was in the adequate care group at two years. Of these 13 women who had been sexually abused as children, 9 were maltreating their children at 6 years of age. Three were physically abusive, 2 were neglectful, and 4 parented children who were being sexually abused. Once again, we find that a parent's history of having been maltreated has significant implications for her own ability to parent. However, the same cautions as were present for physical abuse are also relevant for sexual abuse in that continuity was neither complete nor type to type and there appeared to be a decrease in continuity with the age of the second generation child.

It was surprising that only 9 of the mothers in the sample were judged to have been neglected in childhood. However, the association between neglect as a child and later maltreatment as a parent was also high. Of the 9 mothers neglected as children, 7 were maltreating at 2 years: 3 were cases of severe maltreatment, 4 were questionable caretakers and 2 were adequate. Of these neglected mothers, 4 were also maltreating their children at 6 years of age. At both 2 and 6 years of age the maltreatment of the children by the neglected mothers primarily took the form of neglect. Once again there was neither complete nor type to type transmission of maltreatment, and there appeared to be a decrease in continuity with the age of the second generation child.

This data on intergenerational continuity in maltreatment presents support for the hypothesis that a mother's developmental history, in particular her experience in intimate relationships, is a precursor to her own ability as a caretaker. It is clear that there is evidence that many women maltreated as children have a broad range of difficulties as adult caretakers. We have also made it clear that not all women who have been maltreated also maltreat their children, and there is little evidence for continuity in specific forms of maltreatment.

It is possible that broader definitions of maltreatment in the first generation would result in a higher percentage of continuity across generations because although the childhood experiences of many mothers may not be able to be classified as maltreatment, there is reason to believe that they may have been less than adequate. It is also true that reliance on mothers' recollections of their childhood history may result in low estimates of continuity, as those memories may be less accessible than others due to the age at which childhood maltreatment may have occurred or problems associated with remembering painful experiences (Main and Goldwyn, 1984). In any case, the data does support the conclusion that many maltreating women do have a history of being cared for in an inadequate manner.

Attachment theory has pointed out the extent to which dysfunctional interpersonal relationships may be a result of the types of internal working models of relationships that individuals develop as a consequence of experiences with caretakers (Bowlby, 1977, 1980; Main and Goldwyn, 1984; Sroufe and Fleeson, 1986). This suggests that many of the parental social, cognitive, and personality characteristics found to differentiate maltreating from nonmaltreating parents may be linked to differences in the quality of care they received as children. This hypothesis is supported by evidence for some type of intergenerational continuity in maltreatment, even if such continuity is incomplete.

Interestingly, Egeland, Jacobvitz, and Papatola (1984) report case-study data that suggests that exceptions to intergenerational continuity in this sample can be accounted for by the experience of mild maltreatment as a child or the presence of a loving, nurturing, and supportive parent or parent surrogate. Apparently, somewhere in the developmental history of these women, who experienced poor care but who were adequate caretakers, was the opportunity to experience a healthy, nurturing relationship with an adult. In addition, the exceptions to intergenerational continuity appeared to enjoy healthy relationships with spouses and adult peers (Egeland, Jacobvitz, and Papatola, 1984). These two findings regarding discontinuities in intergenerational transmission are also predictable from an internal working models hypothesis (Bowlby, 1980; Main and Goldwyn, 1984).

The data we have presented from the Mother–Child Project on the antecedents of maltreatment in a disadvantaged sample have led us to hypotheses concerning the role of parents' (especially mothers') internal working models of self and relationships in accounting for the development of maltreatment. This will be a central theme to be discussed in the following section.

Conclusions and discussion

We believe that the main contribution made by our findings to the literature on child maltreatment addresses the extent to which psychological processes involved in mothers' ability to engage in interpersonal relationships serve a central causal role in maltreatment.

Although we have acknowledged and emphasized the multivariate causal framework adopted by the majority of investigators in the area of child maltreatment (Maccoby and Martin, 1983), we have presented findings that suggest a possible hierarchy or integration within this framework. Our analyses of the antecedents of child maltreatment and of the factors that differentiate ongoing from periodic maltreatment suggest that maternal psychological characteristics play a critical role in discriminating among caretaking relationships in which maltreatment will occur and those in which it will not. The most important of these maternal characteristics appeared to be those which tapped mothers' thoughts and feelings about dealing with interpersonal relationships and the extent to which they are able to reflect on those thoughts and feelings. The analyses of ongoing and periodic maltreatment indicated that in the face of high levels of stress and a lack of support the mothers who were characterized as emotionally stable and able to reflect upon their feelings did not maltreat their children. This suggests that stressful experiences and a lack of support may be influential in maltreatment to the extent to which they tax the coping ability of parents, but may not be necessary or sufficient causal factors.

These results are in agreement with the findings of several investigators addressing the role of maternal social cognitive characteristics in maltreatment (Newberger and Cook, 1983; Sameroff and Feil, 1984). However, at this point it would be a mistake to conclude that we are making a case for blaming mothers for the maltreatment of their children. Our close association with these families over the years has led us to the opinion that few, if any, mothers would actively and purposefully maltreat their children; instead, many are the victims of circumstances that lead them to lose control with children, to neglect their children's emotional and physical needs, or to manage households in which children are sexually abused.

We have suggested earlier that one of these circumstances may be a mother's own history of being maltreated as a child. Often women who have been maltreated have suffered significant psychological trauma, which makes it difficult to cope with the demands of close interpersonal relationships, either because they may not understand the necessary cues and transactions or because of emotional lability and instability. These women are enmeshed in cycles of dysfunctional interpersonal relationships, perhaps extending back to their childhood, which were carried forward or validated (Sroufe and Fleeson, 1986) in their inadequate caretaking – problems in intimate relationships with men and insularity. Interestingly, problems in intimate relationships also account for a great deal of the stressful experiences which these women report (Pianta, 1985).

Therefore, it appears that the antecedents of a history of being maltreated as a child, experience of life stress, a lack of support, and maternal characteristics tied to dysfunction in interpersonal relationships all may be integrated within the context of a mother's psychological development and her ability to engage in interpersonal relationships characterized by warmth, affection and security. This hypothesis is supported by Aber and Zigler's (1981) contention that researchers and clinicians need to view the perpetrator, as well as the victim, of maltreatment from a developmental perspective. Attachment theory emphasizes the importance of an individual's history of interpersonal interaction as a child for forming internal working models of self and social relationships (Bowlby, 1969). Several investigators have directed their efforts toward the extent to which a mother's childhood history of interaction with caretakers serves as a foundation for the quality of relationships, including parenting, in which she will engage as an adult (Main and Goldwyn, 1984; Ricks, 1985; Schnieder-Rosen and Cicchetti, 1984; Sroufe and Fleeson, 1986).

Common to these researchers' efforts are a set of propositions that state the manner in which the attachment relationship affects the formation of later relationships. By and large it is proposed that the childhood experiences of parents and their caretaking ability as adults are linked by a pathway that involves the individual's development of a sense of self esteem (Ricks, 1985). Each investigator articulates that the cross-generational effects of attachment on later parenting are carried through a set of feelings and expectations regarding self and close relationships that are learned through the quality of interaction with childhood caretakers. Both Ricks and Sroufe and Fleeson emphasize that these feelings and expectations affect both the individuals' relationships with their own children and their ability to engage in adult–adult relationships. Not surprisingly, difficulties in intimate, supportive relationships with adult peers and as caretakers for dependent children are common characteristics distinguishing maltreating from nonmaltreating parents.

Sroufe and Fleeson emphasize that one proposition of relationships is that the whole relationship resides in each individual. This suggests that individuals who are maltreated in some form as children, either through abuse or rejection experiences, learn not only the role of victim but also the role of victimizer (accounting for their later maltreating parenting behavior). As adults, women who have experienced maltreatment or rejection in attachment relationships are motivated to form relationships that validate their perceptions of themselves and others (Sroufe and Fleeson, 1986). The patterns of thoughts, feelings, and behaviors based on early relationships tend to be validated or replicated when the individual becomes involved in other close relationships at a later time.

For many maltreating women who have histories of being maltreated or rejected, maltreatment of their children tends to contribute to their own already poor self-image and promotes behavior in their children (such as noncompliance) that will tend to elicit maltreating behavior again. Their low sense of self esteem and expectation that they will be victimized in close relationships (based on their childhood experiences) may lead these women to become involved with men who will maltreat them – thus the woman is both victim and victimizer. As Sroufe and Fleeson emphasize, because early relationships shape what individuals understand and know about relationships, later relationships will replicate early ones. Therefore, women who are victimized as children learn to think of themselves as victims and learn the role of victimizer through observation. Both sides of these early relationships become validated when they later remain as victims in peer relationships and become victimizers of their own children as caretakers. The importance of these women's knowledge about relationships may also be one reason why their perspective-taking ability concerning caretaking relationships is such a powerful discriminator of abusing and nonabusing mothers (Newberger and Cook, 1983; Sameroff and Feil, 1984).

There are several reasons to believe that the attachment theory may also help to account for other characteristics that discriminate maltreating and nonmaltreating parents. First, the personality characteristics of emotional reactivity, mistrust, anxiety over competence, and depressed affect found in our sample of maltreating mothers are all consistent with a course of development based upon insecure attachment (Bowlby, 1969). Second, although we have not attempted to empirically establish the link between quality of attachment as a child and later quality of caretaking as a parent, Main and Goldwyn (1984) provide evidence that the characteristics, common to abusing women, of an unsympathetic response to distress, poor control over aggression, and self-isolating tendencies are common consequences of a history of rejection and are found as early as 1–3 years of age in children of maltreated women as well as in children in normal samples who have avoidant attachment relationships consistent with maternal rejection. It is plausible that the roots of many of the personality characteristics exhibited by adult maltreating women may be traced to their own history of interaction when, as children, they were developing an attachment to their own caretakers.

Attachment theorists' research also has implications for altering the internal working models of maltreating parents. Hain and Goldwyn (1984) and Ricks (1985) note that exceptions to intergenerational continuity in maltreatment involved a relearning of self–other concepts and access to the unpleasant emotions resulting from rejection of maltreatment experienced as a child. Ricks notes that even with a history of childhood maltreatment, good outcomes as a parent were possible and involved the reworking of repressed affect. Women who were maltreated as children but who were adequate caregivers as adults were also engaged in strong marriages and had a positive sense of self-esteem according to Ricks. Both of these findings are in agreement with the data presented earlier concerning the exceptions to intergenerational continuity in our sample (Egeland, Jocobvitz, and Papatola, 1984).

Examination of the exceptions to intergenerational continuity in the Minnesota sample (Egeland, Jacobvitz, & Papatola, 1984) as well as the group of mothers who were classified as maltreating at 2 years and not maltreating at 6 years (early maltreatment group) suggests that many of these women had engaged in some form of intervention in the interim period and collectively they were distinguished from maltreating parents by their emotional stability and maturity. From their responses to interview questions regarding the effectiveness of therapy, it appears that the therapeutic relationship afforded them the emotional security necessary for them to gain access to their childhood feelings. Interestingly, Bowlby (1969, 1980) mentions that children often cope with rejection, loss, or maltreatment by using a process of psychological splitting, through which cognitive and affective systems that contain conflicting or painful information are isolated from the systems the child uses to cope with everyday life. It is possible that the access to feelings that occurs through therapy enables sufficient reintegration of these split systems for more healthy behavior patterns to emerge. Thus, for many of these women the value of therapy or intervention was to offer them an experience of an interpersonal relationship that challenged and perhaps reformed their prototypic view of themselves and interpersonal relationships.

It is our conclusion that attachment theory provides a powerful means of integrating the common findings in the maltreatment literature – that maltreating women share similar feelings and thoughts about caretaking, are generally under stress or in stressful relationships, are somewhat isolated, and tend to have experienced inadequate caretaking as children. The power of attachment theory to integrate these findings lies in its emphasis on the importance of the attachment relationship as a prototypic experience for forming an internal model of self and relationships that will be carried forward and validated in later relationships. In the future, attachment and cross-generational research with maltreating samples is likely to converge with intergenerational work with normal samples (Main and Goldwyn, 1984) and make significant contributions to theories of the etiology of child maltreatment.

References

Aber, J. L., and Zigler, D. (1981). Developmental considerations in the definition of child maltreatment. In R. Rizley and D. Cicchetti (Eds.), *New directions in child development: Developmental perspectives in child maltreatment.* San Francisco: Jossey-Bass.

Ainsworth, M., and Bell, S. (1969). Some contemporary patterns of mother–infant interaction in the feeding situation. In J. A. Ambrose (Ed.), *Stimulation in early infancy.* London: Academic Press.

Ainsworth, M., and Wittig, B. (1969). Attachment and exploratory behavior of one year olds in a strange situation. In B. M. Foss (Ed.), *Determinants of infant behavior IV.* London: Methune.

Bayley, N. (1969). *Bayley scales of infant development.* New York: Psychological Corporation.

Bell, R. (1968). A reinterpretation of the direction of effects in studies of socialization. *Psychological Review, 75*, 81–95.

Bell, R., and Harper, L. (1977). *Child effects on adults.* Hillsdale, NJ: Erlbaum.

Belle, D. (1982). The stress of caring. In Goldberger and Breznitz (Eds)., *Handbook of stress.* New York: The Free Press.

Belsky, J. (1980). Child maltreatment. *American Psychologist, 35*, 320–335.

Belsky, J. (1984). The determinants of parenting: A process model. *Child Development, 55,* 83–96.

Bowlby, J. (1969). *Attachment.* New York: Basic Books.

Bowlby, J. (1977). The making and breaking of affectional bonds. *British Journal of Psychiatry, 130,* 201–210.

Bowlby, J. (1980). *Loss.* New York: Basic Books.

Brachfield, S., Goldberg, S., and Sloman, J. (1980). Parent–infant interaction in free play at 8 and 12 months: Effects of prematurity and immaturity. *Infant Behavior and Development, 3,* 289–305.

Brazelton, T. (1973). *A neonatal assessment scale.* Philadelphia: J. B. Lippincott Co.

Breger, L. (1974). *From instinct to identity.* Englewood Cliffs, NJ: Prentice-Hall.

Broussard, E., and Hartner, M. (1971). Further considerations regarding maternal perception of the first born. In Hellmuth, J. (Ed.), *Exceptional infant,* Studies in Abnormalities, Volume II, New York: Brunner and Mazel, Inc.

Brunnquell, D., Crichton, L., and Egeland, B. (1981). Maternal personality and attitude in disturbances of child rearing. *American Journal of Orthopsychiatry, 51,* 680–691.

Caldwell, B., Heider, J., and Kaplan, B. (1966). *The inventory of home stimulation.* Paper presented at the annual meeting of the American Psychological Association, New York, September.

Carey, W. (1970). A simplified method for measuring infant temperament. *Journal of Pediatrics, 77,* 188–194.

Cattell, R. B. (1967). *Sixteen PF.* Champaign, IL: Institute for Personality and Ability Testing.

Cattell, R. B., and Scheier, J. H. (1963). *IPAT Anxiety Scale Questionnaire.* Champaign, IL: Institute for Personality and Ability Testing.

Cicchetti, D., and Aber, L. (1980). Abused children–abusive parents: An overstated case? *Harvard Educational Review, 50,* 244–255.

Cicchetti, D., and Rizley, R. (1980). Developmental perspectives on the etiology, intergenerational transmission, and sequelae of child maltreatment. *New Directions for Child Development, 11,* 31–55.

Cochrane, R., and Robertson, A. (1973). The Life Events Inventory: A measure of the relative severity of psychosocial stressors. *Journal of Psychosomatic Research, 17,* 135–139.

Cohler, B., Weiss, J., and Greenbaum, H. (1970). Child-care attitude and emotional disturbance among mothers of young children. *Genetic Psychology Monographs, 82,* 3–47.

Crnic, K., Greenberg, M., Ragozin, A., Robinson, N., and Basham, R. (1983). Effects of stress and social support on mothers and premature and full term infants. *Child Development, 54,* 209–217.

Egeland, B., Breitenbucher, M., and Rosenberg, D. (1980). Prospective study of the significance of life stress in the etiology of child abuse. *Journal of Consulting and Clinical Psychology, 48,* 195–205.

Egeland, B., and Brunnquell, D. (1979). An at-risk approach to the study of child abuse: Some preliminary findings. *Journal of the American Academy of Child Psychiatry, 18,* 219–235.

Egeland, B., Cicchetti, D., and Taraldson, B. (1976). *Child abuse: A family affair.* Paper presented at the N. P. Masse Research Seminar on Child Abuse, Paris, France.

Egeland, B., and Deinard, A. (1975–1978). *A prospective study of the antecedents of child abuse.* Grant proposal funded by Office of Child Development, HEW.

Egeland, B., Deinard, A., and Sroufe, L. A. (1978–1983). *Early maladaptation: A prospective transactional study.* Grant proposal funded by the Bureau of Maternal and Child Health Service, HEW.

Egeland, B., Deinard, A., and Sroufe, L. A. (1983–1987). *The development of adaptation/maladaptation in early school years.* Grant proposal funded by William T. Grant Foundation, New York, NY, and Office of Special Education, Washington, DC.

Egeland, B., and Erickson, M. F. (1983). *Psychologically unavailable caregiving: The effects on development of young children and implications for intervention.* Paper presented at the International Conference on Psychological Abuse, Indianapolis, IN, August.

Egeland, B., Jacobvitz, D., and Papatola, K. (1984). *Intergenerational continuity of parental abuse.* Proceedings from Conference on Biosocial Perspectives on Child Abuse and Neglect, Social Science Research Council, York, ME, May 20–23.

Egeland, B., and Sroufe, L. A. (1981). Developmental sequelae of maltreatment in infancy. In R. Rizley and D. Cicchetti (Eds.), *New directions in child development: Developmental perspectives in child maltreatment.* San Francisco: Jossey-Bass.

Egeland, B., and Vaughn, B. (1981). Failure of "bond formation" as a cause of abuse, neglect, and maltreatment. *American Journal of Orthopsychiatry, 51,* 78–84.

Erickson, M. F., and Egeland, B. (1984). *An intervention project to improve caretaking in high risk mother-child dyads.* Grant proposal submitted, December.

Fanaroff, A., Kennell, J., and Klaus, M. (1972). Follow-up of low birthweight infants: The predictive value of maternal visiting patterns. *Pediatrics, 49,* 287–290.

Galdston, R. (1965). Observations on children who have been physically abused and their parents. *American Journal of Psychiatry, 122,* 440–443.

Garbarino, J. (1982). *Children and families in the social environment.* New York: Aldine.

Garbarino, J., and Sherman, D. (1980). High risk neighborhoods and high risk families: The human ecology of maltreatment. *Child Development, 51,* 188–196.

Garmezy, N. (1977a). *Parents, patience, and schizophrenia.* Frieda Fromm-Reichman Lecture, Washington, DC.

Garmezy, N. (1977b). On some risks in risk research. *Psychological Medicine, 1,* 1–6.

Gelles, R. (1973). Child abuse as psychopathology: A sociological critique and reformation. *American Journal of Orthopsychiatry, 43,* 611–621.

Gersten, M., Coster, W., Schneider-Rosen, K., Carlson, V., and Cicchetti, D. (1986). The socioemotional bases of communicative functioning: Quality of attachment, language development, and early maltreatment. In M. E. Lamb, A. L. Brown, and R. Rogoff (Eds.), *Advances in developmental psychology* (Vol. 4). Hillsdale, NJ: Erlbaum.

Gil, D. G. (1970). *Violence against children: Physical abuse in the United States.* Cambridge, MA: Harvard University Press.

Horowitz, B., and Wolcock, I. (1981). Material deprivation, child maltreatment and agency interventions among poor families. In L. Pelton (Ed.), *The social context of child abuse and neglect.* New York: Human Sciences Press.

Jackson, D. N. (1967). *Personality research form.* Goshen, New York: Research Psychologist Press, Inc.

Kempe, C. H. (1971). Pediatric implications of the battered baby syndrome. *Archives of Disease in Childhood, 46,* 28–37.

Klaus, M. H., and Kennell, J. (1976). *Mother–infant bonding.* St. Louis, MO: C. V. Mosby.

Light, R. (1973). Abused and neglected children in America: A study of alternative policies. *Harvard Educational Review, 43,* 556–598.

Maccoby, E., and Martin, J. (1983). Socialization in the context of the family: Parent–child interaction. In E. M. Hetherington (Ed.), *Handbook of child psychology* (Vol. 4, Socialization, personality and social development). New York: Wiley.

Main, M., and Goldwyn, R. (1984). Predicting rejection of her infant from mother's representation of her own experience: Implications for the abused–abusing intergenerational cycle. *Child Abuse and Neglect, 8,* 203–217.

Matas, L., Arend, R., and Sroufe, L. A. (1978). Continuity and adaptation: Quality of attachment and later competence. *Child Development, 49,* 547–556.

McCabe, V. (1984). Abstract perceptual information for age level: A risk factor for maltreatment? *Child Development, 55,* 267–276.

McNair, D., Lorr, M., and Droppleman, L. (1971). *Profile of mood states.* San Diego: Educational and Industrial Testing Service.

Mednick, S., and Baert, A. (1981). *Prospective longitudinal research.* Oxford: Oxford University Press.

Newberger, C. M. (1980). The cognitive structure of parenthood: Design a descriptive measure. *New Directions in Child Development, 7,* 45–67.

Newberger, C. M., and Cook, S. J. (1983). Parental awareness and child abuse: A cognitive-developmental analysis of urban and rural samples. *American Journal of Orthopsychiatry, 53,* 512–524.

Newberger, C. M., and Newberger, E. H. (1982). Prevention of child abuse: Theory, myth, and practice. *Journal of Preventive Psychiatry, 1,* 443–451.

Parke, R. D., and Collmer, C. W. (1975). Child abuse: An interdisciplinary analysis. In F. D. Horowitz (Ed.), *Review of child development research.* Chicago: University of Chicago Press.

Patterson, G. (1983). Stress: A change agent for family process. In M. Rutter and N. Garmezy (Eds.), *Stress coping and development in children.* New York: McGraw-Hill, 235–264.

Pianta, R. (1984). Antecedents of child abuse: Single and multiple factor models. *School Psychology International, 5,* 151–160.

Pianta, R. (1985). *The effects of maternal stressful life events on children's developmental outcomes in first grade.* Doctoral dissertation. University of Minnesota.

Radloff, L. (1977). The CES-D Scale: A self-report depression scale for research in the general population. *Applied Psychological Measurement, 1,* 384–401.

Ricks, M. (1985). The social transmission of parental behavior: Attachment across generations. In I. Bretherton and E. Waters (Eds.), *Growing points of attachment theory and research. Monographs of the Society for Research in Child Development, 50* (1–2, Serial No. 209), 211–227.

Rosenbaum, A., and O'Leary, K. (1981). Children: The unintended victims of marital violence. *American Journal of Orthopsychiatry, 51,* 692–699.

Rotter, B. (1966). Generalized expectation for internal versus external control of reinforcement. *Psychological Monographs, 80,* Whole Number 1.

Sameroff, A. J., and Candler, M. J. (1975). Reproductive risk and the continuum of caretaking casualty. In F. D. Horowitz (Ed.), *Review of child development research.* Chicago: University of Chicago Press.

Sameroff, A. J., and Feil, L. A. (1984). Parental concepts of development. In I. Sigel (Ed.), *Parental belief systems: The psychological consequences for children.* Hillsdale, NJ: Erlbaum.

Schaefer, E., and Manheimer, H. (1960). *Dimensions of parental adjustment,* paper presented at Eastern Psychological Association, New York.

Schneider-Rosen, K., and Cicchetti, D. (1984). The relationship between affect and cognition in maltreated infants: Quality of attachment and the development of visual self-recognition. *Child Development, 55,* 648–658.

Shipley, W. C. (1946). *Shipley-Hartford Vocabulary Test.* Shipley Institute of Living Scale.

Sroufe, L. A. 91979). The coherence of individual development. *Child Development, 34,* 834–841.

Sroufe, L. A., and Fleeson, J. (1986). Attachment and the construction of relationships. In W. W. Hartup and Z. Rubin (Eds.), *Relationships and development.* New York: Cambridge University Press.

Steinmitz, S., and Straus, M. (Eds.) (1974). *Violence in the family.* New York: Dodd Mead.

Straus, M. (1983). Ordinary violence, child abuse and wife beating: What do they have in common? In D. Finkelhor, R. J. Gelles, G. T. Hotaling, and M. A. Straus (Eds.), *The dark side of families: Current family violence research.* Beverly Hills, CA: Sage.

Straus, M., Gelles, R., and Steinmitz, S. (1980). *Behind closed doors.* New York: Doubleday.

Terr, L. (1970). A family study of child abuse. *American Journal of Psychiatry, 127,* 665–671.

Thomas, A., and Chess, S. (1977). *Temperament and development.* New York: Bruner-Mazel.

Tonge, W., James, D., and Hillam, S. (1975). Families without hope. *British Journal of Psychiatry, Special Edition #11.* Ashford: The Royal College of Psychiatry.

Vaughn, B., Deinard, A., and Egeland, B. (1980). Measuring temperament in pediatric practice. *Journal of Pediatrics, 96,* 510–514.

Wahler, R., Leske, G., and Rogers, E. (1980). The insular family: A deviance support system for oppositional children. In L. Hamerdynck (Ed.), *Behavioral systems for the developmentally disabled.* New York: Bruner-Mazel.

Wechsler, D. (1955). *Wechsler Adult Intelligence Scale.* New York: The Psychological Corporation.

Wechsler, D. (1967). *Wechsler Preschool and Primary Scale of Intelligence.* New York: The Psychological Corporation.

Weinberg, R. A., Abery, B., and Pianta, R. (1984). *The Minneapolis Crisis Nursery: A report of an external program evaluation.* Report presented to Hennepin County Supervisory Board, Minneapolis, MN, November.

Wolfe, D. A. (1985). Child-abusive parents: An empirical review and analysis. *Psychological Bulletin, 97,* 462–482.

Wooley, P., and Evans, W. (1955). Significance of skeletal lesions in infants resembling those of traumatic origin. *Journal of the American Medical Association, 158,* 539–543.

8 Parental attributions as moderators of affective communication to children at risk for physical abuse

Daphne Blunt Bugental, Susan Madith Mantyla, and Jeffrey Lewis

Current theories of physical child abuse are concerned with the family as an interaction system in which children are both targets and potential elicitors of parental violence. To understand the long-term causes and immediate triggers of physical abuse, researchers now turn to two-way interactive forces operating between all family members as well as between the family and the larger society (e.g., Belsky, 1980; Burgess, 1979; Parke and Collmer, 1975). In the same way, concern for the *effects* of child maltreatment have shifted to consider long-term transactional systems (Aber and Cicchetti, 1984, Cicchetti and Rizley, 1981). In this chapter, we will describe a transactional model of physical abuse that adds to existing models by including cognitions as moderators of affect. Although developmental theorists have consistently attended to the effects of events on children as mediated by their cognitive capacities, less attention has been directed to the mediating role of caregiver cognitions (Goodnow, 1985). If we are to understand the effect of children on adults (as well as the effects of adults on children), it is essential that we concern ourselves with the varying causal constructions that adults make about the caregiving relationship. In this chapter, we are concerned with the role of both adult and child cognitions in the caregiving interaction process. Additionally, attention will be focused on nonverbal communications of affect as mediators of malfunctioning family systems. Clinical observations of abusive family systems have been implicitly concerned with the role of cognitions and affect. What is needed, however, is greater systematic assessment of these processes.

Theories of physical child abuse have followed the general move within the field of socialization toward interactional and transactional models. Socialization processes are no longer understood as simply reflecting the effects of parents on children. Since Bell (1966) first called attention to the presence of two-way effects between parents and children, the literature has yielded countless instances of the effects of children on their own socializa-

254

tion. "Easy" children help to create responsive, affectively positive caregiving environments. "Difficult" children help to create coercive, affectively negative environments (e.g., Bates, 1975; Cantor and Gelfand, 1977). The majority of research on reciprocal influence processes between caregivers and children has focused upon the *behavior* of the interactants. Patterson (Patterson, 1976, 1980; Reid, Patterson, and Loeber, 1981) and his colleagues have documented the escalating cycles in which child unresponsiveness elicits increasingly coercive parental control strategies, which in turn foster and maintain child noncompliance in subsequent interactions. Snow, Jacklin, and Maccoby (1983), in an analysis of parent–child interaction, observed that the mischievous style of play more characteristic of boys than girls is more likely to induce coercive control tactics from fathers. Snow et al.'s research was conducted with 1-year-old infants, indicating the very early origins of parent–child interactions that are likely to foster later child aggressiveness or reduced compliance. Using an experimental analog of family interaction, Vasta and Copitch (1981) have shown that the (apparent) unresponsiveness of a child receiving instruction leads to increased intensity of control tactics by adults. These and many other studies build a picture of the reciprocal effects of "difficult" child behavior and coercive parental responses.

Recently there has been a resurgent interest in the role of caregiver cognitions in this reciprocal influence process. Early concern with parental cognitions focused upon beliefs about caregiving strategies, and research attention was directed to the linear effects of caregiver cognitions on caregiver behaviors. As it became apparent that parents' statements about caregiving and their actual behavior were only weakly related (e.g., Becker and Krug, 1965), research attention shifted away from parental attitudes and beliefs. However, with the subsequent rise of interest in social cognitions, cognitive behavior modification, and so forth, there has been a renewed but altered interest in parental cognitions. Parental cognitions are now more likely to be viewed as assisting in the interpretation of child behavior as well as influencing caregiver behavior, and questions are being raised about the circumstances under which cognitions are more (or less) likely to be related to behavior (e.g., Goodnow, 1985). Cognitions may be thought of as playing a moderator role between the child and the caregiver. Just as adult behaviors differentially influence children as a function of the child's cognitive level, child behaviors differentially influence caregivers as a function of the adult's cognitions.

In our model we are particularly concerned with the moderating role of caregiver *attributions* – that is, beliefs about the causes of caregiving outcomes. For some years now, social psychologists have been interested in the mediating role of attributions in adult interactions. Locus of control and attributional research have converged to give a picture of causal beliefs as sensitizors to and buffers against life experiences. For example, individuals whose causal beliefs about their environment reflect low self-perceived control appear to be more reactive to their environment. As noted in Phares's review of the locus of control literature (Phares, 1976), individuals with an "external" locus of control are more susceptible to social influence than are those with an "internal" locus of control. Additionally, when confronted with stressful life events, "externals" are more likely than "internals" to react with physical illness, anxiety, depression, and so forth (e.g., Johnson and Sarason, 1978; Kobasa, 1979; Lefcourt, Miller, Ware, and Sherk, 1981).

If "difficult" child behavior is reconceptualized as a stressor, it is reasonable to predict that parents with low self-perceived control have a lower threshold for adverse response. On the other hand, high self-perceived control may buffer against the effects of a difficult child. The abuse literature has many examples of child characteristics that set them "at risk" for abuse, and economic and social stresses that increase the probability of abuse. But only *some* of the parents who experience these difficulties respond with violence. It would appear that there are important individual differences between parents that influence how easily physically abusive behavior is triggered. For example, Frodi and Lamb (1978) found that abusive parents were more likely than nonabusive parents to respond negatively to infants as a whole and to infant cries in particular. It is suggested here that caregiver attributions underlie these differential reactions. For example, Affleck, Allen, McGrade, and McQueeney (1982) observed that causal attributions held by mothers of infants with perinatal complications influenced their reaction to the child. Mothers who attributed high blame to themselves for the state of the infant showed less mood disturbances and anticipated more effective coping than did mothers who blamed luck or other people. In an interesting experimental manipulation of infant crying, Donovan and Leavitt (1985) found that inescapable crying acted to produce "learned helplessness" effects. Additionally, mothers who were induced to attribute the crying to a difficult rather than an easy infant were more likely to show performance deficits in stopping the infant crying when given the opportunity.

In our own research, we observed variations in adult response to difficult child behavior as a function of caregiver causal attributions (Bugental, Caporael, and Shennum, 1980; Bugental and Shennum, 1984). We predicted that adults who have "low control" attributions (a) are more reactive to variations in the child's responsiveness or unresponsiveness, and (b) respond more adversely to unresponsive children. To test our predictions, we placed women in interaction with child confederates who behaved in a responsive or unresponsive fashion. In support of our expectations, women with low control attributions showed greater differential reaction to responsive and unresponsive children than did high control women. With unresponsive children, they displayed a pattern of positive affect that could be characterized as condescending and unconvincing. Completing the feedback loop, this communication pattern acted back on child behavior in such a fashion as to support their initial beliefs. That is, if the adult believed she had low control over children, her behavior acted to maintain child unresponsiveness. In contrast, high control caregivers showed little difference in their reaction to responsive and to unresponsive children. Subsequently, unresponsive children came to act more like the responsive children – again, supporting the adult's initial beliefs.

Transactional model of child abuse

It involves only a simple and obvious step to extend the transactional model tested in our earlier research to abusive family systems. The two-way process can be conceptualized as follows:

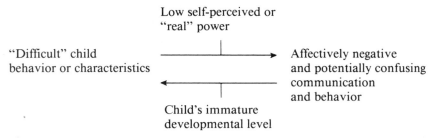

We expect that "hard to manage" child behavior (or characteristics) interact with the parent's self-perceived power (and real power) to influence parental response patterns. "Low power" attributions are predicted to lower the threshold for response to aversive or difficult child behavior. Parents who believe they have little ability to influence children are more sensitive or reactive to potentially threatening interpersonal interactions. Vasta (1982), in similar fashion, proposed that abusive parents are more easily aroused by aversive stimuli, including aversive properties of children. We believe that these easily triggered adults can be characterized by a causal belief system as well as by a physiological response pattern. "High power" attributions, on the other hand, are expected to act as a buffer against the potentially negative impact of difficult child behavior.

It is anticipated that attributions have greater power as moderator variables in ambiguous or unclear settings. If the adult cannot be certain about appropriate caregiving responses (e.g., if the situational demands are unclear), behavior demonstrated is more likely to be mediated by attributions. Social cognitions are accessed as guides to interpret situational demands when that situation fails to provide clear cues.

We predict that parents with a low power belief system react to difficult child behavior (particularly in ambiguous or unclear settings) with a communication pattern likely to produce an escalating spiral of stress. This communication pattern may ultimately culminate in physical abuse. Low power parents are expected to produce a greater amount of negative affect (and lower amount of positive affect) and to produce affectively inconsistent or "confusing" messages. Such messages may contain apparent positive affect along with negative affect or cues to the insincerity of the positive affect (e.g., kidding, sarcasm, condescension). These affectively unclear messages may occur in response to conflict between "true" feelings (e.g., anger) and attempts to play a "good parent" role. Alternately, they may reflect the affective ambivalence experienced by the adult.

The communication style predicted for at risk parents is predicted to maintain or exacerbate the difficult or aversive quality of child behavior. But we also expect that parental communication patterns will have a different impact as a function of the cognitive level of development of the child. Effects of the communication pattern predicted for low power parents are expected to be greater for younger children. Children at a lower level of cognitive development are likely to have difficulty understanding inconsistent or insincere affect and are also more likely to blame themselves for parental displays of negative affect.

Finally, it is anticipated that the family microsystems postulated here are influenced by external forces operating on the family. As theory and research move to increasing concern with the ecological embeddedness of the family, no model of family violence is complete without consideration of the larger social and economic forces operating on the family (e.g., Belsky, 1980; Burgess, 1979; Garbarino, 1977). In our model, we predict that external stresses on the family interact with child characteristics and caregiver attributional patterns to influence family functioning. Maximum levels of stress and abuse are anticipated under the combined conditions of economic and social stress, difficult child behavior, and self-perceived parental powerlessness.

Difficult child behavior

The first component of our model is concerned with the characteristics of the child. Here we are concerned with the question, "What is it about the child that is likely to set him or her at greater risk for physical abuse?" The earliest suggestion that child characteristics might set them at increased risk for abuse came from Milowe and Lourie's (1964) observation that children removed from their home due to abuse were often at disproportionately high risk for subsequent abuse in foster homes. Increasingly, investigators have come to be concerned with the properties of the "abuse-eliciting" child. Beginning in infancy, a child who impinges upon the caregiver's environment in such a fashion as to present an aversive stimulus that demands unusual amounts of attention (and is not readily influenced by caregiver efforts) is more likely to be targeted for abuse. Premature infants whose high-pitched cries are particularly aversive and whose behavioral style is unresponsive (Goldberg, 1979) are more likely to be targets of abuse than full-term infants (Elmer and Gregg, 1967). Research on affective states of abused infants suggests that they may express more negative (and less positive) affect and more ambivalent affect than nonabused infants (Gaensbauer and Sands, 1979; Gaensbauer, Mrazek, and Harmon, 1980). At this point, however, empirical evidence is missing on the extent to which such differences are a result or a cause of maltreatment.

Observations of physically abused children after infancy focus on an assortment of characteristics that might pose difficulty for caregivers. Ounstead, Oppenheimer, and Lindsay (1974) found that abusive mothers were more likely to describe the targeted children as clingy, aggressive, disobedient, and so forth. The developmental histories of such children were more likely to include physical complaints (colic, vomiting), sleeping disturbances, excessive crying, and so on. Friedrich and Boriskin (1976) found that physically or cognitively limited children (Down's syndrome, blind, deaf, or learning handicapped) receive more *severe* abuse than other abused children. De Lissovoy (1979) found that aversive or atypical child behavior (sleeping disturbances, frequent illness, very high activity level, extreme dependence) predicted later parental abuse. In direct home observations of families, Reid et al. (1981) found that physically abused children produced a 50 percent higher frequency of aversive behaviors than did nonabused children. Beyond purely objective differences in targeted children, they are also more likely to be *perceived* in negative ways, for example, as being similar to a disliked parent, spouse, or even the person him- or herself (e.g., Burgess, 1979; Friedrich and Boriskin, 1976; Green, Gaines, and Sandgrund, 1974). In summary, there is a strong body of evidence supporting the notion that abused children are more likely to be seen as difficult. Going along with these findings is the common observation that one child within a family is often disproportionately targeted for abuse (e.g., Friedrich and Boriskin, 1976), suggesting that it may be something about the particular child and/or the perception of the child that sets him or her at risk.

Caregiver characteristics as moderators of child effects

Many children have characteristics that make them more difficult for caregivers to manage, but not all caregivers react with abusive behavior. As transactional approaches to child abuse become more common, there is an increasing interest in determining the characteristics of those parents who do respond to difficult children with elevated stress and ultimate violence. Hunter, Kilstrom, Kraybill, and Loda (1978), for example, conducted a prospective study on premature infants to determine their subsequent histories. They found that 9 of the 10 parents who ultimately maltreated their infant had themselves been abused as children and had an ill-defined, poorly-integrated view of their own experiences. The reactions of adults to premature infants and the cries of such infants are also influenced by such factors as parity (Zeskind, 1980; Lester and Zeskind, 1978), social class, and age (Field, 1980). Adverse reactions appear to be higher with lower levels of caregiver experience and/or knowledge. Frodi and Lamb (1978) assessed differential physiological responses of abusive and nonabusive parents to infant crying; they found that abusive parents were more likely to respond even to normal crying (full-term infant) with elevated levels of arousal and aversive response. Cries of difficult infants are likely to be seen as intentional or demanding by most adults (Boukydis and Burgess, 1982) and are attributed particularly unrealistic psychological complexity by abusive parents (Egeland and Brunnquell, 1978).

Our model predicts (and our past research supports) a moderator role for parental attributions in the adult–child interaction process. Individuals who believe that caregiving outcomes are outside of their own control are particularly reactive to difficult child behavior. Although little research has been directly concerned with the causal beliefs of physically abusive parents, it has been noted (Young, 1964) that neither parent in abusive families takes responsibility for what happens within the family. On the other hand, abusive parents appear to assign unusual amounts of responsibility to children not only for taking care of themselves but also for taking care of the parent (Morris and Gould, 1963). Abusive parents thus appear to perceive that they themselves have very little power to control caregiving outcomes, whereas their children have a great deal of power.

In past application of our attributional model (Bugental and Shennum, 1984), we found that parents who assigned high importance to external, unstable events (luck) and low importance to internal, stable factors (ability) as causes of caregiving success were particularly reactive to aversive, unresponsive children. Their reactivity translated into a communication pattern that led to a deteriorating interaction. On the other hand, adults who attributed high control over positive events to *children* were reactive to *shy* behavior in children. But their reactivity moderated a communication pattern that led to *improved* behavior on the part of the child (shyness). These results suggested that "externality" as a whole (assignment of responsibility for outcomes to external causes) acted to heighten reactivity to unusual child behavior and the probability of "upper limit" or "lower limit" control efforts (Bell, 1966). Possibly, external attributors may respond in a negative fashion to unresponsive (threatening) children but in a positive, supportive way to shy (nonthreatening) children. Although our observations of "synthetic" families (where adults typically produce polite, affectively positive or neutral communications) did not reveal any significant consequences of caregiver attributions about *failure,* we expect to find such consequences in "natural" families where the expression of negative affect is more common (in particular in distressed families). We expect that physically abusive parents are likely to attribute high responsibility to child characteristics as causes of caregiving failure. This extrapunitive belief is predicted to lead to a reduced threshold for negative response to aversive, hard-to-manage child behavior. Just as we observed that the belief in the power of children to create positive interactions acted in a self-fulfilling fashion, we anticipate that the belief in the power of children to create negative interactions also acts to ultimately increase the probability of negative interactions.

We are proposing here that attributional influences increase in unclear settings. If a child poses an interpersonal problem and the environment provides few cues as to reasonable or appropriate responses, the adult may be guided by preexisting causal beliefs about caregiving. If on the other hand, the adult faces a difficult child in a clearly structured situation, caregiving behavior can be guided by environmental cues rather than internal cognitive structures. In support of this notion, our strongest attributional effects (as moderators of child behaviors) have been observed in unstructured interactions (Bugental and Shennum, 1984). When adults and children were simply told to "get to know each other for a few minutes," caregiver attributions had a stronger influence on behavior than in structured play settings.

The attributional measure we have employed in our research, the Parent Attribution Test (PAT), was derived originally from Weiner's (1974) two-dimensional taxonomy of causal attributions. Respondents are asked to assign importance ratings to a series of factors as causes of hypothetical caregiving success and caregiving failure. Half of the items concern adult variables (e.g., adult parenting ability, adult's particular circumstances) and half concern child variables (e.g., child's disposition, child's physical environment). Causes are either internal (e.g., ability, effort) or external (luck, other people), and they are either stable (e.g., ability, other people) or unstable (effort, luck). The content of causal factors in the most recent version of the PAT is drawn from free responses of parents to open-ended questions about the causes of their own caregiving success and failures. The instrument has been analyzed by multidimensional scaling methods in order to determine the dimensional structure that people actually impose upon causes of caregiving outcomes (Bugental and Cruzcosa, 1985). The dimensions obtained were: (a) adult versus child as causal, (b) "good" versus "bad" causes, and (c) controllable versus uncontrollable causes. Since his original formulations, Weiner has added a dimension of "controllability" to his own taxonomy (1980b); both controllability and locus are seen as influencing affect. Parents who make strong attributions to uncontrollable variables (i.e., take low credit) for caregiving success and to controllable variables for the *child* (i.e., assign high blame or responsibility) for caregiving failure are expected to be easily triggered by difficult child behavior.

One could potentially make some generalizations from the learned helplessness literature to our model. According to the Abramson, Seligman, and Teasdale (1978) reformulation of the learned helplessness hypothesis, individuals who make attributions to stable, internal and global causes of failure are more likely to respond in a helpless fashion to uncontrollable events. If we observe that abusive parents attribute unusually high blame to themselves as well as to the child, they could be seen as broadly punitive in their belief system. Research by Diener and Dweck (1978) has suggested that individuals who demonstrate helplessness when confronted with failure are more likely to make causal explanations for their negative outcomes than are "mastery-oriented" individuals. Mastery-orientation was observed to lead to a focus on remedies for failure, whereas helplessness led to a focus on the *causes* of failure. Attributed blame to self or child in our sample can be anticipated to be associated with feelings of helplessness and depression.

Caregiver stress and support as moderators of child effects

In our model we also predict that adverse child effects are greater for parents who have low "real" power (e.g., who have less adequate social support networks and higher life stresses). The literature suggests that physically abusive families often experience high degrees of external stress. These families also tend to isolate themselves from potentially supportive social networks. The presence of economic and other stresses in their lives has also been well-documented (e.g., Garbarino and Crouter, 1978; Steinberg, Catalano, and Dooley, 1981; Justice and Duncan, 1976). Abusive fathers are more likely to have experienced recent unemployment (Gil, 1970), and when they work they are more likely to have low skill, potentially unrewarding jobs (Garbarino and Crouter, 1978). Low income and residence in a generally stressful socioeconomic area are positively associated with higher levels of child maltreatment by both mothers and fathers. Additionally, abusive parents are more apt to have experienced marital discord (Strauss, Gelles, and Steinmetz, 1980). Such factors are expected to act as situational triggers. Just as caregivers with a particular attributional style have a lower threshold for adverse response to difficult children, individuals in an externally imposed state of low power are expected to have a low threshold for response to difficult children. As an indication of the power of external forces on family interaction, Conger, McCarty, Yang, Lahey, and Kropp (1984) found that chronic environmental stressors account for over a third of the variance of emotionally affective behavior of mothers to their children.

The effects of objective sources of reduced power or competence in the exosystem of the family may also be expected to interact with parents' self-perceived power. The parent who is not only confronted with real-world economic and social adversities but also believes him- or herself to be helpless to control life events is likely to be at exceptionally high risk for physical abuse. The presence of a child who is out of control or who places high perceived demands on the parents as caregivers creates an overload on their already depleted personal resources. Lazarus and his colleagues (Folkman, Aldwin, and Lazarus, 1981; Lazarus, 1981) have proposed that general beliefs about control are important determiners of the individual's primary appraisal of potentially stressful or threatening events, and individuals with low perceived control are likely to react to such stresses with ineffective (e.g., emotional rather than problem-solving) coping strategies. For example, job stresses are more likely to result in illness among individuals who lack the personality features (including an internal locus of control) that buffer their impact (Kobasa, 1979). And catastrophic life events are more likely to lead to ineffective coping strategies among individuals who have a low sense of their own control in comparison to individuals with high self-perceived control (Anderson, 1977). In the domain of family interaction, the combination of stresses and threats to power in both the exosystem and the microsystem of the family can be anticipated to interact to produce an overwhelming impact if parents also believe they are helpless to control their world.

Parental communication of affect

Parental communication of affect is predicted to vary as an interactive function of child behavior and parental beliefs about their own power and the power of the child (as well as variations in real power). Weiner (1980a) has given consideration to the affective consequences of different attributions. Here we are concerned with affective states that are elicited by the child – as *moderated* by causal beliefs of the caregivers. For example, an adult who believes that bad caregiving outcomes are under the control of the child may easily respond to unsuccessful caregiving transactions with anger.

The communication pattern expected for low power adults (who attribute low credit to themselves and high blame to others) interacting with difficult children includes:

> high frequency of negative affect;
> low frequency of positive affect;
> affectively inconsistent or "unclear" messages (positive affect accompanied
>   by cues to its managed or ambivalent nature); and
> stress or tension.

It can be noted that these are the same affective patterns that have been observed among abused children themselves. It is maintained here that an assortment of difficult child characteristics can elicit these parental patterns – which in turn are likely to elicit matched patterns in children.

In our experimental research concerning reactions to unresponsive child behavior (Bugental and Shennum, 1984), adults with low self-perceived power were observed to demonstrate two of these patterns. Low power women, in interaction with unresponsive children, expressed negative affect in their tone of voice (judged independently of their verbal content) – that is, their voice quality was relatively monotone or had a rough quality. In view of the relatively nonreactive nature of these particular communication components (i.e., they are relatively hard to manage or control), it can be inferred that such a communication pattern reflects the individual's underlying affective state. These negative internal reactions are translated into a modality over which speakers are unlikely to have much control or awareness (Holzman and Rousey, 1966), but that is very likely to have a strong influence on others (Bugental, 1974; Mehrabian and Weiner, 1967).

As a second general pattern in our experimental research, we observed differences reflecting the potential "credibility" or "sincerity" of positive affect expressed by caregivers. We observed one communication pattern we have now seen in a series of studies, including a clinical population of mothers (Bugental and Love, 1975) interacting with their own difficult children (i.e., children who were referred to a clinic for behavioral or emotional disturbances). Mothers who had low self-perceived power reacted to unresponsive children with relatively elevated voice assertion during neutral content (typically consisting of minor directives) and relatively low voice assertion during statements of approval or positive affect. High power women interacting with unresponsive children or any woman interacting with responsive children showed the opposite pattern – their statements of approval were intoned more assertively than their neutral comments. The pattern observed for low power women with unresponsive children may reflect "leakage" of their feelings of powerlessness. But it may also reflect the insincerity or managed nature of their positive statements – statements made in response to cultural "display rules" (Ekman and Friesen, 1969) rather than to their own internal affective state. Women interacting with children under high observation conditions may be assumed to be operating under a display rule to show positive affect. Any inconsistency between the demands of this rule and actual attitudinal response to the child are likely to be reflected in cues to the deliberate or managed nature of expressed positive affect.

As a second manifestation of potentially insincere positive affect, low power women with unresponsive children demonstrated a high frequency of condescending facial expressions (i.e., facial expressions judged to be typical of communications to a young child – tilting the head to one side, long duration of smiling, bringing their head into a lower and closer position, etc.). This communication pattern can be thought of as simultaneously (a) providing reassurance and (b) suggesting that the target of the message has low capability. Its inappropriate use (e.g., to a competent older child) may be interpreted as a type of power manipulation – it suggests that the child is much less competent than the caregiver. It may, however, be justified by the adult as solicitous, affectively positive behavior.

In our earlier clinical observations of normal versus distressed families (Bugental, Love, Kaswan, and April, 1971), we found one parental communication pattern that was unique to families that included an aggressive child (a group more likely to have experienced a coercive family history). Such parents used a higher frequency of "kidding" comments (i.e., messages in which the parents smiled or laughed and made a negative statement). For example, one parent – noting our procedure for observing different dyadic combinations with the family – commented, "First they took your brother. Then they took your father. Then they'll take me. And then you'll be left all by yourself" (said with a smile). This statement, potentially seen as kidding or bantering by the mother, was a visible source of anxiety to the child. We anticipate that such messages will be disproportionately common among parents with a child they see as unmanageable or hard to control. Teasing, kidding, or taunting reflect communication patterns that can be justified by the parent as positive ("just kidding"), but may actually communicate a very threatening message to the child.

Researchers who have directly observed physically abusive families have noted some of the communication patterns we expect to find. Burgess and Conger (1978), for example, have found that abusive parents direct a higher frequency of affectively negative communications and a lower frequency of affectively positive communications to their children than do nonabusive parents. Reid, Patterson, and Loeber (1982) also noted more coercive parental control tactics (short of abuse) among abusive parents.

In summary, we expect that adults who are at risk to physically abuse their children leak a continuing barrage of negative affect. The negative aspects of such messages may, however, be disguised (mainly from the parents themselves) by an overlay of apparent positive affect.

Interpretation and consequences of parental communication

Communication patterns likely to be manifested by physically abusive parents are predicted to be ineffective. That is, they are expected to maintain or exacerbate the difficult pattern of behavior more typical of the target child. The child may stop one aversive behavior in response to parental communication but then substitute a second aversive behavior or repeat the original behavior at a later time. Observations of coercive family systems by Patterson and his colleagues (Patterson, 1976; Patterson, 1980; Reid, Patterson, and Loeber, 1982) have shown the ways in which escalating parental control and negative affect lead to ultimate maintenance of aversive, noncompliant child behavior.

In the experimental test of our transactional model (Bugental and Shennum, 1984), we found that the adult communication pattern elicited by unresponsive children from low power women acted to maintain the children's impulsive, aversive behavioral style. The communication feature found to be most likely to act back in a negative fashion was that of visual condescension. Women whose positive affect was communicated in a style more appropriate for conversation with a preschooler (our child subjects were aged 7 to 12 years) failed to influence children to behave in a more responsive fashion. Conversely, women who communicated in a more adult fashion influenced the initially impulsive, distractible children to become more socially responsive.

We mentioned earlier that the affectively inconsistent style (kidding) found to be more common among parents of aggressive children (Bugental, Love, Kaswan, and April, 1971) was anecdotally observed to have a negative effect on children. We also conducted systematic judgment studies to determine the ways children perceive affectively inconsistent or noncongruent messages. In our earliest research (Bugental, Kaswan, Love, and Fox, 1970), we found that young children (5 to 8 years) gave little weight to a smiling face accompanying an otherwise neutral message – in particular if the message was delivered by a woman. In a second study (Bugental, Kaswan, and Love, 1970) we found that kidding messages (negative statements accompanied by smiles or laughter) were rated much more positively by adults than by children. It appears that the "managed" positive affect implicit in a smile that is not supported by verbal content is likely to be discounted by children.

More recent research has supported this finding. For example, Volkmar and Siegel (1979) observed that young children tend to discount the positive component of affectively inconsistent messages. The information–integration rule apparently used by children was that of assigning greater weight to the affectively negative component of inconsistent messages. Reilly and Muzekari (1979) compared the decoding of inconsistent messages by children and mentally ill adults. They found that both young children and disturbed adults discounted affectively positive components of inconsistent messages. These authors suggested that young children's decoding of inconsistent messages may reflect their inability to decenter. That is, they focus upon only one part of the message rather than integrating positive and negative components. Saarni's research (1982) has also shown that young children do not understand communication display rules, and only as they acquire higher levels of cognitive competence and cultural training in elementary school are they able to correctly understand the ways in which one is expected to dissimulate or mask particular affects.

It appears, then, that children at a lower level of cognitive maturity and social experience are likely to respond to the more negative portion of unclear or inconsistent messages. In doing so, they may be more accurate than older children or adults. It is something of an anomaly that we have to learn the "politeness norms" (DePaulo and Jordan, 1982) of attending to and believing facial expressions – expressions that are easily managed and more likely to present a false positive image than less manageable communication channels such as tone of voice. If the young child responds to the parent's inconsistent message as if a negative message has been communicated, the stage may be set for a deteriorating interchange.

Developmental factors may also play a part in the child's assignment of responsibility in negative interchanges with parents. It has often been noted that physically abused children are likely to blame themselves as responsible for – and deserving of – not only the punishment they receive but also their parents' misfortunes (e.g., Bender, 1976; Green, 1974; Helfer, 1980; Steele, 1976). This pattern could reasonably be expected to be even more common among younger abused children. Young, cognitively immature children are still prone to illusory control over life events; they believe that they are responsible for events over which they actually have no control. Weisz (1980), for example, found that preschool children believed that they caused the turn of a set of playing cards by "trying," "being smart," etc. Older children, on the other hand, knew that the cards were subject to chance rather than being under their control. Such illusory control may lead young children to blame themselves for events they do not cause. Preschool children are, for example, more likely to blame themselves for catastrophic events such as the divorce of their parents (Wallerstein and Kelly, 1975). Mutually agreed upon and self-maintaining blaming systems are, thus, more likely in families in which a cognitively immature child is targeted for abuse. That is, parents and young children are more likely to concur in the inaccurate assignments of responsibility to the child.

Preliminary test of the model

Design of the study

The transactional model proposed here was tested in an observational study of mothers interacting with children at risk for physical abuse in comparison with their lower-risk siblings. In one study, we are videorecording mother–child interactions among families being seen at CALM[1] (a child abuse prevention and counseling agency in Santa Barbara, California). Half of these parents are "abusive"[2] and half "overdiscipline" their children but are not abusive. In a second study, we are videorecording the interaction of the children from CALM families with strangers (mothers from the general community). Thus, high-risk children and their lower-risk siblings are observed interacting with both their own mother and with an unrelated mother. The sibling control group allows us to determine the specific effects of children targeted for abuse as opposed to effects present within entire families. Observation of target (and nontarget) children with *unrelated* caregivers allows us to determine the generality of their eliciting quality. The design is depicted below.

	Study 1 Target (Difficult) Child	Nontarget (Easier) Sibling		*Study 2* Target Child	Nontarget Sibling
Low power related mother[a]			Low power unrelated mother[a]		
High power related mother			High power unrelated mother		

[a]Maximum negative effects on caregiver communication are expected.

Mothers are videotaped interacting separately with the child (aged 3 to 12 years) they describe as the most difficult in the family and a sibling (matched for sex and age as closely as possible) they describe as relatively easier. Unrelated mothers are brought in from the general community to interact with the two children in exactly the same setting as the related mothers. All videorecording occurs in a pleasant room within CALM House, an attractive older house within a residential area of the community. Dyads are videotaped during four minutes of an unstructured, spontaneous social interaction and eight minutes of a game taught to the child by the adult.

The design of the two companion studies (children with mothers, children with strangers) allows us to test:

- The eliciting characteristics of target versus nontarget children both with their own and an unrelated mother.
- The moderating role of parental attributions. Low power attributions (e.g., high blame to children for caregiving failure) are expected to be more common among abusive mothers than among overdisciplining mothers.[3] For both sets of mothers, attributions are predicted to moderate the effects of child behavior on caregiver communication of affect.
- The moderating role of parental social support and stress. A questionnaire, including questions about the availability and use of social support networks, and an adaptation of the Holmes–Rahe Scale are administered to parents in the clinical sample. It is expected that moderate-risk families will have higher social support and lower stress than high-risk families. Levels of stress and support are predicted to moderate the effects of child behavior on caregiver communication.
- The caregiver communication patterns elicited as an interactive function of child behavior and caregiver attributions. Patterns will be measured (a) across time and (b) in direct response to child eliciting behavior.

  – The consequences of caregiver communication patterns. Changes in child behavior (maintenance or interruption of difficult behaviors) will be measured as a function of caregiver communication patterns.

Communication measures

Measures will focus upon the communication of specific affects, but we will also measure global dimensions such as pleasantness and assertiveness. We are primarily interested in the communication of negative affect and "insincere, inconsistent, or unconvincing" positive affect. Because parents may reasonably be motivated to present themselves in a favorable light, we are particularly interested in leakage of negative affect – negative affect that is revealed through nonverbal components that are difficult to manage (e.g., many aspects of voice quality or very brief facial displays). The caregiver's true attitude or affective response to the child may be revealed by subtle cues or particular combinations of communication components. For example, an insincere smile may fade from the face too quickly; unfelt praise may be expressed in a flat or tense voice.

The facial communication of affect will be assessed by the use of Ekman and Friesen's (1978) FACS (Facial Action Coding System). This neuro-culturally based coding system is the most refined measure of facial affect available. It allows the assessment of the frequency (and often intensity) of facial action units and combinations of units likely to be involved in the communication of specific affects (happiness, surprise, fear, sadness, disgust, anger).

Voice analysis will be of two types: (a) a judgment analysis of the quality of the mother's voice (audio portion of messages routed through a band-pass filter to eliminate intelligibility) and (b) acoustical analysis of the specific prosodic features of the voice (fundamental frequency, variability in fundamental frequency, etc.). (Measures of verbal content and proxemic measures are still being developed and will be described in later papers.)

Pilot findings

As an advance indication of the kind of results that may be anticipated when the study is complete, we conducted a preliminary analysis of global vocal dimensions for the first ten at risk mothers and the first ten unrelated mothers.[4] Both samples were drawn from predominantly Anglo middle-class backgrounds.[5] Typically, at risk mothers were self-referred, for example, members of parent support groups. Unrelated mothers were not, however, matched with at risk mothers for demographic variables. The mean education of unrelated mothers was 15.3 years and the mean education of at risk mothers was 12.6 years. The mean age of unrelated mothers was 38.4 years and the mean age of at risk mothers was 31.4 years. The two groups were equivalent in number of children ($\bar{x}_{unrelated}$ = 2.5; $\bar{x}_{at\ risk}$ = 2.7). These twenty mothers were videorecorded in interaction with 10 target children and their 10 nontargeted siblings. The target group included 7 boys and 3 girls; the nontarget group included 4 boys and 6 girls.[6] The average age in the target group was 8.8 (age range was 4–12). The average age in the non-target group was 7.0 (age range was 5–12).

Maternal messages[7] were precategorized into those that included affectively positive, neutral, or negative *verbal* content. Judges then rated these selected messages on the basis of their vocal *intonation* (through the use of band-pass filter). Ratings were made on the following scales:

Pleasant, friendly |_|_|_|_|_|_|_|_| Unpleasant, unfriendly

Strong, assertive |_|_|_|_|_|_|_|_| Weak, unassertive

Tense (sounds as if |_|_|_|_|_|_|_|_| Relaxed (does not sound
under stress)   as if under stress)

Sounds like speech |_|_|_|_|_|_|_|_| Sounds like speech to a
to an adult   child

Comparisons were made of the voice quality used to target and nontarget children by relatively high power (attributions) and low power mothers (median split) within the two groups (related and unrelated mothers). Voice quality on these four dimensions was compared (within groups) by analyses of variance that included one grouping variable (attributional style) and two repeated measures (target versus non-target child, and affective content of the verbal component of messages).[8]

Child effects were found for unrelated mothers for the dimension of voice assertion. Difficult (target) children elicited weaker voice quality than did their easier siblings $F(1,8)$ = 14.51, p = .005.

Significant effects were observed as a function of attributed blame to children for unsuccessful caregiving. Equivalent attributional effects were found for related and unrelated mothers. High blamers were found to manifest higher stress in their voice quality than did low blamers, $F(1/8)_{unrelated\ mothers}$ = 6.10, p = .04, $F(1/8)_{related\ mothers}$ = 4.75, p = .06. Additionally, high blamers differed from low blamers in their voice affect. Among unrelated mothers, high blamers had an affectively more negative voice quality than did low blamers, $F(1,8)$ = 6.90, p = .03.

A number of provocative interactive trends were found between child status and maternal attributions. For example, high-blaming mothers were more likely to sound negative when talking to the target child than to the nontarget child, $F(1,8) = 4.43$; $p = .07$. Because of the small sample size at this stage of analysis, any interpretation of more complex patterns is premature. When our analyses are based on a larger sample, more secure conclusions can be drawn.

Interaction sequences over time

Although we have not as yet begun our sequential analysis of adult–child interaction (to determine the immediate consequences of difficult child behavior on adult communication, and the reciprocal consequences of adult communication on child behavior), an anecdotal account of one set of interactions may suggest the type of findings we will obtain.

The target child in the illustrative family is a 4-year-old female who has been "beat up" by her mother several times during the last year. The nontarget child is a 7-year-old boy who has been overdisciplined (slapped or spanked frequently) but not abused. The girl's behavior is characterized by restlessness and hyperactivity. She bounces in the chair or rubs the arms of the chair in a constant, rhythmic fashion. She looks older than 4 and often her verbal content seems older than 4. Listed below are excerpts from the mother's interactions with the target child (abused and perceived by the mother as difficult) and the nontarget child (nonabused and seen as relatively easy by the mother). (The important point to note is the differential interactional flow. Static components are less interesting than sequential patterns.)

Mother with target child
Mother: What do you want to have for dinner tonight? I still haven't thought of anything yet. *(looks down while talking)*
Girl: um . . . I want . . . um
Mother: *(protracted yawn)*
Girl: Do we have steak? *(girl rubs arms of chair with heavy pressure)*
Mother: You want steak?
Girl: Yeah.
Mother: Okay . . . that sound good. *(looks at ceiling)*
Girl: *(looks away)* And I . . . t-tomorrow let's have . . . uh . . . buy . . . uh TV dinners. *(continues rubbing arms of chair in a grinding fashion)*
Mother: *(looks down)* Yuck!
Girl: Yeah. *(looking at mother)*
Mother: Yuck!
Girl: For us. Just for us.
Mother: Yuck. Yuck. Yuck.
Girl: Okay? Just for us. *(still rubbing arms of chair)*
Mother: *(lowers head)* All right *(softly)* . . . maybe not tomorrow . . . maybe the next day. Okay? *(looks up)*
Girl: Yeah!
Mother: *(looks down and mumbles something undecipherable and pulls lips tight[9])*
Girl: I'll . . . I'll . . . I'll . . . I'll . . . I'll . . . I'll . . . I'll . . . uh *(child stops rubbing arms of chair)*

Mother: *(looks up)* Think about what you're going to say *(opens eyes wide[10])*
Girl: I know what I'm going to say.
Mother: Okay.
Girl: I'll take the TV dinner out. Okay?
Mother: *(as child is talking, mother bites finger and looks away without response)*
(Throughout the remainder of the interaction, the mother's level of self-manipulation and movement away from the child increases.)

Mother with nontarget child
Mother: What happened to all our games . . . our Monopoly . . . and . . .
Boy: Uh, yeah . . . we have Monopoly.
Mother: Yeah . . . where is it? I haven't seen them.
Boy: They're at our school.
Mother: No, I mean the ones we have at home.
Boy: We don't have Monopoly.
Mother: We did.
Boy: We didn't.
Mother: *(Nods head "yes"; looks down, appears frustrated[11] and speaks softly)* I
        thought we did . . . maybe not.
Boy: I never saw it. The only game I . . . uh . . . I know is . . . uh . . .
        Backgammon.
Mother: You don't know how to play Backgammon! *(speaks sharply and with a con-temptuous facial expression[12])*
Boy: *(softly)* Teach me.
Mother: I know. I will. Then you'll have somebody else to play with.
        (pause)
Mother: It's fun. You'll like it. *(laughs)*
Boy: It looks fun too. *(looks down and speaks very softly)*
Mother: Are you behaving yourself?
Boy: *(nods "yes" and looks down)*
Mother: You're kidding.
Boy: *(looks up quickly at mother and continues looking at her)* Huh?
Mother: You're kidding.
Boy: *(looks down and speaks very softly)* No.
        (after pause, boy shifts topic to discussion of candy)
Boy: Do you like jawbreakers?
Mother: Uh uh. I don't like hard candy.
Boy: You don't? You like soft. I want . . . I want a bag of popcorn.
Mother: *(puts head down, smiles and looks up coyly)* You know what I got in my
        pocket?
Boy: *(looks at mother)*
Mother: *(whispers)* Tootsie Rolls.
Boy: *(draws in a big breath, smiles, bounces, and whispers)* Can I have one?

It can be seen that the mother was initially quite actively negative and sarcastic with the nontarget child. He responded to her behavior, however, with nonverbal submissiveness and verbal redirection. That is, he dropped topics that seemed headed in a bad direction and shifted over to pleasant ones. The consequence was that he succeeded in eliciting affectively positive behavior from her. The girl, on the other hand, pursued topics that were not well-received by her mother. The mother ultimately gave in to her daughter but showed escalating nonverbal signs of agitation and negative affect, even though the start of the interaction included a lot of positive affect.

The interactions between the two children and the *unrelated* mother both began pleasantly with discussions about the child's interests. With the boy, however, the conversation stayed at an animated and pleasant level. With the girl, the mother showed an increasing level of agitation and distress (rubbing her arms, kicking a leg, leaning away from the child). The children behaved in a similar fashion with their mother and the stranger. The boy monitored the conversation closely in both situations, sat quietly and was very responsive. The girl, on the other hand, was in constant motion in both settings. Her activity level took a more restrained form, however, with her own mother – she rubbed the arms of her chair rather than bouncing up and down.

Summary

We have proposed a transactional model of physical abuse that considers not only the effects of reciprocal behavior but also the potential moderating role of *social cognitions* (attributions). Additionally, attention is focused upon the communication of *affect* as a mediating variable in the family transactional system. It was predicted that difficult child behavior elicits affectively negative and unclear/inconsistent messages from caregivers, but more so from caregivers with a low power attributional style (or, in fact, with low real power). Caregivers who take low responsibility or credit for their caregiving successes and who attribute high blame to the child for caregiving failure were seen as more likely to be triggered by aversive, hard to manage child behavior. Attributional effects were expected to be stronger in ambiguous or unclear settings. Our preliminary findings produced effects as a function of attributions, child status (target versus nontarget), and interactive trends between attributions and child status. High blame women (mothers or strangers who attributed relatively high responsibility to children for unsuccessful interaction) were found to be more likely to demonstrate negative affect and tension in their tone of voice. Additionally, target (difficult) children were more likely to elicit vocal unassertiveness from caregivers than were nontarget (easier) children. Finally, trends were found supporting our prediction that difficult children have a more negative impact on low power caregivers than on high power caregivers.

Although we have no systematic evidence on interaction *sequences,* the anecdotal account presented suggested one possible mechanism whereby deteriorating sequences may occur. Target children may persevere in behavior that is potentially annoying to adults. The adult leaks information about her response to this behavior (annoyance and stress), which in turn may lead to escalating stress and negative affect in the child. The child's response to his or her own tension (e.g., restlessness) may then provide an additional stressor to the caregiver.

We hope to be able to demonstrate systematically that communication patterns typical for low power caregivers with difficult children are likely to maintain the child's behavior and elicit expressions of negative or ambivalent affect. This is particularly likely for young children, who have neither the social sophistication nor the cognitive competence to understand the mother's affectively unclear messages. By considering the linkage between social cognitions and affect (as well as behaviors), we believe that much is added to the understanding of the functional dynamics of abusive family systems.

Notes

1 Child Abuse Listening and Mediation.

2 We are using the Conflict Tactics Scale (Strauss, Gelles, and Steinmetz, 1980) as our measure of parental discipline. "Abusive" parents have "beat up, used a knife or gun, punched" or hit one or more of their children. "Overdisciplining" parents have made very frequent use of nonabusive physical discipline limited to spanking, slapping, etc.

3 They are also expected to differ from unrelated mothers. This comparison, however, has less meaning due to the noncomparability of groups. That is, both physically abusive and overdisciplining mothers sought counseling for family problems. Unrelated mothers were recruited in response to ads requesting mothers to interact with children in a play setting.

4 The design of the study calls for 40 related mothers (20 abusive and 20 overdisciplining) and 40 unrelated mothers.

5 A separate study is planned for low SES Hispanic families. In this later endeavor, both maternal groupings (and experimenters) will be bilingual and bicultural.

6 Sex distribution of more recent families is better balanced; sex will, however, be included as a variable in our final analysis. As a preliminary test of sex effects, ANOVA comparisons were made of the voice quality elicited by boys versus girls from their own versus unrelated mothers. Separate comparisons were made for target versus nontarget children. Sex differences were in opposite directions in the two child groupings and did not approach significance, $F_{target}(1,8) = 2.36$, and $F_{nontarget}(1,8) = .68$. In the target group, boys were found to elicit adult voice quality that was more pleasant, $F(1,8) = 4.18$, $p = .08$, and more relaxed, $F(1,8) = 5.68$, $p = .04$. As these findings run counter to the potential confound between sex and target status (i.e., boys are more likely to be difficult and thus elicit more parental stress or negative affect), any differences as a function of child status would not appear to be an artifact of sex. No other significant differences or trends were found as a function of child sex.

7 This initial analysis was limited to messages occurring during unstructured social interaction. Categorization was based on preratings by four judges (mothers themselves) on content affect.

8 Comparisons were made separately for affectively positive, neutral, and negative content. This controls for any differences in voice quality that may have occurred as a function of variations in verbal affect. Messages of all three types were available for related mothers;

for unrelated mothers, however, comparisons were limited to affectively positive and neutral content (few unrelated mothers made negative comments).
9 Action unit #23 (Ekman and Friesen, 1978). Additionally, she presses her lips together (action unit #24) on a regular basis throughout the interaction.
10 Action unit #5.
11 Action unit #14.
12 Action unit #10 combined with "plus face" (Zivin, 1982).

References

Aber, J. L. and Cicchetti, D. (1984). The social–emotional development of maltreated children: An empirical and theoretical analysis. In H. Fitzgerald, B. Lester, and M. Yogman (Eds.), *Theory and research in behavioral pediatrics.* New York: Plenum.

Abramson, L. Y., Seligman, M. E. P., and Teasdale, J. D. (1978). Learned helplessness in humans: Critique and reformulation. *Journal of Abnormal Psychology, 87,* 49–74.

Affleck, G., Allen, D., McGrade, B. J., and McQueeney, M. (1982). Maternal causal attributions at hospital discharge of high-risk infants. *American Journal of Mental Deficiency, 86,* 575–580.

Andersen, C. R. (1977). Locus of control, coping behavior, and performance in a stress setting: A longitudinal study. *Journal of Applied Psychology, 62,* 446–451.

Bates, J. E. (1975). The effects of a child's imitation versus nonimitation on adults' verbal and nonverbal positivity. *Journal of Personality and Social Psychology, 31,* 840–851.

Becker, W. C., and Krug, R. S. (1965). The Parent Attitude Research Instrument: A research review. *Child Development, 36,* 329–365.

Bell, R. Q. (1966). A reinterpretation of the direction of effects in studies of socialization. *Psychological Review, 75,* 81–95.

Belsky, J. (1980). Child maltreatment: An ecological integration. *American Psychologist, 35,* 320–335.

Bender, B. (1976). Self-chosen victims: Scapegoating behavior sequential in battering. *Child Welfare, 55,* 417–422.

Boukydis, C. F. Z., and Burgess, R. L. (1982). Adult physiological response to infant cries: Effects of temperament of infant, parental status and gender. *Child Development, 53,* 1291–1298.

Bugental, D. B. (1974). Interpretation of naturally occurring discrepancies between words and intonation: Modes of inconsistency resolution. *Journal of Personality and Social Psychology, 30,* 125–133.

Bugental, D. B., Caporael, L., and Shennum, W. A. (1980). Experimentally produced child uncontrollability: Effects on the potency of adult communication patterns. *Child Development, 1980, 51,* 520–528.

Bugental, D. B., and Cruzcosa, M. (1985). Causal attributions for caregiving success and failure: A theoretical and methodological analysis. Unpublished paper, University of California, Santa Barbara.

Bugental, D. E., Kaswan, J. W., and Love, L. R. (1970). Perceptions of contradictory messages conveyed by verbal and nonverbal channels. *Journal of Personality and Social Psychology, 16,* 647–655.

Bugental, D. E., Kaswan, J. W., Love, L. R., and Fox, M. N. (1970). Child versus adult perception of evaluative messages in verbal, vocal, and visual channels. *Developmental Psychology, 2,* 367–375.

Bugental, D. B., and Love, L. R. (1975). Nonassertive expression of parental approval and disapproval and its relationship to child disturbance. *Child Development, 46,* 747–752.

Bugental, D. E., Love, L. R., Kaswan, J. W., and April, C. (1971). Verbal–nonverbal conflict in parental messages to normal and disturbed children. *Journal of Abnormal Psychology, 77,* 6–10.

Bugental, D. B., and Shennum, W. A. (1984). "Difficult" children as elicitors and targets of adult communication patterns: At attributional–behavioral transactional analysis. *Monographs of the Society for Research in Child Development, 49* (Serial No. 205, 1).

Burgess, R. L. (1979). Child abuse: A social interactional analysis. In B. B. Lahey, and A. E. Kazdin (Eds.), *Advances in clinical child psychology.* New York: Plenum.

Burgess, R. L., and Conger, R. (1978). Family interaction in abusive, neglectful, and normal families. *Child Development, 49,* 1163–1173.

Cantor, N., and Gelfand, D. (1977). Effects of responsiveness and sex of children on adults' behavior. *Child Development, 48,* 232–238.

Cicchetti, D., & Rizley, R. (1981). Developmental perspectives on the etiology, intergenerational transmission, and sequelae of child maltreatment. *New Direction for Child Development, 11,* 31–55.

Cohn, J. F., and Tronick, E. Z. (1984). Three-month-old infant's reaction to simulated maternal depression. *Child Development, 54,* 185–193.

Conger, R. D., McCarty, J. A., Yang, R. K., Lahey, R. K., and Kropp, J. I. (1984). Perception of child, child-rearing values, and emotional distress as mediating links between environmental stressors and observed maternal behavior. *Child Development, 55,* 2234–2247.

Cruzcosa, M. (1985). Causal attributions as moderators of social facilitation effects. Unpublished manuscript, University of California, Santa Barbara.

de Lissovoy, V. (1979). Toward the definition of "abuse provoking child." *Child Abuse and Neglect, 3,* 341–350.

DePaulo, B. M., and Jordan, A. (1982). Age changes in deceiving and detecting deceit. In R. S. Feldman (Ed.), *Development of nonverbal and behavior in children.* New York: Springer-Verlag.

Diener, C. I., and Dweck, C. S. (1978). An analysis of learned helplessness: Continuous changes in performance, strategy, and achievement cognitions following failure. *Journal of Personality and Social Psychology, 36,* 451–462.

Donovan, W. L. & Leavitt, L. A. (1985). Simulating conditions of learned helplessness: The effects of interventions on attributions. *Child Development, 56,* 594–603.

Egeland, B., and Brunnquell, D. (1978). An at-risk approach to the study of child abuse: Some preliminary findings. Unpublished manuscript, University of Minnesota.

Ekman, P. (1972). Universal and cultural differences in facial expressions of emotion. In J. Cole (Ed.), *Nebraska symposium on motivation.* Lincoln: University of Nebraska Press.

Ekman, P., and Friesen, W. V. (1969). Nonverbal leakage and clues to deception. *Psychiatry, 32,* 88–106.

Ekman, P., and Friesen, W. V. (1978). Manual for the Facial Affect Coding System. Palo Alto, CA: Consulting Psychologists Press.

Ekman, P., Friesen, W. V., and Scherer, K. R. (1976). Body movement and voice pitch in deceptive interaction. *Semiotica, 16,* 23–27.

Elmer, E., and Gregg, G. S. (1967). Developmental characteristics of abused children. *Pediatrics, 40,* 596–602.

Field, T. M. (1980). Interactions of preterm and term infants with their lower- and middle-class teenage and adult mothers. In T. M. Field, S. Goldberg, D. Stein, and A. M. Soster (Eds.), *High-risk infant and children,* New York: Academic Press.

Folkman, S., Aldwin, C., and Lazarus, R. S. (1981). The relationship between locus of control, cognitive appraisal and coping. Paper presented at the meeting of the American Psychological Association.

Friedrich, W., and Boriskin, J. (1976). The role of the child in abuse: A review of the literature. *American Journal of Orthopsychiatry, 46,* 580–590.

Frodi, A. M., and Lamb, M. E. (1978). Child abusers' responses to infants' smiles and cries. *Infant Behavior and Development, 1,* 187–198.

Frodi, A. M., Lamb, M. E., Leavitt, L. A., Donovan, W. L., Neff, D., and Sherry, D. (1978). Fathers' and mothers' responses to the faces and cries of normal and premature infants. *Developmental Psychology, 14,* 490–498.

Garbarino, J. (1977). The human ecology of child maltreatment: A conceptual model for research. *Journal of Marriage and the Family, 39,* 721–736.

Garbarino, J., and Crouter, A. (1978). Defining the community context for patent–child relations: The correlates of child maltreatment. *Child Development, 49,* 604–616.

Gaensbauer, T., Mrazek, D., & Harmon, R. (1980). Affective behavior patterns in abused and/or neglected infants. In N. Frude (Ed.), *The understanding and prevention of child abuse: Psychological approaches.* London: Concord Press.

Gaensbauer, T., and Sands, S. (1979). Distorted affective communications in abused/neglected infants and their potential impact on caretakers. *Journal of the American Academy of Child Psychiatry, 18,* 236–250.

Gil, D. G. (1970). *Violence against children: Physical child abuse in the United States.* Cambridge, MA: Harvard University Press.

Goldberg, S. (1979). Premature birth: Consequences for the parent–child relationship. *American Scientist, 67,* 214–220.

Goodnow, J. J. (1985). Change and variation in ideas about childhood and parenting. In I. E. Sigel (Ed.), *Parental belief systems: The psychological consequences for children* (pp. 235–270). Hillsdale, N.J.: Erlbaum.

Goodnow, J. J. (in press). Parents' ideas about parenting and development: A review of issues and recent work. In M. Lamb, A. Brown, and B. Rogoff (Eds.), *Advances in developmental psychology.* Hillsdale, N.J.: L. & A. Publishers.

Green, A. H. (1974). Self-destructive behavior in battered children. *American Journal of Psychiatry, 135,* 579–582.

Green, A. H., Gaines, R. W., and Sandgrund, A. (1974). Child abuse: Pathological syndrome of family interactions. *American Journal of Psychiatry, 131,* 881–886.

Helfer, R. E. (1980). Developmental deficits which limit interpersonal skills. In C. H. Kempe and R. E. Helfer (Eds.), *The battered child.* Chicago: University of Chicago Press.

Holzman, P. S., and Rousey, C. (1966). The voice as a percept. *Journal of Personality and Social Psychology, 4,* 78–86.

Hunter, R. S., Kilstrom, N., Kraybill, E. N., and Loda, R. (1978). Antecedents of child abuse and neglect in premature infants: A prospective study in a newborn intensive care unit. *Pediatrics, 61,* 629–635.

Johnson, J. H., and Sarason, J. C. (1978). Life stress, depression and anxiety: Internal–external locus of control as a moderator variable. *Journal of Psychosomatic Medicine, 22,* 205–208.

Justice, B., and Duncan, D. G. (1976). Life crisis as a precursor to child abuse. *Public Health Reports, 91,* 110–115.

Kobasa, S. C. (1979). Stressful life events, personality, and health: An inquiry into hardiness. *Journal of Personality and Social Psychology, 37,* 1–11.

Kuiper, N. A. (1978). Depression and causal attribution for success and failure. *Journal of Personality and Social Psychology, 36,* 236–246.

Lazarus, R. S. (1981). The stress and coping paradigm. In C. Eisdorfer, D. Cohen, A. Kleinman, and P. Maxim (Eds.), *Models for clinical psychopathology.* New York: Spectrum.

Lefcourt, H. M., Miller, R. S., Ware, E. E., and Sherk, D. (1981). Locus of control as a modifier of the relationship between stressors and moods. *Journal of Personality and Social Psychology, 41,* 357–369.

Lester, B. M. and Zeskind, P. S. (1979). The organization and assessment of crying in the infant at risk. In T. M. Field, A. M. Sostek, S. Goldberg, and H. H. Shuman (Eds.), *Infants born at risk.* New York: Spectrum.

Mehrabian, A., and Weiner, M. (1967). Decoding of inconsistent communication. *Journal of Personality and Social Psychology, 6,* 109–114.

Milowe, I., and Lourie, R. (1964). The child's role in the battered child syndrome. *Society for Pediatric Research, 65,* 1079–1081.

Morris, M., and Gould, R. (1963). Role reversal. A necessary concept in dealing with the battered child syndrome. In: *The neglected/battered child.* New York: Child Welfare League of America.

Ounstead, C., Oppenheimer, R., and Lindsay, J. (1974). Aspects of bonding failure: The psychopathology and psychotherapeutic treatment of families of battered children. *Developmental Medicine and Child Neurology, 16,* 447–452.

Parke, R. D., and Collmer, C. (1975). Child abuse: An interdisciplinary analysis. In E. M. Hetherington (Ed.), *Review of child development research* (Vol. 5). Chicago: University of Chicago Press.

Patterson, G. R. (1976). The aggressive child: Victim and architect of a coercive system. In L. A. Hamerlynck, L. C. Handy, and E. J. Mash (Eds.), *Behavior modification and families. I. Theory and research.* New York: Brunner/Mazel.

Patterson, G. R. (1980). Mothers: The unacknowledged victims. *Monographs of the Society for Research in Child Development, 45* (Serial No. 186, 5).

Phares, E. J. (1976). *Locus of control in personality.* Morristown, NJ: General Learning Press.

Reid, J. B., Patterson, G. R., and Loeber, R. (1981). The abused child: Victim, instigator, or innocent bystander? In J. Bernstein (Ed.), *Response structure and organization.* Lincoln: University of Nebraska Press.

Reilly, S., and Muzekari, L. (1979). Responses of normal and disturbed adults and children to mixed messages. *Journal of Abnormal Psychology, 88,* 203–208.

Saarni, C. (1982). Social and affective functions of nonverbal behavior: Developmental concerns. In R. S. Feldman (Ed.), *Development of nonverbal behavior in children.* New York: Springer-Verlag.

Snow, M. E., Jacklin, C. N., and Maccoby, E. E. (1983). Sex-of-child differences in father–child interaction at one year of age. *Child Development, 54,* 227–232.

Spinetta, J. J., and Rigler, D. (1972). The child-abusing parent: A psychological review. *Psychological Bulletin, 77,* 296–304.

Steele, B. F. (1976). Violence within the family. In R. E. Helfer and C. H. Kempe (Eds.), *Child abuse and neglect.* Cambridge, MA: Ballinger Publishing Co.

Steele, B. F., and Pollock, D. D. (1968). A psychiatric study of parents who abuse infants and small children. In R. E. Helfer and C. H. Kempe (Eds.), *The battered child.* Chicago: University of Chicago Press.

Steinberg, L. D., Catalano, R., and Dooley, D. (1981). Economic antecedents of child abuse and neglect. *Child Development, 52,* 975–985.

Strauss, M. A., Gelles, R. J., and Steinmetz, S. K. (1980). *Behind closed doors: Violence in the American family.* New York: Anchor.

Vasta, R. (1982). Physical child abuse: A dual-component analysis. *Developmental Review, 2,* 125–149.

Vasta, R., and Copitch, P. (1981). Simulating conditions of child abuse in the laboratory. *Child Development, 52,* 164–170.

Volmar, F. R., and Siegel, A. E. (1979). Young children's responses to discrepant social communications. *Journal of Child Psychology and Psychiatry, 20,* 139–149.

Wallerstein, J. S., and Kelly, J. B. (1975). The effects of parental divorce: Experiences of the preschool child. *Journal of the American Academy of Child Psychiatry, 14,* 600–616.

Weiner, B. (1974). *Achievement motivation and attribution theory.* Morristown, NJ: General Learning Press.

Weiner, B. (1980a). A cognitive (attribution)-emotion-action model of motivated behavior: An analysis of judgments of help-giving. *Journal of Personality and Social Psychology, 39,* 186–200.

Weiner, B. (1980b). *Human motivation.* New York: Holt, Rinehart & Winston.

Weisz, J. R. (1980). Developmental change in perceived control: Recognizing noncontingency in the laboratory and perceiving it in the world. *Developmental Psychology, 16,* 385–390.

Young, L. (1964). *Wednesday's children: A study of child neglect and abuse.* New York: McGraw-Hill, 1964.

Zeskind, P. S. (1980). Adult responses to cries of low and high risk infants. *Infant Behavior and Development, 49,* 580–589.

Zivin, G. (1982). Watching the sands shift: Conceptualizing development of non-verbal mastery. In R. S. Feldman (Ed.), *Development of nonverbal behavior in children.* New York: Springer-Verlag.

9 Perceived similarities and disagreements about childrearing practices in abusive and nonabusive families: intergenerational and concurrent family processes

Penelope K. Trickett and Elizabeth J. Susman

Physical abuse of a child occurs within a family context and yet little is known about many of the processes that may differentiate abusive families from nonabusive families. The evidence that does exist indicates that abusive families differ from nonabusive families in the quality of parent–child interactions (Burgess and Conger, 1978; Reid, 1986; Trickett and Kuczynski, 1986), in parental attitudes and values about childrearing, and in parental perceptions of their children (Susman, Trickett, Iannotti, Hollenbeck, and Waxler, 1985; Trickett, Susman, and Gordon, 1984). However, to understand child development within the context of the family, one must go beyond looking solely at parent–child dyadic interaction to examine other aspects of complex family processes (see, e.g., Bronfenbrenner, 1977).

It is the purpose of this chapter to examine two aspects of family process of particular relevance to the etiology of abuse and to the consequences of abuse for child development. These two areas are: first, parents' perceptions of their own upbringing – a topic that bears on the issue of intergenerational transmission of abuse – and second, parental conflict or disagreement, especially concerning childrearing.

Parental perceptions of their own upbringing

The notion of intergenerational transmission is popularly posited as an important factor in the etiology of child abuse. There is, in fact, considerable empirical evidence that abusive parents are more likely to have experienced aggression, violence, and/or harsh physical punishment during their child-

We are very grateful for the support of the staff of the protective service agencies of Frederick, Montgomery, and Prince George's Counties in Maryland; of Arlington County, Virginia; and of the District of Columbia Superior Court. Without their help this study could never have been completed. We are also grateful to Pauline Kolman for her assistance in the preparation of this manuscript and to Marian Radke Yarrow for her continued support.

hood than nonabusive parents (Parke and Collmer, 1975), although it is also clear that many people with similar backgrounds do not become abusive parents (Cicchetti and Rizley, 1981). The processes that account for the transmission of this specific facet of childrearing from one generation to the next are not well understood. Most hypotheses have been derived from social learning theory. Thus, it is postulated that abused children learn aberrant patterns of parent–child interaction through the principles of observational learning, modeling, and patterns of reinforcement (Barahal, Waterman, and Martin, 1981).

But what are the cognitive processes that may mediate this transmission? Apparently, the only relevant empirical studies are those of Main and Goldwyn (1984) and Hunter and Kilstrom (1979). In a study of normal mothers and their infants, Main and Goldwyn attempted to assess the impact of maternal rejection during childhood on mothers' relations with their own infants. Based on a retrospective interview, ratings of rejection during childhood were derived for each mother. These ratings were found to correlate significantly with the mother being avoided by her own infant following brief separations, suggesting problems in mother–infant attachment. The ratings of maternal rejection during childhood also were found to be positively related to ratings of the degree to which the mothers idealized their own mothers and the degree to which they could not recall their childhood and negatively to ratings of "coherence in discussing childhood." These findings are supported by the results of a psychiatric study that compared abused parents who abuse their own children with abused parents who do not (Hunter and Kilstrom, 1979). These authors found the nonabusive parents (i.e., those who broke the intergenerational transmission cycle) to report more detailed accounts of their own maltreatment and to express more anger about these experiences than abusive parents. Main and Goldwyn speculate that their findings may help to illuminate

our understanding of the distortions in cognitive processes which arise as a result of particular types of child maltreatment; the way in which these distortions in cognitive processes become systematically related to particular types of childhood experience; and the role which these distortions play in determining whether an individual will "repeat" the experience of maltreatment and abuse when he/she becomes a parent. (p. 215)

The present chapter also is concerned with cognitive processes that may mediate the continuation of patterns of maltreatment. The focus here is on two issues: (a) the degree to which abusive and nonabusive parents report themselves to be in agreement with the childrearing styles or values of their own parents and to use their parents as sources of knowledge and support in the rearing of their own children, and (b) the degree to which parental beliefs about their own upbringing are related to their children's development.

Parental disagreement

The second focus of this chapter is on examining disagreement between mothers and fathers in abusive and nonabusive families and to relate this to children's development. It is unknown whether parental disagreement is more prevalent in abusive families than in nonabusive families but, given the frequent characterization of these families as disorganized and chaotic, it is not unreasonable to believe that this may be the case. Parental disagreement in abusive families can be either an etiological factor or a sequelae of abuse. It can be an etiological factor in abuse when a child becomes a scapegoat for disagreement between mother and father. The parents may project their disagreements and conflict on a child in the form of physical abuse in order to avoid expressing their hostility toward each other. Disagreement may be a sequelae of abuse when parents attempt to change longstanding patterns of childrearing as a result of intervention by others or from the general stress of being labeled abusive. Also, if the child develops behavior problems as a result of the abuse and becomes harder to manage, difficult parental demands may increase, inducing disagreement between the parents. However, if child abuse is indeed a family problem, perhaps there is a high degree of agreement between parents at least as far as rearing children is concerned. To date there is no empirical evidence to support either of these contradictory hypotheses.

There is, however, evidence that parental conflict and disagreement can have a deleterious impact on children's development. This evidence comes from research done from two slightly different perspectives. The first has focused on intense marital conflict. Two types of families have been studied, those in which divorce has occurred and those in which there is parental psychopathology. The second perspective has focused explicitly on parental agreement/disagreement about childrearing in nonclinical research samples.

In studies of families where conflict exists or divorce occurs, children have been shown to have a variety of behavior problems (Hetherington, Cox, and Cox, 1978; Rutter, 1971). If a child whose parents divorce has problems, the question is whether the problems are a sequelae of separation from a parent or of the marital conflict that preceded the separation. Evidence supports the latter alternative (Emery, 1982; Hetherington, 1979). Rutter (1971) found that even in the absence of divorce, children from families reporting marital conflict experience more behavior problems than children from families where there is little conflict. In fact, the percentage of boys reporting behavior problems was linearly related to the marital distress reported by their parents. Similar relations were reported for marital discord and conduct disorder problems (McCord and McCord, 1959).

In families with parental psychopathology, children have been shown to have more behavior problems than in families where there is none (e.g.,

Beardslee, Bemporad, Keller, and Klerman, 1983). The association between marital conflict and child problems is stronger in clinic than nonclinic samples (e.g., Oltmanns, Broderick, and O'Leary, 1977; Porter and O'Leary, 1980). However, marital conflict may be more salient in some groups of disordered parents, whereas the nature of the disorder may be more salient in others (Emery, Weintraub, and Neale, 1982). To examine this hypothesis, Emery et al. (1982) compared the association between school problems and marital discord in children of bipolar-depressed, unipolar-depressed, schizophrenic, and normal parents. Marital problems were more strongly related to school problems in the bipolar and unipolar groups and less strongly in the schizophrenic group. Rutter (1971) also showed that marital problems were related to antisocial behavior in the children of both normal and personality-disorder individuals. However, when marriages were harmonious, antisocial personality in the parent was not associated with antisocial behavior in the child.

The problem in all of these studies is that it is difficult to determine the causal direction of the relation between the psychopathology of the parents and behavior problems of the child. In earlier studies, the disturbed person – the schizophrenic or depressed parent – was presumed to have a unique impact on another family member – the child. Recent literature on family systems shows that the disturbed person may have an impact on multiple family systems, all of which may affect individuals within a family or the family as a whole (Margolin, 1981). For instance, a depressed parent may have an adequate parenting style, but depression in one spouse may deleteriously affect the marital relationship which, in turn, has negative consequences for the child.

In nonclinic parents, few studies have examined disagreements between mothers and fathers and their impact on the child. The exception is a longitudinal study by Block, Block, and Morrison (1982) that examined disagreements between mothers and fathers on childrearing values and orientations. The index of disagreement was found to predict divorces in these families and psychological functioning in the children at the time of assessment and four years later. For instance, 7-year-old boys whose parents were low on disagreement four years earlier were described by their teachers as more task oriented, verbally facile, and interesting than boys whose parents were high on disagreement. Seven-year-old girls whose parents were low on disagreement were rated as less inhibited than girls whose parents were high on disagreement. In general, results for boys showed that parental agreement is related positively to ego control and ego resiliency. For girls, parental agreement is related negatively to ego control and is independent of ego resiliency. Block et al. (1982) suggest that agreement between parents creates a more structured and predictable environment than that found in homes characterized by disagreement about childrearing.

The present chapter is concerned with parental disagreement, measured both specifically in terms of childrearing beliefs and, more generally, in terms of the overall family environment. The focus is on two questions: (a) whether disagreement is more prevalent in abusive than in nonabusive families, and (b) whether such disagreement has an impact on children's development.

For both aspects of the family process examined in this chapter (parental perceptions of their own upbringing and parental disagreement), child development is assessed in terms of the prevalence of behavior problems using the Achenbach Child Behavior Checklist (Achenbach and Edelbrock, 1983). As indices we use the two "broad-band" groupings of behavior problems: internalizing problems (fearful, inhibited, overcontrolled behavior), and externalizing problems (aggressive, antisocial, undercontrolled behavior).

To summarize, this chapter addresses the following questions:

1. Do abusive and nonabusive families differ in the degree to which parents report agreeing with the childrearing values of their own parents and using their own parents as sources of knowledge and support?
2. Do abusive and nonabusive families differ in the degree to which mothers and fathers share childrearing values and perceptions of the psychological environment of the home?
3. Is the development of abused and nonabused children related to the degree of perceived similarity and/or disagreement about childrearing between generations and/or between parents?

Description of participants

Participants were all the two-parent families ($N = 34$) who were taking part in a study of the impact of physical abuse on the psychological development of children between the ages of 4 and 11 (Trickett, Susman, and Lourie, 1980). In half of these families the children were physically abused by one or both parents. These families were recruited from protective service agencies located in the Washington, D.C., metropolitan area. For almost all these families, there was a history of reported incidents lasting several months or years. The usual injury incurred by the child was bruising or welts or, in a few cases, fractures. The injury resulted in hospitalization of the child in 15% of the cases. In 18% of the families, both parents were identified as the abuser; in 59% the mother alone was identified as the abuser; and in 23% the father alone was so identified. (Approximately half of the abusing fathers were stepfathers and half were biological fathers.)

The other half of the sample was a control group matched on gender and age of the child, race, and family socioeconomic status as measured by the Four Factor Index of Social Status (Hollingshead, 1975). Table 9.1 sum-

Table 9.1. *Demographic characteristics of participating families*

		Abuse group $n = 17$	Control group $n = 17$
Child's age (mean in months)		85.50	83.17
Child's gender (%)	male	28	33
	female	72	67
Child's ethnic group (%)	white	67	78
	black	33	22
Family SES[1] (mean)		33.53	37.22
Family type (%)	step parent	50	17
	biological parent	50	83

[1]An index of family SES was completed using the Hollingshead 4-factor Index of Social Status (1975). In this measure, for two-parent families, both parents' education scores (which can range from 1 = less than 7th grade education to 7 = graduate degree) are weighted by 3 and averaged. Parents' occupation scores (which can range from 1 = menial service workers/chronically unemployed to 9 = major professionals) are weighted by 5 and averaged. (If the mother is a homemaker, just the father's occupation score is used.) These two scores are then summed to find the family SES figure. In the case of single-parent homes, only the resident parent's education and occupation scores are used. For the Hollingshead Index, scores ranging from 30 to 39 are represented by the occupations of skilled craftsmen, and clerical and sale workers.

marizes the demographic characteristics of the participating families. There are no significant differences between the two groups on any of the characteristics listed in the table.

Parental perceptions of their own upbringing

Parent measures

Information about mothers' and fathers' perceptions of their own parents and upbringing and of the use of their parents as sources of knowledge and support was obtained from an interview administered to each parent separately. This interview lasted about one hour and covered many topics, including a developmental history of the child in the study and many questions on the childrearing attitudes and values of the parent. Embedded in this interview were questions concerning each of the following topics:

Initial childrearing support from parents. Parents were asked, "Think back to just before and just after the birth of your first child – to the time when you were first becoming a parent. How did you learn to be a parent? That is, some people talk to relatives or friends with questions about what babies are like and how to take care of them, some people talk to the doctor or nurse, others read books or go to a parenting class, and others just follow their instincts. What did you do?" For the present analyses, responses were coded in terms of whether participants mentioned their own parents in response to this question.

Amount of current childrearing support received from one's parents. In order to obtain information about the parents' social support networks, participants were asked to list those people whom they considered close and important and then to indicate on a 23-item support checklist whether they received various types of support from each of these people. Five of the items on this checklist concerned childrearing support (e.g., "I get help from this person such as babysitting, picking the kids up from school, etc."). For the present analyses, the number of childrearing supports provided by each parent was tallied. (If the parent was not listed on the network a score of zero was given.) Because the scores for amount of childrearing support received from one's mother and one's father were positively correlated, a combined score indicating amount of childrearing support from both parents was derived (with a possible range of 0 to 10).

Perceived difference from one's own parents. Parents were asked to describe themselves as parents by rating themselves (on a five-point scale) on six pairs of adjectives (strict–lenient, irritable–easy going, inconsistent–consistent, uninvolved–involved, nondemonstrative–demonstrative, and unfair–fair). They were then asked to rate their own mothers and fathers on these same characteristics. Two Perceived Difference Scores were derived by summing the absolute difference scores of the parents' rating of themselves and of their mother and father for each of the six characteristics. Because these scores were positively correlated, they were averaged to derive one Perceived Parental Difference score.

Raising one's child the same or differently from one's own upbringing. Parents were asked, "Overall, do you think you're raising your child(ren) much the same way that you were raised or very differently?" Responses were coded on a five-point scale ranging from 1 (just the same) to 5 (very differently).

Severity of physical punishment parent received as a child. Parents were asked what kinds of punishment were used with them when they were children. Responses were coded on a five-point scale from 1 (no physical punishment) to 5 (abused as a child).

Table 9.2. *Means for parental perception variables for abuse and control groups*

	Abuse group		Control group	
	M	SD	M	SD
Amount of childrearing support from parents	2.17	2.68	3.00	3.32
Perceived difference from own parents	7.75	3.82	7.22	4.93
Raising own child different from own rearing	3.78	1.26	3.55	1.10
Severity of physical punishment received as a child	3.44	1.25	2.89	1.02

Child measure

The Child Behavior Checklist (CBC) (Achenbach and Edelbrock, 1983) was completed by each child's mother. The CBC consists of 113 behavior problems rated on a scale of 0 (not true of my child) to 2 (very true or often true of my child). The items can be scored into two broad-band scores representing the number of internalizing problems (fearful, inhibited, overcontrolled behavior) and the number of externalizing problems (aggressive, antisocial, undercontrolled behavior). Information about the reliability, validity, and standardization of the CBC is available from the Manual (Achenbach and Edelbrock, 1983).

Results and discussion

Group differences. A chi-square was computed to compare the number of parents in the abuse and control groups who mentioned their own parents as one way they learned how to be a parent. Not only was the chi-square nonsignificant, but exactly 38.2 percent of both groups responded affirmatively.

For the remaining measures, group by sex of parent by sex of child analyses of variance were conducted. The means appear in Table 9.2. With one exception, there were no significant main effects or interactions. The exception was that the abusive parents reported receiving harsher physical punishment as children than did the control parents, $F(1,67) = 5.39$, $p = .02$.

It is important to emphasize the potential significance of this lack of differences between the two groups on these measures. This suggests that both groups of parents are equally likely to pass on what they have learned about parenting to their own families. And yet, the abusive parents report an important difference in their own rearing – the use of harsher physical punishment. Putting these two findings together, it is logical to assume that this tendency to use harsh physical punishment is one legacy that is likely to be passed on from generation to generation.

Interrelationships between parent perception variables for the abuse and control groups. Correlations were calculated for all the variables separately for the two groups. (Patterns for mothers and fathers in the two groups were very similar, so all parents were combined.) Table 9.3 illustrates these correlational patterns. There are striking differences in the pattern of relationships for the two groups. For the abuse group, none of the 10 coefficients is significant. For the control group, six of the ten are significant, all at the $p \leq .01$ level or higher. In every case, the difference between the six significant coefficients for the control group and the comparable coefficient for the abuse group is statistically significant (the six z's ranged from 1.98, $p \leq .05$, to 2.76, $p \leq .01$). Briefly, for the control group, parents who reported raising their child differently from the way they were raised were less likely to report learning parenting from their own parents (Initial Parental Childrearing Support) or getting current childrearing support from their parents and more likely to view their parenting style as quite different from that of their own parents. Further, the parents who rated themselves as different from their own parents also were less likely to report learning how to be a parent from their own parents and more likely to report receiving harsh physical punishment as children. None of these relationships was true for the abusive parents.

The difference in the pattern of relationships of these measures for the abuse and control groups is important. For the control group, these form a coherent pattern. Thus, control parents who said they were raising their children differently from the way they were raised also perceived themselves as different from their own parents and were less likely to be currently using their parents for childrearing help. These are all logical relationships that are not present for the abusive parents. This lack of coherence is similar to the Main and Goldwyn (1984) findings discussed earlier in the chapter. Further, the control parents who reported receiving harsh punishment as children were more likely to report that they perceive themselves as different from their own parents and as raising their children differently. This suggests a conscious turning away from their upbringing and an attempt to be different. Again, one does not see this same pattern in the abusive parents.

Relation of parent perception variables to child behavior. In order to assess the impact of these measures on child development, stepwise regression analyses were conducted. Three of the parental perception variables were selected as independent variables (current parental childrearing support, perceived difference from parents, and severity of physical punishment) on a combination of empirical and conceptual grounds. The first two variables

Table 9.3. *Correlations of parental perception measures for abuse and control groups*

	Initial parental childrearing support	Current parental childrearing support	Perceived differences from parents	Raising child differently from own upbringing	Severity of physical punishment from parents
Initial parental childrearing support		.56***	−.46**	−.63***	−.18
Current parental childrearing support	.13	—	−.27	−.45**	−.13
Perceived difference from parents	.14	−.04	—	.60***	.61**
Raising child differently from own upbringing	−.04	.07	.17	—	.25
Severity of physical punishment from parents	−.01	.06	.17	.26	—

Note: Abuse group scores are below the diagonal and control group scores above the diagonal.

*$p < .05$

**$p < .01$

***$p < .001$

were based on scales (rather than one-item measures) and represented different aspects of the intergenerational transmission issue. The third variable, severity of physical punishment, was selected, even though it is based on a one-item scale, because of its special relevance to the issue of intergenerational transmission of physical abuse. Because mothers' scores and fathers' scores were not positively correlated, composite scores were not computed and these three indexes were entered separately into the regression equations for mothers and fathers. The final independent variable was a dummy variable representing abuse- or control-group status. The dependent variables in these analyses were the internalizing and externalizing t scores from the CBC. In reporting the findings, use of the terms predictor, dependent variable, and independent variable does not imply causality. These terms should be interpreted on the basis of their statistical meaning only. A stepwise regression procedure was used in which, first, all the independent variables except the variable of group status were entered as a set and each noncontributing variable was removed in a stepwise fashion. Then, the group status variable was entered. The results of these analyses appear in Table 9.4.

For the internalizing dimension of the CBC, prior to the addition of group, three variables were significant predictors of the children's behavior problems: fathers' current parental childrearing support, mothers' severity of physical punishment, and mothers' parental difference score. When group was added on the last step, it also was a very strong predictor. Also, upon the addition of group to the regression equation, two of the previously significant predictors – mothers' severity of punishment and mothers' parental difference score – were no longer significant.

For the externalizing dimension, prior to the entry of group into the regression, the only significant predictor was fathers' current parental childrearing support. When group was added it was a very significant predictor. Also, upon the entry of group a third variable – fathers' parental difference score – also appeared as a significant predictor.

In these analyses, the strongest predictor of both internalizing and externalizing behavior problems was group membership. This suggests an association of physical abuse with not only acting-out, aggressive types of behavior problems as has been shown in the past (e.g., George & Main, 1979; Reidy, 1977), but also with internalizing problems, which could include social withdrawal, fearfulness, and depression. This finding warrants closer examination. Also, for both types of behavior problems there was one predictor besides group membership that was significant – the fathers' reporting of parental childrearing support. Overall, we have found that fathers in our sample report less childrearing support than mothers do (Trickett and Corse, 1983), which may be because of the lesser role that fathers have traditionally taken in childrearing as compared with mothers. The relation

Table 9.4. *Best regression equations prior to and after the entry of group membership: Parent perception measures*

Dependent variable	Best regression equation for Set 1 variables			Best regression equation for Set 1 and Set 2 variables		
	Variables	Beta	t	Variables	Beta	t
Internalizing behavior problems	Father's parental childrearing support	−.49	−3.45**	Father's parental childrearing support	−.41	−3.35**
	Mother's severity of punishment	.44	2.98**	Group	−.54	−4.39***
	Mother's parental difference score	−.30	−1.99*		$R^2 = .52$	
		$R^2 = .42$			$F = 17.66***$	
		$F = 7.58***$				
Externalizing behavior problems	Father's parental childrearing support	−.33	−2.06*	Father's parental childrearing support	−.27	−2.19*
		$R^2 = .11$		Father's parental difference score	−.26	−2.14*
		$F = 4.24*$		Group	−.61	−4.92***
					$R^2 = .52$	
					$F = 11.78***$	

Note: Predictor variables entered: Set 1: Father's severity of punishment, Mother's severity of punishment, Father's parental childrearing support, Mother's parental childrearing support, Father's parental difference score, Mother's parental difference score. Set 2: Group.
*$p < .05$
**$p < .01$
***$p < .001$

found here between fathers' reporting of parental childrearing support and fewer externalizing and internalizing behavior problems suggests that this variable may reflect the degree to which a father identifies with and is engaged in the parenting role and that such involvement has important, measurable implications for children's development.

One other finding from the regression analyses bears noting: In the analyses with internalizing problems as the dependent variable, two of the mothers' variables – severity of punishment and parental difference score – were significant predictors until the addition of group membership to the regression equation. Even though no main effect for sex of parent or group by sex of parent interaction was found for the severity of punishment variable, this would suggest that the mothers' history of harsh punishment and/or abuse is more closely tied to being in an abusive family than was the fathers' punishment history, which is similar to a finding reported by Hunter and Kilstrom (1979).

Before discussing the practical implications of these findings, the analyses for the other component of family process – parental disagreement – will be presented.

Parental disagreement

Parent measures

Four scores related to parental disagreement were derived, two based on standardized measures and two based on questions contained in the previously described parent interview. These were:

Child Rearing Practices Report (CRPR) disagreement index. The CRPR (Block, 1981) is a 91-item measure of childrearing attitudes and values presented in a *Q*-sort format. Parents sort each item into one of seven piles according to how descriptive the item is of the parent's attitudes, thus resulting in a score of 1 to 7 for each item. The 91 items cover many different areas of childrearing attitudes and values including attitudes about discipline, independence, achievement, and emotional expressiveness. Following the work of Block et al. (1982), an index of parental disagreement in childrearing attitudes was derived by summing the absolute differences of mothers' and fathers' scores for each of the 91 items. In a longitudinal study, Block et al. (1982) found parental disagreement on the CRPR to be predictive of divorce.

Family Environment Scale (FES) disagreement index. The FES (Moos and Moos, 1981) is a 90-item, true–false measure of the psychosocial environment of the home that covers such areas as cohesion, control, expressive-

Table 9.5. *Means for disagreement measures for abuse and control groups*

	Abuse group		Control group	
	M	SD	M	SD
CRPR disagreement index	157.55	27.30	149.33	42.42
FES disagreement index	31.00	4.86	26.35	6.14
Agreement about discipline	3.78	.94	3.67	1.28
Satisfaction with help from spouse	4.12	1.20	4.44	1.15

ness, and moral–religious orientation. An index of parental disagreement about the family environment was derived by summing the absolute differences of mothers' and fathers' scores for each of the 90 items. A similar index of disagreement on this measure developed by Moos (see Moos and Moos, 1981) has been found to yield larger disagreement scores in families in treatment at a psychiatric clinic than normal families and to be correlated with a number of maladaptive behaviors in alcoholic families.

Agreement about discipline. In order to obtain specific information about parents' agreement regarding the discipline of the child in the study, a question included in the parent interview was, "In general do you and your spouse usually agree about how to discipline (child's name)?" Responses were coded on a five-point scale from 1 (always disagree) to 5 (always agree).

Satisfaction with spouse's childrearing help. As another index of presence or absence of parental conflict, a question on the parent interview was, "How satisfied are you with the help you get from your spouse in bringing up the children?" Responses were coded on a five-point scale from 1 (very dissatisfied) to 5 (very satisfied).

Results and discussion

Group differences. Group by sex of child analyses of variance were conducted for the CRPR Disagreement Index and the FES Disagreement Index. The group means appear in Table 9.5. For the CRPR Disagreement Index, there was significantly more disagreement between parents of girls ($M = 175.42$) than between parents of boys ($M = 142.23$), $F(1,33) = 8.00$, $p = .008$. There also was a borderline interaction between group and sex of child, $F(1, 33) = 3.81$, $p < .06$. For the abuse group, there was no difference in amount of disagreement between parents of girls ($M = 164.33$) and parents of boys ($M = 154.36$). For the control group, there was more disagreement between parents of girls ($M = 186.50$) than between parents of boys ($M = 132.09$) and, in fact, control parents of boys had the least disagreement of all four groups.

For the FES disagreement index, there was significantly more disagreement in the abuse than in the control group, $F(1,32) = 5.89$, $p = .02$. There also was an interaction between group and sex of child, $F(1,32) = 4.61$, $p = .04$. For the abuse group there was no difference in the amount of disagreement between parents of boys ($M = 31.27$) and parents of girls ($M = 30.67$). For the control group, there was more disagreement between parents of girls ($M = 31.80$) than between parents of boys ($M = 24.09$). Again, control parents of boys had the least disagreement of all four groups.

For the two variables – agreement about discipline and satisfaction with spouse's childrearing help – group by sex of child by sex of parent analyses of variance were conducted. There were no significant main effects or interactions.

Thus, all these analyses suggest that disagreement between the abuse and control group was most pronounced about the nature of their family environment rather than about childrearing practices, per se. These disagreements about the emotional and social environment of the family may create considerable conflict between husbands and wives, a factor known to be related to deleterious psychological outcomes in children (e.g., Emery, 1982). Conflicts about daily family matters (e.g., social, recreational, and cultural activities) may fragment the relationship between husbands and wives which, in turn, may sever mutual sources of social support outside the family. Failing to participate in activities outside the family may further isolate abusive families from the outside world, which they appear to view as hostile and threatening (Trickett et al., 1984).

In these analyses of variance, the interactions with sex of child suggest that many parents may disagree more about the upbringing of girls than of boys. This disagreement may result from the rapid and pervasive changes regarding the roles of women that have been occurring in the last two decades. Whereas in the past the aim was to prepare girls to assume the role of wife and mother, the aim now is to prepare girls for the multiple roles of wife, mother, employee, and perhaps head of household. Most of the mothers in our sample were employed, which may be a factor in predisposing them to value nontraditional childrearing values for their daughters, such as an emphasis on achievement, independence, and openness to new experience. Fathers may be less inclined to adopt similar nontraditional values because they are less directly involved in the changing roles of women. An implication of the disagreements between mothers and fathers is that girls are reared in an ambivalent environment, which may contribute to role conflicts in women later in the life span. That abusive parents did not show this

Table 9.6. *Correlations of parent disagreement measures for abuse and control groups*

	CRPR disagreement index	FES disagreement index	Satisfaction wtih spouse's childrearing help	Agreement about discipline
CRPR disagreement index[a]	—	.54**	−.02	.06
FES disagreement index	−.07	—	−.27	.04
Satisfaction with spouse's childrearing help	.39*	−.16	—	.13
Agreement about discipline	.25	−.04	.64***	—

Note: Abuse group scores are below the diagonal and control group scores above the diagonal.
[a] For CRPR disagreement index and FES disagreement index the higher the score the higher the disagreement. For agreement about discipline and satisfaction with spouse's childrearing help, the higher the score, the higher the agreement/satisfaction.
*$p < .05$
**$p < .01$
***$p < .001$

greater disagreement about the upbringing of girls than of boys may be another bit of evidence of their inflexibility in childrearing (Susman et al., 1985; Trickett and Kuczynski, 1986).

Interrelations among disagreement indexes. Correlations between the four disagreement indices were calculated separately for the abuse and control groups. The coefficients appear in Table 9.6. As in the previous correlational analyses, there were striking differences in the pattern of relations for the two groups. For the abuse group, parents who reported satisfaction with the help they were receiving from their spouse in childrearing were more likely to report disagreement on the CRPR and higher parental agreement about discipline. For the control group, parents who reported higher disagreement on attitudes and values about childrearing (CRPR disagreement index) also reported higher disagreement about their family environment (FES disagreement index). The correlations of the FES disagreement index with the CRPR Disagreement index for the two groups were significantly different from each other, $z = 2.20$, $p < .05$. Also, the correlations of satisfaction with spouse's childrearing help with agreement about discipline were significantly different for the two groups, $z = 2.45$, $p < .01$.

The different patterns of correlation in the two groups indicate that different processes may mediate parental disagreement and child behavior. For example, even though there were no mean differences for the two groups for agreement about discipline and satisfaction with spouse's help, the relation of these two variables in the abuse group was significantly different from the relation in the control group. For the abuse group, there was a strong positive relation between satisfaction with help from spouse and agreement about discipline. It may be that because discipline is an especially problematic area of childrearing for the abusive families (see Trickett and Kuczysnki, 1986), it is more salient in affecting satisfaction with a spouse's childrearing help than is true for the control families.

Also of significance is the difference in the pattern of correlations for the CRPR disagreement index and the FES disagreement index. On one hand, for the control group, if there was disagreement, it appeared in more than one domain. That is, general disagreement and disagreement specifically about childrearing tended to go together. For the abuse group, on the other hand, although there was more disagreement in general, it did not generalize to disagreement about childrearing.

Relation of parental disagreement to child behavior. To assess the relation between the disagreement measures and the development of the children, stepwise regression analyses were conducted. Two of the parental disagreement measures – CRPR disagreement index and the FES disagreement index – and their interactions with sex of child terms were selected as independent variables. These disagreement indexes were chosen because they are based on standardized measures, one of which has been shown to be related to child outcomes in past studies (e.g., Block et al., 1982). The interaction of the disagreement indices and sex of child were used because of the significant interaction between group and sex of child reported in the group difference analyses. The CRPR disagreement index and the FES disagreement index and their interaction terms were entered as a set into the regression equations. The final independent variable was a dummy variable representing abuse or control group status. The dependent variables in these analyses were the internalizing and externalizing *t*-scores from the CBC.

The results of the regression analyses appear in Table 9.7. For the Internalizing dimension, prior to the addition of Group, the CRPR disagreement by sex of child interaction term and FES disagreement index were significant predictors. For the Externalizing dimension, the results were similar, except that the FES disagreement index was not significant after Group was added to the equation.

Thus, families in which there was disagreement about the general family environment reported a higher incidence of both internalizing and externalizing behavior problems (although for the Externalizing dimension this relationship became nonsignificant when the abuse or control status of the parents was taken into consideration). Based on many previous studies (e.g., Emery, 1982; Rutter, 1971), it was anticipated that in an unpredictable, conflict ridden family environment, children may begin to show externalizing behavior problems. These behaviors may reflect undercontrolled ego devel-

Table 9.7. *Best regression equations prior to and after the entry of group membership: Parent disagreement measures*

	Best regression equation for Set 1 variables			Best regression equation for Set 1 and Set 2 variables		
Dependent variable	Variables	Beta	t	Variables	Beta	t
Internalizing behavior problems	CRPR by sex interaction	.34	2.44*	FES Disagreement index	.36	2.56*
	FES Disagreement index	.60	4.32**	Group	−.45	−3.20**
	$R^2 =$ .40			$R^2 =$ .46		
	$F = 10.92***$			$F = 13.92***$		
Externalizing behavior problems	CRPR by sex interaction	.37	2.50*			
	FES Disagreement index	.50	3.86***	Group	−.63	−4.66***
	$R^2 =$ .32			$R^2 =$ .40		
	$F = 7.65**$			$F = 21.69***$		

Note: Predictor variables entered: Set 1: FES disagreement index, CRPR disagreement index, FES by sex interaction, CRPR by sex interaction; Set 2: Group.
* p .05
** p .01
*** p .001

opment or an inability to control and cope with the conflict that exists in their enduring childrearing environment. What was not anticipated based on previous research was the relationship between parental disagreement and internalizing behavior problems, which are often viewed as a manifestation of overcontrolled ego development. Thus, it appears that both over- and undercontrolled ego development are affected by family conflict.

A second finding of the regression analyses was that, for both dimensions of the CBC, families in which there was disagreement about childrearing and in which there was a male child reported a higher incidence of behavior problems. This was so even though the analyses of variance showed that parental disagreement was higher in parents of girls than in parents of boys. These seemingly inconsistent findings actually are consistent with sexual dimorphic patterns of social and biological development. The higher number of behavior problems in boys from families where there is higher disagreement about childrearing is consistent with the hypothesized heightened biological vulnerability of boys for many mental and physical health problems (Block et al., 1982; Rutter, 1970). For instance, boys experience more deleterious psychological consequences related to marital discord (Rutter, 1971) and divorce (Hetherington et al., 1978) than do girls.

In addition to the vulnerability hypotheses, Block et al. (1982) suggest two other interpretations of the relation between negative quality of parenting and its impact on boys. First, mothers and fathers may be equally salient for boys – the mother by virtue of her caretaking role, the father by virtue of his bond to his son. Fathers may be less salient for girls when they are young. When conflict erupts between parents, boys may be confused and stressed by their conflicted loyalties, whereas girls can align themselves with their mothers. In these families, parental conflict would be expected to create more problems for boys. Second, boys may have a greater need to control events. Conflict contributes to children's perceptions of their inability to control events, which may be more stressful for boys than for girls.

The issues of vulnerability, differential parental saliency, and control as factors in the development of behavior problems in boys may be important psychological processes in mediating the higher incidence of abuse of boys in the preadolescent years. Boys may exhibit behavior problems that are reacted to with harsh physical discipline. In turn, boys may escalate acting out. An escalating pattern of acting out and harsh discipline may eventually lead to parental physical abuse.

Conclusions and implications

We found some support for the notion that intergenerational transmission of attitudes and values about childrearing, particularly as it relates to harsh discipline, may be related to the etiology of child abuse. Consonant with the findings of Hunter and Kilstrom (1979) and Main and Goldwyn (1984), we also found some indication that breaking the cycle of intergenerational transmission may require rejection of the attitudes and values of one's own parents. Control parents who experienced harsh punishment saw themselves as raising their children quite differently from the way they were raised and were less likely to turn to their parents for childrearing help.

Our finding that parental disagreement about childrearing and the nature of the family environment is related to a higher incidence of behavior problems, especially for boys, suggests that such disagreement as a component of the childrearing environment of abusive families is another risk factor in the development of abused children.

In combination, these findings suggest the importance of studying the broader family context in the attempt to understand the processes involved in abuse. An important implication is that both primary prevention programs and intervention programs for abusive families should be concerned not only with the didactics of child management. Also essential is attention to the dynamics of both intergenerational and intragenerational family processes, including the nature of the childrearing experienced by abusive parents, the degree of engagement of the father in the parenting process, and the amount of current parental conflict.

There are a number of important questions that could not be addressed by the current study. First, because of the small sample size, we were unable to investigate how the child's age might be related to the impact of these family variables. It might well be that these family processes have a different impact on children in the early school years than on children entering puberty. Similarly, we were unable to examine the relevance of stepfather or biological father status. Although, in this very small sample, there is no evidence that stepfathers are more prone to being abusive than biological fathers, it may well be that the family processes relevant to abuse differ in stepparent and nonstepparent families. These topics need to be the subject of further research.

Another focus for future research could be on specifying more exactly which aspects of childrearing attitudes and perceptions of the family environment abusive families disagree about most and which areas of disagreement have the greatest impact on child development. As a whole, abusive parents disagree more about the general family environment than about childrearing per se. However, within both of these categories, there may be specific areas of agreement or disagreement of importance. For example, abusive parents may disagree more than nonabusive parents about independence of family members than about degree of family organization or more about the value of emotional expressiveness than about discipline. Such knowledge, added to that of the relevance of the child's age and of stepparent status, would allow for the design of much-needed, more effective, developmentally and ecologically appropriate intervention and prevention programs.

References

Achenbach, T. M., & Edelbrock, C. (1983). *Manual for the Child Behavior Checklist.* Burlington, VT: Queen City Printers, Inc.

Beardslee, W. R., Bemporad, J., Keller, M. B., and Klerman, G. L. (1983). Children of parents with major affective disorders: A review. *American Journal of Psychiatry, 140,* 825–832.

Barahal, R. M., Waterman, J., and Martin, H. P. (1981). The social cognitive development of abused children. *Journal of Consulting and Clinical Psychology, 49,* 508–516.

Block, J. H. (1981). The child-rearing practices report (CRPR): A set of Q items for the description of parental socialization attitudes and values. Unpublished manuscript, University of California, Berkeley.

Block, J. H., Block, J., and Morrison, A. (1982). Parental agreement–disagreement on child-rearing orientations and gender-related personality correlates in children. *Child Development, 52,* 965–974.

Bronfenbrennner, U. (1977). Toward an experimental ecology of human development. *American Psychologist,* 513–531.

Burgess, R. L., and Conger, R. C. (1978). Family interaction in abusive, neglectful, and normal families. *Child Development, 49,* 1163–1173.

Cicchetti, D., and Rizley, R. (1981). Developmental perspectives on the etiology, intergenerational transmission, and sequelae of child maltreatment. In R. Rizley and D. Cicchetti (Eds.), *New Directions for Child Development.* Washington: Jossey-Bass, Inc., pp. 31–56.

Emery, R. E. (1982). Interparental conflict and the children of discord and divorce. *Psychological Bulletin, 92,* 310–330.

Emery, R., Weintraub, S., and Neal, J. M. (1982). Effects of marital discord on the school behavior of children of schizophrenic, affectively disordered and normal parents. *Journal of Abnormal Child Psychology, 10,* 215–228.

George, C., and Main, M. (1979). Social interactions of young abused children: Approach, avoidance, and aggression. *Child Development, 50,* 306–318.

Hetherington, E. M. (1979). Divorce: A child's perspective. *American Psychologist, 34,* 851–858.

Hetherington, E. M., Cox, M., and Cox, R. (1978). The aftermath of divorce. In J. H. Stevens, Jr., and M. Matthews, (Eds.), *Mother–Child, Father–Child Relations.* Washington: National Association for the Education of Young Children.

Hollingshead, A. F. (1975). Four-factor index of social status. Working paper, Department of Sociology, Yale University.

Hunter, H. S., and Kilstrom, N. (1979). Breaking the cycle in abusive families. *American Journal of Psychiatry, 136,* 1320–1322.

Main, M., and Goldwyn, R. (1984). Predicting rejection of her infant from mother's representation of her own experience; Implications for the abused–abusing intergenerational cycle. *Child Abuse and Neglect, 8,* 203–217.

Margolin, G. (1981). The reciprocal relationship between marital and child problems. In J. P. Vincent (Ed.), *Advances in Family Intervention, Assessment, and Theory,* Vol. 2. Greenwich, CT: Jai Press.

McCord, W., and McCord, J. (1959). *Origins of Crime: A New Evaluation of the Cambridge-Somerville Youth Study.* New York: Columbia University Press.

Moos, R. H., and Moos, B. S. (1981). *Family Environment Scale Manual.* Palo Alto, CA: Consulting Psychologists Press.

Oltmanns, T. F., Broderick, J. E., and O'Leary, K. D. (1977). Marital adjustment and the efficacy of behavior therapy with children. *Journal of Consulting and Clinical Psychology, 45,* 724–729.

Parke, R. D., and Collmer, C. W. (1975). Child abuse: An interdisciplinary analysis. In E. M. Hetherington (Ed.), *Review of Child Development Research, Vol. 5,* Chicago: University of Chicago Press.

Porter, B., and O'Leary, K. D. (1980). Marital discord and childhood behavior problems. *Journal of Abnormal Child Psychology, 80,* 287–295.

Reid, J. B. (1986). Social-interaction patterns in families of abused and nonabused children. In C. Zahn-Waxler, E. M. Cummings, and R. Iannotti (Eds.), *Altruism and Aggression: Social and Biological Origins.* Cambridge: Cambridge University Press.

Reidy, T. (1977). The aggressive characteristics of abused and neglected children. *Journal of Clinical Psychology, 33,* 1140–1145.

Rutter, M. (1970). Sex differences in response to family stress. In E. J. Anthony and C. Kompernik (Eds.), *The Child and His Family.* New York: Wiley.

Rutter, M. (1971). Parent–child separation: Psychological effects on the children. *Journal of Child Psychology and Psychiatry, 12,* 233–260.

Susman, E. J., Trickett, P. K., Iannotti, R., Hollenbeck, B. E., and Zahn-Waxler, C. (1985). Child-rearing patterns in depressed, abusive, and normal mothers. *American Journal of Orthopsychiatry, 55,* 237–251.

Trickett, P. K., and Corse, S. J. (1983). Support networks, stress and child-rearing attitudes: Relationships in abusive families. Paper presented at the annual meeting of the American Psychological Association. Anaheim, CA.

Trickett, P. K., and Kuczynski, L. (1986). Children's misbehaviors and parental discipline strategies in abusive and non-abusive families. *Developmental Psychology, 22,* 115–123.

Trickett, P. K., Susman, E. J., and Gordon, M. (1984). The childrearing environment of abusive and nonabusive families. Paper presented at the 92nd annual meeting of the American Psychological Association, Toronto.

Trickett, P. K., Susman, E. J., and Lourie, I. (1980). The impact of the child-rearing environment on the abused child's social and emotional development. Protocol # 80-M-112, National Institute of Mental Health, Bethesda, MD.

Carolyn Moore Newberger and Kathleen M. White

What is parental development, and how is parenthood defined? Is it a biologically based instinct, or a set of behaviors and/or skills learned at a parent's own mother's (and father's) knee? Is the development of parental competence largely a psychological process, or is it a reflection of the capacity of the environment to support or erode the establishment and maintenance of a nurturant home context?

Parental development has been variously defined, and the definitions attached to parenting have had important implications for our understanding of the breakdown in parental functioning represented by child maltreatment. For example, researchers who conceptualize parental development as the acquisition of a set of traits or abilities may fail to examine characteristics of the environment or characteristics of the child in order to explain adequately why some parents sharing certain psychological attributes may abuse a child in their care and others may not. Clinicians who focus exclusively on parental psychological variables may place a child in foster care without recognizing that there is a strong and caring extended family where the child could be placed with a minimum of trauma until the parent's emotional issues can be addressed.

We define parenting as a complex and multidimensional process. As Klaus and Kennell (1976) remark,

A mother's and father's actions and responses toward their infant are derived from a complex combination of their own genetic endowment, the way the baby responds to them, a long history of interpersonal relations with their own families and with each other, past experience with this or previous pregnancies, the absorption of the practices and values of their cultures, and perhaps most importantly how each was raised by his or her own mother and father. (p. 7)

What, then, do we see as the essential components of the parenting process that are necessary to our understanding of child maltreatment? The parent's own characteristics and experiences contribute importantly to the process. For example, a mother's capacity to foster the healthy development of her child may be influenced by her own upbringing, by the kind and amount of nurturing and protection she may have experienced at the hands of her own parents. This capacity is also influenced by such characteristics as her own self-esteem, depression, the quality of her social and physical environment, knowledge of developmental norms, and how she understands the child's needs. Parents bring to the parental role their levels of maturity in a variety of domains (emotional, cognitive, social) as well as their personal histories, attitudes toward childrearing, and personalities. Children also bring their own characteristics to their relationships. Both parents and children are seen as dynamic and interacting individuals whose mutual influence on each other is affected by complex forces, including their own characteristics, their relationships with each other, and the broader contexts (e.g., social, economic, and historical) in which they interact.

Our appreciation for (if not yet understanding of) the complexity of the development and expression of parental care does not in any way limit the importance of developing a fuller understanding of each of the component parts. In focusing in depth on a component of a complex picture, however, we must not lose sight of the eventual need to integrate that component into a broader whole.

In this chapter we will focus on cognitive dimensions of influence on the development of parental care. These cognitive dimensions have been studied as a subcategory of parental personality characteristics. They include attitudes and beliefs about childrearing, parental attributions and expectations of the child, and the development of the cognitive perspectives that parents draw from in order to make sense of the child and to guide their actions in relation to the child.

Parental attitudes and expectations

Although the characterization of parental thinking and its effects on children has generated a large body of literature, until the past ten years research and theory had been primarily concerned with attitudes toward specific childrearing practices and with behavior (Baldwin, Kalhorn, and Breese, 1945; Blank, 1963; Schaefer and Bell, 1958; Sears, Maccoby, and Levin 1957). Parental attitudes, however, have been found to be poor predictors of parental behavior (Becker and Krug, 1965) and of child outcome (Leton, 1958; Yarrow, Campbell, and Burton, 1968). Nowlis (1952) found that different parental interpretations or concepts can underlie similar acts, so that an act can have different meanings for different mothers and, by implication, for their children.

Even though Sears et al. (1957) found interesting and provocative relationships between parental care variables and children's behavior, Yarrow and her colleagues (1968) were not able to replicate the findings. Becker and Krug (1965) and Beckwith (1972) found meaningful relationships between standardized measures of parental attitudes and children's behavior only with middle-class families. Tulkin and Choler (1973) report that relationships between the Maternal Attitude Scale scores and observed maternal behavior were much less clear in the working-class sample than in the middle-class sample.

As parental attitude studies have been based on the belief that there is a "best" way to raise children, with the purpose of research being to find this best way, they do not take into account the possibility that people from diverse backgrounds and circumstances might have different beliefs and different standards from those of the researchers and the standardizing populations. Duvall (1946), for example, found different beliefs about "good" parents and children among mothers from various subcultures. Because particular behaviors and attitudes would have different meaning in subcultures with different beliefs and values, they would be likely to have different effects on children's behavior. In a study of Black mothers, both teen-aged and adult, Field, Windmayer, Stringer, and Ignnatoff (1980) concluded that "Despite the teenage mothers' less optimal perceptions and attitudes, their offspring did not differ from those of adult mothers on developmental assessments. Any expected developmental differences may have been attenuated by family support systems, the greater availability of substitute caregiving (e.g., by the unemployed grandmothers) and the infants' exposure to a wide range of playmates" (p. 433).

In addition to these limitations in research and theory on parental attitudes, there is some suggestion that the relationship between attitudes of both parents toward childrearing and toward each other as caregivers may be importantly implicated in parental competence. A review of a number of relevant studies by Parke, Power, and Gottman (1979) supports the conclusion that "Consensus in childrearing attitudes, the father's perception of the mother's caretaking competence, and other qualities of the husband–wife relationship are all related to maternal involvement or competence" (Parke, Power, and Fisher 1980, p. 99).

Another type of characteristic assumed to be related to parenting behavior is knowledge of and expectations concerning normal child development. In a longitudinal study of 37 young couples who married in high school, DeLissovoy (1973) collected data over a three-year period on a number of marriage and parenting issues, including a questionnaire on developmental norms. According to DeLissovoy, "The responses of both parents revealed that knowledge of basic norms was sadly lacking. The answers were skewed to an unrealistically early expectation of development" (p. 251).

Evidence concerning maternal age and lack of knowledge of developmental norms comes from a study by Epstein (1979) that supports the notion that teenage mothers are deficient in their knowledge of child development and that this lack of knowledge may affect their interactions with their children. Although misperceptions concerning developmental norms have been cited in the literature as related to child maltreatment, the exact nature of this relationship remains unclear.

Parental attributions and child maltreatment

The use of attribution theory to investigate child maltreatment has brought an important new cognitive dimension to the field. With this conceptualization, "a person's perceptions are jointly influenced by a need to objectively understand the environment and by more subjective self-serving needs to enhance or protect self-esteem" (Larrance and Twentyman, 1983, p. 450). Within the bounds of perceived reality, there is flexibility in interpreting the reasons for an individual's actions. In general, investigators have reported that research subjects tend to make positive attributions about their own behavior, and that this tendency toward positive self-attribution is generalized to attributions about others with whom the individual is intimate. As applied to parenting behavior in general and child maltreatment in particular, work has focused on the reasons parents offer for explaining children's specific behavior. These reasons may be related to such factors as motivation ("He's crying because he's upset" or "He's crying because he's bad"), expectations ("She's too young to understand" or "She's old enough to know better"), or situations' influences ("He's tired"). The expectation has been that parents who have maltreated a child in their care will be more likely than control parents to ascribe negative attributions to their children's behavior. For example, a parent who has maltreated a child would be expected to be more likely to attribute a behavior such as breaking a toy to "badness" than to "tiredness."

The results of this approach have been mixed. Several studies matching samples of mothers with protective service histories for having abused and/ or neglected their children with mothers without such histories have found significant differences (e.g., Siracusa, 1985; Larrance and Twentymen, 1983). (As with the majority of studies of child maltreatment, fathers are rarely studied.) In these studies, mothers in the maltreatment groups have had consistently more negative perceptions than mothers in the comparison groups.

In direct contrast, Rosenberg and Reppucci (1983) found no differences in abusive mothers' perceptions of their children's behavior when compared with mothers who had problems with childrearing, but who were not identified as abusive by social workers in the parenting program where they were all enrolled.

A partial explanation for these inconsistencies may be in the different ways parental perceptions were measured and in the differing nature of the control groups employed. In the study (Rosenberg and Reppucci, 1983) with no significant differences, the comparison group consisted of mothers who were receiving help because they had difficulty controlling their children's behavior. That they would view their children's intentions negatively is not surprising. A third comparison group of mothers who did not require intervention for parenting would perhaps have enabled a more differentiated understanding of the relation of parental attributions to parental efficacy in general and to child maltreatment in particular.

Bates, Freeland, and Lounsbury (1979) offer thought-provoking data on the extent to which maternal personality characteristics mediate the ways in which mothers view (and interact with) their babies. In their study, multiparous extroverted mothers tended to rate their babies as "easy." Moreover, there was no evidence that the babies really were easy, as correlations between extroversion and home observation of the babies on variables such as crying and soothability were low. Thus, extroverted mothers tended to *label* their babies as easy despite a wide range of infant behaviors as recorded in the home observations. Noting that mothers who describe themselves as extroverted report a high degree of dominance, Bates, Freeland, and Lounsbury speculate that such mothers may feel that their infants' fussiness is under their control and therefore not difficult. This study raises the important issue of the relation of parental personality characteristics to parental perceptions of the child. Although parental perceptions, attributions, and expectations may all in some way be implicated in child maltreatment, if they covary with parental self-conceptions and emotions, then the limitations of separating the "thought" from the "feeling" are clear.

Parental perspective-taking: a cognitive-developmental view

Emmerich (1969) found that different goals and beliefs can underlie the same surface attitudes, supporting the view that parental attitudes and behavior must be understood within the framework of the parent's own thinking. McGillicuddy-DeLisa, Sigel, and Johnson (1979) propose that parents construct belief systems about their children that provide the basis for predispositions to act certain ways. Sameroff (1975) suggests that mothers' thinking about child development can be grouped into stages that are analogous to Piaget's levels of cognitive development.

Several studies of parental dysfunction have observed relationships between parental conceptions and parental behavior. These investigators have noted that parents who have abused their children frequently lack an awareness of the effects of mistreatment or lack of care on their children (Aldridge, Cautley, and Lichstein, 1974; Berg, 1976; Smith, Hanson, and Noble, 1973). In other words, they fail to comprehend their children's experience from the children's point of view. In a prospective study, Egeland and Brunnquell (1979) found that "the mother's ability to deal with the psychological complexity of the child and childrearing" at 36 weeks gestation accounted for the most variance in a discriminant analysis that predicted dysfunction/nondysfunction status at an 84 percent rate of accuracy.

Such findings have led to a systematic study of the nature and development of parents' conceptions of children and the parental role conducted by the first author. This research on parental awareness, to be described in some detail, has implications for service providers working with families experiencing difficulties in nurturing and protecting their children, as well as for basic researchers interested in family processes with both well-functioning and poorly functioning families.

Parental awareness, parental development, and parental care

During the late 1970s, Carolyn Newberger (1977) initiated a study of parents' conceptions of children, with the goal of drawing on social cognitive-developmental psychology to develop a framework for understanding the process and development of parental understanding of the child and of the parental role. Newberger's work was generated in part from a series of clinical interviews with a group of parents including some mothers and fathers with a clinical history of having abused or severely neglected a child in their care. During the context of these interviews Newberger noted:

How they reasoned appeared to be related to how they behaved as parents. In particular, parents with especially troubled relationships with their children were frequently unable to perceive their children as having needs and rights of their own separate from those of the parent. Other parents understood their children as separate individuals but in a rather stereotyped way, as though one could understand one's own child only through a definition of children offered by others. Yet other parents reasoned about their children as distinct and unique individuals. Stable individual differences in how these parents thought about their children appeared to correspond to descriptions of different cognitive–structural stages in . . . understanding of others' perspectives and personhood as they have been described by cognitive-developmental investigators [Piaget, 1950; Kohlberg, 1969; Selman, 1971]. (C. Newberger, 1980, p. 3)

These observations suggested a developmental progression of understanding in parenthood. This progression was hypothesized to proceed from an egocentric view through a stereotypic view into a more individualized and analytic view of the child and of the parent–child relationship. A study of parental conceptions of children and the parental role was designed in order to develop a methodology to examine parental cognitive process and its development.

Before we describe the study of parental awareness, let us define what we mean by parental cognition from the cognitive-developmental perspective employed in this approach. Cognition can be understood as the logic a person uses to make sense of experience. In other words, cognition is a mental blueprint for how the world operates, which organizes how the individual operates in relation to the world. Social cognition is the logic of thinking about persons and relationships in the interpersonal world. In childhood, the stages through which that social logic progresses proceed from an egocentric view, in which children do not differentiate their own perspectives from those of others, to an increasingly complex and comprehensive awareness of the perspectives and intentions of others as separate from themselves (Selman, 1980). The central question addressed by Newberger's application of social cognitive-developmental theory to the study of parenthood was: Can a developmental process of interpersonal awareness be identified in parental thinking and, if identified, does it bear a relationship to parental functioning?

In order to study the nature and development of parental awareness, Newberger (1977) constructed an interview that explores parental reasoning on a variety of issues requiring parental understanding: interpreting the child's subjective experience, identifying influences on development, defining a "good child," making decisions concerning child discipline, resolving conflict, meeting needs, engendering communication and trust, and learning and evaluating parental performance.

In Newberger's initial study (Newberger, 1977, 1980), 51 families representing a broad cross-section of social and family backgrounds (as defined by the Hollingshead, 1965, two-factor index of social scale) were interviewed. An analysis of the interviews revealed that parental conceptions could be ordered hierarchically into four increasingly comprehensive and psychologically oriented levels. These levels of parental awareness are briefly described as follows:

Level 1: Egoistic orientation. The parent understands the child as a projection of his or her own experience, and the parental role is organized around parental wants and needs.

Level 2: Conventional orientation. The child is understood in terms of externally derived (tradition, culture, "authority") definitions and explanations of children. The parental role is organized around socially defined notions of correct practices and responsibilities.

Level 3: Subjective–individualistic orientation. The child is viewed as a unique individual who is understood through the parent–child relationship, rather than by external definitions of children. The parental role is organized around identifying and meeting the needs of this child, rather than as the fulfillment of predetermined role obligations.

Level 4: Systems orientation. The parent understands the child as a complex and changing psychological self-system. The parent grows in the role . . . and recognizes that the relationship and the role are built not only on meeting the child's needs, but also on finding ways of balancing one's own needs and the child's so that each can be responsibly met (pp. 12–13).

From the interviews, Newberger (1977) constructed a scoring manual for measuring levels of parental awareness. In studies of independent samples of parents, the manual has been found to discriminate among parents, and the reliability between raters has ranged from .88 to .96 (e.g., Cook, 1979; Partoll, 1980; Hofer, 1981; Pita, 1986).

In order to test, in a preliminary way, the relationship between parental awareness and parental functioning, Newberger interviewed a sample of eight parents who presented to a major pediatric hospital with a recent history of having abused or neglected a child in their care. This sample was matched with a comparison sample on race, social status, family size, and age of the index child. Statistically significant differences between the two groups were found in parental awareness level scores ($p < .01$) (Newberger, 1977, 1980).

Although these data suggested a relationship between parental awareness and parental behavior, several limitations of the study constrained the interpretation of the findings. This was a small sample from an urban environment. Furthermore, a subsequent examination of the clinical records of the children in the two groups revealed that all the children in the protective service sample had histories of some sort of physical condition that dated from the neonatal period. These included hearing handicaps, strabismus, and exzema. The review of clinical records suggested the possibility that *both* the development of parental awareness *and* parental care may have been compromised by difficulties in establishing an affectional bond consequent to a medical condition in the child present during the neonatal period.

These issues were addressed with a second controlled study (Cook, 1979). The study sample was recruited from a preschool program for developmentally delayed children in rural Maine. This sampling strategy enabled Cook to match the eight parents in the program who had a history of protective service involvement for child neglect with a comparison sample, not only on the basis of familial and maternal characteristics as in the Children's Hospital study, but also on type and magnitude of developmental delay in the child (Newberger and Cook, 1983). Statistically significant differences ($p < .05$) in parental reasoning were found between the two groups in this sample as well. These findings provide further support for the hypothesis that parental awareness is importantly implicated in parental function and dysfunction.

Further evidence for such a relationship is offered by a recently completed study of childrearing patterns in young mothers. Interactions were observed between 136 adolescent inner city mothers and their one-year-old infants.

Significant relationships were found between level of parental awareness and parental behavior as measured by three widely used rating scales (Flick, 1985).

Developmental parental awareness

One limitation of investigations relying on a measure of parental role variables at a given point in time is that they frequently lack a theoretical framework that enables the investigator to analyze change over time. Several investigators note that parents' behavior and attitudes may change over time and in varying circumstances. Rossi (1968) identified developmental tasks of the parental role analogous to Erikson's tasks of ego development. She identified four stages of a role cycle that can be applied to the parental role: (1) the anticipatory stage; (2) the honeymoon stage; (3) the plateau stage; and (4) the disengagement–termination stage. Each stage is linked to a particular time in the cycle. Because these stages are temporal, rather than functional or developmental, they may serve to identify in a general sense the relationship tasks with which a person is engaged, but do not inform our understanding of the processes within the individual that generate variations in behavior or promote development.

A different approach to parental development is offered by Loevinger (1962). She evolved a test of maternal attitudes that sought basic personality traits from patterns in maternal responses. The Family Problem Scale is composed of a set of dichotomous statements. Each mother was instructed to choose from each pair the statement closest to her way of thinking. Loevinger found that those statements that required a judgment about the inner life of the child assumed a central importance in discriminating personality traits among the respondents. This was interpreted as suggesting that the capacity to conceptualize the child's inner life represents a central maternal personality characteristic. From analyses of patterns in maternal personality types – which she described as (1) resistant to authority; (2) identified with authority; and (3) emancipated from arbitrary authority – Loevinger hypothesized that these personality types represent a developmental sequence, although she did not test the developmental hypothesis in her research.

Further analyses of the parental awareness data (Newberger, 1980) also suggest that parental awareness is a developmental process that unfolds during childhood and continues to develop with parental experience. Initial evidence for the development of parental awareness was derived from two cross-sectional analyses, one of parents with differing years of parental experience, the other of children of different ages. In the parental analysis, a statistically significant relationship ($p < .025$) was found between years of parental experience and level of parental awareness when parents with the same number of children were compared with each other. When 16 children between the ages of 7 and 17 were administered a form of the parental awareness interview adapted for children (questions were revised to read "If you were a parent . . ."), the parental awareness levels were found to be highly related to age ($p < .005$). None of the children achieved Level 4 reasoning, although many parents did (Newberger, 1980).

A follow-up study (Newberger and Cook, 1986) of 13 of the 16 children seven years later revealed that development continued to unfold, with a threshold at Level 3 for these children, who were now all in their late teens or young adulthood. These data suggest that although concepts relating to issues of parenthood appear to develop sequentially commencing in childhood, there may be experiences particular to the parental role that may be necessary (although apparently not sufficient) to stimulate thinking at the highest level. Further research is needed to elucidate how and what kind of experience facilitates development at what time in individuals' lives, and at what stages of development.

That development of parental awareness both continues and can be facilitated in adulthood is suggested by several more recent investigations. In a study of 31 middle-class mothers between 25 and 45 years of age, Partoll (1980) found a significant relationship between parental awareness level and years of parental experience. She also found parental awareness to be related to ego development using Marcia's Ego Identity Interview, a finding that has been recently replicated in a study of the development of parental generativity (Pita, 1986).

Preliminary evidence that parental reasoning is responsive to intervention efforts has also been found. In a small controlled study, Sandy (1982) found a significant increase in parental reasoning following a 12-week parent education program that combined group discussion of childrearing dilemmas with didactic presentation of child development information ($p < .03$). When parents were reinterviewed four months following the completion of the program, further gains, which were statistically significant, were found ($p < .05$). A process of development appears to have been initiated during the intervention that continued in the absence of further intervention. No changes were found over the same interval in a comparison group, who had also signed up for the intervention but who were randomly placed on a waiting list to receive the intervention at the completion of this study.

Conclusions

Cognition in parenthood has been studied from several practical and theoretical vantage points, including attitudes or beliefs about childrearing practices, parental attributions of parent and child behavior and intentions, parental expectations of child development, and the cognitive-developmental structure of parental reasoning about tasks of childrearing.

Research has shown some of these approaches to be more fruitful than others as arenas for the investigation of parental functioning. For example, parental *attitudes* concerning childrearing practices appear to have no strong and consistent relationship with either parental practices (Becker and Krug, 1965) or child outcome (Leton, 1958; Yarrow et al., 1968), or to be related to child outcome only with middle-class families (Beckwith, 1972; Tulkin and Choler, 1973). There is also considerable evidence that sample bivariate studies (e.g., between maternal attitudes and child behavior) are not as useful as those studies providing insights into the contexts in which maternal–child interactions take place. Thus, we learn that maternal personality (Bates, Freeland, and Lounsburg, 1979) and the husband–wife relationship (Parke, Power, and Gottman, 1979) are likely to be of importance in the parenting process, along with social class (Becker and Krug, 1965; Beckwith, 1972; Tulkin and Choler, 1973), which may gain some of its importance through its association with particular forms of support systems that may mediate any relationship between maternal attitudes and child outcomes (Field et al., 1980). (See also Cicchetti and Rizley, 1981, and Sameroff and Chandler, 1975, for discussions of a parent–child–environment transactional model of child maltreatment.)

Attitudes toward childrearing may in some ways reflect fairly superficial cognitions that are strongly influenced by socialization and reflect a concern with social desirability. As we move into "deeper" levels of cognition, where prevailing social values may have less impact, we can discover some research findings with important implications for the role of parental cognitions in the parenting process. For example, there is evidence (particularly where the studies have utilized the most appropriate control groups) that parental *attributions* about their children's behavior are of importance.

Typical measures of parental attitudes focus primarily on the *content* of particular cognitions about childrearing practices. Research aimed at this content level may not be as enlightening as research aimed more at the level of functions and structure in cognition. Research on parental attributions holds promise because of the *function* such attributions play in the parent's efforts to understand the environment and preserve self-esteem. Research on the *structure* of parental cognitions (as in work on parental awareness) has yielded particularly valuable findings on the cognitive foundations of parental care.

The levels of parental awareness are thought to describe *qualitative* differences in the way parents organize their understanding of their children, of the relationship between themselves and their children, and of their role as parents. For example, a shift from a Level 2 awareness – of the child as a "type" of child who is understood from the perspective of the conventional wisdom about children – to a Level 3 awareness – of the child as a unique individual who is understood through personal sharing and communication – is more than a different attitude toward children, or an adding of "unique individual" characteristics onto "character type" characteristics. It represents a qualitative reorientation in how children are known and understood. The qualitative differences are argued to represent *cognitive structures* that operate as mental blueprints through which experience is organized, interpreted, and responded to.

In a structural system, this mental blueprint is consistently applied across different aspects of experience in that system. In the research on parental awareness, this consistency was found in the coherency of responses on interviews (Newberger, 1977). In parent–child relationships, the consistency would be reflected in patterns of childrearing organized around powerful and pervasive world views reflecting a particular cognitive orientation. For example, a conventional orientation might be reflected in a consistent pattern of authoritarian parenting in which the underlying structure is the assumption of an "expert" perspective external to the child, and the more "surface" attitude or belief is that without strict rules children will go "wrong." A limitation of a focus on attitudes is that the attitude (in this example the message of the "expert") may change, but the fundamental orientation of parent toward child might not. In other words, a more critical dimension of parental understanding may be whether the child is related to as a *source* or as an *object* of information, rather than the nature of that information.

Research on parental awareness also offers a developmental perspective on parental thinking and suggests that parental cognition represents an evolving process that begins in childhood and has the potential to continue throughout the lifespan. The process of development, both of understanding and of skills, requires the capacity for both growth and change within the individual, and also the *opportunity* for potential to be realized. This requires attention to the context in which an individual is embedded, the quality of the child's capacity to respond to parental care, and the support available to allow the parent the time and space necessary for growth.

Although much of the important research on the cognitive foundations of care is relatively recent, the findings are of importance to all clinicians and service providers who are concerned with the adequacy of family functioning. Although we would not suggest that attitudinal measures be administered to parents, we would encourage the assessment of deeper levels of cognition. From interviews of parents (ideally, fathers as well as mothers), whether using more structured formal instruments or probing clinical explorations, a sensitive and knowledgeable interviewer can assess how the parent interprets the child's behavior as well as the fundamental reasoning processes underlying parental decisions concerning the handling of discipline, conflict, meeting particular needs, and so forth.

It is clear that any approach limited solely to an assessment of parental cognitions is incomplete. Thus, researchers and practitioners would do well to assess also a variety of other factors that may be of fundamental importance to the adequacy of children's care. These include the consistency between father and mother in their parental conceptions and behavior and how they handle similarities and differences. It is also important to determine the extent to which parents are struggling to cope with acute or chronic stresses, and to remember that parental functioning can break down even in parents with well-developed parental awareness if they are burdened with greater stress than they can handle. Attention to cognitive processes should never replace attention to medical, educational, and social realities of parents and children. Nor should attention to cognitive processes replace attention to the specifics of parental practices and their effects on the child. Rather, parental functioning must be understood as a complex process, influenced by a variety of contextual and internal forces (see Belsky, 1984; Belsky and Vondra, this volume; Cicchetti and Rizley, 1981).

The value of the cognitive approach to the study of parenthood is not that it provides an alternative explanation for parental functioning, but rather that it elaborates a critical dimension of parental competence and development, a dimension that has important implications for parental care and that offers new insights into the formation of the enduring parent–child relationship.

References

Aldridge, M., Cautley, P., and Lichstein, D. *Guidelines for placement workers.* Madison: University of Wisconsin Center for Social Service, 1974.

Baldwin, A., Kalhorn, J., and Breese, F. Patterns of parent behavior. *Psychological Monographs,* 1945, *58,* 1–75.

Bates, J. E., Freeland, C. A. B., and Lounsbury, M. L., Measurement of infant difficultness. *Child Development,* 1979, *50,* 794–803.

Bauer, W. D. and Twentymen, C. T. Abusing, neglectful, and comparison mothers' responses to child-related and non-child-related stressors. *Journal of Consulting and Clinical Psychology,* 1985, *53,* 335–343.

Becker, W. C., and Krug, R. S. The parent attitude research instrument: A research review. *Child Development,* 1965, *36,* 329–365.

Beckwith, L. Relationships between infants' social behavior and their mothers' behavior. *Child Development,* 1972, *43,* 397–411.

Belsky, J. (1984). The determinants of parenting: A process model. *Child Development: Vol. 1,* *55,* 83–96.

Berg, P. Parental expectations and attitudes in child abusing families. *Dissertation Abstracts International,* 1976, *37,* 1889-B.

Blank, M. The mother's role in infant development: A review. *Journal of the American Academy of Child Psychiatry,* 1963, *3,* 89–105.

Button, J. H. and Reivich, R. S. Obsessions of infanticide. *Arch. Gen. Psychiatry,* 1972, *27,* 235.

Cicchetti, D. and Rizley, R. Developmental perspectives on the etiology, intergenerational transmission and sequelae of child maltreatment. *New Directions for Child Development,* 1981, *11,* 32–59.

Cook, S. Parental conceptions of children and childrearing: A study of rural Maine parents. Unpublished master's thesis, Tufts University, Medford, MA, 1979.

DeLissovoy, V. High school marriages: A longitudinal study. *Journal of Marriage and the Family,* 1973, *35,* 245–255.

Duvall, E. Conceptions of parenthood. *American Journal of Sociology,* 1946, *52,* 193–203.

Egeland, B., and Brunnquell, D. An at-risk approach to the study of child abuse: some preliminary findings. *Journal of American Academy of Child Psychiatry,* 1979, *18,* 219–235.

Emmerich, W. The parental role: A functional-cognitive approach. *Monographs of the Society for Research in Child Development,* 1969, *34,* 1–71.

Epstein, A. S., Pregnant teenagers' knowledge of infant development. Paper presented at the biennial meeting of the Society for Research in Child Development, San Francisco, March, 1979.

Field, T. M., Widmayer, S. M., Stringer, S., and Ignnatoff, E. Teenage lower-class, black mothers and their preterm infants: An intervention and developmental follow-up. *Child Development,* 1980, *51,* 426–436.

Flick, L. Personal communication, 1985.

Hofer, C. Sex differences in parental awareness and in the relationship between parents' and children's social cognition: A structural developmental analysis. Unpublished doctoral dissertation, University of Connecticut, Storrs, CT, 1981.

Hollingshead, A. *Two-factor Index of Social Position.* New Haven: Yale University Press, 1965.

Klaus, M. H., and Kennell, J. H., Eds. *Maternal-Infant Bonding.* St. Louis, MO: C. V. Mosby, 1976.

Kohlberg, L. Stage and sequence: The cognitive–developmental approach to socialization. In D. Goslin (Ed.), *Handbook of Socialization Theory and Research.* New York: Rand McNally, 1969.

Larrance, D. T. and Twentyman, C. T. Maternal attributions and child abuse. *Journal of Abnormal Psychology,* 1983, *92,* 544–547.

Loevinger, J. Measuring personality patterns of women. *Genetic Psychology Monographs,* 1962, *65,* 53–136.

Leton, D. A. A study of the validity of parent attitude measurement. *Child Development,* 1958, *29,* 517–520.

McGillicuddy-DeLisi, A., Sigel, I., and Johnson, J. The family as a system of mutual influences: Parental beliefs, distancing behaviors and children's representational thinking. In M. Lewis and L. Rosenblum (Eds.), *This Child and Its Family.* New York: Plenum, 1979.

Newberger, C. M. Parental conceptions of children and child-rearing: A structural developmental analysis. Unpublished doctoral dissertation, Harvard University, Cambridge, MA., 1977.

Newberger, C. M. The cognitive structure of parenthood: The development of a descriptive measure. In R. Selman and R. Yando (Eds.), *New Directions of Child Development: Clinical Developmental Research.* San Francisco: Jossey-Bass, 1980.

Newberger, C. M., and Cook, S. J. Parental awareness and child abuse and neglect: A cognitive-developmental analysis of urban and rural samples. *American Journal of Orthopsychiatry,* 1983, *53,* 512–524.

Newberger, C. M., and Cook, S. J. Becoming the parent: The development of conceptions of parenthood during childhood and adolescence. Unpublished manuscript, Boston, MA, 1986.

Nowlis, V. The search for significant concepts in a study of parent–child relationships. *American Journal of Orthopsychiatry,* 1952, *22,* 286–299.

Parke, R. D., Power, T. G., and Fisher, T. The adolescent father's impact on the mother and child. *Journal of Social Issues,* 1980, *36,* 88–106.

Parke, R. D., Power, T. G., and Gottman, J. Conceptualizing and quantifying influence patterns in the family triad. In M. E. Lamb, S. J. Suomi, and G. R. Stephenson (Eds.), *Social Interaction Analysis: Methodological Issues.* Madison: University of Wisconsin Press, 1979.

Partoll, S. The correlates of parental awareness. Unpublished doctoral dissertation, Boston University, 1980.

Piaget, J. *The Moral Development of the Child.* New York: Harcourt, 1950.

Pita, D. D. Parental generativity development. Unpublished doctoral dissertation, Boston University, 1986.

Rosenberg, M. S. and Reppucci, N. D. Abusing mothers: perceptions of their own and their children's behavior. *Journal of Clinical and Consulting Psychology,* 1983, *51,* 674–682.

Rossi, A. Transition to parenthood. *Journal of Marriage and the Family,* 1968, *30,* 26–39.

Sameroff, A. The mother's conception of the child. Paper presented at the meeting of the International Society for the Study of Behavioral Development, Guildford, Eng., 1975.

Sameroff, A. J. and Chandler, M. J. Reproductive risk and the continuum of caretaking casualty. In F. D. Horowitz, M. Hetherington, S. Scarr-Salopatek, and G. Siegal (Eds.), *Review of Child Development Research,* Vol. 4, 1975, 187–244.

Sandy, L. Teaching child development principles to parents: A cognitive-developmental approach. Unpublished doctoral dissertation. Boston University, 1982.

Schaefer, E. S. and Bell, R. Q. Development of a parental attitude research instrument. *Child Development,* 1958, *29,* 339–361.

Sears, R., Maccoby, E., and Levin, H. *Patterns of Child Rearing.* New York: Row, Peterson, 1957.

Selman R. L. Taking another's perspective: Role-taking development in early childhood. *Child Development,* 1971, *42,* 1721–1734.

Selman, R. L. *The Growth of Interpersonal Understanding: Developmental and Clinical Analyses.* New York: Academic Press, 1980.

Siracusa, A. J. Perception of own and other children by abusive mothers. Paper presented at the Seventh National Conference on Child Abuse and Neglect, Chicago, 1985.

Smith, S., Hanson, R., and Noble, S. Parents of battered babies: A controlled study. *British Medical Journal,* 1973, *17,* 388–391.

Tulkin, S. R. and Choler, B. J. Child rearing attitudes and mother–child interactions in the first year of life. *Merrill-Palmer Quarterly,* 1973, *19,* 95–106.

Yarrow, M., Campbell J., and Burton, R. *Child-Rearing: An Inquiry into Research and Methods.* San Francisco: Jossey-Bass, 1968.

11   Intergenerational continuities and discontinuities in serious parenting difficulties

Michael Rutter

Parental maltreatment of children takes many different forms and has a variety of origins (Mrazek and Mrazek, 1985). Thus, it may involve a pattern of parenting that leads to a nonorganic growth failure or "failure to thrive" disorder in infants and young children; to inadequate or negligent parenting amounting to child neglect; to physical abuse; to sexual abuse; and to deliberately created iatrogenic illness (so-called Munchausen syndrome by proxy). Each of these varieties of maltreatment involves its own specificities but, equally, there is substantial overlap between them with each representing a serious maladaptive distortion of parenting functions and of the parent–child relationship. Accordingly, one way of tackling questions on the antecedents of child abuse is to examine factors associated with serious parenting difficulties more generally. The assumption here is that the occurrence of physical abuse should be seen as just one of several manifestations of aberrant parenting. That is the approach followed in this chapter in the consideration of intergenerational continuities and discontinuities in serious parenting difficulties.

Alternatively, the physical maltreatment of children may be viewed as an example of personal violence that may be linked with violence between husband and wife or violence exhibited outside the home. This approach, too, has validity as shown by the associations between family violence and crime in the community, both violent and nonviolent (White and Strauss, 1981). However, it should be noted that the predictors of violent crime do not differ markedly from the predictors of nonviolent serious crime (Farrington, 1978; Rutter and Giller, 1983). Moreover, the antecedents of adult criminality overlap substantially with the antecedents of nondelinquent social failure and non-antisocial personality disorders (Rutter, 1984a; West, 1982). Thus, a focus on the acts of violence involved in child abuse also leads to attention to variables associated with serious problems in social relationships and in social behavior. It is those variables that will be discussed in the review of possible intergenerational processes in parenting problems.

317

Concepts of parenting

Before turning to the issue of intergenerational continuities and discontinuities in parenting problems, it is appropriate to pause to consider what is
involved in parenting and hence what might be affected in failures of parenting (see Maccoby and Martin, 1983; Rutter, 1975, 1983a; Rutter, Quinton, and Liddle, 1983). First, parenting is a task that is concerned with the
rearing of children; a task that comprises the provision of an environment
conducive to both cognitive and social development (Rutter, 1985a, 1985b)
as well as a task that is concerned with the parental response to children's
distress, social approaches, demands, and disruptive behavior (Dowdney,
Mrazek, Quinton, and Rutter, 1984; Mrazek, Dowdney, Rutter, and Quinton, 1982), and with the resolution of interpersonal conflicts and difficulties
(Shure and Spivack, 1978). Thus, parenting requires "skills" of various
kinds – as reflected in sensitivity to children's cues and a responsiveness to
the differing needs at different phases of development; in social problem
solving and coping with life stressors and adversities; in knowing how to
play and talk with children; and in the use of disciplinary techniques that
are effective in the triple sense of bringing about the desired child behavior,
of doing so in a way that results in harmony, and of increasing the child's
self-control (Rutter, Quinton and Liddle, 1983).

Second, parenting incorporates the parent–child relationship and hence
represents one specific type of social relationship. It has its own particular
qualities and characteristics but nevertheless it forms part of a broader set
of social qualities. The implication is that the upbringing of children needs
to be considered in terms of the enduring 'relationship' aspects of parent–
child interaction, as well as in terms of the features of any interaction with
respect to its qualities as a time-limited interchange focused on some specific social context or demand. Similarly, the parent–child relationship must
be viewed, not only in terms of its dyadic qualities, but also as part of a
more general set of social relationships involving friends, neighbors, and
workmates in addition to the immediate family.

Third, parenting reflects the psychosocial functioning of the mother and
father. Not surprisingly, therefore, it has been found that mental disorder
may interfere with parenting functions (Rutter, 1987a; Rutter and Cox,
1985). Thus, Cox and his colleagues found that mothers with a recurrent or
chronic depressive disorder tended to be less appropriately responsive to
their children, less likely to sustain positive interactions, less able to put
their children's experiences into a personal context, and more often
involved in unsuccessful attempts to control their children (Mills, Puckering, Pound, and Cox, 1985; Pound, Cox, Puckering, and Mills, 1985). Similarly, Davenport, Zahn-Waxler, Adland, and Mayfield, (1984) found that
when one parent had a manic-depressive illness parent–child interaction

was adversely affected; and Näslund, Persson-Blennow, McNeil, Kaij, and Malmquist-Larsson (1984) found an increased rate of insecure attachment between infants and their schizophrenic mothers. It is evident that parenting must be assessed with due attention to other aspects of the parents' functioning as individuals. On occasions, even lethal abuse may be the consequence of parental emotional disturbance rather than of any inherent lack in parenting skills or relationship qualities (Troisi and D'Amato, 1984).

Fourth, parenting is an outcome of the learning involved in the very experience of bringing up previous children. This is evident, for example, in the evidence that parents tend to respond differently to their firstborn compared with the way they deal with later-born children (Rutter, 1981a). It is also apparent in findings from primate studies. Monkeys subjected to social isolation in infancy show a strong likelihood of becoming rejecting, neglectful, or abusing parents of their firstborns; however, some are better mothers with their subsequent offspring (Harlow and Suomi, 1971). It appears that positive experiences with young monkeys do something to activate parenting skills that were damaged or impaired by experimentally imposed early social isolation (Novak, 1979; Novak and Harlow, 1975; Suomi, Harlow, and Novak, 1974).

Fifth, parenting may be influenced by experiences associated with the earlier phases of interaction with the same child (i.e., earlier happenings rather than the effects of child characteristics). This possibility was most dramatically highlighted by Klaus and Kennell's (1976) claim that mother–infant bonding was dependent on skin to skin contact during the neonatal period. The claim has *not* been supported by empirical findings (see Goldberg, 1983). It seems most unlikely that the development of relationships is dependent on a single sensory modality and equally implausible that relationships can arise only during a brief "sensitive period" in the hours after birth. Nevertheless, it may be that the *prevention* of parent–infant interaction in hospital may impair parenting, and that active encouragement of early contact in a supportive atmosphere may well foster feelings of confidence and competence in many parents (Wolkind and Rutter, 1985).

Sixth, parenting must be seen as a dyadic relationship that forms part of a broader social nexus. This means that mother–child interaction is likely to be different when the father is present than when mother and child are together on their own (Clarke-Stewart, 1978). Equally, however, it means that the style of adult–child interaction will vary according to whether one child or several children are present (Schaffer and Liddell, 1984). In polyadic conditions, adults tend to be more peremptory and prohibitive and more likely to ignore children's approaches. However, it is not just a question of the number of people present; it is also a matter of the quality of relationships. Parenting tends to be less adequate when the marital relationship is discordant and disharmonious or when the parent lacks the support of a spouse (Hetherington, Cox, and Cox, 1982; Quinton and Rutter, 1984a, 1984b; Rutter and Quinton, 1984a; Wallerstein, 1983). Moreover, parenting tends to be affected by the presence or absence of effective social supports, perhaps especially at times of stress or when dealing with a difficult child (Belsky, 1984; Cochran and Brassard, 1979; Crockenberg, 1981; Crnic, Greenbert, Ragozin, Robinson, and Basham, 1983; Werner and Smith, 1982). Thus, cross-cultural data (Rohner, 1975; Werner, 1979) seem to suggest that socially isolated mothers who carry the entire burden of shared responsibilities are more likely to become rejecting of their children. That is to say, there must be an *ecological* perspective that recognizes that the family is a functional system, the operation of which will be altered by its internal composition and by external forces (Bronfenbrenner, 1979).

Such a perspective implies attention to parenting in terms of the emotional resources available to the parent. Physical resources, too, are likely to be relevant. Thus, in our studies of families whose children had been received into residential care because their parents could not cope adequately, the families were less likely than those in the general population control group to have received help in looking after the children and more likely to feel the need of such help (Quinton and Rutter, 1984a). Of course, the lack of material support could not be regarded as independent from the families' interpersonal difficulties. To a large extent, their lack of support was a reflection of their less satisfactory primary group relationships, their greater need for emotional and practical support, and probably also a function of their frequent housing moves, which prevented the development of helping relationships with neighbors. Social support is not only a feature of what is available in the environment; it also reflects personality strengths and weaknesses in eliciting or attracting support (Rutter, 1985c; Cohen and Syme, 1985). Nevertheless, in both cases and controls we found that problems in parenting were substantially more frequent when housing conditions were poor and accompanied by other stressors (Quinton and Rutter, 1984b).

Finally, parenting involves a two-way interaction that is affected by the characteristics of the child as well as those of the parent (Maccoby and Martin, 1983). Parenting styles are influenced by the temperamental characteristics of the children as well as by more overt behavioral disturbance and physical or mental handicaps. Longitudinal studies have indicated some of the ways in which these two-way interactions may result in vicious cycles leading to increased parenting difficulties and greater problem behavior in the children.

The implication to be drawn from these considerations of the multifaceted nature of parenting is that parenting cannot be viewed as a unidimensional variable. If intergenerational continuities in parenting are found, it cannot be assumed that the mechanisms of transmission necessarily involve parenting qualities per se; they might involve psychiatric disorder or social support or living conditions - to mention but three alternatives. The demonstration of intergenerational links provides a continuity to be explained; it does not indicate any particular mechanisms.

Issues in intergenerational continuities

In the past it has been assumed that it is common for psychosocial problems to persist from generation to generation and that the root cause of their transmission lies in some kind of failure in parenting. The evidence on this view with regard to serious problems in parenting constitutes the subject matter of this chapter. However, it is clear that as a general concept it is no more than a half-truth; intergenerational discontinuities are at least as striking as continuities, and it would be seriously misleading to view the mechanisms as mainly intrafamilial in origin (Rutter and Madge, 1976). The study of intergenerational transmission raises a number of important conceptual and methodological issues.

To begin, most of the data on intergenerational continuities in parenting behavior look backward rather than forward (Rutter, Quinton, and Liddle, 1983). That is to say, the findings show that many individuals now showing serious parenting problems had an abnormal pattern of upbringing. That observation suggests that the experience of deviant child rearing may constitute one important predisposing factor for later parental abuse or neglect. But, of course, that does not mean that most children who experience deviant rearing will show problems in parenting when they grow up. If intergenerational discontinuities – as well as continuities – are to be investigated, *both* ends of the same stick must be grasped by combining retrospective and prospective research strategies with the same parenting variables.

In that connection, it is crucial to appreciate that intergenerational links necessarily involve at least two parents (three or four is not uncommon as a result of divorce and remarriage), and usually involve several children. Most studies of continuities have examined links between only one parent and one child. However, we need to know whether all children in the same family show the same adult outcome and if not, why not. Equally, it is necessary to ask whether the effects of adverse upbringing experienced by one parent may be accentuated or mitigated by the negative or positive qualities of the other parent.

As implicit in the discussion of the concepts of parenting, it is crucial to determine the extent to which the intergenerational continuities apply to parenting problems as such, as distinct from the manifold psychosocial problems with which they tend to be associated. Many abusing parents show abnormalities in social relationships other than those involved in parenting; many exhibit psychiatric disorder; and many are living in poor socioeconomic conditions (Smith, 1978). Thus, the adverse experiences in childhood may have no direct effect on parenting. Perhaps their main impact is on personality development (with parenting involved only insofar as personality disorders include problems in parenting); alternatively it could be that the childhood adversities are associated with a persistence of social disadvantage that may, in turn, impede good parenting (but, again, with no direct connection between childhood experiences and parenting that is separate from social disadvantage). Of course, it should not be assumed that there will be one overriding explanation; nor can it be expected that the same processes will apply throughout the course of development. Interaction effects of various kinds are common in the course of development (Rutter, 1983b) and in many instances continuities derive from chains of indirect effects (Rutter 1984b, 1984c) rather than from the result of one enduring main effect. The study of the mechanisms involved in intergenerational continuities and discontinuities must take these possibilities into account.

The testing of hypotheses on mechanisms must start with the basic question of whether the statistical associations reflect causal processes. It is all too obvious in the social sciences that causal inferences have sometimes been drawn too readily on the basis of correlations. Nevertheless, there are a variety of ways in which epidemiological/longitudinal data may be used to test causal hypotheses in the absence of experimental data (see Rutter, 1981b; Dooley, 1985). Often the solution lies in the seeking of naturally occurring experiments and in finding ways of manipulating the data to test noncausal alternative explanations (see, e.g., Quinton, Rutter, and Liddle, 1984). With respect to intergenerational transmission of parenting problems, the causal hypothesis has some prima facie plausibility because experimental studies of rhesus monkeys reared in total social isolation have shown that isolation often results in parental abuse or neglect of the next generation (see Rutter, 1981a). The findings provide convincing evidence that experiences in early life may impede parenting. However, these experimental adversities comprised extremely gross distortions of upbringing rarely encountered in humans. As a result it cannot be assumed that the results apply to more ordinary circumstances of aberrant upbringing; nor can the findings in other species be extrapolated to humans without testing to determine that the generalization is justified.

Finally, there is the most important question of the extent to which the ill-effects of seriously adverse experiences in childhood are modifiable or reversible. It is now generally accepted both that there is marked individual variation in responses to stress and adversity and that children who show initial psychosocial impairment may later improve markedly in their functioning or even recover completely (Rutter, 1981a). However, we are only beginning to gather systematic data on the variables associated with resilience in the face of adversity. The few data that are available indicate that, in some circumstances, positive experiences may mitigate the ill-effects of adversity (Rutter, 1985c), and that it is common for adult outcomes to depend on a chain of circumstances rather than any one decisive experience, good or bad (Rutter, 1983b, 1984b, 1987b). A main focus of this chapter concerns the delineation of those chain effects that predispose to continuities and discontinuities.

One aspect of this broad issue concerns the question of whether it is possible for major changes in psychosocial functioning (including parenting) to take place in adult life once serious abnormalities have already been manifest. As already noted, the animal evidence suggests that later experiences of a positive kind can do something to ameliorate the damage inflicted by early social isolation (Novak and Harlow, 1975; Novak, 1979). Few data on humans are available, but Sheridan's (1959) early study of the rehabilitation of seriously neglectful mothers showed that many improved and came to cope satisfactorily. The challenge is to identify the factors that facilitate this occurrence.

Intergenerational links in parenting problems

Looking backward

Early clinical studies of physically abusive parents drew attention to the high proportion who had suffered severely deviant parenting in their own upbringing (Steele and Pollock, 1968; Steele, 1970). There are a variety of problems in these early studies in terms of reliance on retrospective recall, lack of adequate control groups, and other methodological shortcomings (Cicchetti and Aber, 1980). Nevertheless, better controlled studies have tended to confirm the association between severe parenting problems and the experience of serious childhood adversities.

For example, Quinton and Rutter (1984a) used parenting breakdown as an index of serious and persisting parenting difficulties. The cases consisted of a consecutive, epidemiologically based, sample of 48 families with European-born parents who had children admitted to residential care by one inner London borough during a continuous eight-month period (Rutter, Quinton, and Liddle, 1983). In order to exclude cases in which admission occurred because of some short-term crisis, the series was confined to families for which this was at least the second time that a child had been taken into care. Selection was further restricted to those with a child between the ages of 5 and 8 years living at home, so that comparable assessments of parenting could be made. The comparison group consisted of 47 families with a child in the same age group living at home with its mother, but in which no child in the family had ever been taken into care by a local authority. The control sample was drawn randomly from the age and sex registers

Table 11.1. *Family relationships in mothers' early childhood*

	In-care $n = 44$ %	Comparison $n = 43$ %	Statistical significance		
			x^2	df	p
Ever in care	25	7	3.98	1	<0.05
Separation from parents through discord or rejection	44	14	8.12	1	<0.01
Parental marital discord	45	14	8.57	1	<0.01
Hard or harsh paternal discipline	27	10	3.78	1	NS
Hard or harsh maternal discipline	38	10	8.25	1	<0.01

of two general practices in the same inner London borough. Interview data confirmed that mothers with children admitted into residential care (the "in-care" mothers) showed many more parenting difficulties than the control group.

The difference between the two groups in childhood experiences was striking (see Table 11.1). A quarter of the in-care mothers had been in care themselves compared with only 7% of the control group; 44% had been separated from one or both parents for at least one month as a result of family discord compared with 14% of controls; and three times as many suffered harsh discipline (such as frequent beatings with implements or being locked in cupboards or cellars). Altogether 61% of the in-care mothers had experienced 4 or more of these childhood adversities compared with 16% of controls; conversely only 11% (versus 35%) had experienced no more than 1 adversity.

Because many of the in-care women were living in unstable marital circumstances (half were in a single-parent household and, of those with two parents, a third of the mothers' cohabitees were not the father of any of the children), data were often lacking on the childhood experiences of the fathers of the children admitted into residential care. However, the findings for those families for whom information was available showed that in only 11% of cases (as against 59% of the comparison group) did neither parent experience at least two adversities before age 16 years involving admissions into care, harsh parenting, parental marital discord, and parental deviance or psychiatric disorder. In short, intergenerational continuity looking backward was nearly complete (the data on missing cases supports this conclusion). On the other hand, it was striking that quite a high proportion of control families (two-fifths) had also experienced childhood adversities. This suggests that continuity looking forward is unlikely to be as strong.

Two further issues must be considered with respect to intergenerational continuity. First, to what type and degree of parenting problem does this relatively strong continuity apply? Second, what kinds of childhood experiences are associated with parenting breakdown? As already noted, the in-care group was selected on the basis of at least two breakdowns in parenting so that the problems were persistent as well as marked. Nevertheless, other data indicated that the parenting problems were far from the only difficulties shown by these women. Indeed detailed interview measures showed that one in ten of the in-care sample showed no problems in parenting with their 5- to 8-year-old child selected for study (although they had experienced difficulties with other children). However, four-fifths of the in-care mothers showed a current psychiatric disorder (compared with one-fifth of controls) and 44% had received psychiatric in-patient treatment (compared with 2% of controls). Also, most of the in-care group mothers had experienced severe and recurrent marital difficulties; less than half were in a stable cohabitation and, of that half, a third showed severe marital discord. It may be concluded that the high intergenerational continuity applies to multiple-problem families, in which parenting difficulties are associated with multiple other psychosocial disabilities.

Looking forward

Prospective investigations of parenting problems have been of four main types: (1) longitudinal studies of general population samples starting at the time of pregnancy, with retrospective data on the parents' upbringing as children; (2) similar studies of high-risk samples; (3) long-term studies of general population samples beginning when the subjects were children and following them through to adult life and child-bearing; and (4) similar long-term studies of high-risk groups.

The prospective study by Altemeier, O'Connor, Vietze, Sandler, and Sherrod (1982, 1984) of 1400 women followed from the time of pregnancy until the infants were aged 21 to 48 months is an example of the first type. The 23 women who abused their children differed from the remainder in terms of the proportion who experienced foster care as children (17% versus 2%); who did not get along with or separated from their parents (57% versus 25%); and who reported that they received unfair severe punishment (57% versus 30%). The overlap between variables was not reported, but it is evident that adverse experiences in childhood were associated with an increased risk of child abuse. It is also clear, however, that the majority of women with adverse experiences did *not* abuse their children (although the parenting risk following such experiences was greater if failure to thrive and other serious parenting difficulties were included with physical abuse). It was noteworthy that many of the mothers who subsequently abused their children talked or behaved during the pregnancy interview in ways that caused the interviewer to note the situation as already dangerous for the child.

Wolkind and Kruk's (1985) study of women living in inner London illustrates the high-risk strategy applied to women first studied when they were pregnant. Two high-risk groups were chosen: those who had been admitted to residential care as children as a result of parenting breakdown ($n = 33$); and those who had had long-term separations from their parents because of continuing family disharmony or difficulties ($n = 49$). These were compared with a random sample of nonseparated women ($n = 78$), all three groups being followed until the children were aged 42 months. Parenting outcome was assessed from both interview and observation measures. Only small differences were found between the latter two groups, but the group that had experienced foster care as children differed in being less likely to hold the baby for feeding (26% versus 5%) and less likely to experience the baby as enjoyable (41% versus 70%). At 42 months their children were somewhat more likely to show behavioral disturbances (31% versus 13%) and were more likely to have experienced accidents (58% versus 28%) and to have been admitted to a hospital (52% versus 19%). The differences were even more marked in terms of the interviewers' subjective rating of severe concern about parenting (35% versus 11%). The differences in the style of feeding the infant reflects Frommer and O'Shea's (1973a, 1973b) earlier finding from a similar study that women from broken homes were more likely to feed their babies by propping the bottle on a pillow.

The high risk prospective study by Egeland and his co-workers (Egeland, Jacobvitz, and Papatola, 1984) provides rather more extensive data on serious problems in parenting, although it has the limitation that the retrospective data on the mothers' upbringing were not obtained until the children were 4 years of age. On the basis of this information the mothers were subdivided into three groups: (1) those who were emotionally supported as children ($n = 35$); (2) controls without clear support but without experience of abuse ($n = 79$); and (3) those subjected to severe abuse or neglect, including foster-home placement ($n = 47$). The three groups differed markedly in rates of maltreatment of their own children (3%, 9%, and 34%) but there were no differences with respect to borderline or other parenting difficulties (40%, 39%, and 36%). Expressed the other way round, of the 24 children who were maltreated, 16 were being reared by mothers who had themselves experienced abuse or neglect and only 1 was being brought up by a mother who experienced emotional support during childhood. The risks of maltreatment were similarly great for mothers who had been neglected as compared with those subjected to physical or sexual abuse.

Longitudinal studies extending from childhood to parenthood are very few in number. Limited data are available for the British National Survey (Wadsworth, 1985), based on a stratified sample of children born during one week in 1946. The women who experienced family disruption during the preschool years were more likely than those from nondisrupted families to have been divorced or separated by the age of 26 years (11% versus 3%); those experiencing disruption during middle or later childhood were intermediate. Mothers from disrupted homes were more likely as young adults to recall their childhood as unhappy, and those recollections were in turn associated with a somewhat higher rate of reserved relationships with their firstborn (Wadsworth, 1984).

Much the richest body of intergenerational data on general population samples followed from childhood into adult life is that provided by Elder, Caspi, and Downey's (1986) analysis of findings from the Berkeley Guidance Study in California. The data archive includes members of four generations: (1) the subjects born in 1928–29, (2) their parents, (3) their grandparents, and (4) their children. Unstable grandparents (as assessed from retrospective accounts by the parents) were associated with marital tension (r = .28 to .43) and hostility to the child (r = .48 to .55). These parenting patterns in the grandparent generation were in turn associated with similar negative parenting qualities in the parental generation, as well as with similar features of unstable personality (most correlations circa .2 to .4). The children reared in a hostile aversive family environment were more likely to show disturbed behavior in childhood, to show lack of control as adults, and to exhibit marital discord and instability and to manifest ill-tempered parental behavior (correlations again at about the same level). Elder et al. conclude: "Aversive family patterns mediate the influence of unstable parents on offspring, and they were reproduced in the next generation through the development of offspring who are least able to sustain and nurture enduring relationships. . . . The intergenerational cycle of problem behavior and problem relationships resembles a general dynamic across the four Berkeley generations." They go on, however, to caution that the dynamic is highly variable with many turning points and breaks in the intergenerational cycle of transmission of parenting difficulties. They raise the question of what factors buffered children from the deleterious effects of poor parenting and what factors led to a break in the intergenerational cycle – questions that provided the central focus for our own high-risk study of parenting.

Parenting outcome of institution-reared women. High risk was defined in terms of being reared for several years in a residential Children's Home (Quinton, Rutter, and Liddle, 1984; Rutter, Quinton, and Liddle, 1983). The study consisted of a follow-up into early adult life of 94 girls who, in 1964, were in one or the other of two Children's Homes run on group cottage lines – the children having been admitted because their parents could not cope with childrearing. The contrast group of 51 comprised a quasi-random general population sample of individuals of the same age, never admit-

Table 11.2. *Pregnancy and parenting histories of women*

	Ex-care women (n = 81) %	Comparison group (n = 41) %	Statistical significance		
			x^2	df	p
Ever pregnant	72	43	8.50	1	0.01
Pregnant by 19	42	5	16.75	1	0.001
Had surviving child	60	36	5.85	1	0.02
Of those with children	(n = 49) %	(n = 15) %			
Without male partner	22	0	Exact test p = 0.039		
Any children ever in care/fostered	18	0	Exact test p = 0.075		
Temporary or permanent breakdown in parenting	35	0	Exact test p = 0.009		
Living with father of all children	61	100	6.52	1	0.02

Source: Quinton, Rutter, and Liddle, 1984.

ted into care and living with their families in the same general area in inner London. Both groups had their behavior assessed in childhood by means of a standardized teacher questionnaire and both were interviewed at length (2½ to 4 hours) in their mid-twenties using standardized interview techniques. Direct home observations of parent–child interactions were undertaken with cases and controls who had children in the 2- to 3½-year age range.

The parenting outcome of the two groups of women differed markedly, as shown in Table 11.2 by the data on what happened in terms of the pregnancy and the care of the children (Quinton, Rutter, and Liddle, 1984). Nearly twice as many of the institution-reared women had become pregnant and given birth to a surviving child by the time of follow-up; also they were much more likely to have become pregnant while still teenagers. Furthermore, the institution-reared women were much more likely to have parented children while in an unstable marital situation; a fifth were without a male partner at follow-up and only three-fifths (compared with 100% of controls) were living with the father of all their children. Serious breakdowns in parenting were evident only in the institutional group; a third had experienced a temporary or permanent breakdown in parenting and 18 percent had had at least one child fostered or admitted into residential care.

These findings on breakdown are, of course, a function of the willingness of the women to give up their children and the inclination of the authorities to intervene, as well as a reflection of parenting qualities. The latter were

Table 11.3. *Overall observation measure of parenting*

No. areas of difficulty	'Ex-care' women ($n = 23$)	Comparison group ($n = 21$)
None	3	10
1–3	12	11
At least 4	8	0

Note: $\chi^2 = 11 \cdot 746$, df $= 2$, $p < 0.01$
Source: Quinton, Rutter, and Liddle, 1984.

assessed by means of detailed systematic questioning on the care and discipline of the children and on parent–child interactions. On this interview measure of *current* parenting (i.e., ignoring past difficulties or past parenting breakdowns), poor parenting remained much more common in the ex-care group (40% versus 11%). Nevertheless, it should be noted that nearly a third (31%) showed good parenting – emphasizing the marked heterogeneity in outcome. Also, it was apparent that half the comparison group showed some difficulties in parenting. The finding points to the relatively high prevalence of family problems in socially disadvantaged inner city populations – a finding evident in all previous surveys (see Rutter, 1980; Rutter and Madge, 1976).

Inevitably, the interview assessments of parenting could not be made blind to the women's past experiences; however, this was possible for the direct home observations based on systematic time and event samples of discrete behaviors and of sequences of parent–child interaction (Dowdney, Skuse, Rutter, and Mrazek, 1985a; Dowdney, Skuse, Rutter, Quinton, and Mrazek, 1985b). Table 11.3 gives the data for the overall observational assessment based on seven different aspects of parenting (positive affect, negative affect, frequency of distress, frequency of control episodes, ignoring of child initiations, amount of child initiations, amount of joint play). Again, although there was substantial overlap between the groups, widespread parenting difficulties were much more frequent in the institution-reared group (8 out of 23 versus 0 out of 21).

It is evident that all of the prospective studies broadly agree in their findings. They show difficulties in parenting (and especially parenting breakdown) as much more frequent in families where the mother has experienced marked adversities in her own upbringing. However, the same data all indicate very substantial intergenerational *dis*continuity with many women parenting adequately, or even well, in spite of deficiencies and traumas in their own rearing.

In seeking to understand the meaning of this pattern of continuities and discontinuities, there are three key issues that must be addressed. First, what is the nature of the parenting problems that show intergenerational continuity? Second, what types of childhood adversities in upbringing predispose to parenting difficulties in the next generation? And, third, what mix of mechanisms account for the intergenerational continuities and discontinuities?

Nature of parenting problems showing intergenerational continuity

Because most investigations have focused on rather a limited range of outcome measures, few provide data on the specifics of the parenting problems that exhibit intergenerational continuity. However, relevant evidence is available from the Egeland et al. (1984) high-risk study and from our own longitudinal study of institution-reared women and general population controls. Egeland and his collaborators noted that the pattern of maltreatment (n = 44 cases) in the second generation included a wide range of seriously maladaptive parenting, ranging from neglect (n = 24) and psychological unavailability (n = 19) (meaning unemotional detachment, lack of involvement, and unresponsive insensitivity) to hostile, rejecting harassment (n = 19) and physical abuse (n = 24) (meaning frequent intense spanking as well as overt maltreatment of a kind likely to result in court intervention). As is obvious from the numbers, there was considerable overlap between these different varieties of maltreatment. In other words, the maltreatment was as much psychological as physical and, although obviously severe, did not necessarily amount to the degree of battering that would lead to the children's compulsory removal from the home. The maltreating mothers showed many other problems in their social functioning, with life stress and lack of marital support both common and associated with abuse (Egeland, Breitenbucher, and Rosenberg, 1980). Strikingly, as already noted, *no* intergenerational continuity was found for milder levels of parenting problems in the Egeland study.

Our own findings show a closely similar picture. Thus, the between-group differences were at least as strong for psychosocial problems not involving the children as they were for parenting difficulties (see Table 11.4). A quarter of the institution-reared women, but none of the controls, were rated as showing a personality disorder as evidenced by persisting handicaps in interpersonal relationships since the early teens or before; a fifth had a crime record (as assessed from both self-report and official records), and severe marital difficulties were present in over 25% compared with 6% of controls (Rutter and Quinton, 1984b). When these (and other) measures were combined to provide an overall measure of psychosocial functioning or follow-up it was found that 30% of the institution-reared women (versus 0% in

Table 11.4. *Psychosocial outcome of women reared in institutions*

	'Ex-care' women ($n = 81$)	Comparison group ($n = 41$)	x^2	d.f.	p
Personality disorder	25	0	10.37	1	0.01
Criminality (self-report)	22	0	8.59	1	0.02
Criminality (official records)	25	2	8.21	1	0.01
One or more broken cohabitations	38	7	12.70	1	0.001
Marked marital problems (of those cohabiting)	28	6	4.59	1	0.05

Source: Rutter and Quinton, 1984b.

Table 11.5. *Association between current parenting and psychosocial adjustment*

	'Ex-care' women[a] ($n = 42$) %	Comparison group[b] ($n = 27$) %
Good parenting	($n = 13$)	($n = 12$)
Good psychosocial outcome	85	67
Intermediate/poor psychosocial outcome	15	33
Intermediate parenting	($n = 11$)	($n = 12$)
Good psychosocial outcome	45	67
Intermediate/poor psychosocial outcome	55	33
Poor parenting	($n = 18$)	($n = 3$)
Good psychosocial outcome	17	67
Intermediate/poor psychosocial outcome	83	33

[a]Association in 'ex-care' women, $x^2 = 14.07$, df = 2, $p < 0.01$.
[b]Association in comparison group, NS.
Source: Quinton, Rutter, and Liddle, 1984.

controls) had a poor outcome, and 21% showed good functioning (versus 63% of controls).

The overlap between these other psychosocial disabilities and parenting problems was very substantial in the institution-reared sample but *not* in controls (see Table 11.5). Thus, of the 18 ex-care women who showed poor parenting only 3 exhibited good psychosocial functioning. It may be concluded that intergenerational continuity mainly applied to severe and wide-spread problems of psychosocial functioning, of which poor parenting is but one facet. Indeed, the control group findings emphasize (as in the Egeland study) that intergenerational continuity is *not* a feature of less widespread or severe parenting difficulties that are unassociated with general deficits or disabilities in personality functioning. Indeed, intermediate level parenting difficulties in women with good psychosocial functioning were largely a feature of the comparison group (8/28) rather than the ex-care sample (5/42).

It might be thought from these findings that the institution-reared women who showed parenting problems were generally incompetent and uncaring in their parenting. However, our detailed interview and observation data show that this would be a mistaken conclusion in the majority of cases. There were a few women whose relationships with their children (as with other people) seemed grossly maladaptive, and a few of the children had clearly been maltreated (there was one case of infanticide). On the other hand, of the 9 women who had permanently given up one child, 5 had succeeded in keeping and looking after a second child (with varying degrees of skill and responsivity). Moreover, the molecular measures of parenting tended to show a rather complex pattern of strengths and limitations (Dowdney et al., 1985a, 1985b). During the four hours of home observation, the ex-care women were closely similar to the controls in their expression of positive affect (warm comments, affectionate touching, etc.), in their initiation of interactions with their children and in the overall amount of joint play. On the other hand, they exhibited more negative affect (smacking, threats, etc.), were involved in more episodes involving control of disapproved behavior, and were more likely to ignore their children's overtures. The detailed interview measures produced a broadly similar pattern, although the intergroup differences tended to be somewhat greater.

The findings suggest two main inferences. First, most of the institution-reared women were attempting to parent well and were meeting with some degree of success. However, they seemed to lack a certain perceptiveness of their children's cues and they tended to be somewhat maladroit in their handling of minor day-to-day issues in parenting. Their failure to respond promptly and appropriately sometimes led to difficulties that might have been circumvented if they had been handled differently initially. Second, their parenting as observed in relatively unpressured circumstances was rather better than that reported over a longer time span in which they had to cope with the hurly-burly of competing demands and other life stressors and adversities. The history of parenting breakdown indicated that when faced with severe social difficulties they often lacked the personal resources and social supports to cope. Although it would be misleading to view the ex-care women as generally cruel, punitive, or neglectful of their children, they could behave in such ways when severely stressed in adverse circumstances that left them feeling despairing and unable to manage.

Nature of childhood adversities predisposing to parenting difficulties

The second basic question concerns the patterns of rearing that predispose to parenting problems in the next generation. The early clinical reports placed emphasis on the parents' experience of actual physical abuse with the implication that "like begets like." However, all the intergenerational studies that have involved systematic assessment and control groups have found a rather wider range of predisposing experiences, involving a severe lack of love and affection, gross neglect and lack of care, hostility and rejection, and an institutional upbringing. Thus, Egeland et al. (1984) found no differences between neglect, sexual abuse, and foster home placement as predisposing factors to maltreatment of the next generation. It is clear that the risk factors usually involve severe and prolonged disturbances in parent–child relationships rather than acutely stressful experiences or variations in rearing within the normal range. However, it is not evident from these data whether the main risk stems from a lack of affectionate care or from actively hostile, punitive, or cruel parenting. Nor do they indicate whether it matters *when* poor parenting is experienced (for example, whether the risks are greater if it occurs in infancy rather than middle childhood, or vice-versa). We sought to tackle these questions in our study of institution-reared women.

In order to focus on possible age effects we examined adult outcome according to whether or not the ex-care children had experienced disrupted parenting during the first four years of life (defined in terms of short-term admissions into care, multiple separations through parental discord or disorder, persistent family discord, or admission into long-term care before the age of 2 years). The results showed that the proportion with a personality disorder was *much* higher when there had been disrupted parenting in the infancy period (32 percent versus 5 percent) and the proportion with poor parenting was also higher (59 percent versus 29 percent), although the difference was not as great. The implication is that *early* disruptions of parenting may be particularly damaging to personality development; such damage may include ill-effects on parenting, although problems in parenting may arise in other ways as well.

Before that implication can be accepted, however, two other possibilities must be considered. First, it is likely that the children who experienced early family disruption were more likely to have severely deviant parents; accordingly, it is necessary to ask whether the risks stemmed from biological inheritance or experiential adversities. The data did indeed confirm that the women who experienced early disrupted parenting were more likely to have deviant parents (operationally defined in terms of a criminal record in adult life, psychiatric treatment, alcoholism, or dependency on "hard" drugs). A linear logistic analysis showed that there was a massive effect of disrupted parenting on overall psychosocial functioning at follow-up, but no appre-

Table 11.6. *Disrupted parenting in infancy and return home on leaving institutional care*

	Return to non-discordant family (%)	Return to discordant family (%)	No return (%)
Admitted under 2 years ($n = 18$)	6	34	61
Disrupted parenting and admission over 2 years ($n = 41$)	5	49	46
Non-disrupted parenting and admission over 2 years ($n = 21$)	33	29	38

Note: $x^2 = 12.67$, df $= 4$, $p < 0.025$.
Source: Quinton and Rutter, 1985.

ciable effect of parental deviance. Hence, insofar as parental deviance can be taken as a proxy for genetic risk, the inference is that the risk was experiential, not genetic. The pattern was slightly different for personality disorder, in that there were significant effects for *both* parental deviance and disrupted parenting, with a further significant effect from their combination. In other words, the suggestion is that both genetic background and early life experiences were operative in creating a risk for poor functioning in adult life.

The second alternative is that it was not the early occurrence of disrupted parenting that was crucial, but rather its severity and persistence. The data clearly indicated that early life experiences were connected with later ones (see Table 11.6). Thus, a third of the girls admitted to the institution after the age of 2 years who did not experience disrupted parenting during the first four years left the institution in their late teens to go to a nondiscordant family. This applied to 1 in 20 of those with early parental disruption and/ or admission to the Children's Home in infancy. Rather, they went back to a discordant family (usually the same one from whence they had been removed many years before) or they never went back to any family (living independently when they left the institution). It is apparent that the measure of disrupted parenting could not be considered solely in terms of what happened in infancy because what happened then served to influence the girls' circumstances on leaving the institution more than a dozen years later.

Nevertheless, the question remains as to the relative importance of early and late experiences. The pattern proved to be rather different according to the particular outcome considered (see Table 11.7). The home circumstances after leaving the institution were most important with regard to the women becoming pregnant (93 percent of those in discordant families versus 30 percent of those in nondiscordant families). Other evidence showed

Table 11.7. *Circumstances on return home and parenting*

	% Poor social Functioning		% Live Births		% Poor Parenting	
		(Total n)		(Total n)		(Total n)
Remained in care	26	(39)	51	(39)	55	(20)
Characteristics of home life on return						
Nondiscordant	10	(10)	30	(10)	0	(3)
Arguments with parents only	33	(18)	72	(18)	54	(13)
General family discord	50	(14)	93	(14)	46	(13)
Statistical significance of home life trend (1 df)						
x^2	4.15		12.46		NS	
p	<.05		.001			

Source: Quinton and Rutter, 1985.

that many of those in very unhappy homes sought marriage and parenthood as an escape from what they felt to be an intolerable situation. Similar, although weaker, effects were seen for poor psychosocial functioning, but there was no significant effect on parenting. This last negative finding was largely a consequence of the fact that so few women in nondiscordant homes became pregnant; as a result there were only three women with children who were in nondiscordant homes when they left the institution. It seems, then, that both early and late experiences play a part in shaping adult behavior.

The other basic question on the relative importance of active discord as against a lack of loving relationships can best be tackled by focusing on the subgroup of women who were admitted into the institution before the age of 2 years and who remained there throughout their childhood and adolescence. Of course, they are likely to have experienced family discord in early infancy, but such evidence as there is suggests that this is not likely to have major long-term sequelae provided that later experiences are positive and adaptive (see Rutter, 1981a). In most respects, the Children's Homes in which the children were placed provided a high quality of child care, as demonstrated by detailed direct study of the institutions at the time the children were there. King, Raynes, and Tizard (1971) concluded that there was "a system of care geared very closely to the individual needs" of the children. The one crucial respect in which the care was less than would be considered satisfactory today was the high turnover of houseparents.

Unfortunately, the available data lack precise quantification of the number of parent-figures for each child, but a detailed study of another Chil-

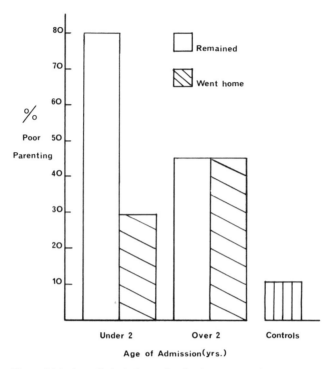

Figure 11.1. Age of admission to institution and quality of parenting. (*Source:* Rutter, Quinton, and Liddle, 1983.)

dren's Home serving a similar population showed that some 50 to 80 caregivers during the preschool years was common (Tizard and Hodges, 1978). The institutions were generally harmonious places with a lot of activities; nevertheless, in keeping with the turnover of caregivers, most of the women in our study looked back on it as a period of their life that lacked personal meaning or affection. Only a minority reported any strong personal attachments to members of the staff.

The findings on parenting outcome are summarized in Figure 11.1 (Rutter, Quinton, and Liddle, 1983). It was striking that the small subgroup of 10 girls who were admitted before 2 years of age and who remained in the Children's Home until 16 years of age later included the highest proportion (80 percent) with poor parenting, although this difference fell short of statistical significance. The finding is particularly striking because the parenting outcome was better for the girls admitted before 2 years of age who returned to their families, where most of them experienced both social disadvantage and severe family discord. The high rate of poor parenting in the group admitted after age 2 who returned home (the subgroup likely to have experienced the most extended exposure to family discord) demonstrates the risks for later parenting associated with active hostility, rejection, and punitiveness. However, the poor outcome for the early admitted, institution-reared group shows the risks associated with a lack of consistent affectionate parenting from caregivers with whom the child develops loving relationships.

That inference assumes that it was indeed the turnover of parent-figures that was damaging in the institution-rearing; it also implies a degree of persistence of effects that is rather unusual in terms of early life experiences generally. Neither feature can be tested directly from our own data. However, evidence from other studies suggests the plausibility of the hypothesized effect. Roy (1983), using direct observations in the classrooms as well as interview and questionnaire measures, compared the behavior of family-fostered children with that of institution-reared children (as well as normal controls). Both groups came from a similar severely disadvantaged background with much parental deviance and disorder; a blind analysis of family backgrounds showed no difference between the family-fostered and institution-reared groups. The institution-reared children differed from both the other groups in being more overactive and inattentive, in displaying more inept social behavior, in seeking attention from teachers, or in being more aggressive and relating less well with peers. It appeared, then, that these deficits were a consequence of some aspect of institutional life.

The next step in the argument is provided by the data from Tizard and Hodges's (1978) study of children in residential nurseries. At 2 years, the institutional children were more clinging and diffuse in their attachments than children brought up in ordinary families; at 4 years they remained less deeply attached but were, in addition, attention-seeking and indiscriminately friendly with strangers; at 8 years they continued to show the combination of affection-seeking and lack of close attachments together with restless, unpopular behavior at school. These two sets of data together with other evidence (Bretherton and Waters, 1985; Hay, 1985) point to a continuity between deficits in early parent–child attachments and later difficulties in social relationships.

The interest in the Tizard and Hodges's study, however, derives even more from the follow-up data on children from the residential nurseries who were adopted after the age of 4 years. Several findings require emphasis. Interviews with the adoptive parents when the children were 8 years of age showed that almost all of the children had developed good, stable affectionate relationships with their adoptive parents and there were few behavior problems at home (Tizard and Hodges, 1978). Evidently, children *can* and do develop strong selective attachments for the first time after the age of 4 years if the conditions are sufficiently good. Nevertheless, the late-adopted children showed similar problems at school to those of the children who remained in the institution. The early lack of bonding opportunities did *not* result in an inability to make true attachments later, but it *did* appear to affect the quality of other social relationships.

Most recently, the same children have been followed up again at age 16 (Hodges and Tizard, in press a and b). Two findings stand out. First, with the majority of behaviors, the *current* family circumstances were most relevant. Thus, the children who left the residential nursery to return to their biological parents experienced much more discord and more social disadvantage than those who were adopted. The effects were evident in the higher rate of delinquency and conduct disturbance in the restored group. Second, even a dozen years after adoption, the adopted children were similar to other institutional and ex-institutional children, and different from controls, in being more indiscriminately friendly but having more difficulty with peer relationships and in being less likely to confide in peers. It seemed that, in spite of general good home circumstances throughout the schoolage years, the early years in the institution had left their mark on the styles and quality of social relationships.

It would not be correct to view these features as a permanent defect in personality functioning both because later experiences affected adult outcome (see next section) and because it was evident that the children *could* form good close relationships (as apparent from those with adopted parents). Nevertheless, the overall pattern of circumstantial evidence suggests that early parent–child relationships may have a particular importance for later relationships with other people. The usual consequence of early adversities is, however, vulnerability and not necessarily a lasting incapacity.

Factors associated with intergenerational continuities and discontinuities

The last issue to be discussed is the central question of the mechanisms involved in intergenerational continuities and discontinuities. As we have seen, there are substantial continuities in parenting behavior. These are stronger looking backward than looking forward. That is to say, it is uncommon for *serious* parenting problems associated with general psychosocial malfunctioning to occur in the absence of important adversities in the upbringing of one or other of the two parents. The experience of bad parenting seems to be an almost necessary condition for these widespread severe parenting difficulties, but they are not a sufficient condition. Current marital support and social circumstances generally are also influential. It should be added that intergenerational continuities are *un*important in the genesis of milder, isolated parenting problems that are *un*associated with generally poor psychosocial functioning.

As noted, intergenerational continuities looking forward are less strong. In other words, although the experience of poor parenting much increases the risk that the individuals concerned will themselves provide poor parenting for the next generation of children, there is marked heterogeneity in outcome. Some women subjected to parental neglect and abuse become ordinary, well functioning adults who are adequate – even good – parents to their children. The challenge is to identify those factors that account for this complex mix of continuities and discontinuities.

Some suggestions are provided by Egeland et al.'s (1984) clinical impressions of their maltreated women who did not go on to abuse their own children. They point to two main variables: (1) the milder the maltreatment experienced by the parents, the less the risk that they will abuse their own children; and (2) the better the marital support in adult life, the less likely it is that abuse will occur. These and other influences were systematically explored through quantitative analyses in our study of institution-reared women.

Early risk factors

Some of the factors associated with a greater risk of a poor outcome in adult life have already been considered. Like Egeland et al. (1984), we found that the greater the overall burden of poor parenting experienced, the greater the risk of poor parenting provided to the next generation of children. It was striking, also, how one adversity tended to lead to another. Thus, parental deviance probably constituted a genetic risk factor of some importance for some outcomes. However, this (possibly) genetic factor also established an environmental risk because the parental deficiencies tended to create a hostile, discordant family environment leading to disrupted parenting and then admission to an institution. The institutional rearing carried its own risks, probably as a consequence of the lack of continuous stable parenting (a risk that was possibly much intensified for these children because of their genetic vulnerabilities and because of their early experiences of disrupted parenting). The early environmental hazards were reactivated in adolescence because they influenced the young people's experiences on leaving the institution. While the children were in residential care, many of the parents continued to show the same psychosocial problems that led earlier to the children being taken into care. Some changed marriage partners but all too often discordant relationships were recreated. As a result, children with the worst early life experiences were the ones least likely to experience a harmonious family environment on leaving the institution. The circumstances in the late teenage years then, in turn, were associated with what happened next. Most of the young women in nondiscordant families did *not* become pregnant quickly; conversely, almost all of those in discordant families *did* become pregnant, often while still teenagers. The timing of the first pregnancy was further associated with later outcomes (Rutter, Quinton, and Liddle, 1983).

Nearly two-thirds of the women who became pregnant by age 18 were rated at follow-up as showing poor parenting, compared with only a third of those who did not have their first baby until later.

Many of those who became pregnant early did so as part of a wish to escape from stressful circumstances. Often this was accompanied by marriage for a negative reason (e.g., to escape or as a result of an unwanted marriage forced by pregnancy). This, too, was related to the women's home circumstances on leaving the institution. Of those returning to a harmonious family, only one-fifth married for a negative reason, whereas over half of those going to a discordant family did so. Not surprisingly, this inauspicious start to marriage frequently resulted in an unhappy marriage to a man with similar psychosocial problems. Such marriages were associated with a much increased risk of poor parenting (see "Later risk and protective factors," below).

It will be appreciated that this cumulative risk stems from a long chain of indirect connections. No one "bad" experience was decisive, but each one created a set of circumstances that made it more likely that another bad experience would occur. Thus, the developmental continuity lies as much in social connections between different forms of adverse environments as in any internal effects on the child's own personality development (Rutter, 1984b, 1984c; 1987b), although the evidence on the social consequences of early institutional rearing suggests that they are present as well. Perhaps, too, this is apparent in the finding that the women's parenting qualities at follow-up were linked with the presence or absence of behavioral disturbance as measured contemporaneously during middle childhood/early adolescence. Thus, of the women with behavioral deviance when young, 64% showed poor parenting and only 4% good parenting; conversely those without such deviance included 41% with poor parenting and the same proportion (41%) with good parenting. As Elder et al. (1986) found in the Berkeley study, childhood problems show some continuity with later family difficulties and parenting qualities. The emphasis up to this point has been on factors leading to continuity; it is necessary now to turn over the same coin to focus on those associated with *dis*continuity.

Later risk and protective factors

Discontinuity is most conveniently studied by considering development in reverse time; that is, by identifying the factors at follow-up most strongly associated with differences in outcome and then working backwards to determine how the favorable circumstances might have been created. With respect to ameliorating factors, there were several variables with weak associations with better outcomes in the institution-reared sample. For example, positive relationships with adults during the teenage years had a nearly significant association with good psychosocial functioning at follow-up, although there was little association with good parenting (Rutter, Quinton, and Liddle, 1983). However, there were only two with major effects; current social circumstances and the marital relationship. The pattern was rather similar for both. First, poor social circumstances (operationally defined in terms of a lack of basic facilities such as a washing machine or telephone, the children having to share a bed or sleep in the parents' room, or over-crowding) were much more frequent in the institution-reared sample (two-fifths of women) than in the comparison group (one in twelve women). Some aspect of the childhood adversities, therefore, predisposed to poor living conditions in adult life. Second, in both cases and controls, poor parenting was much less likely when social circumstances were adequate. Current living conditions, therefore, had an independent effect on parenting. As follows from the first finding, however, although the *effect* was independent, the *occurrence* of poor social circumstances was not (as it was strongly related to childhood experiences). Third, poor parenting was more frequent in the ex-care group after equating for social circumstances. In summary, it seems that rearing patterns are associated with parenting independently of social circumstances, but social conditions exert an additional effect. But, because institutional rearing is associated with an increased likelihood of poor social circumstances, part of the effect of poor living conditions is an indirect outcome of the pattern of upbringing.

The pattern for marriage was similar, but the effect was stronger. Accordingly, the findings will be presented more fully to delineate the ways in which discontinuities in intergenerational transmission develop over time. We start with the findings at follow-up (see Table 11.8). It is apparent that, within the institution-reared group, the quality of parenting was much better if there was a supportive spouse (rated on the basis of a harmonious marriage and a warm confiding relationship) or if the spouse was free of serious psychosocial problems (defined in terms of psychiatric disorder, criminality, a drink or drug problem, or longstanding difficulties in personal relationships). This last association is the more striking because the two measures largely came from different informants (parenting from the woman and psychosocial problems from the spouse). The results strongly suggest that a good marital relationship with a nondeviant man provides a powerful protective effect that to a substantial extent counteracts the ill-effects stemming from disrupted parenting and an institutional upbringing. Of course, it could be an artifact resulting from a tendency for the better functioning women to be more likely to make harmonious marriages. However, the evidence indicated that this had not occurred; there was no significant association between the women's own behavioral disturbance and their choice of spouse (Quinton, Rutter, and Liddle, 1984). This lack of assortative mating may appear rather surprising at first sight. However, it is probably a function

Table 11.8. *Spouse's characteristics and quality of mother's current parenting ('ex-care' mothers)*

	Quality of parenting			Statistical significance		
	Good (%)	Intermediate (%)	Poor (%)	x^2	df	p
Spouse support						
Nonsupportive						
($n = 13$)	0	38	62	10.07	2	0.01
Supportive						
($n = 21$)	52	19	29			
Spouse deviance[a]						
With problems						
($n = 16$)	6	19	75	14.53	2	0.001
Without problems						
($n = 17$)	53	35	12			

[a]Deviance rating was not known for one spouse in this group.
Source: Quinton, Rutter, and Liddle, 1984.

of the fact that, on leaving the institution, the girls were scattered widely to a variety of settings different from those in which they had been reared – a circumstance that is very different from that applicable to girls brought up by their biological parents and one likely to introduce a degree of randomness in the choice of potential marriage partners.

That negative finding leaves unanswered the crucial question of why some girls made successful marriages whereas others did not. In order to tackle that issue, we obtained more detailed data on the circumstances of the marriage. In particular, we sought to determine whether the girls had in some sense chosen their marriage partners as part of a broader attempt to plan their lives. "Planning" was rated as having occurred if the women had known their future spouse for at least six months before cohabitation *and* if the reasons for living together were positive – that is, they involved a clear positive decision without succumbing to outside pressures (such as an unwanted pregnancy or a desire to escape from an unhappy home).

The findings showed both that planners were twice as likely to choose nondeviant first spouses (76% versus 35% of nonplanners) and that planners were much less common in the ex-care group (56% versus 81% in controls). It seemed that the lack of planning among the institution-reared women was one of the main reasons for their increased likelihood of marrying men with psychosocial problems. There was some evidence that this tendency to plan or not plan was a more general feature and not restricted to marriage; the

Table 11.9. *Positive school experiences and planning for marriage for ex-care women*

	Positive school experiences	
	No	Yes
Nonplanners	26	5
Planners	23 (47%)	17 (77%)

Note: $x^2 = 4.50$, df $= 1$, $p < 0.05$

findings on planning for employment were very similar (Quinton and Rutter, 1988). On the other hand, planning was *not* equivalent to a generally better level of social adjustment; there was no significant association with behavioral deviance as assessed in early adolescence (Quinton, Rutter, and Liddle, 1984).

A similar issue arises in relation to a possible artifact regarding the supposed protective effect of marital support. If planning was associated with choice of spouse and if spouse characteristics were related to parenting outcome, perhaps the whole association was a reflection of the women's own personality characteristics. The data showed that this was not so. The protective effect of marital support applied to both planners and non-planners. Thus, within planners, poor parenting occurred in 0% of those with marital support but in 53% of those without support; within nonplanners the comparable figures were 25% and 83%. Planning made a successful marriage more likely, but if a nonplanner happened to strike lucky the protective effect of marital support still applied; conversely, if, in spite of planning, planners lacked marital support they were likely to show poor parenting.

The identification of the important role of planning, of course, simply pushes the question on the origins of discontinuity back one stage further. Why did some ex-care women plan their lives, whereas others seemed just to drift from adversity to adversity without any attempt to alter their life situations? The findings (see Table 11.9) pointed to the protective role of positive school experiences. School experiences were rated as positive if the girls had two or more of the following: exam success, a markedly positive assessment of school work and/or relationships with peers, and a clearly positive recall of three or more areas of school life (such as sport, drama, arts and crafts, or academic work). The ex-care women were only slightly less likely to have positive school experiences but such experiences were much less likely to include exam success (24% versus 67% in the control group). The data showed that these positive school experiences had a significant association with outcome in the ex-care group but not in controls (illustrating the finding that often positive experiences exert a buffering or protective effect only in the presence of stress or adversity – Rutter, 1985c). Further analyses suggested that positive school experiences had a beneficial effect on outcome because they increased the likelihood of planning (planning was present in 47% of those without positive school experiences but in 77% with such experiences).

The fact that planning was present in nearly half of the women who lacked positive school experiences indicates that it is most unlikely that this constituted the only protective factor of note. However, perhaps what is important is not so much the specifics of protective influences but rather their mode of operation. Other research suggests the importance of feelings of self-esteem and self-efficacy. It may be that the girls acquired a sense of their own worth and of their ability to control their destinies as a result of their pleasure, success, and accomplishments in a few specific areas of their lives. Certainly it is a common observation that many people with multiple psychosocial problems suffer because they act as if they can do nothing about their plight. Our evidence suggests that the experience of some form of success or accomplishment may be important, not because it dilutes the impact of unpleasant happenings, but because it serves to enhance confidence and competence to deal with the hazards and challenges of everyday life.

Conclusions

The evidence from a variety of studies has been consonant in its demonstration of both intergenerational continuities and discontinuities in parenting problems. The finding of continuities is important in alerting us to the long-term risks for the upbringing of the next generation that can flow from this generation's experience of neglect, abuse, or even just lack of loving relationships during the growing years. The finding of strong discontinuities, however, is equally crucial in its reminder of large individual differences in people's response to serious stress and adversity. Sometimes these differences are dismissed as just variations in biological vulnerability about which we can do nothing. The evidence on the ways in which continuities and discontinuities come about shows how mistaken is this predestination view. There is very little that is unalterable even with respect to the sequelae of severe and prolonged maltreatment in childhood. Good experiences as late as early adult life can make an important difference in outcome. However, it would be misleading to see such experiences as a matter of chance or good luck. In part, later experiences arise as a result of earlier circumstances, but also individuals can do much to shape their lives, and it is the possibility of this positive action to break cycles of transmitted deprivation that provides the opportunity for preventive and therapeutic interventions.

References

Altemeier, W. A., O'Connor, S., Vietze, P., Sandler, H., and Sherrod, K. (1982). Antecedents of child abuse. *Journal of Pediatrics, 100,* 823–829.

Altemeier, W. A., O'Connor, S., Vietze, P., Sandler, H., and Sherrod, K. (1984). Prediction of child abuse: A prospective study of feasibility. *Child Abuse and Neglect, 8,* 393–400.

Belsky, J. (1984). The determinants of parenting: A process model. *Child Development, 55,* 83–96.

Bretherton, I., and Waters, E. (Eds.) (1985). Growing points of attachment theory and research. *Monographs of the Society for Research in Child Development, 50,* Nos. 1–2. Serial No. 209.

Bronfenbrenner, U. (1979). *The ecology of human development: Experiments by nature and design.* Cambridge, MA: Harvard University Press.

Cicchetti, D., and Aber, J. L. (1980). Abused children – abusive parents: An overstated case? *Harvard Educational Review, 50,* 244–255.

Clarke-Stewart, K. A. (1978). And daddy makes three: The father's impact on mother and young child. *Child Development, 49,* 446–478.

Cochran, M. M., and Brassard, J. A. (1979). Child development and personal social networks. *Child Development, 50,* 601–616.

Cohen, S. and Syme, L. S. (Eds.) (1985). *Social support and health.* New York: Academic Press.

Crockenberg, S. B. (1981). Infant irritability, mother responsiveness, and social support inferences on the security of infant–mother attachment. *Child Development, 52,* 857–865.

Crnic, K., Greenbert, M. T., Ragozin, A., Robinson, N., and Basham, R. (1983). Effects of stress and social support on mothers and premature and full-term. *Child Development, 54,* 209–217.

Davenport, Y. B., Zahn-Waxler, C., Adland, M. L. and Mayfield, A. (1984). Early child-rearing practices in families with a manic-depressive parent. *American Journal of Psychiatry, 141,* 230–235.

Dooley, D. (1985). Causal inference in the study of social support. In S. Cohen and L. S. Syme (Eds.), *Social support and health.* New York: Academic Press.

Dowdney, L., Mrazek, D., Quinton, D., and Rutter, M. (1984). Observation of parent–child interaction with two- to three-year-olds. *Journal of Child Psychology and Psychiatry, 25,* 379–407.

Dowdney, L., Skuse, D., Rutter, M. and Mrazek, D. (1985a). Parenting qualities: Concepts, measures and origins. In J. Stevenson (Ed.), *Recent research in developmental psychopathology.* Journal of Child Psychology and Psychiatry Monograph No. 4. Oxford: Pergamon, pp. 19–42.

Dowdney, L., Skuse, D., Rutter, M., Quinton, D., and Mrazek, D. (1985b). The nature and qualities of parenting provided by women raised in institutions. *Journal of Child Psychology and Psychiatry, 26,* 599–625.

Egeland, B., Breitenbucher, M., and Rosenberg, D. (1980). Prospective study of the significance of life stress in the etiology of child abuse. *Journal of Consulting and Clinical Psychology, 48,* 195–205.

Egeland, B., Jacobvitz, D., and Papatola, K. (1984). Intergenerational continuity of abuse. Paper presented at the Social Science Research Council Conference on Child Abuse and Neglect, York, Maine, May 20–23.

Elder, G. H., Caspi, A., and Downey, G. (1986). Problem behavior and family relationships: Life course and intergenerational themes. In A. Sorensen, F. Weinert, and L. Sherrod (Eds.), *Human development and the life course: Multidisciplinary perspectives.* Hillsdale, NJ: Erlbaum.

Farrington, D. P. (1978). The family backgrounds of aggressive youths. In L. A. Hersov, M. Berger and D. Shaffer (Eds.), *Aggression and antisocial behaviour in childhood and adolescence.* Oxford: Pergamon, pp. 73–93.

Frommer, E. A., and O'Shea, G. (1973a). Antenatal identification of women liable to have problems in managing their infants. *British Journal of Psychiatry, 123,* 149–156.

Frommer, E. A., and O'Shea, G. (1973b). The importance of childhood experience in relation to problems of marriage and family-building. *British Journal of Psychiatry, 123,* 157–160.

Goldberg, S. (1983). Parent–infant bonding: Another look. *Child Development, 54,* 1355–1382.

Harlow, H. F., and Suomi, S. J. (1971). Social recovery by isolation-reared monkeys. *Proceedings of the National Academy of Science, 68,* 1534–1538.

Hay, D. (1985). Learning to form relationships in infancy: Parallel attainments with parents and peers. *Developmental Review, 5,* 122–161.

Hetherington, E. M., Cox, M., and Cox, R. (1982). Effects of divorce on parents and children. In M. E. Lamb (Ed.), *Non-traditional families.* Hillsdale, NJ: Erlbaum, pp. 233–288.

Hodges, J., and Tizard, B. (in press, a). IQ and behavioural adjustment of ex-institutional adolescents. *Journal of Child Psychology and Psychiatry.*

Hodges, J., and Tizard, B. (in press, b). Social and family relationships of ex-institutional adolescents. *Journal of Child Psychology and Psychiatry.*

King, R. D., Raynes, N. V., and Tizard, J. (1971). *Patterns of residential care: Sociological studies in institutions for handicapped children.* London: Routledge & Kegan Paul.

Klaus, M. H., and Kennell, J. H. (1976). *Maternal–infant bonding: The impact of early separation or loss on family development.* Saint Louis, MO: C. V. Mosby.

Maccoby, E. E., and Martin, J. A. (1983). Socialization in the context of the family: Parent–child interaction. In E. M. Hetherington (Ed.), *Socialization, personality, and social development, Vol. 4, Mussen's handbook of child psychology (4th edition).* New York: Wiley, pp. 1–101.

Mills, M., Puckering, C., Pound, A., and Cox, A. (1985). What is it about depressed mothers that influences their children's functioning? In J. Stevenson (Ed.), Recent research in developmental psychopathology. *Journal of Child Psychology and Psychiatry,* Monograph Supplement No. 4. Oxford: Pergamon.

Mrazek, D., Dowdney, L., Rutter, M., and Quinton, D. (1982). Mother and preschool child interaction: A sequential approach. *Journal of the American Academy of Child Psychiatry, 21,* 453–464.

Mrazek, D., and Mrazek, P. (1985). Child maltreatment. In M. Rutter and L. Hersov (Eds.), *Child and adolescent psychiatry: Modern approaches* (2nd edition). Oxford: Blackwell Scientific, pp. 679–697.

Näslund, B., Persson-Blennow, I., McNeil, T., Kaij, L., and Malmquist-Larsson, A. (1984). Offspring of women with nonorganic psychosis: Infant attachment to the mother at one year of age. *Acta Psychiatrica Scandinavica, 69,* 231–241.

Novak, M. A. (1979). Social recovery of monkeys isolated for the first year of life. II. Long term assessment. *Developmental Psychology, 15,* 50–61.

Novak, M. A., and Harlow, H. F. (1975). Social recovery of monkeys isolated for the first year of life: I. Rehabilitation and therapy. *Developmental Psychology, 11,* 453–465.

Quinton, D., and Rutter, M. (1984a). Parents with children in care: I. Current circumstances and parenting. *Journal of Child Psychology and Psychiatry, 25,* 211–229.

Quinton, D., and Rutter, M. (1984b). Parents with children in care: II. Intergenerational continuities. *Journal of Child Psychology and Psychiatry, 25,* 231–250.

Quinton, D., and Rutter, M. (1985). Parenting behaviour of mothers raised 'In care.' In A. R. Nicol (Ed.), *Longitudinal studies in child psychology and psychiatry: Practical lessons from research experience.* Chichester: Wiley, pp. 157–201.

Quinton, D., and Rutter, M. (1988). *Parenting breakdown.* Aldershot, Eng.: Gower Publishing.

Quinton, D., Rutter, M., and Liddle, C. (1984). Institutional rearing, parenting difficulties and marital support. *Psychological Medicine, 14,* 107–124.

Pound, A., Cox, A., Puckering, C., and Mills, M. (1985). The impact of maternal depression on young children. In J. Stevenson (Ed.), Recent research in developmental psychopathology. *Journal of Child Psychology and Psychiatry,* Monograph Supplement No. 4. Oxford: Pergamon.

Rohner, R. P. (1975). *They love me, they love me not: A worldwide study of the effects of parental acceptance and rejection.* Human Relations Area Files, Inc., New York.

Roy, P. (1983). Is continuity enough?: Substitute care and socialization. Paper presented at the Spring Scientific Meeting, Child and Adolescent Psychiatry Specialist Section, Royal College of Psychiatrists, London, March.

Rutter, M. (1975). *Helping troubled children.* Harmondsworth, Eng.: Penguin. (1976, New York: Plenum.)

Rutter, M. (1980). *Changing youth in a changing society: Patterns of adolescent development and disorder.* Cambridge, MA: Harvard University Press.

Rutter, M. (1981a). *Maternal deprivation reassessed (2nd edition).* Harmondsworth, Eng.: Penguin.

Rutter, M. (1981b). Epidemiological/longitudinal strategies and causal research in child psychiatry. *Journal of the American Academy of Child Psychiatry, 20,* 513–544.

Rutter, M. (1983a). *A measure of our values: Goals and dilemmas in the upbringing of children.* London: Friends Home Service Committee.

Rutter, M. (1983b). Statistical and personal interactions: Facets and perspectives. In D. Magnusson and V. Allen (Eds.), *Human development: An interactional perspective.* New York: Academic Press, pp. 295–319.

Rutter, M. (1984a). Psychopathology and development: I. Childhood antecedents of adult psychiatric disorder. *Australian and New Zealand Journal of Psychiatry, 18,* 225–234.

Rutter, M. (1984b). Psychopathology and development: II. Childhood experiences and personality development. *Australian and New Zealand Journal of Psychiatry, 18,* 314–327.

Rutter, M. (1984c). Continuities and discontinuities in socio-emotional development: Empirical and conceptual perspectives. In R. Emde and R. Harmon (Eds.), *Continuities and discontinuities in development.* New York: Plenum, pp. 41–68.

Rutter, M. (1985a). Family and school influences on behavioural development. *Journal of Child Psychology and Psychiatry, 26,* 349–368.

Rutter, M. (1985b). Family and school influences on cognitive development. *Journal of Child Psychology and Psychiatry, 26,* 683–704.

Rutter, M. (1985c). Resilience in the face of adversity: Protective factors and resistance to psychiatric disorder. *British Journal of Psychiatry, 147,* 598–611.

Rutter, M. (1986). Meyerian psychobiology, personality development and the role of life experiences. *American Journal of Psychiatry* (143). 1077–1087.

Rutter, M. (1987a). Parental mental disorder as a psychiatric risk factor. In R. E. Hales, and A. J. Frances, (Eds.), *American Psychiatric Association's annual review, Vol. 6.* Washington: American Psychiatric Association.

Rutter, M. (1987b). Continuities and discontinuities from infancy. In J. Osofsky, (Ed.), *Handbook of infant development (2nd edition).* New York: Wiley.

Rutter, M., and Cox, A. (1985). Other family influences. In M. Rutter and L. Hersov (Eds.), *Child and adolescent psychiatry: Modern approaches* (2nd ed.). Blackwell Scientific, Oxford, pp. 58–81.

Rutter, M., and Giller, H. (1983). *Juvenile delinquency: Trends and perspectives.* Harmondsworth, Eng.: Penguin.

Rutter, M., and Madge, N. (1976). *Cycles of disadvantage.* London: Heinemann Educational.

Rutter, M., and Quinton, D. (1984a). Parental psychiatric disorder: Effects on children. *Psychological Medicine, 14,* 853–880.

Rutter, M., and Quinton, D. (1984b). Long-term follow-up of women institutionalized in childhood: Factors promoting good functioning in adult life. *British Journal of Developmental Psychology, 2,* 191–204.

Rutter, M., Quinton, D., and Liddle, C. (1983). Parenting in two generations: Looking backwards and looking forwards. In N. Madge (Ed.), *Families at risk.* London: Heinemann Educational, pp. 60–98.

Schaffer, H. R., and Liddell, C. (1984). Adult–child interaction under dyadic and polyadic conditions. *British Journal of Developmental Psychology, 2,* 33–42.

Sheridan, M. D. (1959). Neglectful mothers. *Lancet, i,* 722–723.

Shure, M. B., and Spivack, G. (1978). *Problem-solving techniques in child rearing.* San Francisco: Jossey-Bass.

Smith, S. M. (Ed.) (1978). *The maltreatment of children.* Lancaster, Eng.: MTP Press.

Steele, B. F. (1970). *Working with abusive parents from a psychiatric point of view.* U.S. Department of Health, Education, and Welfare, Washington, DC.

Steele, B., and Pollock, V. (1968). A psychiatric study of parents who abuse infants and small children. In R. Helfer and C. H. Kempe (Eds.), *The battered child.* Chicago: University of Chicago Press.

Suomi, S. J., Harlow, H. F., and Novak, M. A. (1974). Reversal of social deficits produced by isolation rearing in monkeys. *Journal of Human Evolution, 3,* 527–534.

Tizard, B., and Hodges, J. (1978). The effect of early institutional rearing on the development of eight-year-old children. *Journal of Child Psychology and Psychiatry, 19,* 99–118.

Troisi, A., and D'Amato, F. R. (1984). Ambivalence in monkey mothering: Infant abuse combined with maternal possessiveness. *Journal of Nervous and Mental Disease, 172,* 105–108.

Wadsworth, M. E. J. (1984). Early stress and associations with adult health, behaviour and parenting. In N. R. Butler and B. D. Corner (Eds.), *Stress and disability in childhood: The longterm problems.* Bristol: Wright, pp. 100–104.

Wadsworth, M. E. J. (1985). Parenting skills and their transmission through generations. *Adoption and Fostering, 9,* 28–32.

Wallerstein, J. (1983). Children of divorce: Stress and developmental tasks. In N. Garmezy and M. Rutter (Eds.), *Stress, coping, and development in children.* New York: McGraw-Hill, pp. 265–302.

Werner, E. E. (1979). *Cross-cultural child development: A view from the planet Earth.* Monterey, CA: Brooks/Cole.

Werner, E. E., and Smith, R. S. (1982). *Vulnerable but invincible: A longitudinal study of resilient children and youth.* New York: McGraw-Hill.

West, D. (1982). *Delinquency: Its roots, careers and prospects.* London: Heinemann.

White, S. O., and Straus, M. A. (1981). The implications of family violence for rehabilitation strategies. In S. E. Martin, L. B. Sechrest, and R. Redner (Eds.), *New directions in the rehabilitation of criminal offenders.* Washington, DC: National Academy Press, pp. 255–288.

Wolkind, S., and Kruk, S. (1985). From child to parent: Early separation and that adaptation to motherhood. In A. R. Nicol (Ed.), *Longitudinal studies in child psychology and psychiatry: Practical lessons from research experience.* Chichester, Eng.: Wiley, pp. 53–74.

Wolkind, S., and Rutter, M. (1985). Sociocultural factors. In M. Rutter and L. Hersov (Eds). *Child and adolescent psychiatry: Modern approaches* (2nd ed.). Oxford: Blackwell Scientific, pp. 82–100.

12   The construct of empathy and the phenomenon of physical maltreatment of children

Norma Deitch Feshbach

Introduction

Empathy and child abuse, seemingly disparate concepts, are both topics of contemporary concern to professionals and lay individuals. Although each has its own extensive history, current interest in the two topics revived in the sixties and has grown dramatically since then.

The composition and functions of the empathic response were once questions that philosophers and artists debated. With the development of Rogerian theory and therapy, the psychotherapeutic role of empathy was discussed and efforts were initiated to assess this complex psychological dimension (Dymond, 1949; Rogers and Truax, 1967). During the sixties and seventies, developmental and personality theorists broadened the arena of discourse and, more importantly, developed situational and self-report measures of empathy (Borke, 1971; Chandler, 1973; Feshbach and Roe, 1968; Hogan, 1969; Mehrabian and Epstein, 1972) that substituted for the earlier approaches that were more difficult to interpret.

It was also during the decade of the sixties that Kempe and his colleagues reminded us of the plight of the maltreated child, especially the physically abused child, with his papers on the battered child syndrome (Kempe, Silverman, Steele, Droegemueller, and Silver, 1962). The writings of de Mause (1974) and others sadly attest to the fact that child abuse is an age-old malpractice rather than a current aberration. Yet research findings, public concern, and the frequency of reported cases of child abuse have only really become salient during the last twenty years.

There is an anomaly in the fact that empathy and child abuse are simultaneously dominant themes of interest for the professional and for the pub-

Special thanks are extended to Professor Carolee Howes, the codirector of the UCLA project on Child Abuse/School of Education, and Child Help, U.S.A., who supported, in part, the project and the preparation of this chapter

349

lic. Empathy connotes a sharing, a perspective-taking, a sensitive, an other-centered attitude. Child abuse, on the other hand, connotes an impulsive, an egocentric, an aggressive, and an antisocial style of interaction. Is the absence of the former – empathy – the occasion for the appearance of the latter – child abuse? Is early experience of the latter – abuse in childhood – responsible for a later void in the former – adult empathy?

These and related questions will be posed in this chapter, which is addressed to the overall issue of the relationship between the personal attribute of empathy and the malpractice of child abuse. But first a few caveats. The category of maltreatment considered in this chapter will be primarily physical abuse. In referring to extant literature, reviews employing the criteria of physical abuse will be utilized (nonaccidental physical injury directed by parents and guardians toward children, as ascertained by a protective service agency and/or clinical interview by a researcher). Existing data covering harsh parental discipline practices, but not physical abuse, will not be included. Issues and data involved in the relationship between empathy and sexual abuse or neglect will similarly not be considered. (However, there are only a few studies directed toward understanding the role of empathy in any category of maltreatment.) This review also does not address constructs and behaviors related to empathy such as nurturance, caring, and helping. Because the construct of empathy is sometimes viewed cognitively, affectively, or integratively, both the theoretical analysis and literature review will represent these varied perspectives.

The chapter is organized in the following way: A brief overview of prevalent orientations and measures of empathy will be presented. This will be followed by a theoretical analysis of the relationship between empathy and physical maltreatment. The scant literature on empathy in perpetrators and in the abused will be summarized and reviewed, followed by a presentation of the procedures and findings from a major project on physical abuse, carried out in our laboratory at UCLA, in which parental empathy was an important factor. A discussion of possible directions for research and intervention programs will conclude the chapter.

Empathy

Background

Empathy is generally acknowledged to occupy a key role in the social development of an individual. What is less universally agreed upon are conceptions of empathy, its functions, its antecedents, procedures for its optimal assessment, and its role in the evolutionary survival of a species.

Prior to the 1970s there were only sporadic efforts to systematically evaluate some of the complex issues surrounding empathy. However, the construct itself was a subject of historical and clinical interest. A number of reviews published during this decade (Deutsch and Madle, 1975; N. Feshbach, 1975, 1979; Hoffman, 1975, 1977) present the early history of discourse on empathy. Interest in the process began with the British associationists, German introspectionists, and early American psychologists. Latter-day interest in children's empathy was manifested by the Piagetians and contemporary psychologists concerned with children's prosocial and emotional development.

Conceptions of empathy have varied greatly. What empathy is, does, and relates to is a function of a particular theoretical position and, frequently, of a particular procedure of measurement. Empathy is sometimes conceived of as a sympathetic reaction to distress and also, more broadly, as a reflection of social understanding and emotional identification. Although there are a number of different versions of affective approaches to empathy, the requirement of an affective correspondence between the emotional experience of an observer and the observed is a critical dimension of the empathic response, distinguishing the affective approaches to empathy from those employing predominantly cognitive criteria (Berger, 1962; Feshbach, 1975; Feshbach and Roe, 1968; McDougall, 1960; Stotland, 1969; Sullivan, 1953).

An early formulation of empathy in predominantly cognitive terms appeared in the writings of George Herbert Mead (1974). A critical element in his theorizing was the acquisition of social empathy through role taking and imitation. For Mead, empathy facilitated social interaction, because through this process a person could anticipate another's actions and be alerted with an appropriate response. Although Mead suggested that empathy involved feeling as well as thinking, it was the latter component that was predominant in his conceptualization of the term. Mead's attention to the activity of role playing anticipated an essential feature of cognitive definitions and explanations of the phenomenon of empathy. This account was also conducive to the conception of the empathic process as a mechanism for predicting the attitudes and behaviors of other people.

Focus on the empathy of the therapist – the therapeutic sharing of a client's emotional state – which was studied in the sixties and early seventies (Rogers and Truax, 1967; Truax, 1961, 1967, 1972), also had a strong cognitive flavor. Empathy in the Rogerian framework, like the psychoanalytic framework, stresses cognitive sensitivity to the client's feelings, attitudes, and desires (Feshbach, 1978).

Latter-day cognitive definitions conceptualize empathy in terms of role taking, perspective taking, or social comprehension. These formulations and descriptions of more situational measures are found in the writings of Borke (1971), Chandler (1973), Chandler and Greenspan (1972), Chandler, Greenspan, and Barenboim (1974), Deutsch and Madle (1975), Hogan (1969), and Shantz (1975).

Integrative approaches to empathy

The debate of the 1970s regarding the nature of the internal response, whether cognitive or affective, has subsided, and the general consensus appears to be that empathy entails both affective and cognitive elements, the relative role of each varying with the situation and the age and personality of the child or adult (Feshbach, 1973, 1978, 1982; Hoffman, 1977, 1982). According to N. Feshbach, although empathy is defined as a shared emotional response between observer and stimulus person, it is contingent upon cognitive factors. Thus, in this integrative–affective model, the affective empathy reaction is postulated to be a function of three component factors: (1) the cognitive ability to discriminate affective cues in others, (2) the more mature cognitive skills entailed in assuming the perspective and role of another person, and (3) emotional responsiveness – that is, the affective ability to experience emotions (Feshbach, 1973, 1975, 1978; Feshbach and Kuchenbecker, 1974; Feshbach and Feshbach, 1969; Feshbach and Roe, 1968). Implicit in this and other models of empathy is the critical requirement of differentiation of self from object.

Hoffman's (1977) subsequent developmental model of empathy also has three components – cognitive, affective, and motivational – and focuses on empathic responses to distress in others as the motivation for altruistic behaviors. For Hoffman, empathic arousal is already reflected in infant behavior, and although empathic behavior is primarily affective, it subsequently becomes transformed when the cognitive system of the child develops and is afforded a strong role (Hoffman, 1977).

Prosocial behavior and empathy

Although there appears to be a theoretical and empirical relationship between empathy and prosocial behavior (Feshbach, 1982; Feshbach and Feshbach, 1987), empathy is distinct and not synonymous with helping, caring, sharing, and other prosocial or altruistic behaviors. The need for this important theoretical and empirical distinction relates to whether empathy invariably serves as the motivation for altruistic behavior. Prosocial behaviors, especially altruism, can be mediated by factors other than empathy. And I would also contend that when empathy is aroused, altruism does not inevitably follow (N. Feshbach, 1982). Although overall, extant research findings reflect a positive relationship between empathy and prosocial behavior, the direction and strength of the findings vary as a function of the manner in which empathy is defined and measured and the specific prosocial behavior being evaluated (N. Feshbach, 1982; Feshbach and Feshbach, 1987).

Aggression and empathy

The findings bearing on the relationship between empathy and the converse of prosocial behavior – aggression – reflect a more stable association. A number of studies report an inverse relationship between empathy and aggression across a wide age range using a variety of assessment techniques (Chandler, 1973; N. Feshbach, 1983; Feshbach and Feshbach, 1969, 1982; Mehrabian and Epstein, 1972; Rothenberg, 1970). These findings led to a series of training studies in which a curriculum based on the three-component model of empathy was developed and implemented with elementary school children for the purpose of regulating aggression and promoting prosocial behaviors (N. Feshbach, 1979; 1983; Feshbach, Feshbach, Fauvre, and Ballard-Campbell, 1983). In general, the data from this program indicated that participating in an empathy training program resulted in reduced aggressive behaviors and an enhancement of self-esteem as well as a greater number of prosocial behaviors. The pattern of correlations of individual measures obtained in the study indicated that children high in empathy manifested more prosocial behavior and other related cognitive competencies than did children low in empathy. There were some sex differences in the pattern of these correlations. Cognitive correlates of empathy, such as social comprehension, reading, and vocabulary skills, were more pronounced for boys than for girls, and correlations of empathy with prosocial behavior and self-concept were significantly higher for girls than for boys.

Empathy and characteristics of personal adjustment

A number of investigators have studied the relationship between empathy and characteristics indicative of psychological adjustment (Andrews, Wormith, Daigle-Finn, Kennedy, and Nelson, 1980; Grief and Hogan, 1973; Kupfer, Drew, Curtis, and Rubinstein, 1978; and Speilberger, Gorsuch, and Luschene, 1970). A consistent finding in personality studies in which the Hogan Scale has been used to assess empathy is that persons high in empathy are low on anxiety and less depressed and appear better adjusted than individuals low in empathy. Similarly, empathy and neuroticism are shown to be inversely correlated when the Mehrabian and Epstein Empathy Scale has been used (Eysenck and Eysenck, 1978; Eysenck and McGurk, 1980).

Measurement

The difficulties inherent in the conceptualization of empathy are reflected in the methodological problems entailed in its assessment. Although there has been an expansion in the number of available instruments for assessing empathy, there is still a paucity of measures. Also, given the internal, multidimensional nature of the construct, a precise assessment of empathy continues to be an ideal we strive for rather than a reality we can achieve immediately.

Measures that assess empathy in children are varied and include methods that can be categorized along several theoretical dimensions as primarily affective (e.g., Bryant, 1982) or primarily cognitive (e.g., Borke, 1973; Chandler, 1973); as primarily integrative (N. Feshbach, 1980; Feshbach and Roe, 1968); as predictive (Dymond, 1949; Hogan, 1969); or as situational (Borke, 1973; N. Feshbach, 1968, 1980; Mood, Johnson, and Shantz, 1978). Additionally, empathy measures differ in several aspects of the method of assessment: on the basis of stimulus modality such as stories (Borke, 1973); audiotapes (Deutsch and Madle, 1975; Rothenberg, 1970); cartoons (Chandler, 1973); paper and pencil (Bryant, 1982); the inclusion of slides and narration (Feshbach and Roe, 1968) and audiovideo tapes (N. Feshbach, 1980, 1982); and type of response modality – verbal, physiological, or gesture.

At the adult level there are a number of paper and pencil measures that attempt to assess empathy. These include the Chapin Social Insight Test (Chapin, 1942); the Kerr and Speroff Empathy Test (Kerr and Speroff, 1954); and the more widely used Hogan (1969) and Mehrabian and Epstein (1972) Empathy Scales. The latter procedure, entitled the Questionnaire Measure of Emotional Empathy (QMEE), is clearly oriented to the assessment of emotional empathy. The other measures, however, are designed to tap social insight, ability to put oneself in another's place, role taking, and social sensitivity, and fall within cognitive orientations to the study of empathy.

Summary

A brief overview of the field of empathy has been presented. Although interest in empathy has had a long history, its salience as a major theoretical construct in psychology and significant area of empirical inquiry has occurred only during the last two decades. Traditional beliefs regarding whether empathy is primarily affective or cognitive have been supplanted by integrative models combining both dimensions. Although research in this area has recently burgeoned, there is still a wide gap between the critical theoretical role afforded to empathy in regard to development, personality functioning and psychopathology, and the empirical data base that provides information on many theoretical and developmental issues. Overall, empathy appears to be positively related to prosocial behaviors and negatively related to both antisocial behaviors and personality characteristics indicative of poor social adjustment. Assessing empathy is a very difficult task. A variety of procedures, varying in modality and orientation, have been developed.

Empathy and child abuse: theoretical considerations

Parent empathy – parent maltreatment

The previous discussion of the relationship between empathy and prosocial behavior and empathy and aggression suggests that the abusive parent should be low in empathy and that the abused child should also manifest a lack of empathy. Empathy appears to be a desirable psychological attribute, facilitating positive social behaviors. One would not expect an adult who physically abuses a child to be empathic with that child nor would one expect a history of physical abuse to be conducive to the development of empathy. However, it would be too facile to conceive of empathy as an all-embracing good such that the abusive adult and his or her victim must be deficient in this quality. A closer analysis of the construct of empathy and its theoretical properties provides a framework for identifying the specific variables that may influence the relationship between parent empathy and physically abusive behavior and its effects.

The anticipated relationship between empathy and the commission of abusive acts is relatively straightforward in contrast to the effects of being abused on empathy. Empathy, according to the three-dimensional model proposed by N. Feshbach, has significant cognitive features. Each of the cognitive components, discrimination of affective cues and perspective, or role taking, implies that an empathic parent will manifest greater understanding of a child with whom he or she interacts than would a nonempathic parent. The empathic parent is better able to identify a child's feelings (discrimination) and to appreciate a child's perception of a situation (role taking). An empathic adult is less likely to misunderstand a social situation, thus reducing the likelihood of conflict-induced abuse.

Misunderstandings are not the only antecedents of child abuse. A child may be unwanted, a parent may be inadequate and lack the skills necessary to modify a child's aversive behavior, a parent may be impulsive and lack self-control, a household may be burdened with short- or long-term problems, creating high levels of stress. The significance of the cognitive components of empathy in reducing the likelihood of child abuse becomes less salient when these other factors are present. However, the functions of empathy are not limited solely to its cognitive features. There is also a critical emotional element that becomes manifested in the vicarious sharing of another's feelings. The empathic parent is likely to experience some degree of the pain and distress of a child who has been subjected to physical assault.

Consequently, this empathic response should function to inhibit abusive behaviors that not only pain the child but, by virtue of empathy, also pain the adult.

Thus, an empathic parent is likely to be upset by a maltreated child's distress as well as understand a child's feelings and the situation that gives rise to these feelings and behavior. One would expect an empathic parent to develop a repertoire of positive social behaviors and disciplinary alternatives to physical abuse. However, empathic inhibition, or these alternative constructive behaviors, may be insufficient to inhibit abuse if the individual has a low frustration tolerance and is impulsive. For the impulsive abuser, empathy may be evoked after the fact and contribute to regret and remorse, rather than function to prevent the abusive act from occurring.

Personal characteristics such as impulsiveness, low nurturance, and child-rearing incompetence are factors that attenuate the anticipated inverse relationship between empathic disposition and the tendency to maltreat a child. A factor that might conceivably even reverse the relationship is the degree of separation between self and other. Mature or true empathy should not reflect the merging of observer and object, but should derive from the individual's ability to assume the perspective and share the feeling of the other.

Empathy requires the maintenance of boundaries between self and the environment. When these boundaries are blurred, the individual is reacting as if the other person's experience were happening to him- or herself. The emotional response under these circumstances is likely to be exaggerated rather than modulated and mediated by cognitive factors. An individual with an ambiguous self-definition can be expected to be very variable in responding to a child, sometimes being overly protective and other times abusive. Individuals who lack a sense of self are basically narcissistic and self-referent and are unlikely to see another's, including the child's, perspective. The distress of a child may not inhibit the narcissistic parent, but may serve to intensify feelings of anger and frustration, raising, not reducing, the probability of an abusive act. Ideally, we should employ measures that would enable us to distinguish individuals who manifest true "empathy" from those individuals who merely manifest the same emotion as that of another.

Parent maltreatment: child empathy

When we turn to the question of the effects of physical abuse upon the child's development of empathy, the theoretical possibilities are more complex. The abusing parent serves as a model for identification. The salience of the parent as a model for identification and imitation may be greater for maltreated youngsters. Abusive families tend to be more isolated and less integrated into social networks. This is a family system that provides less opportunity for the child to be exposed to surrogate models. In addition, the child is likely to have fewer opportunities to interact with peers, an important factor in the development of role-taking skills and empathy.

Moreover, being the object of abuse elicits negative feelings in the child with which he or she must cope. The nature of the relationship with the abusing parent is both a context for and a consequence of the coping mechanisms that the child develops. In addition, the child's attitudes toward the source of abuse will influence the degree and nature of the child's identification with the abuser. To understand how the experience of physical maltreatment may affect the development of empathy, one must consider a matrix of reciprocally interacting influences of identification, the relationship with the abuser, and the child's understanding of the abusive act and his or her methods of adjusting to the physical and psychological pain that abuse engenders, the social context of the family, and the relative wealth or dearth of social support outside the family of origin.

Data bearing on the socialization antecedents of empathy (Feshbach, 1975) suggest that the identification process may be a useful entrée into this constellation of interacting factors. In a study examining the antecedents and correlates of aggression and empathy, striking sex differences were found in maternal and paternal childrearing behavioral correlates of empathy in their 6- to 8-year-old offspring. For girls, empathy appears to be related to maternal behaviors reflecting a positive and nonrestrictive relationship with their daughters, and facilitative of identification. Thus, empathy in girls is positively correlated with maternal tolerance and permissiveness and negatively correlated with maternal conflict, rejection, punitiveness, and excessive control. No significant relationships were obtained between fathers' childrearing attitudes and practices and their daughters' empathic responsiveness. Extrapolating from these data to physical abuse by significant adult caretakers, one would predict that, for girls, physical abuse by maternal figures is much more disruptive of empathy development than physical abuse by paternal figures. Conceivably, physical abuse by a paternal figure, in the context of a nonabusive, positive maternal figure, might sensitize a young girl to experiences of pain in others as well as herself, and enhance empathic responsiveness to distress in others.

For boys, empathy proved to be only weakly associated with socialization antecedents. The only significant relationship was an inverse one: Low levels of empathy were found among sons whose fathers tended to foster competitive behavior. Degree of punitiveness by father or mother was unrelated to boys' empathy. It may be noted that empathic responsiveness, apart from its correlates, appears to be sex linked, with girls manifesting greater empathy than boys (Feshbach, 1982; Hoffman, & Levine, 1976). Also, there are data indicating that empathy in boys is more strongly related to various cognitive skills than it is for girls. It is as though empathy in girls develops through identification, normative role adaptation, and positive childrearing experiences, whereas the routes to empathy in boys are more diverse. Another way of phrasing this sex difference is that in western culture, empathy is ego- or role-syntonic for girls and less so for boys (Feshbach, 1980).

Consequently, it is more difficult to predict the consequences of abuse for the development of boys' than for girls' empathy. If identification is not a major antecedent of empathy in boys, the difference between a nonabusive and abusive caretaker will be less important for boys. The distress in the child caused by abuse might foster sensitivity to distress in others. However, abuse also elicits anger, defensiveness, and egocentric reactions that would be incompatible with an empathic disposition. Perhaps physical abuse of brighter boys, with cognitive skills that are requisites for empathy, may heighten empathy in these children but have an opposite effect on boys that are lower in intelligence, resulting in decreased empathy in these boys.

This theoretical analysis suggests that the relationship between a history of physical abuse and the degree of empathy manifested by a child will depend upon the interaction of sex of the abuser, sex of the child, the cognitive competence of the child, and the child's relationship to the nonabusing caregiver. It is unlikely that extant research has taken into account this multiplicity of factors and, consequently, one can expect that the research literature will reflect diverse relationships between caregiver abuse and the degree of empathy manifested by the child as a function of these complex interactions.

Empathy and child abuse: literature review

Acknowledging the multidimensional antecedents of abuse that include individual, familial, and ecological factors, one approaches the empirical literature with two basic questions: "Are individuals who physically abuse children – parent or caretaker – low in empathy?" and "Are children who have been subjected to physical abuse low in empathy?" Obviously, there are other questions one would like to add, such as whether these relationships are consistent across both sexes, across ages, and for various socioeconomic groups. However, the literature relating these two phenomena is quite sparse and does not provide the basic information that we seek.

The little research that has been carried out suggests that empathy or the lack of empathy in a parent or surrogate is related to propensity to abuse, and that children exposed to abusive parenting develop deficits in this important attribute.

Physical abuse of child and empathy of the perpetrator

Recent reviews of personality attributes in child abusing parents or surrogates do not reveal any consistent pattern or profile (Starr, 1982; Wolfe,

1981). A number of individual studies reflect characteristics that are indicative of greater mental distress in abusing parents, especially mothers (Mash, Johnston, Kovitz, 1983; Milner and Wimberley, 1980). There are also a number of studies that indicate that abusing parents/surrogates manifest behavioral repertoires that can be considered correlates of low empathy, such as: anger (Spinetta, 1978); aversive behavior with other family members (Reid, Taplin, and Lorber, 1981); and low sense of competence (Mash, Johnston, and Kovitz, 1983).

Interestingly, although empathy is conceptualized as having affective as well as cognitive components, indices of greater affectivity are more characteristic of the abusing rather than the nonabusive adult. When Frodi and Lamb (1980) compared the responses of child abusers with a matched sample of nonabusers who were observing crying and smiling infants on videotapes, a number of physiological differences were obtained. Abusers manifested greater skin conductance responses and greater increments in heart rate than nonabusers. Wolfe (1981) similarly found greater skin conductance and respiration changes (but no differences in heart rate) in an abuse group than in a nonabuse group when viewing stressful and nonstressful parent and child interactions on videotapes. The physiological differences manifested by abusive as contrasted to nonabusive adults reflect the greater emotional lability of the abusive group and, perhaps more importantly, also indicate that emotional reactivity and empathy are not the same process. This distinction is pertinent to our theoretical understanding of empathy and also to guidelines for intervention programs.

In the same Frodi and Lamb (1980) study, the abusive group had difficulty in discriminating the crying infant scenes from the smiling infant scenes. This finding suggests that abusers show less discrimination of emotional cues than nonabusers, and discrimination of cues is an important, if rudimentary, cognitive facet of empathy. Of even greater significance is that the abusive parent sample showed more anger and less sympathy than the control group when they observed the videotapes of crying infants, demonstrating low general empathy.

In another study, focusing on the relationship between empathy and physical abuse in mothers, Letourneau (1981) found that the two measures of empathy used in the study were better predictors of abuse than was a life stress measure. The Hogan Scale (1969) classified 80 percent of the abusive mothers correctly, whereas the Mehrabian and Epstein measure (1972) identified 63 percent of the abusive mothers. In this same study, it was found that the abusive parents were less nurturant and more aggressive than nonabusing mothers and that, overall, empathy and aggression were inversely related. In a study exploring personality characteristics of moderately physically abusive mothers (a group warranting protective case work but not immediate court action) and a nonabusive comparison group, Evans (1980) found that nonabusive mothers as compared to abusive mothers were more likely to give TAT responses rated as trusting, empathic, and supportive of children's needs.

Empirical studies directly exploring the relationship between empathy and physical abuse are few and tend to be inconclusive. The limited extant data that permit generalizations indicate that, overall, low empathy in caretakers and adults reflects greater likelihood of physical maltreatment of children. Cognitive aspects of empathy appear to have stronger links to reduced incidence of child abuse than affective components. Abusive parents also manifest personal attributes that are correlates of low empathy such as anger, conflict ridden behavior, and low sense of competence, and they appear more emotionally reactive or labile.

Physical abuse of child and child empathy

Data from studies that focus on the relationship between parent physical abuse and empathy in children are important. The information garnered would provide developmental insights into the array of negative effects of abuse and would also be pertinent to questions regarding intergenerational patterns of child abuse. These insights would suggest directions for successful intervention projects. In general, it is expected that children who have been subjected to parental physical abuse are less empathic than children without the abusive history for the reasons suggested in the theoretical analysis and review of parent data. Unfortunately, when we turn to existing research we find only a few studies that bear directly upon that relationship.

In one study, physically abused children between 5 and 10 years of age, mostly boys, were compared to same age nonabused children on empathy, aggression, and emotional adjustment (Straker and Jacobson, 1981). In this study an abused child was defined as a child who had been subjected to repeated physical injuries resulting in bone fractures, contusions, abrasions, cuts, or burns inflicted by a parent or caretaker. The Feshbach and Roe (1968) Affective Situation Test, a picture/story measure, was used to assess empathy. The findings from this study clearly showed that abused children were significantly less empathic than the controls. Interestingly, the abused children did not differ from the controls on aggression, the latter attribute assessed on a number of family aggression measures. Perhaps the physical abuse functioned to inhibit aggression in the family situation.

Barahal, Waterman, and Martin (1981) investigated the social cognitive aspects of empathy in matched groups of abused and nonabused children, mostly males, between 6 and 8 years of age. The authors predicted that the abused children would be less socially sensitive to the emotional states of others, would demonstrate more egocentric perspective-taking styles, and exhibit less advanced social role concepts. The abused children included in the study had experienced documented physical maltreatment that had occurred more than one year previously. The Audio-tape measure of social sensitivity developed by Rothenberg (1970) was used to assess the accuracy of children's labeling of specific affects portrayed on the tapes. The measure of perspective-taking used in the study required the children to tell a story that lacked essential elements (Flavell, Botkin, Fry, Wright, and Jarvis, 1968), whereas the measure of understanding of social role concepts was derived from puppet play with three puppets (Watson, 1977). The authors' predictions were confirmed in all areas that related to empathy. Abused youngsters were less sensitive and were less able to identify appropriate feelings in others. Not only were the abused group less accurate in labeling the emotions of others, but they were also less articulate in describing the social and interpersonal causes of the specific emotions. Nonabused children were better in perspective-taking skills, manifesting views that were not as egocentric as the views of the abused children. The control children were also more effective in comprehending increasingly complex social roles than were abused children.

In another study, generally related to this overall topic, the empathic ability of boys and girls aged 4 and 5 whose mothers had been the target of conjugal violence was compared to that of same age children who came from nonviolent homes (Hinchey and Gavelek, 1982). Four measures assessed the empathic abilities of the children: a role-enactment task; a social inference task that required understanding how the social other felt (Borke, 1971); and a role-taking measure that required the child to examine a situation from another person's perspective and to discriminate between more or less socially appropriate responses. The fourth measure was a social behavioral measure that included cooperative play, positive facial expression, personal initiative, and conversation ability, In this study, the children from violent households manifested less competence on three of the four measures, Role-enactment, Social Conference, and Role Taking.

Observation studies

Several observational studies of preschool children's behaviors carried out in child care settings reflect a variety of significant differences in behavior that are related to empathy or may be the precursors to empathy. In an early study, George and Main (1979) found that abused toddlers were more aggressive to caretakers and more avoidant of peers than a matched group of nonabused children. In a later paper, these same children's response to distress in agemates was analyzed (Main and George, 1985). The authors found highly significant differences between the abused and nonabused groups. Although five of the nine nonabused children showed concern, sadness, or empathy at least once in response to distress in a peer, not one abused toddler ever exhibited a concerned response. Moreover, the children in the abused group responded negatively to distress in peers with eight out of nine abused toddlers in comparison to only one of the nine control children responding with fear, physical attack, or anger to the crying of other children. The authors interpret the children's patterns of behavior as similar to those of abusing caretakers.

Data from a major research endeavor carried out at UCLA under the overall direction of Professor Carollee Howes and myself showed that in newly formed play groups abused toddlers and preschool children were less socially skilled than a matched group of nonabused children (Howes and Espinosa, in press). The former group expressed fewer positive and negative behaviors to peers, initiated social interaction less often and engaged in fewer play behaviors than normal children. The reactions of the children to the distress of a peer found in this study, which included a larger and broader subject population, were similar to the findings of Main and George (1985) and differentiated the abused and nonabused children. Howes and Espinosa found that abused children, in contrast to the nonabused children, responded more aggressively to signs of distress (mostly crying) of peers in both a free play and a structured situation.

The implications drawn from these studies, in conjunction with the earlier research of Radke-Yarrow and Zahn-Waxler (1982) on nonabusive young children's helping responsiveness to distressed individuals in the environment, strongly suggest that the experience of physical abuse poses a major threat to the child's emotional and behavioral development, including the development of precursors to empathy and/or empathy itself.

Summary

Suggestive rather than definitive conclusions can be drawn from extant research exploring the relationship between empathy and physical maltreatment of children. Methodological shortcomings and criticisms that characterize much of the research on child maltreatment – small subject samples, inadequate measuring instruments, unidimensional approaches – also apply to the literature on empathy and abuse. Nevertheless, the overall findings indicate that perpetrators and nonperpetrators differ on an important dimension – empathy – a psychological process that has important implications for interpersonal experiences and relations. The child data bearing on the relationship between physical abuse and empathy suggests that an antecedent for the dysfunctional pattern observed in perpetrators may arise chronologically early in the context of being abused.

Abused children do not respond to their social environment in the same way that nonabused children do. Like the perpetrators, abused children have difficulty in assessing social cues, in social role-taking, and in socializing with peers. In regard to emotional reactivity, both abusers and abused show a propensity to overrespond to negative emotional stimuli in the environment – a finding that has implications for understanding and preventing abuse, and a finding that has implications for understanding the construct of empathy and using empathy as a tool in preventing abuse.

The UCLA School of Education Project on Child Abuse

The literature relating parental empathy and parental maltreatment of children, while suggestive, is incomplete, A major reason for the paucity of research as well as the status of research in this area is the absence of measures that have been specifically designed to assess parental or adult empathy with a child as the object. One of the major goals of the UCLA Project on Child Abuse carried out by Professor Carollee Howes and myself was to develop an instrument to assess empathy that would specifically be concerned with empathy for the child (see Feshbach and Caskey, 1985).

The UCLA project was multifaceted, with parental empathy comprising one major focus. We were interested in the social behaviors of abused and high-risk children (Howes and Espinosa, in press); in the compliance and self-control of these young children, and in the relationship between these behaviors and parent empathy, stress, and social support (Howes, Feshbach, Gilly, and Espinosa, 1985). We were conscious of the methodological problems limiting this area of research and we strove to avoid them. Thus, our abuse sample was restricted to physically abusive families and did not include children and families whose problem was sexual abuse or neglect. The age range of the children was limited to the toddler and early preschool period. We used two control groups, a mental health clinic sample and a normative sample, in an effort to have a wider range in comparison groups. Our data base included peer interactions, parent–child interactions, and an array of self-report measures believed to be psychologically relevant and psychometrically valid. A recently developed empathy measure designed to assess parent and partner empathy (Feshbach and Caskey, 1985) was used in the study.

Subjects

The total sample included 336 participants: 219 mothers and 117 children. Of the mother–child pairs, 26 consisted of physically abused children and their abusing mothers. These pairs were selected from child guidance clinics and were identified by the agency as well as the dependency court as documented cases of physical abuse. Twenty-five of the mother–child pairs were also clients of child guidance clinics but had no history of abuse, nor were they suspected by therapists of abuse. A sample of 66 mother–child pairs were obtained from day care centers and parent education classes. The families were predominantly middle class and moderately well educated. The total sample also included two additional abuse mothers, three additional

Table 12.1. *Examples of items with high loading on the four factors of the Parent/Partner Empathy scale*

	Factor loading
Factor 1: Cognitive	
I have trouble understanding my spouse (or partner)	−.74
I have trouble figuring out what my child wants	−.68
I have difficulty understanding how my child feels	−.69
I am able to figure out what my spouse (or partner) wants for a present	.62
Factor 2: Affect expression	
I like my child to keep his (her) feelings to themselves	−.76
I think it's important to know how my child feels	.73
I do not like my child to hug and kiss in public	−.70
Children should be seen and not heard	−.68
Factor 3: Partner empathy	
My spouse (or partner) complains that I am not very sympathetic	−.57
Even when I don't agree with my spouse (or partner), I try to understand their point of view	.56
My spouse (or partner) and I have the same feelings about things	.51
I can tell when my spouse (or partner) is anxious	.46
Factor 4: Empathic distress	
I find it hard to be in a good mood when my child is sad	.62
When my child is disappointed, I feel some of his (her) disappointment	.62
I get upset when I see an animal in pain	.58
When I see sad things, I feel like crying	.55

clinic mothers, and 163 additional mothers in the control group. About eighty percent of the families were anglo, the remaining families were Hispanic, black and Asian. All of the mothers spoke English.

In spite of our concerted efforts there were some demographic differences between the three groups. Children in the control groups were younger, and their parents had more years of schooling. And there were significantly more divorced and separated parents in the abuse and clinic than in the control group.

Empathy scale

All the parents were administered the newly developed Parent/Partner Empathy Scale constructed by N. Feshbach and Caskey (Feshbach and Caskey, 1985). This paper and pencil self-report inventory is designed to assess a parent's empathy toward his or her child and empathy toward the spouse or partner. The measure consists of 40 statements presented in a Likert format in which a respondent indicates whether the statement is always, usually, sometimes, or never true. The measure is based on N. Feshbach's con-

Table 12.2. *A comparison of mean scores of control, high-risk and child abuse groups on Parent/Partner Empathy Measure and its factorial components*

	Total empathy	Cognitive F1	Affect expression F2	Partner empathy F3	Empathic distress F4
Mean scores					
Control	131.7	42.3	35.2	30.3	21.8
Clinic	124.8	38.8	34.2	28.8	21.6
Abuse	122.8	39.2	34.1	27.2	20.2
	$p < .001$	$p < .001$	$p < .05$	$p < .05$	$p < .05$
Planned comparisons					
Control versus					
Clinic	$t = 3.46$	$t = 4.4$	$t = 1.99$	$t = 3.38$	NS
	$p < .01$	$p < .0001$	$p < .05$	$p < .001$	
Control versus					
Abuse	$t = 4.17$	$t = 3.8$	$t = 1.97$	$t = 4.48$	$t = 2.18$
	$p < .0001$	$p < .0001$	$p < .05$	$p < .0001$	$p < .05$
Clinic versus abuse	NS	NS	NS	NS	$t = 1.5$
					$p = .14$

ceptual model of empathy (Feshbach, 1975; Feshbach, 1978). Individual items were designed to assess parental and spousal/partner discrimination of affective cues, role-taking skills, emotional expressiveness, and general empathy. A factor analysis of this scale yielded four factors: The first factor, labeled Cognitive, includes 13 parental and partner discrimination and role-taking items. The second factor, labeled Affect expression, includes 10 items about one's own expressiveness and attitudes about others' expressiveness. Most of the items on this factor are directed toward children. The third component is a Spouse/partner empathy factor and includes 9 cognitive, affective, and general empathy items with the object as the spouse. The fourth factor, labeled Empathic distress, consists of 7 items reflecting shared reactions to distress and discomfort in others. One item that did not load on any of the four factors was retained for the total measure for the purpose of maintaining a relatively even balance between parent and partner items. Examples of items with high loadings on the four factors of the Parent/Partner Empathy scale are presented in Table 12.1.

Findings

The results of a one-way analysis of variance and of planned comparisons of the total Empathy scores and the four factors scores are presented for the three comparison groups in Table 12.2 (Feshbach and Caskey, 1985).

Although the total Empathy scores of both the clinic and child abuse groups were significantly lower than the mean score of the control groups, the mean score of the two clinical groups was not significantly different. In addition, as Table 12.2 indicates, the means of the control group for the first three factors (Cognitive, Affect–expression, and Partner empathy) were significantly different from those of the clinic and child abuse groups. The differences on these three factors between the two latter groups were again small and insignificant. However, for Empathic distress (Factor 4), the means of the control and clinic parents were comparable, both means being higher than that obtained by the child abuse parent group. The difference between the controls and the child abuse group was significant at the 5 percent level of confidence, whereas the difference between the clinic and child abuse groups fell short of statistical significance, most likely because of the much smaller sample sizes of these groups as compared to the controls.

The Empathy subscales, with the exception of the Empathic distress factor, significantly discriminated between parents of a control sample of children and parents of emotionally disturbed or physically abused children. The latter groups of parents reported less empathy with their child and less empathy with their spouse. The Empathy scales did not, however, discriminate between the two clinical groups, although the Empathic distress factor may be a possible exception. The controls were similar to the clinic group on this factor, differing significantly only from the abuse group. It seems quite possible that with a larger sample the difference between the clinic and abuse groups would attain a satisfactory level of significance.

The Empathic Distress factor did not discriminate between the control parents and the clinic parents, nor did it manifest a similar pattern of correlations to that obtained with the other Factor scales (Feshbach and Caskey, 1985). Yet for some theorists (Hoffman, 1977), empathic distress is the core of empathy. There is one facet of the findings that is consistent with this view – namely, the lower scores obtained by the child abuse group on this factor.

Overall, these data suggest the following theoretical possibility. The cognitive, role-taking skills that are central components of empathy are less salient for the dimension of empathic distress. Empathy, because it entails sensitivity to another's affective state and perspective, can be a significant element in the maintenance of positive interpersonal relationships. Empathic distress that involves sympathetic distress reactions to another's pain appears to be a less important factor with regard to the quality of social relationships, but may be more closely linked to distress reducing behaviors that inhibit abuse. Thus, empathic distress, although only peripherally related to social relationships, may enhance the likelihood of sympathetic responses to someone who is in physical pain, of sharing responses to someone who is in need, or of restraints on physical punishment because of the pain it inflicts on the child. This empathic distress factor appears similar, in a number of important respects, to the conception of egocentrically based empathy as contrasted to a sympathetic, other-centered empathy (Batson, O'Quin, Fultz, Vanderplas, and Isen, 1983).

The parent–child interaction situation

A laboratory session including four tasks was carried out with a subset of mother–child pairs (abuse pair $n = 26$, clinic pair $n = 25$, control pair $n = 66$). This situation yielded a number of child behavior indices including compliance, self control, expression of positive affect, and expression of negative affect. In addition, a number of maternal behaviors were measured. These included parent involvement in child compliance, parent investment in child's compliance, parent expression of positive affect, and parent expression of negative affect. A partial correlation analysis was performed (controlling for social support and stress) in order to examine the hypotheses that mothers with high parental empathy are highly invested and involved in their children's performance, and that their children have well developed capacities for compliance and self control.

Across all three groups of mother–child pairs, total Empathy was positively related to child self-control (.49), parent investment (.67), involvement (.51), and positive affect (.39) and negatively related to child (−.27) and mother negative affect (−.39) with the effects of social support and stress partialled out. Interestingly, with one exception of maternal negative affect, the pattern of correlations obtained between the distress factor and these mother–child behavioral indices in this interactive situation is similar to that found for the total empathy score.

These data, reflecting systematic behavior correlates of the empathy measure in conjunction with the group comparisons, provide evidence of the construct validity of the empathy measure. Of equal importance, these findings suggest that parental empathy is a relevant factor in the matrix of variables that influence child abuse.

Directions for research and prevention

The principal thesis of this chapter has been that the psychological process and dimension of empathy has theoretical properties that are relevant to the prevention and reduction of the phenomenon of child abuse. The data that have been reviewed are consistent with this thesis. Although empathy is acknowledged to be only one of a large number of variables that constitute the psychological and contextual antecedents of child abuse, empathy appears to have a special potential for the regulation of physical violence toward children. Parents who have not abused their children are significantly more empathic than parents with a history of abusive practices. Non-abusive parents are also more empathic than parents of emotionally disturbed children. However, there also appear to be subcomponents of empathy that are specific to the control of child abuse.

The inverse relationship found in parents between empathy and physical abuse of an offspring is consonant with the inverse relationship that has been reported between empathy and aggression in children and young adults. The latter finding has given rise to prevention and intervention programs that are designed to reduce the frequency or development of aggression (Feshbach, Feshbach, Fauvre, and Ballard-Campbell, 1983; Feshbach, 1984). The relative success of these programs suggests that empathy training is a promising avenue to explore in intervention and prevention planning oriented to the amelioration and reduction of physical maltreatment of children. However, one cannot automatically assume from the evidence of success of empathy training with children that such training will be equally effective with adults or that training that reduces aggressive responses will also reduce the particular and severe form of aggression that constitutes child abuse. The empathy training exercises that have been utilized with children need to be adapted for adult and caretaker use. Adults have to be challenged and engaged by training procedures no less than children do. Sophisticated types of role taking and subtle forms of emotional sensitivity exercises, strategies used in the Empathy Child Training Program, will be required by the adult programs. In addition, transfer to the specific child abuse situation will be facilitated if the empathy exercises focus on the parent–child relationship and parent–child interactions.

The effort to apply empathy training procedures to adult groups requires systematic research evaluation. The findings from program evaluation have implications for application and for research. Evaluations of empathy training programs can contribute to our understanding of the empathy process itself; that is, applied research in this area can provide a context for basic research on empathy. The richness and relevance of this type of applied research is enhanced if the training procedures and training innovations are theoretically based. From my perspective, a productive route for future research on empathy is the development and evaluation of empathy training programs for adult clinical groups.

The data bearing on the factorial structure and construct validity of the Parent/Partner Empathy Scale reflect the interplay between theory and potential application. The Feshbach three-component model of empathy provided the basis for the initial construction of the scales, sets of items being included to assess discrimination and sensitivity to emotional cues, role taking and emotional expression as well as general empathy. The factor analysis and the correlates of the factors introduce some modification in the three-component structure in that, for this adult population discrimination of emotional cues or emotional sensitivity is integrated with perspective and role taking and, to a lesser extent, with emotional expression. In addition, although empathic responsiveness appears to be a general disposition in that partner empathy is related to empathy components that involve the child, there is also evidence of specificity so that the parent who is highly empathic with his or her child is not necessarily empathic with his or her partner. The abusive parent obtains low scores on all of the components of empathy, suggesting that the abusive parent has interpersonal difficulties or deficits that extend beyond the interaction with the child who is the object of abuse.

At the same time, the relative independence of the empathic distress component from the other empathy factors, the different pattern of correlates obtained for the distress factor, and the finding that the distress factor differentiated between the control and abusive parents but not between the control and clinic parents suggest that empathic distress may have a unique function in the management of child abuse. Abusive parents appear more indifferent to emotional pain in others than do the control or psychiatric parents. Further research is needed both to confirm this suggested relative indifference and to determine the underlying mechanism. It may be that these parents do not fully appreciate the pain their child is experiencing, or they are not responsive to the pain because they are angry at the child or feel that the infliction of physical pain is merited, or have learned to inhibit or block their empathic reaction to distress in others. Exploration of empathic distress in abusive parents is another research direction that merits pursuit.

The empathy training programs that have been suggested for abusive parents should also be provided for abused children if the cycle of abuser – abused – abuser is to be effectively interrupted. The review of the research literature, particularly the studies by George and Main (1979), Main and George (1985), and Howes and Espinosa (in press) indicate that children who have been physically abused have difficulties in role taking or related social interaction skills that mediate or are mediated by empathy. Although the experience of being abused may not inevitably result in diminished empathy – some children perhaps develop heightened empathy – the prevailing response for most physically abused children is likely to be a relative lack of empathy and difficulty in empathy related components. These children, in our judgment, could profit from the kinds of systematic, guided experiences in perspective and role taking, in affective discrimination, and in affective expression that an empathy training program provides.

We are not suggesting that empathy training is a panacea that will completely reduce child abuse and heal the effects of having been subjected to abuse. There may be abusive adults and children who have been abused for whom empathy is not a problem. In addition, much research is needed to extend empathy training programs to abusive adult populations and to enhance its effectiveness for the abused child. However, previous research suggests that empathy and its related components are responsive to psychoeducational training programs, and, given the problems that abuser and abused have in this important interpersonal dimension, empathy training, its development, variation, implementation, and evaluation should be a fruitful approach for researchers and practitioners working in the area of child abuse.

References

Andrews, D. A., Wormith, J. S., Daigle-Finn, W. J., Kennedy, D. J., and Nelson, S. (1980). Low and high functioning volunteers in group counseling with anxious and non-anxious prisoners: The effects of interpersonal skills on group process and attitude change. *Canadian Journal of Criminology* (22), 443–456.

Barahal, Robert M., Waterman, J., and Martin, H. P. (1981). The social cognitive development of abused children. *Journal of Consulting and Clinical Psychology, 49* (4), 508–516.

Batson, C. D., O'Quin, K., Fultz, J., Vanderplas, M., and Isen, A. M. (1983). Influence of self-reported distress and empathy on egoistic versus altruistic motivation to help. *Journal of Personality and Social Psychology, 45* (3), 706–718.

Berger, S. M. (1962). Conditioning through vicarious instigation? *Psychological Review, 69,* 450–456.

Borke, H. (1971). Interpersonal perception of young children: Egocentrism or empathy. *Developmental Psychology, 5* (2), 263–269.

Borke, H. (1973). The development of empathy in Chinese and American children between three and six years of age. *Developmental Psychology, 9,* 102–108.

Bryant, B. (1982). An index of empathy for children and adolescents. *Child Development, 53,* 413–425.

Chandler, M. J. (1973). Egocentrism and antisocial behavior: The assessment and training of social perspective-taking skills. *Developmental Psychology, 9* (3), 326–332.

Chandler, M., and Greenspan, S. (1972). Ersatz egocentrism: A reply to Borke. *Developmental Psychology, 7,* 104–106.

Chandler, M., Greenspan, S., and Barenboim, C. (1974). The assessment and training of role-taking and referential communication skills in institutionalized emotionally disturbed children. *Developmental Psychology, 10* (4), 546–553.

Chapin, F. S. (1942). Preliminary standardization of a social insight scale. *American Sociological Review, 7,* 214–225.

Davis, M. H. (1983). Measuring individual differences in empathy: Evidence for a multidimensional approach. *Journal of Personality and Social Psychology, 44,* 113–126.

de Mause, L. (Ed.) (1974). *The history of childhood.* New York: Psychohistory Press.

Deutsch, F., and Madle, R. (1975). Empathy: Historic and current conceptualizations, measurement, and a cognitive theoretical perspective. *Human Development, 18,* 267–287.

Dymond, R. F. (1949). A scale for the measurement of empathic ability. *Journal of Consulting Psychology, 13,* 127–133.

Evans, A. L. (1980). Personality characteristics and disciplinary attitudes of child-abusing mothers. *Child Abuse and Neglect, 4,* 179–187.

Eysenck, S. B. G., and Eysenck, H. J. (1978). Impulsiveness and venturesomeness: Their position in a dimensional system of personality description. *Psychological Reports, 43,* 1247–1255.

Eysenck, S. B. G., and McGurk, B. J. (1980). Impulsiveness and venturesomeness in detention center population. *Psychological Reports, 47,* 1299–1306.

Feshbach, N. D. (1973). Empathy: An interpersonal process. In W. Hartup, *Social understand-*

ing in children and adults: Perspectives on social cognition. Symposium presented at the meeting of the American Psychological Association, Montreal, August.

Feshbach, N. D. (1975). Empathy in children: Some theoretical and empirical considerations. *The Counseling Psychologist, 4* (2).

Feshbach, N. D. (1978). Studies of empathic behavior in children. In B. A. Maher (Ed.), *Progress in experimental personality research, 8.* New York: Academic Press.

Feshbach, N. D. (1979). Empathy training: A field study in affective education. In S. Feshbach and A. Fraczek (Eds.), *Aggression and behavior change: Biological and social processes* (pp. 234–249). New York: Praeger.

Feshbach, N. D. (1980). *The psychology of empathy and the empathy of psychology.* Presidential Address, 60th annual meeting of the Western Psychological Association, Honolulu, Hawaii, May.

Feshbach, N. D. (1982). Sex differences in empathy and social behavior in children. In N. Eisenberg (Ed.), *The development of prosocial behavior.* New York: Academic Press.

Feshbach, N. D. (1983). Learning to care: A positive approach to child training and discipline. *Journal of Clinical Child Psychology, 12* (3), 266–271.

Feshbach, N. D. (1984). Empathy, empathy training and the regulation of aggression in elementary school children. In R. M. Kaplan, V. J. Konecni, and R. Novoco (Eds.), *Aggression in children and youth* (pp. 192–208). The Hague, Netherlands: Martinus Nijhoff Publishers.

Feshbach, N. D., and Caskey, N. (1985). *A new scale for measuring parent empathy and partner empathy: Factorial structure, correlates and clinical discrimination.*

Feshbach, N., and Feshbach, S. (1969). The relationship between empathy and aggression in two age groups. *Developmental Psychology, 1,* 102–107.

Feshbach, N. D., and Feshbach, S. (1982). Empathy training and the regulation of aggression: Potentialities and limitations. *Academic Psychology Bulletin, 4,* 399–413.

Feshbach, S., and Feshbach, N. D. (1987). Aggression and altruism: A personality perspective. In C. Zahn-Waxler, M. Chapman, and M. Radke-Yarrow (Eds.), *Aggression and altruism: Biological and social origins.* New York: Cambridge University Press.

Feshbach, N. D., Feshbach, S., Fauvre, M., and Ballard-Campbell, M. (1983). *Learning to care: A curriculum for affective and social development.* Glenview, IL: Scott, Foresman & Company.

Feshbach, N. D., and Kuchenbecker, S. (1974, September). *A three-component model of empathy.* Symposium presented at the meeting of the American Psychological Association, New Orleans.

Feshbach, N. D., and Roe, K. (1968). Empathy in six and seven year olds. *Child Development, 39,* 133–145.

Flavell, J. H., Botkin, P. T., Fry, C. I., Wright, J. W., and Jarvis, P. E. (1964). *The development of role-taking and communication skills in children.* New York: Wiley.

Frodi, A. M., and Lamb, M. E. (1980). Child abusers' responses to infant smiles and cries. *Child Development, 51,* 238–241.

George, C., and Main, M. (1979). Social interactions of young abused children: Approach, avoidance and aggression. *Child Development, 50,* 306–318.

Greif, E. B., and Hogan, R. (1973). The theory and measurement of empathy. *Journal of Counseling Psychology, 20,* 280–284.

Hinchey, F. S., and Gavelek, J. R. (1982). Empathic responding in children of battered mothers. *Child Abuse and Neglect, 6,* 395–401.

Hoffman, M. L. (1975). Developmental synthesis of affect and cognition and its implications for altruistic motivation. *Developmental Psychology, 11,* 607–622.

Hoffman, M. L. (1977). Empathy, its development and prosocial implications. In C. B. Keasey (Ed.), *Nebraska symposium on motivation, 25.* Lincoln: University of Nebraska Press.

Hoffman, M. L. (1982). Development of prosocial motivation: Empathy and guilt. In N. Eisenberg (Ed.), *The development of prosocial behavior* (pp. 281–311). New York: Academic Press.

Hoffman, M. L., and Levine, L. E. (1976). Early sex indifferences in empathy. *Developmental Psychology, 6,* 557–558.

Hogan, R. (1969). Development of an empathy scale. *Journal of Consulting and Clinical Psychology, 33,* 307–316.

Howes, C., and Espinosa, M. P. (in press). The consequences of child abuse for the formation of relationships with peers. *International Journal of Child Abuse and Neglect.*

Howes, C., Feshbach, N. D., Gilly, J., and Espinosa, M. (1985). *Compliance and self control in young children from varying family context: Relationships with parent empathy, stress, and social support.* A paper presented at the American Psychological Association Meetings, Los Angeles, California.

Kempe, C. H., Silverman, F. N., Steele, B. B., Droegemueller, W., and Silver, H. K. (1962). The battered-child syndrome. *Journal of the American Medical Association, 181,* 17–24.

Kerr, W. A., and Speroff, B. J. (1954). Validation and evaluation of the empathy test. *The Journal of General Psychology, 50,* 269–276.

Kupfer, D. J., Drew, F. L., Curtis, E. K., and Rubinstein, D. N. (1978). Personality style and empathy in medical students. *Journal of Medical Education, 53,* 507–509.

Letourneau, C. (1981). Empathy and Stress: How they affect parental aggression. *Social Work, 26,* 383–389.

Main, M., and George, C. (1985). Responses of abused and disadvantaged toddlers to distress in agemates: A study in the day care setting, *Developmental Psychology, 21* (3), 407–412.

Mash, E. J., and Johnston, C., and Kovitch, K. (1983). A comparison of mother–child interaction of physically abused and non-abused children during play and task situations. *Journal of Clinical Psychology, 12* (3), 337–346.

McDougall, W. (1960). *An introduction to social psychology.* New York: Barnes & Noble. (Originally published, 1908.)

Mead, G. H. (1974). *Mind, self, and society.* Chicago: University of Chicago Press. (Originally published, 1934.)

Mehrabian, A., and Epstein, N. (1972). A measure of emotional empathy. *Journal of Personality, 40* (4), 525–543.

Milner, J. S., and Wimberley, R. C. (1980). Prediction and explanation of child abuse. *Journal of Clinical Psychology, 36,* 875–884.

Mood, D. W., Johnson, J. E., and Shantz, C. U. (1978). Social comprehension and affect-matching in young children. *Merrill-Palmer Quarterly, 24,* 63–66.

Radke-Yarrow, M., and Zahn-Waxler, C. (1982). Roots, motives and patterns in children's prosocial behavior. In J. Reykowski, J. Karylowski, D. Bar-Tel, and E. Staub (Eds.), *The development and maintenance of prosocial behaviors: National perspectives.* New York: Plenum.

Reid, J. B., Taplin, P. S., and Lorber, R. (1981). A social interactional approach to the treatment of abusive families. In R. B. Stuart (Ed.), *Violent behavior: Social learning approaches to prediction, management, and treatment* (pp. 83–101). New York: Brunner/Mazel.

Rogers, C. R., and Truax, C. B. (1967). The therapeutic conditions antecedent to change: A theoretical view. In C. R. Rogers (Ed.), *The therapeutic relationship and its impact: A study of psychotherapy with schizophrenics.* Madison: University of Wisconsin Press.

Rothenberg, B. B. (1970). Child's social sensitivity and the relationship to interpersonal competence, intrapersonal comfort and intellectual level. *Developmental Psychology, 2* (3), 335–350.

Shantz, C. U. (1975). The development of social cognition. In E. M. Hetherington (Ed.), *Review of child development research, 5.* Chicago: University of Chicago Press.

Spielberger, C. D., Gorsuch, R., and Luschene, R. E. (1968). *State-trait Anxiety Inventory.* Palo Alto, CA: Consulting Psychologists Press.

Spinetta, J. J. (1978). Parental personality factors in child abuse. *Journal of Consulting and Clinical Psychology, 46,* 1409–1414.

Starr, R. H., Jr. (1982). A research-based approach to the prediction of child abuse. In R. H. Starr, Jr. (Ed.), *Child abuse prediction: Policy implications.* Cambridge, MA: Ballinger.

Stotland, E. (1969). Exploratory investigations of empathy. In L. Berkowitz (Ed.), *Advances in experimental social psychology, 4.* New York: Academic Press.

Straker, G., and Jacobson, R. S. (1981). Aggression, emotional maladjustment, and empathy in the abused child. *Developmental Psychology, 17* (6), 762–765.

Sullivan, H. S. (1953). *The interpersonal theory of psychiatry.* New York: W. W. Norton.

Truax, C. B. (1961). A scale for the measurement of accurate empathy. *Psychiatric Institute Bulletin.* Wisconsin Psychiatric Institute, University of Wisconsin, *1*, 12.

Truax, C. B. (1967). A scale for the rating of accurate empathy. In C. R. Rogers (Ed.), *The therapeutic relationship and its impact: A study of psychotherapy with schizophrenics.* Madison: University of Wisconsin.

Truax, C. B. (1972). The meaning and reliability of accurate empathy ratings: A rejoinder. *Psychological Bulletin, 77* (6), 397–399.

Watson, M. (1977). *A developmental sequence of role playing.* Paper presented at the meeting of the American Psychological Association, San Francisco.

Wolfe, R. (1981). Origins of child abuse and neglect within the family. *Child Abuse and Neglect, 5*, 223–229.

Zahn-Waxler, C., Radke-Yarrow, M., and King, R. A. (1979). Child rearing and children's prosocial initiations toward victims of distress. *Child Development, 50*, 319–330.

Part III

The developmental consequences of child maltreatment

13 How research on child maltreatment has informed the study of child development: perspectives from developmental psychopathology

Dante Cicchetti

Introduction

Throughout the past decade, a growing number of investigators have focused their theoretical formulations and empirical research on the normal processes of ontogenesis in the social, emotional, social-cognitive, cognitive, and linguistic domains and on the relation between functioning in childhood and later developmental outcome (Lewis, Feiring, McGuffog, and Jaskir, 1984; Main, Kaplan, and Cassidy, 1985; Sroufe, 1979a, 1983). Much of this work has been guided by the organizational perspective on development (Cicchetti and Schneider-Rosen, 1984, 1986; Cicchetti and Sroufe, 1978; Sroufe, 1979b; Sroufe and Waters, 1976; Werner, 1948) and has been conducted in order to expand our knowledge of the normal developmental process. The study of children who are at high risk for developmental deviation and psychopathology can contribute greatly to our extant theories of normal development (Cicchetti, 1984; Werner, 1948). For example, the empirical investigation of populations where divergent patterns of socioemotional,

The writing of this chapter was supported in part by grants from the Foundation for Child Development Young Scholars Program, the John D. and Catherine T. MacArthur Foundation Network on Early Childhood, the National Center on Child Abuse and Neglect, the National Institute of Mental Health, the Smith Richardson Foundation, Inc., and the William T. Grant Foundation. I wish to thank the staff of the Harvard Child Maltreatment Project and the Mt. Hope Family Center for all of their hard work, dedication, and invaluable suggestions, most notably Drs. J. Lawrence Aber, Marjorie Beeghly, Vicki Carlson, Jan Gillespie, Laura McCloskey, Ross Rizley, Sheree Toth, and Joan Vondra and Joe Allen, Douglas Barnett, Judy Bigelow, Karen Braunwald, Ann Churchill, Wendy Coster, Michelle Gersten, Kevin Hennessy, Joan Kaufman, Amber Keshishian, Carol Kottmeier, Jody Todd Manly, Kristi King, Michael Lynch, Diana Meisberger, Kurt Olsen, Gerald Rabideau, Carolyn Rieder, Karen Schneider-Rosen, Susan Shonk, Kathryn Staggs, Mimi Wetzel, and Jennifer White. I would like to extend my appreciation to Sheree Toth and to Jennifer White for the helpful feedback that they have given to me on this manuscript. Finally, I would like to acknowledge my grandmother, Josephine Butch, and my friend, Heidi Mitke, for their encouragement, help, and support over the years.

cognitive, linguistic, and social-cognitive development may be expected as a consequence of the pervasive and enduring influences that characterize the transaction between the child and the environment, such as is the case with maltreated children and their families, provides the appropriate basis for affirming and challenging current developmental theories. Additionally, the study of the developmental organization of high risk children simultaneously allows for the formulation of a more integrative theory of development that can account for the nature of the interrelations among the social, emotional, linguistic, and cognitive/social-cognitive domains (Cicchetti and Schneider-Rosen, 1984; Hesse and Cicchetti, 1982).

Developmental psychopathology

Although it has been only during the past two decades that developmental psychopathology has crystallized as a new interdisciplinary science with its own integrity, it nonetheless has historical roots within a variety of areas and disciplines (Cicchetti, 1984, in press; Kaplan, 1966, 1983; Rutter and Garmezy, 1983).

The field of developmental psychopathology has been built upon the assumption that a developmental approach could be applied to any unit of behavior or discipline and to all cultures or populations, normal or otherwise (Werner, 1948). Working within diverse disciplines, including embryology, the neurosciences, and clinical and experimental psychology and psychiatry, researchers have utilized atypical, pathological, high risk and psychopathological populations to elucidate, expand, and affirm further the basic underlying principles of their developmental theories (A. Freud, 1965; S. Freud, 1955a, 1955b; Goldstein, 1939, 1940; Inhelder, 1943/1968; Jackson, 1958; Kaplan, 1966; Twitchell, 1951, 1970; Waddington, 1957, 1966; Weiss, 1969b; Werner, 1948).

Developmental psychopathology emphasizes the argument put forth by many of the great synthetic thinkers in the behavioral and neurosciences that we can learn more about the normal functioning of an organism by studying its pathology and, likewise, more about its pathology by studying its normal condition (Cicchetti, 1984). By virtue of its interdisciplinary nature, the field of developmental psychopathology requires that multiple domains of development be studied, including cognitive, socioemotional, linguistic, and biological processes (Achenbach, in press; Cicchetti, 1984, in press; Rutter and Garmezy, 1983).

The organizational perspective on development

The organizational approach to development is based upon a set of regulative principles that can guide research into and theorizing concerning human behavior (Santostefano and Baker, 1972; Sroufe and Rutter, 1984).

According to the organizational perspective, development may be conceived as a series of qualitative reorganizations among and within behavioral systems, which occur through the processes of differentiation and hierarchical integration. Variables at many levels of analysis determine the character of these reorganizations: genetic, constitutional, neurobiological, biochemical, behavioral, psychological, environmental, and sociological. Furthermore, these variables are viewed as being in dynamic transaction with one another.

The qualitative reorganizations characteristic of development are conceived as proceeding in accordance with the orthogenetic principle (Werner, 1948), which states that the developing organism moves from a relatively diffuse and globally undifferentiated state, by means of differentiation and hierarchical integration, to a state of greater articulation and organized complexity. The orthogenetic principle may be seen as a solution to the problem of the individual's continuous adaptation to the environment and to the question of how integrity of functioning may be maintained via hierarchical integration despite rapid constitutional changes and biobehavioral shifts (Block and Block, 1980; Emde, Gaensbauer, and Harmon, 1976; Sackett, Sameroff, Cairns, and Suomi, 1981; Sroufe, 1979b).

The organizational approach to normal development views it in terms of a series of interlocking social, emotional, cognitive, and social-cognitive competencies (Cicchetti and Schneider-Rosen, 1984). When competence occurs at one level, it allows environmental adaptation and prepares the way for future competence (Sroufe and Rutter, 1984). Normal development is marked by the integration of earlier competencies into later modes of functioning. It follows, then, that early adaptation tends to promote later adaptation and integration.

In contrast, pathological development is perceived as a lack of integration of the social, emotional, cognitive, and social-cognitive competencies that underlie adaptation at a particular developmental level (Cicchetti and Schneider-Rosen, 1984, 1986; Kaplan, 1966; Sroufe, 1979a). Because early structures often are incorporated into later structures, an early disturbance in functioning may ultimately cause much larger disturbances to appear later on.

Goals of this chapter

The organizational developmental psychopathology perspective, with its emphasis on the study of developing systems and on uncovering the relation between normal and deviant forms of ontogenesis, provides an excellent theoretical framework for conducting research with maltreated children and their families. We believe that the study of maltreated children can make many significant contributions to the understanding of normal developmental processes. When there are prominent and pervasive disturbances in the parent–child–environment transaction, such as is the case with child mal-treatment, the child is at a greater risk for suffering the negative conse-quences of the "continuum of caretaking casualty" (Sameroff and Chandler, 1975). Given the negative impact that poor quality parent–child relation-ships can exert on the development of children from "normal" families (Ainsworth, Blehar, Waters, and Wall, 1978; Main, Kaplan, and Cassidy, 1985; Sroufe, 1979a, 1983), it is not surprising that maltreated children manifest disturbances in the resolution of stage-salient developmental issues (Cicchetti and Olsen, in press, b) and in the organization of their ontogenetic systems (Aber and Allen, 1987; Aber and Cicchetti, 1984; Schneider-Rosen and Cicchetti, 1984). In this chapter, we illustrate how the study of the causes, intergenerational transmission, and consequences of child abuse and neglect can enhance our knowledge about several important theoretical issues in normal developmental theory. Conversely, we demonstrate how a developmental approach to the investigation of maltreated children and their families can elucidate our understanding of the maltreatment process. A developmental scheme is necessary for tracing the roots, etiology, and nature of maladaptation so that treatment interventions may be appropri-ately timed and guided. Moreover, a developmental perspective will prove useful for uncovering the nature and etiology of the maladaptation, the development of compensatory mechanisms in the face of deficiencies, and the interrelations between maladaptation and abuse and neglect.

The transactional model

Prior to the 1970s, the majority of the existing developmental models were "linear/main effects" in nature (Reese and Overton, 1970). According to the main-effects model, developmental outcomes are the direct and inevitable result of some specific early pathogenic experience or process or of an inher-ent biochemical/biological dysfunction. In parallel, most of the early etio-logical models of child abuse and neglect were also main effects conceptual-izations. The most prevalent example is the psychiatric model (Parke and Collmer, 1975), which holds that parental personality characteristics, devel-oped in response to their childhood upbringing, inevitably bring about abu-sive incidents. Other examples of equally simplistic causal models are the assertion that factors associated with low-socioeconomic status, such as poverty, social isolation, and stress, are necessary and sufficient to produce child abuse (Belsky, 1980; Cicchetti, Taraldson, and Egeland, 1978; Parke and Collmer, 1975). Although interactional models of development and of child abuse evolved in response to the glaring deficiencies of main effects theorizing (e.g., the belief that *both* parental personality characteristics and stress interact to cause child abuse), in the mid-seventies, Arnold Sameroff and Michael Chandler described a revolutionary new framework for the study of development – the transactional model (Sameroff and Chandler, 1975).

Sameroff and Chandler proposed a psychobiological model of development that was transactional in that it took into account the interrelations among dynamic systems and the processes characterizing system breakdown. Moreover, they explained the mechanisms by which compensatory, self-righting tendencies (Waddington, 1966) were initiated whenever higher level monitors detected deviations in a subsystem. Thus, a transactional model viewed the multiple transactions among environmental forces, caregiver characteristics, and child characteristics as dynamic, reciprocal contributions to the events and outcomes of child development. Sameroff and Chandler decried the efficacy of simple, linear "cause–effect" models of etiology and suggested that it was impossible to understand a child's development by focusing on single pathogenic events. Rather, Sameroff and Chandler argued that it was necessary to analyze the ways in which the environment responded to a particular child's characteristics at a particular point in time.

The transactional model presents the environment and the child as exerting a dynamic mutual influence on each other. Thus, if a child demonstrates deviant development across time it is assumed that the child has been involved in a *continuous* maladaptive process. The continued manifestation of maladaptation depends on environmental support, whereas the child's characteristics, reciprocally, determine the nature of the environment.

Sameroff and Chandler's proposal that investigators consider a child's position on both the "continuum of reproductive casualty" and the "continuum of caretaking casualty" has obvious applications to the study of the causes, intergenerational transmission, and developmental sequelae of child maltreatment. The transactional developmental perspective makes it plausible to view maltreatment phenomena as expressive of an underlying dysfunction in the parent–child–environment system, rather than solely as the result of aberrant parental personality traits, environmental stress, or deviant child characteristics.

The application of a transactional model of development to child maltreatment requires that one consider the specific risk factors associated with its occurrence. Child maltreatment is a heterogeneous problem. In mode of maltreatment, etiology, and sequelae, there are subtle and complex differences of type and severity. The influx of developmental theorizing into the field of child maltreatment has resulted in the formation of appropriately complex etiological models and a rich framework for conceptualizing the effects that maltreatment has upon adaptive and maladaptive ontogenetic processes.

Focusing on the concept of "risk factors," Cicchetti and Rizley (1981) extended Sameroff and Chandler's (1975) transactional model to examine

Table 13.1. *Risk factors for child maltreatment: impact on probability of maltreatment*

Temporal dimension	Potentiating factors	Compensatory factors
Enduring Factors	Vulnerability factors: enduring factors or conditions which increase risk.	Protective factors: enduring conditions or attributes which decrease risk.
Transient Factors	Challengers: transient but significant stresses.	Buffers: transient conditions which act as buffers against transient increases in stress or challenge.

Source: Cicchetti and Rizley, 1981.

the etiology and intergenerational transmission of child maltreatment (see Table 13.1). Cicchetti and Rizley (1981) classify risk factors into two broad categories: *potentiating factors,* which increase the probability of maltreatment, and *compensatory factors,* which decrease the risk of maltreatment. Under each category, two subgroupings are distinguished: *transient,* fluctuating, "state" factors and more permanent, *enduring* conditions or attributes.

Enduring vulnerability factors include all relatively long-term factors, conditions or attributes that serve to potentiate maltreatment. These may be biological (e.g., physical or behavioral anomalies that make childrearing unrewarding or difficult), historical (e.g., a parent with a history of being maltreated), psychological (e.g., parental or child psychopathology, personality attributes such as poor frustration tolerance, or high trait levels of aggression and anger), and/or ecological (e.g., high stress levels, inadequate social networks or chaotic neighborhoods, and maltreatment-promoting societal values; see Belsky, 1980).

Transient challengers include the short-term conditions and stresses that confront families and that may cause a predisposed parent to maltreat his or her child (e.g., physical injury or illness, legal difficulties, marital or family problems, discipline problems with children, the emergence of a child into a new and more difficult developmental period).

Long-term protective factors comprise those relatively enduring or permanent conditions or attributes that decrease the risk of maltreatment or its transmission across generations (e.g., a parent's history of good parenting and a secure quality of intimate relationships between the parent figures).

Transient buffers include factors that may protect a family from stress, thereby reducing the probability of maltreatment and its transmission (e.g., sudden improvement in financial conditions, periods of marital harmony, a child's transition out of a difficult developmental period).

Cicchetti and Rizley (1981) argue that it is necessary to examine both positive and negative risk factors in order to understand the occurrence of maltreatment and the specific forms it will take. According to the transactional model, maltreatment is expressed only when potentiating factors override compensatory ones. It is then that an act of abuse is committed or a maltreatment condition is allowed to begin. Furthermore, Cicchetti and Rizley (1981) contend that the intergenerational transmission of maltreatment can best be understood by examining the transmission of risk factors. Cross-generational transmission must operate by either increasing vulnerability or by decreasing protective factors.

Schneider-Rosen, Braunwald, Carlson, and Cicchetti (1985) have extended Cicchetti and Rizley's model to account for the processes leading to the formation and current state of the mother–child attachment relationship. Schneider-Rosen et al.'s model, which can be applied more broadly to the study of any maltreatment sequelae, highlights an ongoing transaction between a variety of factors that may serve to support or to inhibit competent behavior at any point in time. Following Cicchetti and Rizley (1981), within this model there are two broad categories that influence a competent developmental outcome: (1) *potentiating factors,* which increase the probability of manifesting incompetence, and (2) *compensatory factors,* which increase the likelihood of manifesting competent behavior. Potentiating factors include the enduring influence of vulnerability factors (longstanding psychological, environmental, sociocultural, or biological factors that may inhibit competence) and the transient influence of challengers such as stressful life events. Similarly, compensatory factors include enduring protective factors and transient buffers.

The Schneider-Rosen et al. (1985) elaboration of the Cicchetti and Rizley model provides a way of conceptualizing developmental outcome not only in a population of children from maltreating families but in all populations of children from normal or high-risk families. It is assumed that the current quality of adaptation represents neither enduring nor transient factors alone, but a variety of factors that must be considered in combination with one another in order to account for a specific developmental outcome. It then becomes possible to explain the finding that not all maltreated children manifest developmental failure or maladaptation. Rather than assuming that this is impossible, the transactional model illustrates the multiplicity of influences on the child's quality of adaptation and allows for the identification of factors (e.g., severity and duration of maltreatment, when maltreatment occurred, the quality of a family's social networks, life stress –

both perceived and actual) that support or inhibit the successful resolution of stage-salient development tasks and promote or undermine the adaptive developmental process.

Increasingly, as many of the chapters in this volume epitomize, researchers investigating maltreatment phenomena are being guided by the transactional model. In keeping with one of the basic tenets of developmental psychopathology, through the application of an influential model of normal development, we have seen how the developmental perspective can inform the study of high-risk populations. Likewise, extending this transactional etiological model of normal and pathological development to the study of the sequelae of maltreatment, we have illustrated how the study of maltreatment can enhance our knowledge of normal developmental processes.

Additionally, Cicchetti and Toth (1987) have shown how the transactional risk model could be applied successfully to intervening with multirisk maltreating families. Because the parent–child–environment system is viewed as exerting reciprocal influence among all components, attempts to intervene in a maladaptive process by focusing on one component of dysfunction in a multirisk family are likely to result in frustration and failure. Cicchetti and Toth show how the transactional approach guides the intervention philosophy of Mt. Hope Family Center, a mandated center for the prevention and treatment of child abuse in Rochester, New York. The goal of the program is to intervene in order to reduce the magnitude of family risk factors while increasing protective factors and buffers. Moreover, Cicchetti, Toth, Bush, and Gillespie (1988) have illustrated that it is possible to utilize developmentally derived research in order to address the intervention needs of maltreated children and their families. For example, as we will describe in a later section, there are disturbances in internal-state (or emotion) language usage in maltreated children (Cicchetti and Beeghly, 1987). Therapies enhancing recognition of, and verbalization about, personal emotions should help such children develop better impulse control and self regulation (Cicchetti et al., 1988), especially when carried out in conjunction with work done with the caregiver that sets the stage for the acceptance of such open expression of feelings (Cicchetti, Toth, and Bush, in press).

The effects of maltreatment on the negotiation of stage-salient issues: implications for developmental theory

Influenced by the appearance of these more sophisticated developmental models, research on the developmental sequelae of child maltreatment has improved significantly during the past decade. Child maltreatment, as a true "experiment in nature" (Bronfenbrenner, 1979), presents an excellent opportunity to answer important questions in developmental theory that, on ethical grounds alone, would be impossible to manipulate experimentally. We proceed by first assessing the impact that maltreatment experiences have on the child's ability to resolve successfully the stage-salient issues of early development.

Agreement has coalesced regarding the presence of a series of stage-salient issues that are characteristic of child development (Erikson, 1950; Sroufe, 1979a). Rather than construe the ontogenetic process as a series of unfolding tasks that need to be accomplished and then decrease in importance, we perceive development as consisting of a number of important age and stage-appropriate tasks which, upon emergence, remain critical to the child's continual adaptation, although decreasing somewhat in salience relative to other newly emerging tasks (see Table 13.2). For example, we do not perceive of attachment as a developmental issue of the first year of life alone; rather, once an attachment relationship develops, it continues to undergo transformations and reintegrations with subsequent accomplishments such as emerging autonomy and entrance into the peer world. As a result, children are continually renegotiating the balance between being connected to others and being independent and autonomous (see, e.g., Aber and Allen, 1987; Aber, Allen, Carlson, and Cicchetti, this volume). Consequently, each issue represents a life-span developmental task that requires ongoing coordination and integration in the individual's adaptation to the environment. Furthermore, there are corresponding roles for caregivers that increase the probability that their children will successfully resolve each stage-salient issue (Sroufe, 1979a).

The investigation of maltreated children's abilities to negotiate these issues provides an interesting opportunity to test the underlying assumptions of how competent resolution of these tasks is fostered. Because more elaborate presentations have been presented in several chapters throughout this volume, we will keep our treatment focused on the contributions that studies of these issues can make to the formulation of an integrative developmental theory.

The development of a secure attachment

The development of a secure attachment relationship with the primary caregiver is considered to be the stage-salient developmental issue between the ages of 6 and 12 months (Sroufe, 1979a; Sroufe and Rutter, 1984; Waters and Sroufe, 1983). It is marked by increased attention and attunement to interpersonal interactions (Stern, 1985). Although the capacity for attachment originates in earlier stages, overt manifestations of this issue reach ascendancy in the latter half of the first year of life. Dyadic interactions, marked by relatedness and synchrony, resiliency to stress, and appropriate affective interchange, are associated with successful adaptation during this

Table 13.2. *Stage-salient issues for conceptualizing the ontogenesis of competence*

Stage-salient developmental issue	Approximate age			
	0–12 months	12–30 months	30 months–7 years	7–12 years
Attachment	Modulation of arousal Physiological regulation Formation of secure attachment relationship with primary caregiver Differentiation and integration of emotional reactions			
Autonomy and self-development		Differentiation of persons Awareness of self as distinct entity Exploration of environment Regulation and control of emotional reactions Problem solving, pride and mastery motivation Capacity to delay gratification and to tolerate frustration Awareness of standards Development of language and communicative skills		

Establishing peer relationships

Hierarchical integration of attachment, autonomy, and peer relationships

- Development of sense of efficacy and pride
- Awareness of social roles
- Ego-resiliency and ego control
- Sex role development
- Integration into peer groups and social support networks
- Development of emotional bonds with peers
- Role taking
- Empathy and prosocial behavior
- Capacity to take initiative
- Self-regulation
- Development of criteria for evaluating one's performance
- Hierarchization of plans

- Hierarchization of social networks and multiple attachment figures
- Formation of feelings of volition and agency of the self
- Awareness of and ability to express multiple emotions
- Internalization of standards of right and wrong and development of morality
- Capacity to assume responsibilities and to accomplish tasks
- Awareness of internal psychological processes

Source: Cicchetti and Schneider-Rosen, 1986.

stage (Sroufe, 1979a). Inadequate response-contingent stimulation from the caregiver is likely to exert a negative impact on the infant's ability to master the tasks of this stage. In the absence of regular contingent responsivity, neither infant nor caregiver develop feelings of efficacy and the development of a secure attachment relationship may be impeded (Ainsworth et al., 1978).

The study of attachment relationships in high-risk and psychopathological populations is necessary for the same reasons that cross-cultural research on attachment is necessary. Both kinds of studies can tell us what developmental sequences are logically necessary and what alternate pathways of development are possible, as well as provide evidence on which factors accounting for relationship formation, maintenance, and dissolution are most important (e.g., sociocultural, cognitive, sociocognitive, socioemotional).

Several investigators have documented that maltreated infants and toddlers are significantly more likely to form insecure attachment relationships with their primary caregivers than are infants drawn from well-matched, lower-socioeconomic status comparison groups (Carlson, Cicchetti, Barnett, and Braunwald, this volume; Crittenden, 1988; Crittenden and Ainsworth, this volume; Egeland and Sroufe, 1981; Schneider-Rosen et al., 1985). Estimates of insecurity range from approximately 70 percent to 100 percent across studies. Moreover, over time, there is a striking tendency for these attachments to become avoidant in quality (see Egeland and Sroufe, 1981; Schneider-Rosen et al., 1985). Because there are many enduring, problematic characteristics of the home environments where maltreatment has occurred, such as emotional or physical rejection, aggression or hostile management, threatening affective or verbal assaults, or lack of or inappropriate responsivity (Crittenden, 1981; Crittenden and Ainsworth, this volume), it is hardly surprising to find such a high degree of pathological relationships between maltreated youngsters and their caregivers.

Given the unpredictable, chaotic environments often characteristic of maltreating families (Egeland, Breitenbucher, and Rosenberg, 1980; Garbarino and Gilliam, 1980; Gil, 1970; Pelton, 1978) and the strong likelihood that the parents in these families had insecure attachment relationships with their own parents (DeLozier, 1982; Main and Goldwyn, 1984), it is not surprising that Carlson and her colleagues (this volume) found that nearly 80 percent of a sample of 12-month-old infants from maltreating families manifested Type D (disorganized/disoriented) attachment relations (cf. Main et al., 1985; Main and Solomon, 1986).

These studies on attachment and maltreatment, akin to the early nonhuman primate studies of Harlow and his colleagues (see Ruppenthal, Arling, Harlow, Sackett, and Suomi, 1976, for a review; see also Reite and Caine, 1983), demonstrate that maltreated human youngsters do form attachments to their caregivers despite receiving inadequate care. As predicted by the Bowlby–Ainsworth theory, we saw that the quality of these relationships was poor.

In addition to being a possible sequelae of child maltreatment, attachment dysfunction may be a prime etiological factor for the occurrence of maltreatment as well as for its continuation across generations. Bowlby (1980), Bretherton (1985, 1987), and Sroufe (1988) have all underscored that "internal working models" of relationships can change. With the advent of formal operational thought, it is possible for adults to re-represent their relationship experiences into a more secure, hierarchically integrated model of attachment relationships. Main and Goldwyn (1984) have shown how adults who were maltreated as children may distort their early experiences and describe their caregivers in an exaggeratedly positive fashion – a form of defensive idealization. When viewed alongside Hunter and Kihlstrom's (1979) findings that adults who broke the cycle of maltreatment, despite their own history of abuse, were characterized by having open and angry recollections about their early childhood, one can readily see how continuing anomalies of attachment could play an influential role in the intergenerational transmission of child maltreatment. As Kaufman and Zigler (this volume) have noted, not all abused children become abusive parents (see also Cicchetti and Aber, 1980). The reworking of existing poor quality internal representational models of attachment relationships, alone and/or in therapy (see Cicchetti, Toth, and Bush, in press), seems like an effective prescription for preventing the occurrence, recurrence (within a family), and intergenerational transmission of child abuse and neglect.

Even though child maltreatment is not listed as a diagnostic entity in the *Diagnostic and Statistical Manual III – Revised* (American Psychiatric Association, 1987), we think that maltreatment should be conceived as a "relational psychopathology" – that is, the result of a dysfunction in the parent–child–environment transactional system. Historically, a number of infant classification schemes have focused on such relational pathologies. For example, Spitz's (Spitz and Wolf, 1946; Spitz, 1965) classic research on hospitalism and anaclitic depression, Bowlby's (1951) work on the effects of maternal deprivation (see also Rutter, 1972/1981), and Provence and Lipton's (1962) studies on the effects of institutionalization upon infant development provide exemplars of how dysfunctions within the caretaker–child–environment system may result in disturbances in infant functioning. We believe that, other than the pervasive developmental disorders and the organic forms of mental retardation, the vast majority of the disorders of the early years of life can best be characterized as transactional "relational pathologies" and not as disorders arising solely "within the child" (cf. Cicchetti and Braunwald, 1984; Greenspan and Porges, 1984; Sroufe and Fleeson, 1986).

Development of an autonomous self

Following the consolidation of the attachment relationship during the second year of life, the emergence of autonomous functioning reflects the increasing differentiation between self and others (Lewis and Brooks-Gunn, 1979). The development of an autonomous self is considered to be one of the stage-salient issues between the ages of 18 and 36 months (Lewis and Brooks-Gunn, 1979; Sroufe, 1979b). The gradual process of differentiation between self and others is thought to be influenced by the infant's relationship with the caregiver and to be affected by social experience (Lewis and Brooks-Gunn, 1979; Mahler, Pine, and Bergman, 1975; Mead, 1934). An emerging awareness of one's capabilities, goals, activities, feelings, and actions is believed to be facilitated by the security of this early relationship (Sroufe, 1988). The evolution of this ability enables the toddler to understand environmental occurrences more fully. Moreover, a well-differentiated sense of self provides the toddler greater comprehension of personal functioning as a separate and independent entity. Caretaker sensitivity and ability to tolerate the toddler's strivings for autonomy, as well as the capacity to set age-appropriate limits, are integral to the successful resolution of this issue.

The examination of the impact of early maltreatment on subsequent adaptation necessitates the consideration of the specific developmental systems that may be most at risk for developmental deviations or delays at particular ages (cf. Cicchetti and Rizley, 1981). Consequently, it is crucial that we investigate the impact of specific social experiences on toddlers' developing self-knowledge.

One such relationship of major theoretical significance is that between the quality of mother–child attachment and the emergence of visual self-recognition (Lewis and Brooks-Gunn, 1979). Specifically, the security of the attachment relationship promotes a movement toward other objects and people and a developing sense of effectance and mastery of the social and nonsocial environments (Sroufe 1979b, 1988). Those youngsters who have developed a secure attachment to their caregivers will have a greater likelihood of exploring their environment with confidence and trust in the caregiver's accessibility (Ainsworth et al., 1978; Lamb, 1982). Their exploration of new objects and persons in the environment and their affective growth will promote the emergence of the skills that underlie the capacity for visual self-recognition. Therefore, securely attached toddlers should evidence this capacity earlier than insecurely attached youngsters.

In an examination of a sample of maltreated and matched lower-socioeconomic status comparison toddlers, Schneider-Rosen and Cicchetti (1984) demonstrated the importance of the quality of the early attachment relationship for explaining individual differences in the development of the capacity for visual self-recognition. Forty-one percent of the sample of 19-month-old youngsters displayed visual self-recognition as assessed by the standard mirror-and-rouge paradigm (Lewis and Brooks-Gunn, 1979). In this procedure, infants observe their reflections in a mirror for a brief period of time in the presence of their mothers and an experimenter. After this short inspection, the experimenter surreptitiously wipes a dot of rouge on the infant's nose. The presence of visual self-recognition is inferred from the infant touching his/her nose while simultaneously watching him/herself in the mirror. When data for the entire sample of infants was analyzed, it was found that those infants who recognized themselves were significantly more likely to be securely attached to their mothers. However, a separate analysis of the maltreated and comparison groups of infants revealed a different pattern of results. Ninety percent of the comparison infants who recognized themselves were securely attached to their caregivers. In contrast, for those maltreated infants who recognized themselves, there was no significant relationship between this capacity and qualitative differences in the security of attachment.

In another study on the development of self differentiation in maltreated toddlers, Egeland and Sroufe (1981) employed a tool-use/problem-solving paradigm to assess 24-month-old toddlers' emerging autonomy, independent exploration of the environment, and ability to cope with frustration. These investigators found that physically abused maltreated children were more angry, frustrated with the mother, noncompliant, and less enthusiastic than controls. Furthermore, they exhibited a higher frequency of positive affect. In contrast, the neglected maltreated children expressed less positive and more negative affect and obtained higher noncompliance, frustration, and anger scores than the controls.

Longitudinal research will also help to determine the developmental consequences of individual differences in the capacity for visual self-recognition, self-regulation, and other early aspects of self-development. Whether the relationship between security of attachment and visual self-recognition will influence the development, quality, or stability of emerging self-cognitions is an empirical question that warrants future investigation. Will those toddlers who demonstrate an earlier emergence of visual self-recognition develop a more stable and secure concept of the self? Will those toddlers with better self-regulatory skills be less likely to manifest problems in peer relationships? Will the quality of one's early self-cognitions affect later adaptation and adjustment? Future research should address these and related questions and be directed toward clarifying the effect of individual differences in the emergence of aspects of early self-system processes (cf. Harter, 1983) on the subsequent development of self-knowledge and on later adaptation.

These early deviations in the "self-system" of maltreated youngsters vividly illustrate the deleterious impact that a maltreating environment can have upon the separation–individuation process and demonstrate the importance of the "vicissitudes of parenting" (cf. Mahler et al., 1975) for promoting the successful fulfillment of this issue. Difficulties with separation–individuation may be a risk factor for later maladaptation in these children. In particular, maltreated children are in grave danger of being "parentified" and, as a result, becoming enmeshed with their parents. One outcome of such an enmeshment might be the development of a "caretaker" relationship with the mother (cf. Main et al., 1985). By becoming caretakers, maltreated children may come to expect their future offspring to treat them similarly. Consequently, maltreated children may themselves transmit maltreatment across generations. Another possible outcome is that these maltreated children may grow up to choose mates who do not take care of them. Even if these children do not become adult perpetrators of maltreatment, they may become victimized in their adult relationships (Sroufe and Fleeson, 1986). Moreover, many of these adults will undoubtedly form relationships that endanger the safety of their children – either through having the children observe interspousal violence (Rosenberg, 1987) or through forming a relationship with a partner who may physically and/or sexually abuse one or more of the children (Daly and Wilson, 1981).

Although, at present, caretaker type of attachments cannot be assessed prior to the early years of life (Cassidy and Marvin, in collaboration with the MacArthur Foundation Working Group on Attachment, 1987; Main et al., 1985), they are associated with the disorganized/disoriented Type D attachments. Thus, it may be noteworthy that Carlson et al. (this volume) reported such a high base-rate of these "disorganized" attachment relationships in maltreated infants. Conceivably, these infants may be highly likely to become victims and/or victimizers in their future relationships.

Empathetic and prosocial acts also begin to emerge during toddlerhood, again a manifestation of the realization that the self can have an impact on others (Zahn-Waxler and Radke-Yarrow, 1982). Main and George (1985) examined previously collected behavioral protocols for instances of peer upsets when in close proximity to the physically abused and nonabused youngsters in their sample. They made ratings of the focus of toddlers' responses to these upsets and found that the physically abused toddlers were significantly more likely to respond negatively or aggressively to their peers' naturally occurring distress than were comparison youngsters. In contrast to the nonabused children, who were likely to respond to peer distress with simple interest, concerned empathy, or sadness, the physically abused children demonstrated a clear lack of empathetic concern for their peers in distress. Hoffman-Plotkin and Twentyman (1984) observed 14 abused, 14 neglected, and 14 matched comparison preschool children. From codings of behavioral observations during free play, they found that neglected children interacted less with peers and were less prosocial to them. Abused children, though they interacted with other children at the same rate as the nonabused children, were more aggressive (i.e., antisocial) with peers. The preponderance of aggression toward peers by physically abused youngsters has been well-documented in the literature (Mueller and Silverman, this volume). It appears that maltreated children show early deviations in the development of prosocial behavior. Given the reported linkages, both retrospective and prospective, between child maltreatment and later delinquency (Lewis, Mallouh, and Webb, this volume; Rutter and Giller, 1983; Wilson and Herrnstein, 1985), the paucity of empathic acts and the preponderance of aggressive incidents in physically abused youngsters may suggest a possible etiological pathway from maltreatment to delinquency.

Symbolic representation and further self–other differentiation

Between 24 and 36 months, toddlers develop the ability to construct even more differentiated mental representations of animate and inanimate objects (Greenspan and Porges, 1984). Investigations in the areas of play, language, and cognition have burgeoned in recent years (Bretherton, 1984; Rubin, Fein, and Vandenberg, 1983). In addition, the use of language and play to represent early conceptions of self and other is an age appropriate manifestation of children's growing awareness of self and other. As Slade (1987) has pointed out, the Genevan school (Piaget, 1962; Sinclair, 1970) has exerted a powerful influence upon this resurgent interest in symbolic activity. For example, Piaget (1962) contended that symbolic competencies such as the acquisition of language or the unfolding of pretend play proceed according to the exact rules that govern other domains of development, most notably cognition. Thus, for example, Piaget stated that linguistic acquisition could be comprehended only by paying *particular* attention to what was known about cognitive development, though he did also note that advances in our understanding of symbolization could be aided by examining our parallel knowledge of social and affective growth (Cicchetti and Hesse, 1983; Hesse and Cicchetti, 1982; Piaget, 1981; Sinclair, 1970). Because Piaget imputed more causal power to the cognitive/maturational aspects of symbolization, he paid very little attention to socioemotional or environmental influences upon symbol formation. Moreover, he was not as concerned about individual differences in functioning across symbolic domains or across contexts.

In contrast to the Genevan viewpoint, the organismic-developmental theorists Werner and Kaplan (1963) stated that symbolization emerged within the context of the mother–child relationship, or what Werner and Kaplan (1963) referred to as the "interpersonal matrix." Guided by the orthogenetic principle (Werner, 1957), Werner and Kaplan (1963) theorized that with the child's development, the "primordial sharing experience" between the mother, child (self), and object of reference proceeded from a state of relative undifferentiation and globality, to one characterized by increasing differentiation and hierarchic integration. Furthermore, Werner and Kaplan (1963) claimed that the motivation to engage in symbolic activity emanated from the desire to share experiences with the other social partner.

More recently, Bruner (1975) has argued along similar lines, stating that, through dyadic interactions with the caregiver, the child develops linguistic knowledge. The dual processes of joint action and joint reference between child and mother are thus viewed as critical for the acquisition of language because they help provide cognitive structure for the child (see also Vygotsky, 1978).

Another way in which the mother can contribute to the ontogenesis of the child's growing symbolic capacities is through her supportive presence (Matas, Arend, and Sroufe, 1978) or emotional availability (Egeland and Sroufe, 1981; Sorce and Emde, 1981). Through her sensitive responsiveness, the mother provides the child with a sense of security that fosters exploration of the inanimate and animate object worlds (cf. Slade, 1987). The child's ability to explore while using the mother as a "secure base" enhances the child's autonomy (i.e., self–other differentiation) and the growth of representational thought. For example, Stern (1985) has described how the caregiver's attunement or emotional intensity calibration with the child plays a crucial role in the unfolding and differentiation of the self system. Moreover, from different theoretical perspectives, Ainsworth (1973) and Mahler (Mahler et al., 1975) both have theorized that infants and toddlers who can be confident in their mother's availability will feel free to explore the world and to devote themselves more fully and enthusiastically to interacting with others. As a consequence, these children are expected to have a more highly differentiated sense of self.

To date no studies have been published on other aspects of symbolic representation in maltreated children, though several longitudinal studies on the relation among play, attachment, and language are ongoing in our laboratory. Investigations of the further differentiation of the self system in maltreated children have been conducted by researchers interested in internal state language.

The ability to share information about intentions, cognitions, and feelings is crucial for the regulation of human interaction. Although infants produce and comprehend nonverbal emotional signals by the end of the first year, it is only after mastering verbal internal state labels that young children can communicate about past or anticipated feelings, goals, intentions, and cognitions. Moreover, the ability to use internal state language allows companions to clarify misunderstandings and misinterpretations during ongoing interactions.

Previous research in middle-class samples has shown that internal state words first emerge during the second year and burgeon during the third. By 28 months, the majority of children master verbal labels for perception (i.e., the five senses), physiological states, volition, and ability. More than half discuss emotions, moral conformity, and obligation, whereas only a few begin to talk about cognition (i.e., thought processes). Children also become increasingly able to use internal state labels for both self and others, reflecting a growing awareness of self as distinct from other (Bretherton and Beeghly, 1982). Cicchetti and Beeghly (1987) investigated internal state language in 30-month-old maltreated and nonmaltreated toddlers from welfare-dependent homes interacting with their mothers in the laboratory. In addition, maternal reports of children's internal state language were compared to similar reports by middle class mothers.

Although maltreated and nonmaltreated children did not differ significantly in receptive vocabulary, Cicchetti and Beeghly (1987) found significant group differences on productive and internal state language variables. Maltreated toddlers used proportionately fewer internal state words, showed less differentiation in their attributional focus, and were more context-bound in their use of internal state language than their nonmaltreated peers. In contrast, the maltreated and nonmaltreated children did not differ significantly in the categorical content of their internal state language (e.g., words about perception, volition, etc.), with two exceptions. Nonmaltreated children produced proportionally more utterances about physiological states (hunger, thirst, state of consciousness) and more utterances about negative affect (hate, disgust, anger, bad feelings). For the most part, the distribution of words in each category was markedly similar to that seen in middle-class 28-month-olds. Children spoke most about volition and perception, and least about cognition.

Analyses of the maternal interview data yielded similar patterns of results. Maltreating mothers reported that their 30-month-olds produced fewer internal state words and attributed internal states to fewer social agents than did nonmaltreating mothers, corroborating the observational findings. In addition, maternal reports concerning the categorical content of their children's language did not differ by child group. In support of the validity of the interview, data for use with low socioeconomic status mothers reported child internal state language was significantly correlated with observed child internal state language production (average $r = .50$).

The results of the maternal language interview revealed that, with very few exceptions, the maltreated toddlers produced far fewer internal state words than did middle class nonmaltreated youngsters of the same age (Bretherton and Beeghly, 1982). In contrast, the percentages of *nonmaltreated* children reported to use different categories of internal state language were markedly similar to that reported for middle-class children. Similar patterns of results were observed for children's ability to use internal state words for both self and other. That is, maltreated toddlers lagged greatly behind their nonmaltreated comparisons in the use of internal state words about the self and other individuals. The lower-socioeconomic status non-maltreated children were very similar in this capacity to nonmaltreated middle-class youngsters.

The tendency for maltreated toddlers to use fewer internal state words may stem from parental disapproval of the expression of affect or of a certain class of affects. In effect, these children may become "overcontrolled" in efforts to meet parental demands. A recent study conducted by Kropp and Haynes (1987) supports this hypothesis. These authors found that abusive mothers had more difficulty decoding specific emotion signals. In particular, they were significantly more likely than comparison mothers to label negative affect as positive affect. Interestingly, Cicchetti and Beeghly's (1987) results on emotional language usage fit nicely with the findings of Kropp and Haynes (1987). Specifically, Cicchetti and Beeghly (1987) found that maltreated toddlers spoke less about negative emotions than did non-maltreated comparison youngsters. One plausible interpretation of these results is that maltreating mothers' socialization of affect interferes with the usage of certain affects, prevents maltreated children from being in touch with their correct feelings, and leads to problems with the development of emotional control. A study by Camras and her colleagues (Camras, Grow, and Ribordy, 1983), which found that abused children were less skilled in decoding facial expressions of emotion, lends credence to these ideas. Given the decreased affective responsiveness and sensitivity of maltreating care-givers (Crittenden, 1981; Crittenden and Ainsworth, this volume; Egeland and Sroufe, 1981), it is not surprising that maltreated youngsters show delays and deviations in the acquisition of emotional control.

In a related vein, Cummings, Zahn-Waxler, and Radke-Yarrow (1981) found that expressions of anger by normal infants' caregivers frequently caused distress in the infants. Repeated exposures to anger between the parents increase the likelihood of a negative emotional reaction by the infants, as well as the active involvement of the infants in their parents' conflict. By approximately 1 year of age, infants not only were aware of angry interactions between persons important to them, but also were likely to evidence an emotional reaction to them. These results suggest that infants' sense of security and feelings about the self, as well as their capacity to display certain positive and negative emotional responses, may be affected by either constant strife or harmony in their environment.

Recent work (Goodman and Rosenberg, 1987; Rosenberg, 1987) in the area of emotional maltreatment has demonstrated that children who witness violence in the home (e.g., screaming, repeated beatings, chokings, assaults with weapons, property destruction, suicide and homicide attempts) are highly likely to develop a myriad of emotional and social-cognitive difficulties. For example, children who are exposed to interparental violence may develop problematic coping and interpersonal problem-solving strategies that may interfere with their relationships with family members (parents, siblings) and peers or with their school performance (Goodman and Rosenberg, 1987). Further research on the role that background anger has on the ability of maltreated children to control their emotions is clearly warranted.

Development of peer relations

As noted in Table 13.2, peer relations are conceived to be a stage-salient developmental issue during the preschool and early school-age period. The salience of the peer system for promoting successful adaptation is apparent. Maltreated children may be regarded as an especially high-risk target group to examine in this domain for a variety of reasons (e.g., parental childrearing histories and practices – Trickett and Susman, this volume; familial stress and disorganization – Garbarino and Gilliam, 1980; the presence of persistent poverty – Pelton, 1987; social isolation and family discord – Gil, 1970). Those children who perform poorly with peers, especially when their total ecology is unsupportive (Bronfenbrenner, 1979), are likely to experience continued incompetence and maladaptation.

Disturbed interpersonal relationships are strongly associated with psychiatric disorders in children and in adults. In childhood, both sociometric and clinical studies have shown that youngsters who fail to make friends, who are not liked by others, and who are socially rejected or isolated have a much increased risk of psychiatric problems (Garmezy, 1974; Kohlberg, LaCrosse, and Ricks, 1972; Rolf and Garmezy, 1974; Rutter, 1972/1981). For example, Rutter, Tizard, and Whitmore (1970/1981) found that the description "*not* much liked by other children" was a powerful indicator of current psychiatric disturbance. Moreover, other investigators (cf. Garmezy and Streitman, 1974; Cowen, Pederson, Babigian, Izzo, and Trost, 1973) have demonstrated that poor quality peer relationships possess not only concurrent, but also predictive validity for later interpersonal difficulties. Furthermore, even among an entire group of children characterized by psychiatric disturbances, those who had the most disturbed peer relationships had the worst prognosis (Sundby and Kreyberg, 1969).

However, success with peers may be a prophylactic device for ensuring competence in the face of adversity despite seemingly deleterious biologic and environmental circumstances. Conceivably, a supportive peer culture could allay somewhat the harmful consequences of an unharmonious, stress-laden environment. Such a restitutive function may help these children "self-right" toward the development of social competence (cf. Sameroff and Chandler, 1975; Waddington, 1966).

Thus, there is a strong basis for suggesting that the study of peer relations might be important in the search for the antecedents of social competence, coping skills, and adaptation. Although the direction of causality eludes us at present (that is, are children made vulnerable to stress by poor peer relations? or, alternatively, do behaviors associated with vulnerability to psychiatric disturbance also "turn off" other children?), the domain of social skills, friendships, and peer relations – social support systems for the child – is a salient developmental issue and warrants extensive study in any search for the correlates of competence or maladaptation in maltreated children.

The peer relations of preschool and school-aged maltreated children have been studied using a variety of measures (e.g., observations, interviews, peer nominations, teacher ratings) and in several different settings (e.g., the laboratory, at school, in a summer camp). Taken in tandem, the results of these studies demonstrate that maltreated children have grave difficulties with peer relations (Mueller and Silverman, this volume).

When viewed in light of the literature on the high percentage of insecure attachments in maltreated infants and toddlers, these data are quite compelling. Bowlby (1973) describes working models as a person's conscious or unconscious mental representation of the world and of him- or herself in it, through the aid of which the person perceives events, forecasts the future, and constructs plans. Two of the most important parts of these working models are: (1) children's conceptions of their attachment figures, their whereabouts, and their likely response to the child's behavior; and (2) children's conceptions of how acceptable or unacceptable they are in the eyes of their attachment figures (i.e., their self-image).

These working models are constructed out of children's own actions, the feedback they receive from these actions, and the actions of caregivers. They include affective, "appraising" components as well as cognitive components (Bretherton, 1985). As such, there will be wide variations across individuals in working models, and individuals' working models will fairly accurately reflect their own experience as well as cognitive, linguistic, and behavioral skills. Finally, these internal working models, once organized, tend to operate outside conscious awareness and resist dramatic change (Bowlby, 1980). Changes that occur during childhood will usually be in response to changing (concrete) experiences, whereas during and after adolescence, "formal operations" may enable individuals to alter somewhat their working models through sophisticated thought processes (Hunter and Kilstrom, 1979; Main and Goldwyn, 1984; Main et al., 1985). For example, Hunter and Kilstrom (1979) have demonstrated how the healthy "re-representation" of one's childhood experiences (e.g., a history of physical abuse) can result in a breakage of the intergenerational transmission of child abuse (see Kaufman and Zigler, this volume).

The high preponderance of insecure infant–mother attachments found in maltreated samples obviously puts maltreated children at high risk for having a more generalized poor-quality working model of the self and of the self in relation to others. In an important study relevant to this issue, Dean, Malik, Richards, and Stringer (1986) examined the consequences of parental maltreatment on the development of school-aged children's conceptions of interpersonal relationships between peers and between adults and children. Dean and her colleagues found that younger maltreated children (aged 6–8), asked to tell stories about kind or unkind child to child, adult to child, or child to adult initiatives and then relay what the recipient would do next, told more stories in which children reciprocated the kind acts of adults; however, nonmaltreated children related more stories in which adults or peers reciprocated the kind acts of children. In addition, Dean and her collaborators found that maltreated children across all ages studied (ages 6–14) justified their parents' unkind acts on the basis of their own misbehavior.

Moreover, the environments of maltreated children show a striking continuity of inadequate caretaking on numerous counts. Accordingly, the influence of a debilitating environment and an insecure mother–child attachment may make it more difficult for the working models of maltreated youngsters to change, at least prior to formal operations, in the absence of intervention (Cicchetti et al., in press). Consequently, these children may manifest a striking difficulty with relationship formation, maintenance, and consolidation that persists over time and that extends to other adults as well as to peers. Such continuity of maladaptation would bode poorly for their later outcomes, especially because impaired peer relations portend later social emotional problems.

The organization of development

Questions concerning the interrelation among ontogenetic domains in maltreated children have just begun to capture the attention of developmentalists. Research on the organization of development in maltreated children has both clinical and theoretical relevance. For the most part, intervention services are being provided in the absence of sufficient empirical data (Cicchetti and Toth, 1987; Zigler, 1976). In addition, research on the organization of development in maltreated toddlers will elucidate our understanding of the normal developmental process. For example, we will illustrate how the study of maltreated children will make important contributions to elucidating the nature of the relation between cognition and emotion and will generate information crucial to resolving the longstanding controversy concerning the role that socioemotional factors play in language acquisition.

The relation between emotion and cognition in maltreated
children

The empirical study of emotional development in maltreated children is a relatively recent phenomenon (Aber and Cicchetti, 1984). This state of affairs is not unique to the field of child maltreatment. The study of emotional phenomena has important implications for understanding the development and organization of the processes underlying abnormal ontogenesis. Even though theoreticians and clinicians have stressed the role that emotions play in the etiology and sequelae of many forms of child and adult psychopathology (cf. Arieti, 1967; Bleuler, 1911/1950; Cleckley, 1941/1976; Kanner, 1943; Kraepelin, 1919/1971), until recently there has been a paucity of experimental inquiry conducted on the nature of the relation between affect and cognition in adult and child clinical populations (cf. Cicchetti and Sroufe, 1976, 1978; Hobson, 1986; Knight, Roff, Barnett, and Moss, 1979; Schneider-Rosen and Cicchetti, 1984).

One of the theoretical consequences of the investigation of emotional development in high-risk populations is that it underscores the importance of constructing a model of normal emotional development in order to distinguish between abnormal and well-adjusted emotional development. Only if we know which kinds of emotions and emotional patterns children express nonverbally and in their reasoning at different points in development, and what kinds of processes they utilize for the acquisition of new nonverbal emotional expressions, emotional language, and different types of reasoning about emotions, will we be able to help children, such as those who have been maltreated, who are often deficient in the encoding (Gaensbauer and Sands, 1979) and decoding (Camras et al., 1983) of nonverbal expressions, in the production of emotional language (Cicchetti and Beeghly, 1987), and in their reasoning about emotions (Dean et al., 1986; Smetana and Kelly, this volume). Knowing the processes used for normal emotional development will allow us to derive training procedures for the children expressing abnormalities in their emotional development. For example, now that we are beginning to learn more about the strategies employed in normal language acquisition (Bretherton, Fritz, Zahn-Waxler, and Ridgeway, 1986), we will soon be able to create situations in therapy that will facilitate the acquisition of emotional language and be better able to control the acting-out behaviors manifested in nonverbal emotional expressions (Cicchetti et al., 1988).

The theoretical and practical impact of the investigation of emotional development is also important with respect to the formulation of an integrated theory of development. Only if we know, for example, how emotions relate to the other aspects of knowledge we have about people's development will we be able to specify the necessary and/or sufficient conditions necessary to bring about change in the emotional domain.

Influenced by the organizational perspective (Cicchetti and Sroufe, 1978; Sroufe, 1979b; Sroufe and Waters, 1976), research on normal emotional development has burgeoned during the past two decades (Izard, 1977; Izard, Kagan, and Zajonc, 1984; Lewis and Michalson, 1983). Contemporary conceptions of the nature of this relation are based upon the sequence or emergence of new cognitive or affective qualities or characteristics (Cicchetti and Hesse, 1983). Emotions may be regarded as developing ontogenetically earlier than cognition, thereby providing the context within which cognitive development may occur *(cognitive epiphenomenalism)*. The emergence of new emotions may be dependent upon cognitive advances that must be made before various emotions may be expressed *(emotional epiphenomenalism)*. Emotions may develop along a separate pathway from cognitive advances so that the sequence, rate, and quality of change must be considered distinctly within each domain *(parallelism)*. Finally, emotions may emerge in interaction with cognitive advances, thereby suggesting a progression that necessitates a consideration of developmental changes that occur across domains and that exert a reciprocal influence upon each other *(interactionism)*.

Schneider-Rosen and Cicchetti's (1984) study on the relation between quality of infant–mother attachment and the emergence of visual self-recognition in maltreated youngsters sheds light on the nature of the relation between emotion and cognition. An analysis of the infants' affective responses to their rouge-marked noses indicated that maltreated infants possess a differential understanding of this event and tend to be developmentally delayed or impaired in their affective reactions to their mirror images. After observing themselves in the mirror, similar to the findings obtained with middle-class toddlers (Lewis and Brooks-Gunn, 1979), a significantly greater percentage of the nonmaltreated lower-socioeconomic status comparison infants (74 percent) showed an increase in positive affect following the application of rouge, whereas a greater proportion of the maltreated infants (78 percent) showed neutral or negative reactions. It is interesting to note here that toddlers with Down's syndrome, an organic form of mental retardation, show positive affect to their images once they have attained the concept of visual self-recognition (Mans, Cicchetti, and Sroufe, 1978), whereas autistic children predominantly show neutral affect upon mirror self-regard (Spiker and Ricks, 1984).

The findings of the Schneider-Rosen and Cicchetti (1984) study provide relevant information for the understanding of those environmental variables (e.g., the experience of early maltreatment by the primary caregiver) that may interact with organismic and constitutional factors to influence development. These results further suggest that maltreated toddlers either attempt to mask their feelings or experience themselves in mainly negative ways. Finally, because there were no differences in performance on the object permanence subscale of the Uzgiris-Hunt (1975) ordinal scales of infant development, the results suggest that cognition is necessary, but not sufficient, for the emergence of the capacity for self-recognition, thereby providing compelling evidence for the interactive nature of the relation between affective and cognitive development in the maltreated toddler.

In the area of cognitive control development, the study of maltreated children has also elucidated the interdependence of affective and cognitive development. First formulated by George Klein (Klein, 1951, 1954; Klein and Schlesinger, 1949), the concept of cognitive controls has been used to explain the way in which individuals coordinate information from the external environment – with the affects, fantasies, and motives from the internal environment – in order to remain in control of the information (Santostefano, 1978). Cognitive controls mediate between the influences of personality and motivation, on the one hand, and cognitions, on the other, and evolve as enduring aspects of the individual's cognitive functioning and adaptive style while continuing to exert influence over subsequent cognitive experiences (Rieder and Cicchetti, in press). Rieder and Cicchetti demonstrated that a history of maltreatment was related to cognitive control development in preschool and early school-age children. Maltreated children were found to be delayed in their cognitive control functioning during the assessment of cognitive controls in a relatively neutral, nonaggressive context. Moreover, maltreated children were found to assimilate aggressive stimuli more readily and with less distortion. Rieder and Cicchetti argued that the requirements (call for action) of aggressive fantasies of maltreated children prescribed a coordination/balance that called for the ready assimilation (sharpening) of aggressive stimuli. In nonmaltreated children, in contrast, the requirements of aggressive fantasies prescribed a coordination/balance between fantasy and stimuli, resulting in avoidance (leveling) of aggressive stimuli. Rieder and Cicchetti hypothesized that the requirements of a maltreating environment encouraged the development of a hypervigilance and ready assimilation of aggressive stimuli as an adaptive coping strategy. In addition, Rieder and Cicchetti noted that the problems in the cognitive–affective balance of maltreated children may lead them to be overly attuned to interpret ambiguous stimuli in the environment as threatening and aggressive. Delays in cognitive control functioning and a readiness to assimilate aggressive stimuli could lead children to experience difficulty in their peer interactions (Dodge, Murphy, and Buchsbaum, 1984). These results point to the importance of environmental factors upon the development of the affective–cognitive balance and suggest that there may be negative ramifications for maltreated children's social development.

Moreover, the tendency for maltreated children to assimilate aggressive stimuli more readily is compatible with the earlier discussions about internal working models of relationships. Whereas Dodge and colleagues (Dodge, Murphy, and Buchsbaum, 1984) have posited deficits in the social information processing capacities of children who interpret ambiguous social stimuli as having aggressive intent, such assumptions may be congruent with the negative expectations maltreated children have formed about interpersonal relations.

The relation between socioemotional and linguistic development

For the past two decades, a large body of investigators have directed their research toward identifying aspects of the social environment that contribute to the ontogenesis of language. The majority of this work can be placed into two categories. A plethora of investigators have focused on uncovering associations between parental verbal input and variables in child linguistic output (Clarke-Stewart, 1973; Cross, 1978; Nelson, 1973, 1977; Snow and Ferguson, 1977). Although there is some evidence to support the contention that language acquisition is enhanced by verbal input that provides responsive and contingent feedback to children's signals and is heavily weighted to the here and now (Snow and Gilbreath, 1983), many of the assumptions of sociolinguists have yet to be confirmed (Gleitman, Newport, and Gleitman, 1984).

In addition, a number of studies have been conducted to ascertain the relation between language development and the quality of the infant–caregiver relationship. In particular, there have been several empirical reports attempting to link differences in the quality of mother–infant attachment as measured in the "Strange Situation" (Ainsworth and Wittig, 1969) to variations in linguistic growth (Clarke-Stewart, 1973; Connell, 1976; Greenberg and Marvin, 1979; Main, 1973; Pentz, 1975). Because differences in interactive style have been shown to be related to individual differences in attachment (Ainsworth, Blehar, Waters, and Wall, 1978), one might logically expect that the securely attached infant's linguistic development would be enhanced by sensitive, high quality social input emanating from the caregiver. However, just as was the case for the studies investigating the relation between maternal verbal input and the child's linguistic output, research that has attempted to link qualitative differences in the attachment relationship to language development has also yielded inconsistent results (see Bretherton, Bates, Benigni, Camaioni, and Volterra, 1979, for a review).

In a review article of the social bases of language literature, Bates, Bretherton, Beeghly-Smith, and McNew (1982) noted the many impediments to isolating the nature of the social inputs and their respective contributions to linguistic growth. Based on the current empirical findings, some researchers have argued that language development is buffered against a wide range of experiential variability; however, Bates et al. (1982) have noted that a number of conceptual and methodological limitations in the existing literature render this conclusion premature. For example, they stated that it was conceivable that the small homogeneous groups from which subjects of child language studies are drawn (i.e., white, normal, middle-class volunteer mothers and their children) yield too small a range of variability in attachment, maternal speech patterns, and language development to uncover significant interrelations among these domains. Bretherton et al. (1979) have hypothesized that a threshold effect may be operating, with most middle-class children receiving a sufficient amount of quality social input to ensure that language moves forward at its expected rate. Thus, perhaps the best way to demonstrate the relation between social input and language acquisition may be through the study of clinical populations who receive substantially different amounts and/or quality of social input. Since on ethical grounds alone it would be impossible to manipulate experimentally the lower limit of the social input threshold required for language development to unfold, the best available alternative for illuminating the relation between various aspects of social interaction and language development appears to be the study of "experiments in nature" (Bates et al., 1982; Bronfenbrenner, 1979).

Contributions of the study of maltreated children to the understanding of the social bases of language

Child maltreatment, as a true "experiment in nature," presents an opportunity to investigate the relation between attachment status and communicative development. Moreover, the study of maltreated children may elucidate our understanding about whether deviations in social input (e.g., inconsistent responsivity, noncontingent feedback, a paucity of stimulation, misattunement) impede linguistic growth.

Observational studies of mother–child interaction in maltreating families

Observational studies comparing maltreating and nonmaltreating mother–child dyads have consistently yielded differences in interactive behavior along dimensions critical to the ontogenesis of communicative competence. Burgess and Conger (1978), in a home study investigating the communication patterns of abusive, neglectful, and nonmaltreating families, found that maltreating mothers conversed less with their children than did the comparison mothers. Furthermore, neglectful and abusive mothers were more negative, more controlling, and less positive than the nonmaltreating mothers in their verbalization.

Aragona and Eyberg (1981) found that in a laboratory play session, neglecting mothers gave less verbal praise and acknowledgment and more criticism and commands than did mothers of behavior problem, nonmaltreated children. Bousha and Twentyman (1984) showed that the rate of mother–child interaction was much lower for neglecting than for comparison mothers. Although this result was not especially surprising, it is noteworthy that the incidence of maternal verbal instructional interaction was especially suppressed in neglecting mothers. Likewise, Wasserman, Green, and Allen (1983) reported that abusive mothers were significantly less likely to initiate play interactions with their infants, far more likely to ignore them, and less likely to employ verbal means to instruct the infant about his/her environmental surroundings.

In one of the few studies relating the maltreated toddler's communicative development to the mother's verbal style, Westerman and Haustead (1982) compared the conversations between an abused child and the natural mother to those of the abused child and the foster mother. These investigators found that the abusive natural mother was less able than the foster mother to utilize linguistic forms that facilitate communication, thereby placing excessive burdens upon the child for managing the dialogue.

The confluence of the findings gleaned from observational studies of mother–child interaction in maltreating families implies that maltreated children are brought up in an unresponsive environment that fails to foster communicative exchanges. If communicative development is affected by the quality and quantity of conversational input, then maltreatment should have a deleterious effect upon linguistic development.

Because most maltreated infants and toddlers have insecure relationships, attachment theory would predict that, as a group, maltreated youngsters are at high risk for developing communicative problems. Moreover, because not all maltreated children have an insecure attachment relationship with their primary caregivers, securely attached maltreated children should be highly represented in the group of maltreated children who develop adequate linguistic skills.

Communicative behavior in 25-month-old maltreated toddlers

Gersten, Coster, Schneider-Rosen, Carlson, and Cicchetti (1986) studied 40 toddlers, 20 who were identified as having been legally maltreated and 20 who were matched lower-socioeconomic status nonmaltreated comparison youngsters. These toddlers were observed at 24 months with their mothers in the "Strange Situation" (Ainsworth and Wittig, 1969). One month later, the toddlers participated in a 30-minute structured free-play and a 20-minute unstructured free-play observation with their mothers. Coders blind to attachment classification and maltreatment status transcribed the entire videotaped mother–child free-play interactions. Independent coders, unaware of the toddlers' maltreatment and attachment status, rated the linguistic performance and communicative behavior of the youngsters. The speech and concomitant nonverbal behaviors of both members of the dyad were recorded as well (see Gersten et al., 1986, for details). The coding system devised for functional communication of the toddlers is presented in Table 13.3.

Contrary to expectations, Gersten et al. (1986) found no significant differences between the two groups in their communicative behavior. In light of the current debate over the role of environmental influences on developing language skills, the failure to document a relation between the experience of maltreatment and communicative functioning is noteworthy. Two interpretations of these data may be offered. The first is that early language development is so highly canalized that variations in interactive experience are of little consequence. This interpretation is consistent with the view that language acquisition may proceed on the basis of minimal environmental input, thereby unaffected by variations in social experience. It may be that the evolutionary fit between mothers and children is so good that all mothers do what must be done in order to get communication under way (Bates et al., 1982). However, this interpretation does not preclude the possibility that *later* developments in language may be adversely affected by environmental conditions. The effects of environmental variations on language development may not show up until language is better established. Correlations of language variables with environmental factors might appear if social aspects of language usage (e.g., discourse ability and the expression of internal states) in older children were studied. Support for this interpretation may be found in the large numbers of school-age maltreated children who have been described as having communicative difficulties, particularly with their discourse skills (e.g., Blager and Martin, 1976). Furthermore, it is possible that the influence of maltreatment on communicative behavior may become more apparent as the child attempts to achieve autonomy during the third or fourth years. At that time, certain patterns of communicative behavior may emerge that reflect coping mechanisms used to deal with the maltreating environment. Studies indicate that the maltreated child may adopt compromise solutions to his or her caregiving environment. For example, Schneider-Rosen et al. (1985) describe how some maltreated children avert gaze, minimize face-to-face contact or physical closeness, and rarely initiate social exchanges with an unresponsive or unpredictable caregiver. Similarly, the child may adopt styles of communicative behavior that reduce the likelihood of prolonged interaction or subsequent abuse. For instance, an abused girl in the Gersten et al. (1986) sample directed almost all of her utterances to a doll or toy rather than to an overtly hostile mother. Others displayed a pattern of speaking only when a response was clearly

Table 13.3. *Functional communication coding system*

	Type of communication	Description	Example
I. Categories of functional acts	0. Unclassifiable	Uncomprehensive vocalizations as well as transcribed utterances that cannot be categorized by a specified functional type.	
	1. Imitation	Partial or complete repetitions of the mother's immediately prior communication, with or without change in intonational contour, which do not *add* new information.	M: "What a big big fish." C: "Big fish."
	2. Self-repetition	Exact repetition of prior communication, either spontaneous or in response to clarification request.	C: "What dis, mommy?" M: (No answer) C: "What dis mommy?"
	3. Conversational devices	Words and phrases serving primarily to mark conversational boundaries or maintain conversational flow without adding substantively to the discourse.	"yeah", "OK", "uh uh", "huh?"
	4. Exchange	Utterances that accompany acts of giving and receiving objects.	"oh here", "dis for you", "here"
	5. Attentional	Utterances that serve to elicit the mother's attention, usually by specifying the attentional object.	"look it", "see that", "watch that"
	6. Routines and social speech	Ritualized or stereotyped expressions and verbal games.	"Thank you"; "vroom vroom" (pushing truck); "whoops"; "hooray"
	7. Action requestives	Attempts to regulate the behavior of a person or plaything, as in demands, action requests, suggestives, and directives.	"do this"; "gimme dat"; "lemme go"
	8. Information requests	Attempts to solicit specific verbal responses including requests for labels or for permission, and questions seeking explanations or descriptions.	"What's that?"; "Want more?"; "Where dis go?"
	9. Naming	Statements that make reference to an object or person by name only.	"car"; "Lisa"; "dis a ball"

Table 13.3. *(Cont.)*

Type of communication	Description	Example
10. Description	Statements that encode relationships of qualification or specification about an object, person, or event.	"nother truck"; "dis is broke"; "dolly in bed"
11. Discusses others	Statements that describe the psychological states (thoughts, feelings, actions) of others, including pretend animate beings.	"baby hungry"; "he tired"
12. Discusses self action	Utterances describing an act the child is performing or has just performed.	"I did it"; "making a snowman"
13. Internal report	Utterances that express sentiments, emotions, intents, and other internal states.	"can't do it"; "gotta go"; "want more"
1. Object	Utterances made while acting on, gazing at, or manipulating objects if not also actively interacting with the mother.	C says "dis goes in here, dat goes dere" in a sing-song fashion while putting furniture in a doll house.
2. Social	Words or phrases used to imitate, interact, or respond to another person or prior to vocalizations. By definition, relevant answers to maternal questions, requests for information, exchanges, and behavior.	

II. Context
The contextual category is designed to capture the extent to which the child utilizes vocalizations to communicate interpersonally or to explore the environment.

Source: Gersten, Coster, Schneider-Rosen, Carlson and Cicchetti, 1986.

demanded or for instrumental purposes (e.g., asking the mother to take her to the bathroom). Viewed in this light, the communicative deficits noted in populations of maltreated school children may stem from socioemotional rather than linguistic difficulties.

Quality of attachment, maltreatment, and language

In contrast, Gersten et al. (1986) found that attachment security was highly related to variations in language performance. Table 13.4 shows how strong and consistent were relations between attachment and language.

Securely attached toddlers as a group consistently demonstrated a more elaborate vocabulary, as measured by total number of words and total number of different words in each of the five categories examined (nouns, verbs, pronouns, adjectives, and social expressives; see Table 13.4). The securely attached toddlers also talked more, as seen in the differences in total utterances. Mean length of utterance (MLU) was examined to provide an index of the structural complexity of the child's language (Brown, 1973). Securely attached toddlers were found by this measure to be using syntactically more complex language than insecure toddlers (mean MLU: secure = 1.83, insecure = 1.50; see Table 13.4).

The relative reliance on particular *types* of communication by the two groups was examined using the fundamental categories of utterances. Resulting analyses revealed differences on four of the separate categories and on one of the composite categories. Securely attached toddlers used a significantly greater proportion of nominals (e.g., truck, ball); descriptors (e.g., pretty doll, blue block); and utterances describing the activities and feelings of other persons (e.g., you sad mommy?; you make a house). In contrast, insecurely attached toddlers used a greater proportion of "exchanges" and "fillers." These types of utterances are relatively content free and serve primarily to mark turns during conversation without supplying novel information (see Table 13.4).

The data suggest that the verbalizations of securely attached toddlers contained proportionately more content language. These infants referred more often to objects, events, themselves, and others than did insecurely attached infants. In contrast, insecurely attached toddlers used proportionately less content language, relying instead on a communicative strategy requiring minimal involvement on the part of the child. They filled their conversational turns with utterances like "hmm," "did," "which," and "here" significantly more often than did the securely attached children.

These results cannot be explained merely on the basis of differences in overall cognitive ability. A group by attachment (2×2) analysis of variance was carried out using scores on the mental scale of the Bayley Scales of Infant Development (Bayley, 1969) as dependent variables. There were no

Table 13.4. *Comparisons on language variables: Secure and insecure groups*

Variable[a]	Secure (n = 22) M	Insecure (n = 18) M	F(df = 1, 39)
MLU	1.83	1.50	7.69**
	(.54)	(.33)	
Total words	405.64	248.33	6.23*
	(257.12)	(171.81)	
Total different			
words	84.45	52.67	11.53**
	(37.36)	(29.87)	
nouns	23.54	13.78	9.26.**
	(11.95)	(9.84)	
pronouns	10.14	7.11	10.15**
	(4.00)	(3.55)	
verbs	19.54	10.94	7.29**
	(12.16)	(7.40)	
social expressives	15.54	11.83	8.59**
	(5.66)	(4.97)	
Adjectives	14.86	7.28	14.00***
	(8.27)	(4.35)	
Total utterances	300.09	220.17	8.08**
	(106.94)	(101.47)	
Total unclassifiable utterances	34.54	27.33	6.88**
	(25.70)	(21.02)	
Imitation	.09	.09	.01
	(.06)	(.09)	
Self repetitions	.18	.24	1.76
	(.07)	(.11)	
Conversationals	.13	.14	.00
	(.06)	(.09)	
Exchanges	.02	.04	6.85**
	(.02)	(.03)	
Attentionals	.04	.06	1.03
	(.04)	(.05)	
Routines	.09	.10	.16
	(.09)	(.07)	
Action requests	.07	.08	.42
	(.04)	(.07)	
Information requests	.06	.05	1.16
	(113)	(.05)	
Names	.13	.08	5.32*
	(.09)	(.04)	
Describes	.09	.04	21.07***
	(.03)	(.04)	
Discuss others	.02	.01	5.05*
	(.02)	(.01)	

Note: All conversational category variables are proportions.
[a]All variables are proportion scores that have been transformed using arcsine square root.
*Variables significant at $p < .05$.
**Variables significant at $p < .01$.
***Variables significant at $p < .001$.
Source: Gersten, Coster, Schneider-Rosen, Carlson, and Cicchetti, 1986.

significant group differences found either between maltreated and comparison toddlers or between securely and insecurely attached toddlers. (See Gersten et al., 1986, for a fuller description and discussion of these data.)

Communicative behavior in 31-month-old maltreated toddlers

As we have noted, despite the high percentage of insecure attachments in the maltreated group and the association of insecure attachment with less mature forms of communication, Gersten et al. (1986) did not find a relation between maltreatment and linguistic competence in the 25-month-old toddlers they studied. Because it is conceivable that the effects of adverse environmental influences may only appear once the basic communicative patterns have been more firmly established (Bretherton et al., 1979), we chose to study a group of maltreated children at a more advanced stage of early language development to ascertain if these toddlers may begin to manifest deviations in their communicative processes.

Coster, Gersten, Beeghly, and Cicchetti (in press) studied two groups of 31-month-old toddlers and their mothers in the same interactional paradigms utilized in the Gersten et al. (1986) study. One group was comprised of 20 legally identified maltreated children, the other was made up of 20 toddlers in a well-matched lower-socioeconomic comparison group. Transcriptions and codings occurred according to the exact procedures described in the Gersten et al. (1986) study. In addition, coders were blind to the diagnostic status of the toddlers. In contrast to the Gersten et al. (1986) findings, many compelling statistically significant findings emerged in the linguistic behavior between the two groups of maltreated and nonmaltreated youngsters.

Maltreated toddlers had lower MLUs and were lower on all measures of expressive vocabulary as well as on total number of different words utilized. Since the maltreated and nonmaltreated toddlers did not differ on the total number of utterances they employed, the expressive language differences obtained cannot be attributed to differences in linguistic output. Coster et al. (in press) found no differences between the two groups on receptive language. Thus, the 31-month-old maltreated youngsters had less well developed expressive language than the nonmaltreated toddlers.

In addition to assessing the expressive language of the maltreated toddlers, Coster and her colleagues found that maltreated children likewise showed deficits in their discourse abilities. For example, maltreated toddlers used significantly more "conversational devices" and fewer descriptive utterances than their nonmaltreated comparisons. Moreover, the maltreated youngsters talked considerably less about their own activities and made fewer requests for information. Furthermore, the maltreated toddlers utilized far less decontextualized speech than their nonmaltreated comparisons. Specifically, the maltreated youngsters made fewer references to persons or events outside the "here and now."

Finally, Coster et al. (in press) compared the communicative behavior of the mothers of the maltreated and nonmaltreated youngsters. Correlations between the child's MLU and mother's total utterances, as well as proportion of utterances discussing others were examined; however, no statistically significant differences occurred.

The findings from this investigation show that major differences in the communicative behavior of maltreated and nonmaltreated youngsters exist by 31 months of age. Recall that in the Gersten et al. (1986) study, when a cross-sectional group of 25-month-old toddlers was examined, no differences emerged. An inspection of the linguistic performance of the 25- and 31-month-old toddlers revealed, not surprisingly, much more elaborate language abilities in the latter group of youngsters. Thus, it may be that communicative functioning may be more of a stage-salient developmental issue at 31 months than at 25 months. Of course, what are needed at this point are longitudinal studies. For example, it would be especially interesting to ascertain if the insecurely attached toddlers in the Gersten et al. (1986) study do show linguistic deficits at a later point in time.

The confluence of findings that has emerged from these studies has contributed to our understanding of many of the most important theoretical questions extant in the acquisition of language. For example, as predicted by a number of attachment and object relations theorists (Ainsworth et al., 1978; Mahler et al., 1975), securely attached youngsters show a more hierarchically organized and integrated self system (e.g., affective and cognitive indices reveal marked coherence). In addition, securely attached youngsters, regardless of their diagnostic status, use more "self" language. Furthermore, maltreated toddlers use fewer internal state words, another sign that their self systems are impaired from a very early age. And by approximately 30 months there are striking differences between the language performance of maltreated and matched lower-socioeconomic status nonmaltreated comparisons. Taken in tandem, even though additional research must be conducted on the social bases of language, we believe that these investigations provide compelling support for theorists who claim that social and emotional factors play important roles in the development of language. Presently, we are embarking on a series of cross-sectional/longitudinal studies, the purpose of which is to further our understanding of the development of representational processes and of the respective contributions of cognitive, play, language, and socioemotional development to the domain of representation.

A final implication of the work on language functioning and development in maltreated children deserves mention here. Historically, there has been a major debate as to whether factors independent of those risk factors commonly associated with lower-SES membership differentiate maltreated from nonmaltreated children (cf. Aber and Cicchetti, 1984; Elmer, 1977). Not only does the study of the communicative development of maltreated children inform this issue; the study of nonmaltreated and maltreated youngsters' communication skills provides insight on the impact of poverty on linguistic development (Feagans and Farran, 1982; Hess and Shipman, 1968). An additional way of disentangling the factors of lower-socioeconomic status and maltreatment on linguistic development would be to compare groups of lower- and middle-SES maltreated and lower- and middle-SES nonmaltreated children.

Implications of the research findings on the sequelae of maltreatment and on the organization of development for the development of psychopathology

Developmental psychopathologists are interested not only in investigating deviant ontogenesis, but also in uncovering the prototypes of, or precursors to, what may later become a psychopathological disorder (Cicchetti and Aber, 1986; Trad, 1986). Moreover, they focus on charting the course of individual differences in adaptation, both normal and psychopathological. Additionally, they are concerned with identifying the circumstances that render certain individuals vulnerable and others protected with respect to life's vicissitudes (Garmezy, 1983; Rolf, Masten, Cicchetti, Neuchterlein, and Weintraub, in press). Finally, developmental psychopathologists seek to ascertain the factors underlying the capacity of the organism to utilize environmental and inner resources (e.g., social supports, superior immune system functioning, effective coping skills, etc.) in an adaptive and competent fashion (cf. Waters and Sroufe, 1983).

Before developmental psychopathology could emerge as a distinct discipline, the science of normal development needed to mature and a broader basis of firm results had to be acquired. In addition to the empirical advances within developmental psychology, increasingly sophisticated theoretical contributions made the developmental approach more viable. One very important example is the principle of equifinality, which refers to the observation that a very large number of paths is available to the same outcome within a particular system (von Bertalanffy, 1968; Weiss, 1969a, 1969b; Wilden, 1980). Consequently, the breakdown as well as the maintenance of a system's function, can occur in a large variety of ways, especially when taking into account environment–organism interaction. To predict the pathology or health of a system based on any single component is not possible, according to this formulation. Thus, the principle of equifinality

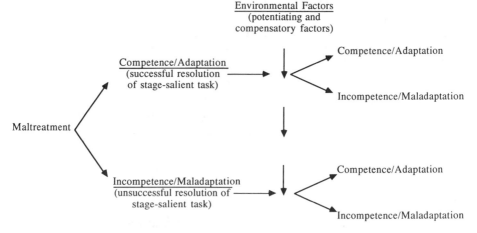

Figure 13.1. A schematic model of the relationship between early maltreatment and later developmental outcome.

offers a more complex and realistic approach to understanding the course of psychopathological disorders and anticipates the failure to identify unique predictors or correlates of psychopathology.

The principle of multifinality (Wilden, 1980) provides another important theoretical tool. This principle states that the effect on functioning of any one component's value may differ in different systems. Actual effects will depend on the conditions set by the value of additional components with which it is structurally linked. Thus, pathology or health of a system must be identified in terms of how adequately its essential functions are maintained (Silvern, 1984). In other words, a particular adverse event should not be seen as necessarily leading to the same psychopathological or nonpsychopathological outcomes in every individual. Together, these principles exemplify significant theoretical progressions within developmental approaches to understanding psychopathology.

As a consequence, psychopathology cannot be conceived according to a linear, main-effects model, but rather through a dynamic transactional one (Sameroff and Chandler, 1975). As depicted in Figure 13.1, early maltreatment may lead to either later competence or incompetence. However, while competence at one stage in life may be predictive of competence at a later stage, this is not necessarily the case. There are many factors that may mediate between early and later adaptation or maladaptation that may allow alternative outcomes to occur. For example, early successful resolution of developmental tasks may be interfered with by environmental factors that inhibit competence at a later stage. Conversely, early problems or deviations in the successful resolution of a developmental task may be countered by major changes in the child's experience that could result in the ultimate successful negotiation of this and subsequent developmental tasks.

As we have seen, maltreated youngsters manifest disturbed functioning on each of the stage-salient developmental issues of the early years of life. Specifically, dysfunctional internal working models (Bowlby, 1980), both in relationships with primary attachment figures and with regard to the self, deviations in self-system processes (Harter, 1983), difficulties in the production and usage of language, and problematic peer relationships were found in maltreated children. These disruptions bode poorly for later adaptation.

Proponents of attachment theory have claimed that many types of psychopathology may be brought about by deviations in the development of the attachment behavioral system (Bowlby, 1977; Guidano and Liotti, 1983). Bowlby believed that parental threats to abandon a child and to commit suicide both would have pathogenic effects on the attachment system. Clearly, maltreated children – especially neglected and emotionally mistreated youngsters – are exposed to such statements (cf. Rosenberg, 1987). In addition, advocates of the attachment theory perspective have argued that there are strong causal relationships between individuals' experiences with their parents and the later capacity to form and to sustain emotional bonds (Bowlby, 1944, 1977; Sroufe and Fleeson, 1986). Furthermore, a number of problems have been implicated as associated with poor quality early parent–child relations, including marital difficulties, the transmission of dysfunctional parenting, personality disorders, neurotic symptoms, and severe psychopathology (Bowlby, 1977; Henderson, 1982; Rutter, this volume; Sroufe and Fleeson, 1986).

Even though attachment is a stage-salient issue primarily during the mid- to late-infancy periods, attachment relations are important across the lifespan. As the attachment system becomes more differentiated, maltreated children continue to display difficulties with relationships (Aber and Allen, 1987; Aber, Allen, Carlson, and Cicchetti, this volume; Dean et al., 1986). Thus the poor-quality attachment relationships of maltreated youngsters are likely to have both predictive and concurrent relations with other developmental domains and stage-salient issues.

During the preschool period, several pathological conditions emerge for the first time during ontogeny – most notably, childhood borderline disorders, attention deficit disorders, and childhood depression (American Psychiatric Association, 1987; Bemporad, Smith, Hanson, and Cicchetti, 1982; Cicchetti and Olsen, in press, a; Kovacs, Feinberg, Crouse-Novak, Paulauskas, and Finkelstein, 1984). Likewise, epidemiological studies suggest that behavior problems are prevalent during the preschool period (Greenberg and Speltz, 1988). As is the case for adult disorders, the problems that occur during the preschool years are often accompanied by relational difficulties (cf. Cicchetti and Schneider-Rosen, 1986; Greenberg and Speltz, 1988). For example, Bemporad and colleagues (1982) have speculated that the particular nature of the relational pathology of the childhood borderline syndrome, a condition associated with severe problems in the separation–individuation process, may be a pathognomonic symptom of this disorder. The "self-system" disturbances of maltreated children place them at great risk for current and later psychopathology. As a final illustration of how failure of a stage-salient issue might predispose maltreated children to develop psychopathology, the poor quality of peer relationships of these children portend later maladaptive functioning.

Retrospective studies of children and adults with psychiatric disorders frequently reveal histories of maltreatment (see, for example, Bemporad et al., 1982; Bryer, Nelson, Miller, and Krol, 1987; Rogeness, Amrung, Macedo, Harris, and Fisher, 1986). Concurrent and follow-up studies of maltreatment often also reveal the presence of psychopathology in these children and their parents, in particular depression and conduct disorders/delinquency (Burgess, Hartman, and McCormack, 1987; Kaplan, Pelcovitz, Salzinger, and Ganeles, 1983; Kazdin, Moser, Colbus, and Bell, 1985; Lewis et al., this volume; Oates, 1984; Rutter and Giller, 1983; Salzinger, Kaplan, Pelcovitz, Samit, and Krieger, 1984; Wilson and Herrnstein, 1985). The presence of parent–child psychopathology, in conjunction with the "stress-laden ecologies" frequently linked with maltreatment (Bronfenbrenner, 1979; Egeland, Breitenbucher, and Rosenberg, 1980; Garbarino, 1977), contribute to disturbances in the parent–child–environment transactional system.

Although not all maltreated children who manifest problems in the resolution of stage-salient issues develop subsequent psychopathology, future disturbances in functioning are likely to occur. In addition, not all children who evidence difficulties with a particular issue (e.g., the formation of secure attachments) will exhibit the same psychopathological disorder. Prospective longitudinal studies are required in order to ascertain the relation between incompetence and the specific form of psychopathology that may eventuate, as well as on the processes whereby psychopathology does not occur even against the backdrop of incompetent functioning.

Future prescriptions

Despite the extreme problems associated with conducting research with maltreating families (Cicchetti and Todd-Manly, in press), we strongly believe that the knowledge gained – both in terms of enhancing our understanding of the causes, intergenerational transmission, and sequelae of maltreatment, and in its impact upon elucidating major issues in normal developmental theory – far outweighs the risks and hard work that are inherent to this process. To date, intervention and policy making have most frequently been guided by a combination of clinical knowledge, lore, and assumptions, as opposed to by empirical knowledge of the scientific strengths and vulnerabilities, and the competencies and incompetencies, that these children and families manifest over time (Zigler, 1976). Outcomes of comprehensive longitudinal studies such as these will enhance the development of services that meet the specific psychological needs of maltreated children and will enable interventions to be appropriately timed and guided (Cicchetti and Toth, 1987; Cicchetti et al., 1988). Moreover, these findings will lead to improvements in treatment, prevention, service planning and evaluation, and policy-making efforts aimed at reducing the tragic long-term effects of maltreatment (cf. Aber and Cicchetti, 1984; Cicchetti and Aber, 1980; Cicchetti and Toth, 1987; Dubowitz and Newberger, this volume; Kaufman and Zigler, this volume; Olds and Henderson, this volume; Wald, Carlsmith, and Leiderman, 1988).

We close this chapter by proposing a series of prescriptions for improving the existing state of research knowledge on maltreating families. We firmly believe that these endeavors will likewise enhance our knowledge about maltreating children and their families as well as contribute to the unraveling of many unanswered questions in basic developmental theory.

> 1. *More large-scale longitudinal research on the etiology, intergenerational transmission, and sequelae of child maltreatment must be conducted.*

Of course, this is labor intensive work (Cicchetti and Todd-Manly, in press) and requires the commensurate support it deserves from funding agencies.

> 2. *Rather than focusing upon isolated areas of functioning, maltreatment investigators must emphasize increasingly the importance of multidisciplinary research.*

In keeping with an organizational developmental psychopathology perspective, child maltreatment should be studied from a variety of perspectives, not merely from the egocentric viewpoint of the investigative team. We believe that the integration of these various disciplinary contributions into a coherent framework (e.g., anthropology – Korbin, 1981; descriptive psychopathology (clinical psychology and psychiatry) – Kaplan et al., 1983; developmental psychology – Egeland and Sroufe, 1981; ecology – Garbarino, 1977; epidemiology – Deykin, Alpert, and McNamara, 1985; experimental psychology – McCabe, 1984; neuropsychology – Tarter, Hegedus, Winston, and Alterman, 1984; pediatrics – Martin, 1976; primatology – Reite and Caine, 1983; psychophysiology – Frodi and Lamb, 1980; social learning theory – Patterson, 1982; Reid, Patterson, and Loeber (1981); social work – Nelson, 1984; sociobiology – Daly and Wilson, 1981; Trivers, 1974; and sociology – Gil, 1970) will result in major advancements in our understanding of child abuse and neglect. It is our contention that the discipline of developmental psychopathology can serve as the overarching framework or macro-paradigm (cf. Achenbach, in press) capable of integrating these interdisciplinary efforts into a coherent whole.

> 3. *Research in the area of child maltreatment should proceed hand-in-hand with studies and theories of normal development. In the absence of an over-arching developmental theory, potentially critical findings may appear uninterpretable* (cf. Aber and Cicchetti, 1984).
> 4. *Additional studies should be carried out in the many varied contexts in which maltreated children spend their lives (e.g., day-care, out-of-home care, after-school care programs).*

With just a few exceptions, most empirical studies of the socioemotional development of maltreated children have been conducted either in developmental laboratories or in the children's homes. This is natural enough for the study of young children. For infants and toddlers, the home is *the* major natural environment of their lives and the laboratory can serve as a well-controlled environment for the detailed study of family interactional processes. But as children grow older, the natural context of their lives rapidly expands beyond the confines of the home and the family and so can no longer be reasonably well-approximated in the lab. If researchers wish to focus on stage-salient developmental tasks (Aber and Cicchetti, 1984; Cicchetti and Rizley, 1981), future studies of maltreated children need to follow older maltreated children into their enduring environments outside their homes and the laboratory. Theorists and researchers should begin to recognize more fully and to study the increasingly important roles of peer relationships, school, and community life in the adaptation of maltreated children. Because school is the focus for much of peer and community life of children from the preschool years through adolescence, it may be an especially important environment in which to study the socioemotional development of maltreated children.

Future studies would benefit from a research strategy that explicitly attempted to study the same underlying developmental processes and issues of maltreated children in the laboratory and/or in several natural environments like the school or camp setting. As Block and Block (1980) have argued, researchers can be much more confident of findings confirmed by both experimental test-level and naturalistic observation-level data on the same underlying psychological construct.

Future studies of maltreated children that assess the children in the natural environments of their lives can begin to address such questions as whether characteristics of maltreated children identified in laboratory studies – for instance, excessive dependency upon or physical avoidance of novel adults (Aber and Allen, 1987; George and Main, 1979) – may interfere with a child's competent adaptation to the school.

5. *Research must be conducted comparing the various traditional and alternative care arrangements for maltreated children (e.g., home care versus foster care versus home care with additional supplemental care). Now that so much is known about normal socioemotional and social-cognitive development and about contextual effects on behavior, we are in a better position to undertake these critical "experiments in nature" (cf. Wald et al., 1983, 1988).*
6. *As longitudinal studies of large representative samples of maltreating families appear more frequently, researchers should focus on identifying competent ("resilient") maltreated children. In addition, some disadvantaged non-maltreated comparison children are also highly likely to be resilient (cf. Pavenstedt, 1965). The study of the processes whereby children "make it" in the face of extreme adversity should also teach us about alternate pathways inherent to the normal development of coping.*

We would like to exert a word of caution here. Like all developmental constructs, "resiliency" should not be treated as a static and/or a dichotomous ("resilient" versus "vulnerable") entity. Some children may look resilient when studied cross-sectionally (e.g., securely attached maltreated children). However, when followed over time, many of these children may no longer be functioning adaptively (cf. Schneider-Rosen et al., 1985). The situation becomes further complicated once new coding schemes (e.g., Main et al.'s, 1985, "D" attachment classification category) are implemented and recodings of collected data reveal that initial estimates of competence were incorrect (cf. Carlson et al., this volume; Crittenden, 1988). Farber and Egeland (1987) have recently concluded that very few abused and neglected children appear invulnerable from the effects of abuse. However, in keeping with our transactional viewpoint, they do not believe that these effects are irreversible. Nonetheless, they caution against using the term "invulnerable" when describing maltreated children lest the impression be given that these children do not need help and are immune to the adverse experiences to which they have been exposed.

We believe that with increasingly differentiated development in a variety of domains, some maltreated children may turn out to be resilient. However, we would not be surprised to find some continuing latent vulnerabilities even in resilient maltreated children. That is, resilient maltreated children may manifest islets of difficulties in some domains while performing competently or better in many (or most) other areas. We do think that all maltreated children will "pay a price" for their misfortune, though we believe that, through therapy and/or adaptive re-representation of their experiences, many maltreated children will go on to lead productive lives. Obviously, these speculations can only be confirmed through rigorous longitudinal investigations.

7. *More research needs to be conducted documenting the effects that persistent poverty conditions exert upon child and family development.*

The study of maltreated children can be very helpful here. Because maltreated children often come from backgrounds characterized by persistent poverty, the comparison samples likewise must be drawn from the lower-socioeconomic status. Consequently, we can gain valuable information about the sequelae of poverty in the context of experimentally sound research in the area of child maltreatment (see Kaufman and Cicchetti, in press). Akin to our discussion of resiliency above, the study of disadvantaged children from poverty samples may likewise result in the identification of children who cope well with adverse conditions.

8. *Researchers should study the relationship between maltreatment and current and future psychopathology.*

9. *Studies focusing on maltreating parents from a developmental perspective are needed to complement the proportionately larger knowledge base on the maltreated children* (cf. Newberger and White, this volume).

10. *Additional studies need to be implemented that investigate how the community context affects the dynamics of child maltreatment* (cf. Garbarino, 1977; Garbarino and Gilliam, 1980).

11. *Research needs to be conducted comparing lower-socioeconomic status maltreating and nonmaltreating families to middle-socioeconomic status maltreating and nonmaltreating families. These studies will enable researchers to separate out the independent main effects of both maltreatment and social-class membership on child development and family functioning.*

12. *Because virtually no empirical work has been conducted with maltreating fathers or father-figures, we believe that such work should be accorded a high priority by researchers and funders.*

Research in child development (Lamb, 1976) and in family systems theory (Cicchetti, Cummings, Greenberg, and Marvin, in press; L'Abate, 1985) has shown that father-presence and father-absence (Hetherington, 1979) exert powerful impacts upon developmental functioning. Because maltreating families contain a variety of fathers or father-figures (Cicchetti and Todd-Manly, in press), the study of the role of males in maltreating families should contribute major information to the fields of child maltreatment and child development.

13. *In order to better understand the intergenerational aspects of child maltreatment, more research is needed on the extended family (e.g., grandparents, parents' siblings).*

14. *Additional work must be conducted in order to develop a psychometrically robust nosology of child maltreatment. This nosology should include explicit, reliably differentiable criteria for discriminating among the subtypes of maltreatment, as well as a scheme for conceptualizing the chronicity and severity of each maltreatment incident and subtype throughout the life course* (cf. Aber and Zigler, 1981; Besharov, 1981; Cicchetti and Barnett, in press; Cicchetti and Rizley, 1981).

15. *Developmental knowledge of maltreated children and their parents gathered from research programs should be used to guide clinical decision making*

and social policy formation (cf. Cicchetti et al., 1988; Wald et al., 1983, 1988).

16. *To date, very little experimentally sound preventive research/interventions have been conducted in the area of child maltreatment. Additional work clearly needs to be done on this important topic.*

References

Aber, J. L., and Allen, J. P. (1987). The effects of maltreatment on young children's socioemotional development: An attachment theory perspective. *Developmental Psychology, 23,* 406–414.

Aber, J. L., and Cicchetti, D. (1984). Socioemotional development in maltreated children: An empirical and theoretical analysis. In H. Fitzgerald, B. Lester, and M. Yogman (Eds.), *Theory and research in behavioral pediatrics,* Vol. II. New York: Plenum.

Aber, J. L., and Zigler, E. (1981). Developmental considerations in the definition of child maltreatment. *New Directions for Child Development, 11,* 1–29.

Achenbach, T. (in press). What is developmental about developmental psychopathology? In J. Rolf, A. Masten, D. Cicchetti, K. Neuchterlein and S. Weintraub (Eds.), *Risk and protective factors in the development of psychopathology.* New York: Cambridge University Press.

Ainsworth, M. (1973). The development of infant–mother attachment. In B. Caldwell and H. Ricciutti (Eds.), *Review of child development research, Volume 3.* Chicago: University of Chicago Press.

Ainsworth, M. D. S., Blehar, M. C., Waters, E., and Wall, S. (1978). *Patterns of attachment: A psychological study of the strange situation.* Hillsdale, NJ: Erlbaum.

Ainsworth, M., and Wittig, B. A. (1969). Attachment and exploratory behavior of 1-year-olds in a strange situation. In B. M. Foss (Ed.), *Determinants of infant behavior, 4,* New York: Wiley.

Alvy, K. T. (1975). Preventing child abuse. *American Psychologist, 30,* 921–928.

American Association for Protecting Children (AAPC) (1986). *Highlights of official child neglect and abuse reporting 1984.* Denver: The American Humane Association.

American Psychiatric Association Committee on Nomenclature (1987). *Diagnostic and Statistical Manual of Mental Disorders, III (Revised).* Washington, DC: American Psychiatric Association.

Aragona, J. A., and Eyberg, S. M. (1981). Neglected children: Mothers' report of child behavior problems and observed verbal behaviors. *Child Development, 52,* 596–602.

Ariès, P. (1962). *Centuries of childhood.* New York: Vintage Books.

Arieti, S. (1967). *The intrapsychic self.* New York: Basic Books.

Bates, E., Bretherton, I., Beeghly-Smith, M., and McNew, S. (1982). Social bases of language development: A reassessment. In H. Reese and L. Lipsitt (Eds.), *Advances in child development and behavior* (Vol. 16). New York: Academic Press.

Bayley, N. (1969). *The Bayley scales of infant development.* New York: Psychological Corporation.

Belsky, J. (1980). Child maltreatment: An ecological integration. *American Psychologist, 35,* 320–335.

Bemporad, J., Smith, H., Hanson, C., and Cicchetti, D. (1982). Borderline syndromes in childhood: Criteria for diagnosis. *American Journal of Psychiatry, 139,* 596–602.

Besharov, D. (1981). Toward better research on child abuse and neglect: Making definitional issues an explicit methodological concern. *Child Abuse and Neglect, 5,* 383–389.

Bertalanffy, L. von (1968). *General systems theory: Foundations, development, applications.* New York: Braziller.

Blager, F., and Martin, H. P. (1976). Speech and language of abused children. In H. P. Martin (Ed.), *The abused child.* Cambridge, MA: Ballinger.

Bleuler, E. (1911/1950). *Dementia praecox or the group of schizophrenias.* New York: International Universities Press.

Block, J. H., and Block, J. (1980). The role of ego-control and ego resiliency in the organization of behavior. In W. A. Collins (Ed.), *Minnesota Symposium on Child Psychology,* Vol. 13. Hillsdale, NJ: Erlbaum.

Bousha, D. M. and Twentyman, C. T. (1984). Mother–child interactional style in abuse, neglect, and control groups: Naturalistic observations in the home. *Journal of Abnormal Psychology, 93,* 106–114.

Bowlby, J. (1944). *Fourty-Four Juvenile Thieves.* London: Bailliere, Tindall and Cox.

Bowlby, J. (1951). *Maternal care and mental health.* (WHO Monograph No. 2). Geneva: World Health Organization.

Bowlby, J. (1977). The making and breaking of affectional bonds. *British Journal of Psychiatry, 130,* 201–210.

Bowlby, J. (1979). *The making and breaking of affectional bonds.* London: Tavistock Publications.

Bowlby, J. (1980). *Attachment and loss: Loss, sadness, and depression.* New York: Basic Books.

Bretherton, I. (Ed.) (1984). *Symbolic Play.* Orlando, FL: Academic Press.

Bretherton, I. (1985). Attachment theory: Retrospect and prospect. In I. Bretherton and E. Waters (Eds.), Growing points of attachment theory and research. *Monographs of the Society for Research in Child Development, 50* (1–2, Serial No. 209).

Bretherton, I. (1987). New perspectives on attachment relations. In J. Osofsky (Ed.), *Handbook of infant development,* Second Edition (pp. 1061–1100). New York: John Wiley and Sons.

Bretherton, I., Bates, E., Benigni, L., Camaioni, D., and Volterra, V. (1979). Relationships between cognition, communication, and quality of attachment. In E. Bates, L. Benigni, I. Bretherton, L. Camaioni, and V. Volterra (Eds.), *The emergence of symbols: Cognitions and communication in infancy.* New York: Academic Press.

Bretherton, I., and Beeghly, M. (1982). Talking about internal states: The acquisition of an explicit theory of mind. *Developmental Psychology, 18,* 906–921.

Bretherton, I., Fritz, J., Zahn-Waxler, C., and Ridgeway, D. (1986). Learning to talk about emotion: A functionalist perspective. *Child Development, 57,* 530–548.

Bronfenbrenner, U. (1979). *The ecology of human development: Experiments by nature and design.* Cambridge, MA: Harvard University Press.

Brown, R. (1973). *A first language: The early stages.* Cambridge, MA: Harvard University Press.

Bruner, J. S. (1975). The ontogenesis of speech acts. *Journal of Child Language, 2,* 1–19.

Bryer, J., Nelson, B., Miller, J. B., and Krol, B. (1987). Childhood sexual and physical abuse as factors in adult psychiatric illness. *American Journal of Psychiatry, 144,* 1426–1430.

Burgess, A., Hartman, C., and McCormack, A. (1987). Abused to abuser: Antecedents of socially deviant behaviors. *American Journal of Psychiatry, 144,* 1431–1436.

Burgess, R., and Conger, R. (1978). Family interaction in abusive, neglectful and normal families. *Child Development, 19,* 1163–1173.

Camras, L., Grow, J. G., and Ribordy, S. (1983). Recognition of emotional expression by abused children. *Journal of Clinical Child Psychology, 12,* 325–328.

Cassidy, J., and Marvin, M., in collaboration with the MacArthur Working Group on Attachment Beyond Infancy (1987). *Attachment organization in three- and-four-year-olds: Coding Guidelines.* Unpublished manual.

Children's Defense Fund (1979). *Children without homes: An examination of public responsibility to children in out-of-home care.* Washington, DC: Children's Defense Fund.

Cicchetti, D. (1984). The emergence of developmental psychopathology. *Child Development, 55,* 1–7.

Cicchetti, D. (in press). An historical perspective on the discipline of developmental psychopathology. In J. Rolf, A. Masten, D. Cicchetti, K. Neuchterlein, and S. Weintraub (Eds.),

Risk and protective factors in the development of psychopathology. New York: Cambridge University Press.

Cicchetti, D., and Aber, J. L. (1980). Abused children – abusive parents: an overstated case? *Harvard Educational Review, 50,* 244–255.

Cicchetti, D., and Aber, J. L. (1986). Early precursors to later depression: An organizational perspective. In L. Lipsitt and C. Rovee-Collier (Eds.), *Advances in infancy, Vol. 4.* Norwood, NJ: Ablex.

Cicchetti, D., and Barnett, D. (in press) Toward the development of a scientific nosology of child maltreatment. In D. Cicchetti and W. Grove (Eds.) *Thinking clearly about psychology: Essays in Honor of Paul E. Meehl.* Minneapolis: University of Minnesota Press.

Cicchetti, D., and Beeghly, M. (1987). Symbolic development in maltreated youngsters: An organizational perspective. In D. Cicchetti and M. Beeghly (Eds.), *Atypical Symbolic Development.* San Francisco: Jossey-Bass.

Cicchetti, D., and Braunwald, K. (1984). An organizational approach to the study of emotional development in maltreated infants. *The Journal of Infant Mental Health, 5,* 172–183.

Cicchetti, D., Cummings, E. M., Greenberg, M. T., and Marvin, R. (in press). An organizational perspective on attachment beyond infancy: Implications for theory, measurement, and research. In M. T. Greenberg, D. Cicchetti, and E. M. Cummings (Eds.), *Attachment in the preschool years: Theory, research, and intervention.* Chicago: University of Chicago Press.

Cicchetti, D., and Hesse, P. (1983). Affect and intellect: Piaget's contributions to the study of infant emotional development. In R. Plutchik and H. Kellerman (Eds.), *Emotion: Theory, research and experience,* Vol. II. New York: Academic Press.

Cicchetti, D., and Olsen, K. (in press, a). Borderline disorders in childhood. In M. Lewis and S. Miller (Eds.), *Handbook of developmental psychopathology.* New York: Plenum.

Cicchetti, D., and Olsen, K. (in press, b). The developmental psychopathology of child maltreatment. In M. Lewis and S. Miller (Eds.), *Handbook of developmental psychopathology.* New York: Plenum.

Cicchetti, D., and Rizley, R. (1981). Developmental perspectives on the etiology, intergenerational transmission, and sequelae of child maltreatment. *New Directions for Child Development, 11,* 31–55.

Cicchetti, D., and Schneider-Rosen, K. (1984). Theoretical and empirical considerations in the investigation of the relationship between affect and cognition in atypical populations of infants: Contributions to the formulation of an integrative theory of development. In C. Izard, J. Kagan, and R. Zajonc (Eds.), *Emotions, cognition and behavior.* New York: Cambridge University Press.

Cicchetti, D., and Schneider-Rosen, K. (1986). An organizational approach to childhood depression. In M. Rutter, C. Izard, and P. Read (Eds.), *Depression in young people, clinical and developmental perspectives.* New York: Guilford.

Cicchetti, D., and Sroufe, L. A. (1976). The relationship between affective and cognitive development in Down Syndrome infants. *Child Development, 47,* 920–929.

Cicchetti, D., and Sroufe, L. A. (1978). An organizational view of affect: Illustration from the study of Down's syndrome infants. In M. Lewis and L. Rosenblum (Eds.), *The development of affect.* New York: Plenum.

Cicchetti, D., Taraldson, B., and Egeland, B. (1978). Perspectives in the treatment and understanding of child abuse. In A. Goldstein (Ed.), *Perspectives for child mental health and education.* New York: Pergamon.

Cicchetti, D., and Todd-Manly, J. (in press). Problems and solutions to conducting research in maltreating families: An autobiographical perspective. In I. Sigel and G. Brody (Eds.), *Research on families.* New York: Academic Press.

Cicchetti, D., and Toth, S. (1987). The application of a transactional risk model to intervention with multi-risk maltreating families. *Zero to Three,* Vol. VII, 1–8.

Cicchetti, D., Toth, S., and Bush, M. (in press). Developmental psychopathology and incompetence in childhood: Suggestions for intervention. In B. Lahey and A. Kazdin (Eds.), *Advances in clinical child psychology.* New York: Plenum Press.

Cicchetti, D., Toth, S., Bush, M. A., and Gillespie, J. F. (1988). Stage-salient issues: A transactional model of intervention. *New Directions for Child Development, No. 39,* 123–145.

Clarke-Stewart, K. A. (1973). Interactions between mothers and their young children: Characteristics and consequences. *Monographs of the Society for Research in Child Development, 38,* Serial no. 153.

Cleckley, H. M. (1941/1976). *The mask of sanity.* St. Louis, MO: The C. V. Mosby Company.

Connell, D. (1976). *Individual differences in attachment behavior: Long term stability and relations to language development.* Unpublished doctoral dissertation, Syracuse University.

Coster, W., Gersten, M., Beeghly, M., and Cicchetti, D. (in press). Communicative functioning in maltreated toddlers. *Developmental Psychology.*

Cowen, E., Pederson, A., Babigian, H., Izzo, L., and Trost, M. (1973). Long-term follow-up of early detected vulnerable children. *Journal of Consulting and Clinical Psychology, 41,* 438–446.

Crittenden, P. M. (1981). Abusing, neglecting, problematic, and adequate dyads: Differentiating by patterns of interaction. *Merrill-Palmer Quarterly, 27,* 201–208.

Crittenden, P. M. (1988). Relationships at risk. In J. Belsky and T. Nezworski (Eds.), *Clinical implications of attachment theory.* Hillsdale, NJ: Erlbaum.

Cross, T. G. (1978). Motherese: Its association with rate of syntactic acquisition in young children. In N. Waterson and C. Snow (Eds.), *The development of communication: Social and pragmatic factors in language acquisition.* London: Wiley & Sons.

Cummings, E. M., Zahn-Waxler, C., and Radke-Yarrow, M. (1981). Young children's responses to expressions of anger and affection by others in the family. *Child Development, 52,* 1274–1282.

Daly, M., and Wilson, M. (1981). Child maltreatment from a sociobiological perspective. *New Directions for Child Development, 11,* 93–112.

Dean, A., Malik, M., Richards, W., and Stringer, S. (1986). Effects of parental maltreatment on children's conceptions of interpersonal relationships. *Developmental Psychology, 22,* 617–626.

DeLozier, P. (1982). Attachment theory and child abuse. In C. M. Parkes and J. Stevenson-Hinde (Eds.), *The place of attachment in human behavior.* London: Tavistock Publications.

Derdeyn, A. (1977). Child abuse and neglect: The rights of parents and the needs of their children. *American Journal of Orthopsychiatry, 47,* 377–387.

Deykin, E., Alpert, J., and McNamara, J. (1985). A pilot study of the effect of exposure to child abuse or neglect on adolescent suicidal behavior. *American Journal of Psychiatry, 142,* 1299–1303.

Dodge, K., Murphy, R., and Buchsbaum, K. C. (1984). The assessment of intention-cue detection skills in children: Implications for developmental psychopathology. *Child Development, 55,* 163–173.

Dubowitz, H. (1986). *Child maltreatment in the United States: Etiology, Impact and Prevention.* Background paper prepared for the Congress of the United States, Office of Technology Assessment.

Dubowitz, H., and Newberger, E. (in press). Pediatrics and child abuse. In D. Cicchetti and V. Carlson (Eds.), *Child maltreatment: Theory and research on consequences of child abuse and neglect.* New York: Cambridge University Press.

Egeland, B., Breitenbucher, M., and Rosenberg, D. (1980). Prospective study of the significance of life stress in the etiology of child abuse, *Journal of Consulting and Clinical Psychology,* Vol. 48, 195–205.

Egeland, B., and Sroufe, L. A. (1981). Developmental sequelae of maltreatment in infancy. *New Directions for Child Development, 11,* 77–92.

Elmer, E. (1977). *Fragile families, troubled children.* Pittsburgh, PA: University of Pittsburgh Press.

Emde, R. N., Gaensbauer, T., and Harmon, R. (1976). *Emotional expression in infancy: A biobehavioral study.* New York: International Universities Press.

Erikson, E. (1950). *Childhood and society.* New York: Norton.

Fanshel, D., and Shinn, E. G. (1972). *Dollars and sense in the foster care of children: A look at cost factors.* New York: Child Welfare League of America.

Farber, E., and Egeland, B. (1987). Invulnerability among abused and neglected children. In E. J. Anthony and B. Cohler (Eds.), *The invulnerable child* (pp. 253–288). New York: Guilford Press.

Feagans, L., and Farran, D. (Eds.) (1982). *The language of children reared in poverty.* New York: Academic Press.

Freud, A. (1965). *Normality and pathology in childhood: Assessments of development.* New York: International Universities Press.

Freud, S. (1955a). Fetishism. In J. Strachey (Eds.), *The standard edition of the complete psychological works of Sigmund Freud* (Vol. 21). London: Hogarth. (Originally published, 1927.)

Freud, S. (1955b). Analysis terminable and interminable. In J. Strachey (Ed.), *The standard edition of the complete works of Sigmund Freud* (Vol. 23). London: Hogarth. (Originally published, 1937.)

Frodi, A., and Lamb, M. (1980). Child abusers' responses to infant smiles and cries. *Child Development, 51,* 238–241.

Gaensbauer, T. J., and Sands, S. K. (1979). Distorted affective communications in abused/neglected infants and their potential impact on caretakers. *Journal of the American Academy of Child Psychiatry, 18,* 236–250.

Garbarino, J. A. (1976). A preliminary study of some ecological correlates of child abuse: The impact of socioeconomic stress on mothers. *American Journal of Orthopsychiatry, 47,* 372–381.

Garbarino, J. (1977). The human ecology of child maltreatment: A conceptual model for research. *Journal of Marriage and the Family, 39,* 721–732.

Garbarino, J., and Gilliam, G. (1980). *Understanding abusive families.* Lexington, MA: Lexington Press.

Garmezy, N. (1974). The study of competence in children at risk for severe psychopathology. In E. J. Anthony and C. Koupernik (Eds.), *The child in his family.* New York: Wiley.

Garmezy, N. (1983). Stressors of childhood. In N. Garmezy and M. Rutter (Eds.), *Stress, coping, and development in children.* New York: McGraw-Hill.

Garmezy, N., and Streitman, S. (1974). Children at risk: The search for the antecedents of schizophrenia. Part I: Conceptual models and research methods. *Schizophrenia Bulletin, 1*(8), 14–90.

George, C., and Main, M. (1979). Social interactions of young abused children: Approach, avoidance, and aggression. *Child Development, 50,* 306–318.

Gersten, M., Coster, W., Schneider-Rosen, K., Carlson, V., and Cicchetti, D. (1986). The socioemotional bases of communicative functioning: Quality of attachment, language development, and early maltreatment. In M. E. Lamb, A. L. Brown and B. Rogoff (Eds.), *Advances in developmental psychology,* Vol. 4. Hillsdale, NJ: Erlbaum.

Gil, D. B. (1970). *Violence against children: Physical child abuse in the United States.* Cambridge, MA: Harvard University Press.

Gleitman, L. R., Newport, E. L., and Gleitman, H. (1984). The current status of the motherese hypothesis. *Journal of Child Language, 11,* 43–79.

Goldstein, J., Freud, A., and Solnit, A. (1973). *Beyond the best interests of the child.* New York: Free Press.

Goldstein, K. (1939). *The organism.* New York: American Book Company.

Goldstein, K. (1940). *Human nature in the light of psychopathology.* Cambridge: Harvard University Press.

Goodman, G. S., and Rosenberg, M. S. (1987). The child witness to family violence. In D. J. Sonkin (Ed.), *Domestic violence on trial: Psychological and legal dimensions of family violence.* New York: Springer.

Greenberg, M., & Marvin, R. (1979). Attachment patterns in profoundly deaf preschool children. *Merrill-Palmer Quarterly, 25,* 265–279.

Greenberg, M. T., and Speltz, M. (1988). Attachment and the ontogeny of conduct problems.

In J. Belsky and T. Nezworski (Eds.), *Clinical implications of attachment.* Hillsdale, NJ: Erlbaum.

Greenspan, S. I., and Porges, S. W. (1984). Psychopathology in infancy and early childhood: Clinical perspectives on the organization of sensory and affective–thematic experience. *Child Development, 55,* 49–70.

Gruber, A. R. (1978). *Children in foster care.* New York: Human Science Press.

Guidano, V. F., and Liotti, G. (1983). *Cognitive processes and emotional disorders.* New York: Guilford.

Harter, S. (1983). Developmental perspectives on the self system. In E. M. Hetherington (Ed.), *Handbook of child psychology.* New York: Wiley.

Henderson, S. (1982). The significance of social relationships in the etiology of neurosis. In C. M. Parkes and J. Stevenson-Hinde (Eds.), *The place of attachment in human behavior.* London: Tavistock Publications.

Hess, R., and Shipman, V. (1968). Maternal influences upon early learning: The cognitive environments of urban preschool children. In R. Hess and R. Bear (Eds.), *Early education: Current theory, research, and action.* Chicago: Aldine.

Hesse, P., and Cicchetti, D. (1982). Perspectives on an integrated theory of emotional development. In D. Cicchetti and P. Hesse (Eds.), *New Directions for Child Development, 16, Emotional Development* (pp. 3–48).

Hetherington, E. M. (1979). Divorce: A child's perspective. *American Psychologist, 34,* 851–858.

Hobson, R. P. (1986). The autistic child's appraisal of expression of emotion. *Journal of Child Psychology and Psychiatry, 27,* 321–342.

Hoffman-Plotkin, D., and Twentyman, C. T. (1984). A multimodal assessment of behavioral and cognitive deficits in abused and neglected preschoolers. *Child Development, 55,* 794–802.

Hunter, R. S. and Kilstrom, N. (1979). Breaking the cycle in abusive families. *American Journal of Psychiatry, 136,* 1320–1322.

Inhelder, B. (1943/1968). *The diagnosis of reasoning in the mentally retarded.* New York: John Day.

Izard, C. (1977). *Human emotions.* New York: Plenum.

Izard, C., Kagan, J., and Zajonc, R. (Eds.) (1984). *Emotions, cognition, and behavior.* New York: Cambridge University Press.

Jackson, J. H. (1958). Evolution and dissolution of the nervous system. In J. Taylor (Ed.), *The selected writings of John Hughlings Jackson* (Vol. 2). New York: Basic Books (Originally published, 1884).

Juvenile Justice Standards Project (1977). *Standards relating to abuse and neglect.* Cambridge, MA: Ballinger.

Kanner, L. (1943). Autistic disturbances of affective contact. *Nervous Child, 2,* 217–250.

Kaplan, B. (1966). The study of language in psychiatry: The comparative developmental approach and its application to symbolization and language in psychopathology. In S. Arieti (Ed.), *American handbook of psychiatry.* New York: Basic Books.

Kaplan, B. (1967). Meditations on genesis. *Human Development, 10,* 65–87.

Kaplan, B. (1983). Genetic-dramatism: Old Wine in New Bottles. In S. Wapner and B. Kaplan (Eds.), *Toward a Holistic Developmental Psychology.* Hillsdale, NJ: Erlbaum.

Kaplan, S. J., Pelcovitz, D., Salzinger, S., and Ganeles, D. (1983). Psychopathology of parents of abused and neglected children and adolescents. *Journal of the American Academy of Child Psychiatry, 22,* 238–244.

Kaufman, J., and Cicchetti, D. (in press). The effects of maltreatment on school-aged children's socioemotional development: Assessments in a day camp setting. *Developmental Psychology.*

Kazdin, A. E., Moser, J., Colbus, D., and Bell, R. (1985). Depressive symptoms among physically abused and psychiatrically disturbed children. *Journal of Abnormal Psychology, 94,* 298–307.

Kempe, C. H. and Helfer, R. E. (1972). *Helping the battered child and his family.* Philadelphia: Lippincott.

Kempe, C. H., Silverman, F. N., Steele, B. B., Droegemueller, W., and Silver, H. K. (1962). The battered child syndrome. *Journal of the American Medical Association, 181,* 17–24.

Kempe, R., and Kempe, C. H. (1978). *Child abuse.* London: Fontana/Open Books.

Klein, G. S. (1951). The personal world through perception. In R. R. Blake and G. V. Ramsey (Eds.), *Perception: An approach to personality.* New York: Ronald Press.

Klein, G. S. (1954). Need and regulation. In M. R. Jones (Ed.), *Nebraska symposium on motivation* (Vol. 2). Lincoln: University of Nebraska Press.

Klein, G. S., and Schlesinger, H. J. (1949). Where is the perceiver in perceptual theory? *Journal of Personality, 18,* 32–47.

Knight, R., Roff, J., Barnett, J., and Moss, J. (1979). Concurrent and predictive validity of thought disorder and affectivity: A 22-year follow-up. *Journal of Abnormal Psychology, 88,* 1–12.

Kohlberg, L., LaCrosse, J., and Ricks, D. (1972). The predictability of adult mental health. In B. Wolman (Ed.), *Manual of child psychopathology.* New York: John Wiley & Sons.

Koocher, G. P. (Ed.) (1976). *Children's rights and the mental health professions.* New York: Wiley-Interscience.

Korbin, J. (Ed.) (1981). *Child abuse and neglect: Cross-cultural perspectives.* Berkeley: University of California Press.

Kovacs, M., Feinberg, T., Crouse-Novak, M., Paulauskas, S., and Finkelstein, R. (1984). Depressive disorders in childhood: I. A longitudinal prospective study of characteristics and recovery. *Archives of General Psychiatry, 41,* 229–237.

Kraepelin, E. (1919/1971). *Dementia praecox and paraphrenia.* New York: Robert E. Krieger Publishing Company, Inc.

Kropp, J., and Haynes, O. M. (1987). Abusive and nonabusive mothers' ability to identify general and specific emotion signals of infants. *Child Development, 58,* 187–190.

L'Abate, L. (Ed.) (1985). *The handbook of family psychology.* Homewood, IL: Dorsey Press.

Lamb, M. E. (Ed.) (1976). *The role of the father in child development.* New York: Wiley.

Lamb, M. (1982). Individual differences in infant sociability. In H. Reese and L. Lipsitt (Eds.), *Advances in child development and behavior.* New York: Academic Press.

Lewis, M., and Brooks-Gunn, J. (1979). *Social cognition and the acquisition of self.* New York: Plenum Press.

Lewis, M., Feiring, C. McGuffog, C., and Jaskir, J. (1984). Predicting psychopathology in six-year-olds from early social relations. *Child Development, 55,* 123–136.

Lewis, M., and Michalson, L. (1983). *Children's emotions and moods: Developmental theory and measurement.* New York: Plenum.

Lynch, M. (1985). Child abuse before Kempe: An historical literature review. *Child Abuse and Neglect, 9,* 7–15.

Mahler, M., Pine, F., and Bergman, A. (1975). *The psychological birth of the human infant.* New York: Basic Books.

Main, M. (1973). *Play, exploration and competence as related to child-adult attachment.* Unpublished doctoral dissertation, The John Hopkins University.

Main, M., and George, C. (1985). Response of abused and disadvantaged toddlers to distress in agemates: A study in the day care setting. *Developmental Psychology, 21,* 407–412.

Main, M., and Goldwyn, R. (1984). Predicting rejecting of her infant from mother's representation of her own experience: Implications for the abused–abusing intergenerational cycle. *Child Abuse and Neglect, 8,* 203–217.

Main, M., Kaplan, N., and Cassidy, J. C. (1985). Security in infancy, childhood and adulthood: A move to the level of representation. In I. Bretherton and E. Waters (Eds.), *Growing Points of Attachment Theory and Research: Monographs of the Society for Research in Child Development, 50* (Serial No. 209), Nos. 1–2, 66–104.

Main, M., and Solomon, J. (1986). Discovery of a disorganized disoriented attachment pattern.

In T. B. Brazelton and M. W. Yogman (Eds.), *Affective development in infancy*. Norwood, NJ: Ablex.

Main, M., and Solomon, J. (in press). Procedures for identifying infants as disorganized/disoriented during the Ainsworth Strange Situation. In M. Greenberg, D. Cicchetti, and M. Cummings (Eds.), *Attachment during the preschool years*. Chicago: University of Chicago Press.

Mans, L., Cicchetti, D., and Sroufe, L. A. (1978). Mirror reactions of Down's syndrome infants and toddlers: Cognitive underpinnings of self-recognition. *Child Development, 49,* 1247–1250.

Martin, H. P. (Eds.), (1976). *The abused child: Multidisciplinary approach to developmental issues and treatment*. Cambridge, MA: Ballinger.

Matas, L., Arend, R., and Sroufe, L. A. (1978). Continuity in adaptation in the second year: The relationship between quality of attachment and later competence. *Child Development, 49,* 547–556.

McCabe, V. (1984). Abstract perceptual information for age level: A risk factor for maltreatment? *Child Maltreatment, 55,* 267–276.

Mead, G. H. (1934). *Mind, self, and society: From the standpoint of a social behaviorist*. Chicago: University of Chicago Press.

Mnookin, R. (1973). Foster care: In whose best interest? *Harvard Educational Review, 43,* 599–638.

Nelson, K. (1973). Structure and strategy in learning to talk. *Monographs of the Society for Research in Child Development*. Serial no. 149, Vol. 38.

Nelson, B. (1984). *Making an Issue of Child Abuse*. Chicago: University of Chicago Press.

Nelson, K. E. (1977). Facilitating children's syntax acquisition. *Developmental Psychopathology, 13,* 101–107.

Oates, R. K. (1984). Personality development after physical abuse. *Archives of Diseases of Childhood, 59,* 147–150.

Parke, R. D., and Collmer, C. W. (1975). Child abuse: An interdisciplinary analysis. In E. Mavis Hetherington (Eds.), *Review of Child Development Research,* Vol. V, 509–590.

Patterson, G. (1982). *Coercive family process*. Eugene, OR: Castalia.

Pavenstedt, E. (1965). A comparison of the child-rearing environment of upper-lower and very low-lower class families. *American Journal of Orthopsychiatry, 35,* 89–98.

Pelton, L. (1978). Child abuse and neglect: The myth of classlessness. *American Journal of Orthopsychiatry, 48,* 608–617.

Pentz, T. (1975). *Facilitation of language acquisition: The role of the mother*. Unpublished doctoral dissertation, Johns Hopkins University.

Piaget, J. (1962). *Play, dreams and imitation in childhood*. New York: W. W. Norton.

Piaget, J. (1981). *Intelligence and affectivity: Their relationship during child development*. Palo Alto, CA: Annual Reviews. (Originally published, 1954).

Polier, J. W. (1975). Professional abuse of children: Responsibility for the delivery of services. *American Journal of Orthopsychiatry, 45,* 357–362.

Provence, S., & Lipton, R. (1962). *Infants in institutions*. NY: International Universities.

Radbill, S. X. (1968). A history of child abuse and infanticide. In R. E. Helfer and C. H. Kempe (Eds.), *The battered child*. Chicago: University of Chicago Press.

Reese, H., and Overton, W. (1970). Models of development and theories of development. In L. R. Goulet and P. Baltes (Eds.), *Life span developmental psychology: Research and theory*. New York: Academic Press.

Reid, J., Patterson, G., and Loeber, R. (1981). The abused child: Victim, instigator, or innocent bystander? *Nebraska Symposium on Motivation*. University of Nebraska Press.

Reite, M., and Caine, N. (Eds.) (1983). *Child abuse: The nonhuman primate data*. New York: Alan R. Liss, Inc.

Rieder, C., and Cicchetti, D. (in press). An organizational perspective on cognitive control functioning and cognitive-affective balance in maltreated children. *Developmental Psychology*.

Rodham, H. (1973). Children under the law. *Harvard Educational Review, 43,* 487–514.

Rogeness, G., Amrung, S., Macedo, C., Harris, W., and Fisher, C. (1986). Psychopathology in abused and neglected children. *Journal of the American Academy of Child Psychiatry, 25,* 659–665.

Rolf, J., and Garmezy, N. (1974). The school performance of children vulnerable to behavior pathology. In D. F. Ricks, T. Alexander, and M. Roff (Eds.), *Life history research in psychopathology, vol. 3.* Minneapolis: University of Minnesota Press.

Rolf, J., Masten, A., Cicchetti, D., Neuchterlein, K., and Weintraub, S. (in press). *Risk and protective factors in the development of psychopathology.* New York: Cambridge University Press.

Rosenberg, M. S. (1987). New directions for research on the psychological maltreatment of children. *American Psychologist, 42,* 166–171.

Ross, C. (1980). The lessons of the past: Defining and controlling child abuse in the United States. In G. Gerbner, C. Ross, and E. Zigler (Eds.), *Child abuse: An agenda for action.* New York/Oxford: Oxford University Press.

Rubin, K., Fein, G., and Vandenberg, B. (1983). Play. In P. Mussen (Ed.), *Handbook of child psychology, Vol. 4: Socialization.* New York: Wiley.

Ruppenthal, G., Arling, G., Harlow, H., Sackett, G., and Suomi, S. (1976). A 10-year perspective of motherless mother monkey behavior. *Journal of Abnormal Psychology, 85,* 341–349.

Rutter, M. (1972/1981). *Maternal deprivation reassessed.* Harmondsworth, Eng.: Penguin Books.

Rutter, M., and Garmezy, N. (1983). Developmental psychopathology. In P. Mussen (Ed.), *Handbook of child psychology.* vol. IV. (pp. 775–911). New York: Wiley and Sons.

Rutter, M., and Giller, H. (1983). *Juvenile delinquency.* New York: Guilford Press.

Rutter, M., Tizard, J., and Whitmore, K. (1970/1981). *Education, health and behavior.* Krieger: Huntington, NY. (Originally published, 1970, London, Longmans).

Sackett, G., Sameroff, A., Cairns, R., and Suomi, S. (1981). Continuity in behavioral development: Theoretical and empirical issues. In K. Immelmann, G. Barlow, L. Petrinovich, and M. Main (Eds.), *Behavioral development.* Cambridge: Cambridge University Press.

Salzinger, S., Kaplan, S., Pelcovitz, D., Samit, C., and Krieger, R. (1984). Parent and teacher assessment of children's behavior in child maltreating families. *Journal of the American Academy of Child Psychiatry, 23,* 458–464.

Sameroff, A., and Chandler, M. (1975). Reproductive risk and the continuum of caretaking causalty. In F. Horowitz (Ed.), *Review of child development research* (Vol. 4). Chicago, IL: University of Chicago Press.

Santostefano, S. (1978). *A bio-developmental approach to clinical child psychology.* New York: Wiley.

Santostefano, S., and Baker, H. (1972). The contribution of developmental psychology. In B. Wolman (Ed.), *Manual of child psychopathology* (pp. 1113–1153). New York: McGraw-Hill.

Schneider-Rosen, K., Braunwald, K., Carlson, V., and Cicchetti, D. (1985). Current perspectives in attachment theory: Illustration from the study of maltreated infants. In I. Bretherton and E. Waters (Eds.), *Monographs of the society for research in child development, 50,* (Serial No. 209), 194–210.

Schneider-Rosen, K., and Cicchetti, D. (1984). The relationship between affect and cognition in maltreated infants: Quality of attachment and the development of visual self-recognition. *Child Development, 55,* 648–658.

Silvern, L. (1984). Emotional–behavioral disorders: A failure of system functions. In E. Gollin (Ed.), *Malformations of development* (pp. 95–152). New York: Academic Press.

Sinclair, H. (1970). The transition from sensory-motor behavior to symbolic activity. *Interchange, 1,* 119–126.

Slade, A. (1987). A longitudinal study of maternal involvement and symbolic play during the toddler period. *Child Development, 58,* 367–375.

Snow, C., and Ferguson, C. (1977). *Talking to children.* Cambridge: Cambridge University Press.

Snow, C. E. and Gilbreath, B. J. (1983). Explaining transitions. In R. M. Golinkoff (Ed.), *The transition from prelinguistic to linguistic communication.* Hillsdale, NJ: Erlbaum.

Sorce, J., and Emde, R. N. (1981). Mother's presence is not enough: Effect of emotional availability on infant exploration. *Developmental Psychology, 17,* 737–745.

Spiker, D., and Ricks, M. (1984). Visual self-recognition in autistic children: Developmental relationships. *Child Development, 55,* 214–225.

Spinetta, J. J., and Rigler, D. (1972). The child-abusing parent: A psychological review. *Psychological Bulletin, 77,* 296–304.

Spitz, R. (1965). *The first year of life: A psychoanalytic study of normal and deviant object relations.* New York: International Universities Press.

Spitz, R., and Wolf, K. (1946). Anaclitic depression: An inquiry into the genesis of psychiatric conditions in early childhood, II. *Psychoanalytic Study of the Child, 2,* 313–342.

Sroufe, L. A. (1979a). Socioemotional development. In J. Osofsky (Ed.), *Handbook of infant development.* New York: Wiley.

Sroufe, L. A. (1979b). The coherence of individual development. *American Psychologist, 34,* 834–841.

Sroufe, L. A. (1983). Infant–caregiver attachment and patterns of adaptation in preschool: The roots of maladaptation and competence. In M. Perlmutter (Eds.), *Minnesota Symposium on Child Psychology, 16.*

Sroufe, L. A. (1988). The role of infant-caregiver attachment in development. In J. Belsky and T. Nezworski (Eds.), *Clinical implications of attachment,* Hillsdale, NJ: Erlbaum.

Sroufe, L. A., and Fleeson, J. (1986). Attachment and the construction of relationships. In W. Hartup and Z. Rubin (Eds.), *Relationships and development.* Hillsdale, NJ: Erlbaum.

Sroufe, L. A., and Rutter, M. (1984). The domain of developmental psychopathology. *Child Development, 55,* 1184–1199.

Sroufe, L. A. and Waters, E. (1976). The ontogenesis of smiling and laughter: A perspective on the organization of development in infancy. *Psychological Review, 83,* 173–189.

Steele, B. F. and Pollock, C. B. (1968). A psychiatric study of parents who abuse infants and small children. In R. E. Helfer and C. H. Kempe (Eds.), *The battered child.* Chicago: The University of Chicago Press.

Stern, D. (1985). *The interpersonal world of the infant: A view from psychoanalysis and developmental psychology.* New York: Basic Books.

Straus, M. A., and Gelles, R. J. (1986). Change in family violence from 1975–1985. *Journal of Marriage and the Family, 48,* 465–479.

Sundby, H., and Kreyberg, P. (1969). *Prognosis in child psychiatry.* Baltimore: Williams and Wilkens.

Tarter, R., Hegedus, A., Winston, M., and Alterman, A. (1984). Neuropsychological, personality, and familial characteristics of physically abused delinquents. *Journal of the American Academy of Child Psychiatry, 23,* 668–674.

Trad, P. V. (1986). *Infant depression: Paradigms and paradoxes.* New York: Springer-Verlag.

Trivers, R. L. (1974). Parent–offspring conflict. *American Zoologist, 14,* 249–264.

Twitchell, T. E. (1951). The restoration of motor function following hemiplegia in man. *Brain, 74,* 443–480.

Twitchell, T. E. (1970). Reflex mechanisms and the development of prehension. In K. J. Connolly (Ed.), *Mechanisms of motor skill development.* New York: Academic Press.

Uzgiris, I., and Hunt, J. (1975). *Assessment in infancy.* Urbana: University of Illinois Press.

Vygotsky, L. S. (1978). *Mind in society.* Cambridge, MA: Harvard University Press.

Waddington, C. H. (1957). *The strategy of genes.* London: Allen and Unwin.

Waddington, C. H. (1966). *Principles of development and differentiation.* New York: Macmillan.

Wald, M. S. (1975). State intervention on behalf of neglected children: A search for realistic standards. *Stanford Law Review, 27,* 985–1040.

Wald, M. S., Carlsmith, J. and Leiderman, P. H. (1988). *Protecting abused/neglected children: A comparison of home and foster placement.* Stanford, CA: Stanford University Press.

Wald, M. S., Carlsmith, J., Leiderman, P., and Smith, C. (1983). Intervention to protect abused and neglected children. In M. Perlmutter (Ed.), *Minnesota Symposium on Child Psychology*, Vol. 16. Hillsdale, NJ: Erlbaum.

Wasserman, G., Green, A., and Allen, R. (1983). Going beyond abuse: Maladaptive patterns of interaction in abusing mother–infant pairs. *Journal of the American Academy of Child Psychiatry, 22,* 245–252.

Waters, E., and Sroufe, L. A. (1983). Competence as a developmental construct. *Developmental Review, 3,* 79–97.

Weiss, P. A. (1969a). The living system: Determinism stratified. In A. Koestler and J. Smythies (Eds.), *Beyond reductionism*. Boston: Beacon Press.

Weiss, P. A. (1969b). *Principles of development*. New York: Hafner.

Werner, H. (1948). *Comparative psychology of mental development*. New York: International Universities Press.

Werner, H. (1957). The concept of development from a comparative and organismic point of view. In D. Harris (Ed.), *The concept of development*. Minneapolis: University of Minnesota Press.

Werner, H., and Kaplan, B. (1963). *Symbol formation: An organismic–developmental approach to language and the expression of thought*. New York: Wiley.

Westerman, M., and Haustead, L. F. (1982). A pattern-oriented model of caretaker–child interaction, psychopathology and control. In K. Nelson (Ed.), *Children's language,* Vol. 3. Hillsdale, NJ: Erlbaum.

Wilden, A. (1980). *System and structure*. London: Tavistock.

Wilson, J., and Herrnstein, R. (1985). *Crime and human nature*. New York: Simon and Schuster.

Zahn-Waxler, C., and Radke-Yarrow, M. (1982). The development of altruism: Alternative research strategies. In N. Eisenberg (Ed.), *Development of social behavior*. New York: Academic Press.

Zigler, E. (1976). Controlling child abuse: An effort doomed to failure? In W. A. Collins (Ed.), *Newsletter of the Division on Developmental Psychology, American Psychological Association,* February, 17–30.

14   Child maltreatment and attachment theory

Patricia M. Crittenden and Mary D. S. Ainsworth

The study of child maltreatment has grown exponentially in the years since the identification of the "battered child syndrome" (Kempe, Silverman, and Steele, 1962). In that time the area has experienced many of the conflicts and missteps to be expected in an emerging field. Underlying these problems is the lack of a single, comprehensive theoretical approach to child maltreatment (Newberger, Newberger, and Hampton, 1983). It is the purpose of this chapter to examine attachment theory in regard to its adequacy in accounting for the existing data on child abuse and child neglect.

Because child abuse was identified as a social issue earlier than child neglect, it will be discussed first. However, in regard to the early literature, the dichotomy is difficult, and sometimes impossible, to make because cases of neglect or abuse-with-neglect were included indiscriminately under the rubric of abuse. One goal of this chapter will be to disentangle the conditions and consider separately how relevant attachment theory is to understanding them.

The first studies of child abuse focused on identifying the characteristics of abusers. Although abusers were not usually found to be mentally ill, they were often described as more aggressive, punitive, domineering, and inconsistent than nonabusing parents. As more cases of less severe child abuse were reported and investigated, the incidence of clear parental deviance decreased while the evidence for cultural and child influence increased. The societal variables associated with abuse included unemployment, job dissatisfaction, single-parent families, and social isolation of low-income, multiproblem families. More recently, there has been a focus on those charac-

This work was supported in part by grant #90–CA–844 from the National Center on Child Abuse and Neglect to the first author.

teristics of children that may make them targets for abuse. Premature, handicapped, and temperamentally difficult children have all been identified as at risk for abuse (Maden and Wrench, 1977; National Center on Child Abuse and Neglect, 1978; Parke and Collmer, 1975).

Eventually, broader definitions of abuse and increases in both the data base and the types of hypotheses being tested lead to two general conclusions: (1) that all "bad" things were related to abuse (low income, stress, abuse as a child, impoverished neighborhoods, unemployment, infant birth complications or handicapping conditions, limited parental education, and the cultural value placed on physical punishment) and (2) that abusers were not easily distinguishable from nonabusers.

An early attempt by Helfer (1973) to integrate all of this information resulted in the explanation that abuse occurred when a deviant parent of an at risk child was in an especially stressful situation (within a society that encourages violence). Not only has this hypothesis never been tested under conditions that independently assess the several factors, but also very little attention has been given to the probability that these factors are causally interrelated. Neither has the relative influence of the correlates of abuse been investigated satisfactorily. Furthermore, the research has not adequately explained the large numbers of families with one or more risk conditions who do *not* abuse their children. The emphasis has largely been one of identifying as many cases as possible and seeking linear, additive explanations for their etiology.

Our knowledge about neglect is considerably more scant (Wolock and Horowitz, 1984). However, there is evidence that failing to provide adequate care for children (as opposed to providing inappropriate care) is associated with extreme poverty, maternal depression, social isolation, and maternal retardation (Polansky, Chalmers, Buttenwieser, and Williams, 1981; Polansky, Hally, and Polansky, 1976). However, it is not clear that these conditions *cause* neglect. There is certainly evidence that not all low-income or retarded mothers are neglectful, as well as evidence that some economically advantaged and higher IQ mothers are unresponsive to their children's needs. Again, one contribution that a theoretical perspective could offer would be to tie these conditions together logically in ways that would predict and explain the pattern of occurrence of neglect.

More recently, investigators have pursued a more sophisticated approach than the single- or additive-cause models described above. Both Garbarino (1977) and Belsky (1980) have proposed comprehensive ecological models of maltreatment. However, such models replace naive simplicity with infinite complexity. Total specification of the necessary, sufficient, and contributing causes of maltreatment in even one case may be impossible; for large numbers of cases, it becomes unrealistic. What is needed is a way to narrow our view to a workable model that can both explain the pattern of occurrences and nonoccurrences of maltreatment and describe the process by which maltreatment is transmitted from one person to another (Aber and Zigler, 1981; Cicchetti and Rizley, 1981). Such a model should also be sufficiently focused that it has implications for intervention.

There is a need to focus on the "critical causes" of maltreatment – that is, those causes which, if changed, would lead to improvements in the other detrimental conditions and, thus, to improved family functioning. Because simply undoing the situation that caused maltreatment might not be the most effective or feasible way to correct it, such causes might imply one thing for the prevention of maltreatment and another for the amelioration of existing maltreatment.

The thesis of this chapter is that anxious (or insecure) attachment is a critical concept in regard to both the origin of family maltreatment and the rehabilitation of families. There are many advantages of such a hypothesis. First, it permits an integration of much of the existing knowledge about maltreatment around a single, although not simple, concept while concurrently permitting the differentiation of abuse from neglect. Second, because attachment theory is a developmental theory, it is responsive to differences in the nature and effects of anxious attachment at different points in the lifespan. As others have pointed out, it is impossible to develop appropriate diagnostic and treatment procedures without an awareness of developmentally salient issues (Cicchetti and Rizley, 1981; Sroufe and Rutter, 1984). Third, this lifespan approach is very compatible with a family perspective on maltreatment and, in fact, is incompatible with an approach focused entirely on individuals. Fourth, attachment theory also permits the integration of "external" (i.e., environmental) conditions and events with interpersonal conditions as interlocking influences upon the development of attachment. The advantage of combining these perspectives in the context of a focus on attachment is that risk status can be considered to vary across both families and time depending upon individuals' past experiences, current contextual factors, and developmental processes as well as random (or unexpectable) events without collapsing the model into an overly simplistic everything-is-interconnected approach. Finally, although issues regarding maltreatment are not generally open to testing by experimental means, attachment theory does facilitate the posing of specific hypotheses that can be tested with maltreating samples. Moreover, the extent to which attachment-related concepts account for the data may be compared to that of other theoretical approaches. Thus, attachment theory is compatible with ecological theory and also provides a specific focus and predicted hierarchy of influences.

This chapter will first consider some of the basic concepts of attachment theory and, then, apply those ideas specifically to maltreatment, considering the extent of empirical support for those propositions.

Attachment theory

Attachment theory is a relatively new, open-ended theory with eclectic underpinnings. Intended as a revision of psychoanalytic theory, particularly Freudian instinct theory and metapsychology, it has been infused by present-day biological principles with an emphasis on ethology and evolutionary theory, as well as by control-systems theory and cognitive psychology. Although it began with an attempt to understand the disturbed functioning of individuals who had experienced traumatic losses or early separations, it is a theory of normal development that offers explanations for some types of atypical development (Bowlby, 1969, 1973, 1980). Since Bowlby's preliminary formulation (Bowlby, 1958), it has stimulated research into socioemotional development and the growth of interpersonal relationships and has been responsive to the findings of such research with continuous clarifications, refinements, and extensions of applications. For example, it suggests a causal relationship between anomalies of attachment in the parent and abuse of the child (Ainsworth, 1980).

Ethological theory proposes that there are species-characteristic patterns of behavior that have evolved because they function to promote species survival – or to be more specific, gene survival. The propensity to develop these behaviors is transmitted genetically and evoked by specific and expectable internal and environmental conditions. Attachment theory applies this principle to the almost universal occurrence of infant attachment to the parent and of parental caregiving to the infant, as well as to attachment components in close relationships between adult partners (Ainsworth, 1985, Bowlby, 1969, 1979).

Attachment as a developmental construct

Bowlby (1969) proposed that the survival of humans and, especially, human infants is best ensured when proximity to an attachment figure is maintained. Such proximity is initially accomplished through complementary maternal and infant patterns of behavior. Infant signals such as crying tend universally to attract mothers into closer proximity. Such infant behaviors tend to be elicited by alarming situations, such as those involving loud noises, looming objects, strange persons or objects, and being left alone, as well as by internal discomfort or pain. Once close bodily contact is attained, aversive signals such as crying tend to be terminated and other behaviors, such as smiling, clinging, and vocalizing, function to maintain contact with and/or proximity to the mother.

Thus the "predictable" outcome of an infant's attachment behavior is the attainment of proximity to a trusted person (Bowlby, 1969). Subjectively, this outcome usually brings a feeling of security. Attachment behavior may be activated also by undue time or distance away from an attachment figure, even though there may be no perception of external threat and no other experience of internal discomfort. Such behavior, however, is not peculiar to the young infant. Although the tolerable time periods and distances increase with age and experience, most older children and adults feel lonely and anxious when separated from their loved ones either inexplicably or for too long, and they too seek the support of an attachment figure during periods of stress (Bowlby, 1979).

An infant's primary attachment(s) develop through three phases in the course of the first year, clear-cut attachment usually being achieved about the middle of the first year with the emergence of behaviors such as locomotion that enable the baby to take initiative in keeping proximity and seeking contact. Most attachment research has been devoted to this third active phase, but it gradually gives way to a fourth and much more sophisticated phase, beginning sometime after a child's third birthday, with the development of what Bowlby (1969) termed a "goal-corrected partnership" between child and mother. This advance is made possible both by the increased effectiveness of communication between the partners through the child's burgeoning language skills and by his or her increased ability to see the world through the perspective of another. As the child becomes more able to understand that the mother has motivations, feelings, and plans of her own, and as he or she becomes better able to communicate motivations, feelings, and plans to her, they, as partners, become able to negotiate differences in plans and often reach mutual agreement about them (Marvin, 1977; Marvin and Greenberg, 1982). Meanwhile the child's competence has increased, and he or she has become able to sustain confidence in the attachment figures across increasingly long periods of absence from them. The upshot of all of this is that a child's sense of security no longer depends so much on the actual presence of the attachment figure as upon the mutual trust and understanding that has been built up in the partnership. However, should the parent herself (or himself) be handicapped either in perspective-taking or in being able to communicate motivation, feelings, and plans to the child, the child's latent capacities for perspective taking and for clearer communication may well remain undeveloped or, if developed, be likely to fail in producing mutual understanding and trust. Nevertheless, normally, a partnership will be established based on mutual understanding and trust that each partner will be vigilant in regard to the other's perception of danger and will seek proximity whenever time, distance, or other relevant conditions cause a reduction in felt security.

By adolescence, attachments can be maintained without actual physical proximity for increasingly long periods of time. During absences, distal modes of communication, such as letters and phone calls, can temporarily replace proximity and contact. Furthermore, adolescents become active in a search for new attachments outside the family, and more consciously accept some of the responsibility for being an attachment figure to new partners.

Even in adulthood, stable, affectionate relationships are wanted and needed by most people. A parent, of course, is expected not only to manage a reciprocal attachment with his or her partner, but concurrently to be a caring and nurturant attachment figure in the nonsymmetric relationship with his or her child. According to Bowlby, attachment – first to the parents and later to a partner or spouse – is basic to the security of all.

Attachment as a behavioral system

The attachment system is but one of the important species-characteristic behavioral systems that forward survival. The individual's overt behavior in any one set of circumstances depends upon the relative strength of activation of his behavioral systems, with the most intensely activated having the most effect. Whereas some systems may often act in synchrony – as, for example, when fear leads both to the avoidance of the object feared and to seeking contact with an attachment figure – other systems are usually antithetical, so that when one is intensely activated the other is at least temporarily submerged.

In infancy the two behavioral systems that chiefly compete with the attachment system are the exploratory and affiliative systems. As long as the infant's attachment system is the more highly activated and his behavior is primarily functioning to ensure proximity to an attachment figure, he or she is not free to explore the environment. If an infant feels secure in his relationship with his mother, however, he can use her as a secure base from which he can become acquainted with his world and the other people in it (Ainsworth, 1967). This antithetical arrangement itself has survival value, for it is critical to an infant's cognitive, language, and social development that he have experience with his physical and social environment. Because he gains his experience while sustaining reasonable proximity to a caregiving figure, the experience is not gained under risky conditions.

Although older children and adults normally require much less proximity to their attachment figures than do infants, much the same principle pertains to them. Although they, too, enjoy being with those to whom they are attached, much of the time they feel free to respond to other demands on their time and attention and to follow up other interests and activities. However, as Bretherton (1980) suggested, the attachment system functions primarily as a security-maintenance system. Throughout life, attachment behavior is most intensely activated under stressful conditions that evoke alarm or anxiety. Yet the development of knowledge about the world, competence, and self-reliance are fostered by feeling secure about the availability of attachment figures when needed. Thus, the nature of the conditions that elicit attachment behavior is modified by each person's own experience, particularly the nature or quality of his or her past and present relationships with attachment figures.

Attachment as a qualitative construct

The principal quantitative dimension of an attachment is the degree to which it is characterized by feelings of security or insecurity. However, qualitative distinctions are equally important. These indicate the various ways in which a person organizes his or her behavior, thoughts, and feelings toward an attachment figure. In infancy, three major patterns, together with eight subpatterns, have been distinguished and are especially highlighted in a laboratory situation called the "Strange Situation" (Ainsworth, Blehar, Waters, and Wall, 1978). The major patterns are indicative of (1) secure attachment, with four subpatterns, (2) anxious/avoidant attachment, with two subpatterns, and (3) anxious/ambivalent or anxious/resistant attachment, also with two subpatterns. The discussion below will focus on the relation between maternal behavior and infant pattern of attachment, the antecedents of maternal insensitivity or unresponsiveness, and adjustments to the classificatory system made to account for the behavior of disturbed children, including maltreated children.

Maternal behavior and infant pattern of attachment. Infant patterns of attachment are believed to be closely related to the behavior of the attachment figure in question, although the chief evidence of this so far pertains to mothers as attachment figures. Such evidence stems from the work of Ainsworth et al. (1978), although subsequently other studies have yielded confirmatory evidence (e.g., Belsky, Rovine, and Taylor, 1984; Egeland and Farber, 1984; Grossmann, Grossmann, Spangler, Suess, and Unzer, 1985).

An infant whose mother is sensitive in her responsiveness to infant signals usually displays positive affect in interaction with her and cries relatively little even in little everyday separations from her. When his attachment behavior has been intensely activated (for example, by separation from her under unaccustomed circumstances), he tends to be easily reassured and comforted by her close presence, and is soon ready again to pursue his activities. Such an infant is judged to be securely attached to his mother.

However, an infant whose mother tends to be inaccessible, unresponsive, or inappropriately responsive to his behavioral cues is likely to emerge as insecure or anxious in his attachment to her. Because his bids for proximity and contact tend often to be frustrated, attachment behavior persists and tends to intensify and to become mingled with anger. Consequently, when his mother does respond, he behaves ambivalently and is hard to soothe. Since he cannot rely on her to be accessible, he is vigilant for any indications of decreased proximity and displays more distress at little everyday separations or threats thereof. Such behavior is characteristic of the anxious/ambivalent pattern of attachment.

Infants showing an anxious/avoidant pattern of attachment have experienced interaction with mothers who are also inaccessible, unresponsive, or inappropriately responsive to their behavioral cues. These infants behave at home much as the anxious/ambivalent babies do. When the stress is relatively high, however, as in the Strange Situation, they behave quite differently. They show little stress upon separation and upon reunion they display avoidance of the mother rather than seeking proximity to her. Others display a mingling of avoidance and proximity seeking upon reunion. This avoidance has been identified as a defensive maneuver, similar to the detachment shown by young children after long, depriving separations from their mothers.

The mothers of these anxious/avoidant babies differ from the mothers of anxious/ambivalent babies in Ainsworth's sample in that the latter are merely inconsistent in their responsiveness and accessibility, whereas the former were more rejecting and angry, whether overtly or covertly. Because these mothers manifested an aversion to close bodily contact, it appeared that this rejection was most likely to be expressed by rebuffing or withholding close bodily contact when the baby most needed it – for example, when his attachment behavior was activated at high intensity. This implies that the baby experiences a severe approach/avoidance conflict whenever he most wants to be close to his mother, for he not only feels angry because he expects her to be unresponsive, but he also fears he may be painfully rebuffed. The avoidant defense seems to enable him to disconnect his attachment behavior from the situational cues that usually activate it. Consequently, he interprets neither his mother's departure nor her return as cues for wanting close contact with her. He avoids both the contact-seeking and the anger that seem likely to evoke rebuff. Recently, Grossmann et al. (1985) reported that a disproportionate number of their sample of North German infants showed an anxious/avoidant pattern, which they attributed to cultural pressure to encourage independence as early as the middle of the first year (rather than to maternal attitudes of rejection). This suggests that in infancy it is the withholding of close bodily contact – with or without rejecting attitudes – that accounts for the anxious/avoidant pattern.

The antecedents of maternal insensitivity or unresponsiveness. There are a number of situations that can result in maternal insensitivity. If a mother herself is securely attached to no one, it is expected that it will be difficult for her to respond to her child in such a way that he can become securely attached to her (Bowlby, 1973). Indeed, if she has had a history of anxious attachment herself, there is increased likelihood that her own attachment behavior will be in conflict with her infant's. Because even normal infant signals may seem overdemanding to her, the angry, escalated attachment behavior of a child whose attachment to her has already become anxious may be highly noxious. She may delay or avoid responding or become angry at his demands. Thus, a pattern of anxious attachment may be communicated and passed on to a child from its parent. Evidence that a mother's unresolved distress resulting from childhood experiences with her own parent can affect the quality of her relationship with her infant has been demonstrated in a study comparing the results of an Adult Attachment Interview given to the mothers (George, Kaplan, and Main, 1985) with the Strange Situation classifications of the children in infancy as well as their attachment as assessed at 6 years of age (Main, Kaplan, and Cassidy, 1985). Mothers in that study who were accepting of their relationships with their own parents tended to have securely attached infants and children. This does not mean that the secure infants and children necessarily had mothers whose childhood relationships were similarly secure. Rather, it suggests that those mothers who acknowledged and accepted the reality of their own difficult childhood situations, often even forgiving their mothers, were best able to mitigate the expected negative effects of their previous insecure relationships and to provide their children with a sensitive and responsive attachment figure. In some cases their means for doing so may have included the development of a secure relationship with a surrogate attachment figure and successful counseling or psychotherapy.

Other situations that are especially likely to result in extremes of unresponsiveness or inappropriate responsiveness on the part of an adult in interaction with his or her child include unresolved traumatic separations from or permanent loss of attachment figures. In two samples, parents who had suffered loss of a significant attachment figure in childhood were particularly likely to have anxiously attached infants whose behavior did not fit the Ainsworth classificatory system (Ainsworth and Eichberg, in press; Main, Kaplan, and Cassidy, 1985). Periods of depression or other severe emotional or mental disturbance for the parent, recent death of a significant figure, and childhood experiences of abuse, including sexual abuse, may interfere with normal reactions to close contact. Such situations can result in either inconsistencies in the parental patterns of caregiving or in persistent distortions; the effects of these two conditions are expected to be somewhat different.

Adjustments to the classificatory system. Although all 56 of the infants in the original samples used to develop the classificatory system could be classified in one of the three major patterns, it was believed from the beginning that the behavior of some infants would not fit this classificatory scheme. Indeed, a number of investigators have identified infants whose behavior does not fit comfortably into any of three patterns described by Ainsworth (Crittenden, 1985 a, 1985b; Main and Weston, 1981; Radke-Yarrow, Cummings, Kuczynski, and Chapman, 1985; Spieker and Booth, in press). Two approaches to expanding the classificatory system have been taken. One grew out of attempts to better describe the behavior of a number of apparently normal children whose behavior in the Strange Situation could not be satisfactorily classified using the Ainsworth criteria (Main and Weston, 1981). The other approach was the result of studies of samples of maltreated or low birthweight infants and infants of severely depressed mothers.

The children identified by Main and Weston as unclassified were later classified as "disorganized/disoriented" (Main and Solomon, in press). It was not assumed that this constituted a fourth pattern. Indeed it seemed that each of these infants showed disorganization of one of the three major patterns previously identified. Such disorganizations did tend to imply even more extreme insecurity than the basic patterns of which they were variations.

In otherwise normal families, a disorganized pattern of infant attachment appears to result from inconsistency of maternal behavior rather than persistent distortion. This inconsistency is not the day-to-day mixture of sensitivity and unresponsiveness that is associated with mothers of infants with an anxious/ambivalent pattern. Rather, it appeared to occur when the mother has first been consistent for a sufficiently extended period of time that the infant has formed expectations about her behavior. This consistency is then interrupted by the sudden interjection of quite different behavior. Such violations of expectations are especially frightening to the child if the unexpected maternal behavior is itself threatening or if the mother herself appears frightened (Main and Hesse, in press).

In contrast, when the mother's behavior is thought to be consistently and severely distorted, the child has both a basis for developing expectations and a need to adapt to bizarre and unsatisfying conditions. This situation has led to the second approach to expanding the classificatory system. The behavior in the Strange Situation of many children of such mothers does not fit the classificatory system devised by Ainsworth. Although the behavioral markers she described are present, they are organized differently than in the normal samples used for the development of the classificatory system. Children of these consistently insensitive mothers may show in one observation period all of the major types of behavior described by Ainsworth: the high proximity seeking usually indicative of secure or anxious/ambivalent attachment, the high avoidance indicative of avoidant attachment, and the high resistance indicative of ambivalent attachment (Crittenden, 1985 a, 1985b; Radke-Yarrow et al., 1985.) In addition, many of the children showed the stereotypic behaviors described by Ainsworth for one of the secure subpatterns. Both the Crittenden and Radke-Yarrow research groups classified the children showing this pattern as avoidant/ambivalent (A/C). The Crittenden observations are particularly relevant here because they pertain to maltreated children. In two separate samples, maltreated children who had experienced abuse or abuse-and-neglect were frequently classified as A/C_1 or A/C_2 – avoidant and openly resistant or avoidant and overwhelmingly passive – respectively. Both groups of children were very distressed, an observation supported by the presence, in many cases, of clinically relevant indicators of stress (i.e., stereotypic behaviors such as huddling and rocking on the floor, wetting). Furthermore, these patterns were not only apparent in infants, but also in preschool-aged maltreated children, for whom the Strange Situation would ordinarily be expected to provide little stress.

Although the disorganized category of infant Strange Situation behavior described by Main is currently thought of as a disorganized form of one of the standard patterns, Crittenden views the avoidant/ambivalent classification as representing a separate pattern – that is, another organization of the behaviors identified by Ainsworth as relevant to the assessment of security of attachment. The behavior of maltreated children in the Crittenden samples seems better described as organized around resolving the conflict between the child's needs for proximity to the mother and his expectations of his mother's reactions to his behavior. That is, the maltreated child needs proximity and contact with his mother following separation as much as other children do. In fact, his experiences of previous maltreatment heighten his distress during the brief separation of the Strange Situation, making the need for contact more imperative. However, the maltreated child also has learned to expect that his bids for contact will be ignored, rebuffed, or possibly punished. The ability of such children to maintain avoidance following the stress of separation together with their ability to limit their resistance to noncontextual aggression directed away from the mother and their use of distal and circumspect means of achieving proximity would suggest a highly controlled, or organized, pattern of behavior.

Although the relation of the disorganized category and the avoidant/ambivalent pattern to each other and to the original Ainsworth patterns in infancy is as yet unclear, there is some evidence that the disorganization observed in Main's sample of infants had been resolved by the age of 6 years into an organized pattern. Similarly both Radke-Yarrow's and Crittenden's samples included preschool-aged children who showed the (organized) A/C pattern. The suggestion is that young children organize their behavior most easily if the mother's behavior is predictable regardless of how sensitive or appropriate it is, but that older children who have had to cope with major inconsistencies eventually integrate that information into their set of expectations and develop an organized pattern of responding. The nature of that integration awaits further research.

Anxious attachments may occur at any age. Some of the indications of anxious attachment in older children and adults resemble the indications of anxious attachment in infancy: undue preoccupation with the whereabouts of the attachment figure and undue difficulty in separating from him or her, lack of trust in the attachment figure, chronic anger and resentment toward him or her, inability to seek or use support from the attachment figure when such support is needed, or absence of feeling toward him or her. Other indications that are less likely to be observed in infancy are: compulsive compliance to the wishes of the attachment figure, compulsive caregiving, or an excessive sense of self-reliance and emphasis on independence from any need for an attachment figure. The conditions leading to such anxiety include traumatic or depriving separation from an attachment figure or permanent loss thereof, unresponsiveness of an attachment figure, or inappropriate responsiveness. These conditions can have impact at any time throughout the life span. However, they are more influential when they occur earlier in life, if only because previous experiences influence the way later experiences are perceived and interpreted.

Attachment as a representational construct

Over time, the developing infant's repeated experiences with his mother lead him to form expectations regarding the nature of future interactions. This set of expectations is the basis for the infant's development of internal representational models of his mother and of himself (Bowlby, 1969). If his mother has been consistently responsive and sensitive to his signals, he forms a representational model of her as responsive and accessible and of himself as competent in eliciting her response and worthy of it. Such an infant is considered securely attached to his mother (Ainsworth et al., 1978). Some infants' experience, however, is of a mother who either does not respond to signals of need or who does not respond appropriately, whether she is rejecting (or unduly interfering) or inconsistent. The representational model formed by one of these infants of the mother figure reflects the particular nature of the behavior his experience with her has led him to expect. In any case he cannot trust her to give the kind of response he wants or needs. Moreover, he forms an image of himself as ineffective in obtaining her cooperation and as unworthy of it.

In similar fashion, an infant forms a representational model of his father and/or other caregiving figure(s) who constitute a prominent part of his social world. It is believed that at first the models of such figures, as well as the complementary models of self, are independent of each other. Although it is not clear how or when in the course of development it happens, these independent models of attachment figures become more or less loosely integrated into a generalized model of attachment figures. As the child continues his relationship with his parents and establishes new relationships with others, he assimilates his new experiences into his models of attachment figure and of self and to some extent alters his model accordingly. Thus, at any given time, the model is an "open model" more or less open to new input and consequent adjustment based on additional experience, or (perhaps not until adolescence or adulthood) rethinking of previous experience. Nevertheless, it is in terms of the current model that the individual tends to perceive his social world, and to seek out some persons and situations and avoid others.

For the infant and young child whose experiences with attachment figures have been secure on the whole, the task of integrating experiences into a generalized set of working models is relatively simple. Occasional experiences of disappointment, frustration, or anxiety do not loom large enough to interfere with the generally positive nature of the models. However, for the infant and young child whose experiences have led to anxious attachment(s), the task of integration is more difficult. Bowlby (1973, 1980) suggests that multiple models of even one attachment figure are likely to be formed. Thus, a mother who is inconsistent, sometimes offering close comfort when the child needs it, yet often failing to do so, may lead a child to form two models of her, one of a responsive mother and another that is quite antithetical, and similarly two models of self, one of a person who is effective and love-worthy and another of a person who is incompetent and unworthy. These two sets of models may alternate with one being uppermost sometimes and sometimes the other.

However, the picture is likely to be complicated by another consideration as development proceeds, verbal communication improves, and the child becomes cognitively more competent. No longer are the models based solely on the sequence of episodes of experience, but integration and generalization may be aided by conceptual processes, so that the conceptual formulations come to replace the actual episodes of experience that gave rise to it. Furthermore, this conceptual formulation may be much influenced by ready-made generalizations provided by the parent. Thus, a child who is frequently told that he is bad, and is being deprived or punished entirely for his own good by a mother who has only his best interests at heart, is likely to have a model of his mother as a wonderful person and of himself as generally bad and unworthy. It is this set of models that are likely to be most accessible to consciousness, whereas his other model of his mother as harsh, rejecting, and unresponsive to his needs and his model of himself as a love-seeking child justifiably resentful of unfair treatment tend to be disconnected from further conscious processing, even though based on repeated episodes of actual experience.

As implied above, defensive processes are particularly likely to interfere with the task of constructing models that are accurately based on experience and, perhaps more important, open to new input and consequent adjustment. Thus, the child who as an infant was anxious and avoidant in his attachment to his mother, and who defends himself from demanding closeness when he most needs it, tends to close himself off from new experiences, whether with his mother or with others, that might invalidate his expectation of rebuff and weaken his feeling of distrust of closeness.

Child maltreatment considered in the light of attachment theory

Even this necessarily brief synopsis of attachment theory provides several related postulates from which hypotheses can be drawn that may explain the behavior of maltreated children and maltreating parents. First, attachment relationships are important for individual functioning at all ages, although the specific nature of attachments changes as a consequence of development. Second, the primary function of attachments is to promote the protection and survival of the young, which is precisely what is at risk in cases of maltreatment. Third, whereas humans are genetically predisposed to exhibit certain patterns of behavior, an individual's actual behavior in a specific situation is determined by an interplay of environmental/ situational factors and previous experience with similar situations. The previous experience is encoded as internal representational models of the other(s) and of the self, including the emotional flavor associated with experience of the relationship. Fourth, actual patterns of attachment behavior affect the direction of children's developmental courses (rather than arresting development at a problematic stage). Fifth, the effect of the internal representational models that underlie anxious attachments is to change behavior in a way that makes current attachments more stressful and future attachments less likely to be secure. Finally, attachment problems are not best defined in terms of one person's psychopathology. Rather, they are defined in terms of how successful a relationship is in providing sufficient security such that individuals are freed to attend to other aspects of their lives.

Using these concepts, it is possible to predict and understand many seemingly unrelated or even paradoxical aspects of abuse and neglect. In the following discussion, a number of hypotheses drawn from attachment theory will be presented together with the research relevant to them. The intent is not to "prove" the validity of the theoretical perspective offered, but rather to establish an empirical basis for considering it seriously. The hypotheses cover the following aspects of individual and dyadic functioning: (1) anxious attachment, (2) internal conflict, (3) child strategies for coping with parents, (4) child strategies for coping with the environment, (5) niche-picking, and (6) adaptation.

In each case the tie between the theory and the predicted outcomes is the internal representational model of relationships. To the extent that the behavior of individuals in maltreating families provides a basis for inferring the nature of the inner models, those models can serve as the basis for predicting the nature of other relationships. Indeed, information on the nature of mother–infant interaction in maltreating and adequate families has been used to infer the nature of the underlying representational models and to predict both the nature of the child's attachment to his or her mother and the mother's relationships with network members and professionals (Crittenden, 1985b, 1988a, b). These models will be used in the present discussion as the basis for a broader set of hypotheses.

Based on that work, abusing mothers are expected to have working models tied to issues of conflict, control, and rejection. Their expectations of others will tend to center around the idea that others will attempt to dominate them to meet the needs of the other and reject them when they press to have their own needs met. Their model of themselves will be tied to the idea that others have, and will not willingly give up, needed psychological or physical resources. Consequently, coercion and victimization will be central to the mothers' perceptions of themselves. The accompanying affect will be one of anger.

Neglecting mothers are expected to have models centering around the concept of helplessness. They will not perceive others as having, or being able to give them, what they need. Neither will they see themselves as effective at eliciting the help and support of others. The affect accompanying their relationships will be one of emptiness and depression.

Adequate mothers, by contrast, will have models centered around ideas of competence and reciprocity. They will perceive others as helpful and responsive. They will perceive themselves as capable of obtaining help and support when it is needed and also of providing support to others. The accompanying affect will be one of satisfaction (Crittenden, 1985b).

Discussed below are several hypotheses, based on attachment theory and drawn from the above working models, regarding the behavior of maltreated children and maltreating parents.

Anxious attachment

Individuals in maltreating families will be expected to form anxious attachments with family members. For maltreated children, this would mean anxious attachment to the parent(s). For maltreating adults, this would include anxious attachments to the adults' parents, to their partners, and to their children. Underlying these anxious attachments would be distorted internal representational models of the self and other(s). The quality of previous relationships is expected to influence, but not wholly determine, the nature of later relationships.

Abuse. The clearest evidence that relationships in abusing families are anxious comes from investigations using the Strange Situation procedure (Ainsworth et al., 1978) to assess the quality of the child's relationship to the parent. Abused children, ranging in age from 1 to 4 years, have been found to be anxiously attached to their mothers (Crittenden, 1985a, 1985b; Egeland and Sroufe, 1981; Gaensbauer and Harmon, 1982; Schneider-Rosen, Braunwald, Carlson, and Cicchetti, 1985) and to show the anxious/avoidant pattern in particular. Nonlaboratory derived evidence of anxious attachment between abusing mothers and their children comes from a study of mothers' and children's response to protective daycare (Crittenden, 1983).

It is also possible to infer quality of attachment from observations of parent–child interaction. As previously noted, maternal insensitivity (i.e., interference and/or unresponsiveness) in interaction with the child has been associated with child anxiety in the Strange Situation (Ainsworth et al., 1978; Belsky, Rovine, and Taylor, 1984; Crittenden, 1985a; Sroufe, 1985). There is substantial evidence that abusing mothers are more harsh, interfering, controlling, and negative when interacting with their children (Burgess and Conger, 1978; Crittenden, 1981, 1985; Crittenden and Bonvillian, 1984; Dietrich, Starr, and Weisfeld, 1983; Mash, Johnson, and Kovitz, 1983; Robinson and Solomon, 1979; Wasserman, Green, and Rhianon, 1983). Such evidence is based on observations of children across the full range of childhood and supports the inference that maltreated children of all ages will tend to be anxiously attached to their parents.

Evidence regarding the nature of adult attachments to parents, partners, and children is derived primarily from family history data regarding the duration and nature of such relationships. Based on the inferred nature of abusing mothers' models of relationships, it would be expected that mother–partner relationships would be non-egalitarian (i.e., composed of a dominant and a submissive partner) and that there would be conflict over these roles. The evidence is generally consistent with this hypothesis in terms of distressed marriages, broken marriages, and, especially, wife abuse (Baldwin and Oliver, 1975; Herrenkohl and Herrenkohl, 1981; Johnson and Morse, 1968; National Institute of Mental Health, 1977; Perry, Wells, and Doran, 1982; Starr, 1982; Wolfe, 1985). Moreover, following a separation, many abusing mothers choose another abusive partner or remain single, whereas nonabusing mothers are more likely to remain with the children's father or a relative (Burgess, Anderson, Schellenbach, and Conger, 1981; Friedman, 1976; Hunter and Kilstrom, 1979; Kotelchuck, 1982). This suggests an inability on the part of the abusing parents to incorporate new information into existing models, thus increasing the likelihood of the repetition of previous problems.

Following the popularization of the concept of maternal bonding to the neonate, there have been numerous suggestions that maltreating mothers may not bond properly to their children (Helfer, 1976; Hurd, 1975; Lynch and Roberts, 1977). Although there is no formal assessment of the presence or absence of bonding, it seems reasonable to assume that a mother who keeps and nurtures her infant sufficiently to maintain life has formed a bond. However, it is quite possible that the nature of that bond is different for maltreating mothers than for adequate mothers. One study that has examined this issue has reported that mothers who later abused or neglected their children differed in their attitudes toward the pregnancy, in their behavior with the infant immediately following delivery, and in their behavior in the postpartum period (Gray, Cutler, Dean, and Kempe, 1977). However, another study with less subjective measures found no evidence of bonding failure in maltreating mothers (Egeland and Vaughn, 1981). Studies that have evaluated the effectiveness of interventions to improve bonding have reported mixed results such that it is unclear whether or not extended contact in the hospital and/or home visitation are helpful (Gray et al., 1977; Siegal, Bauman, Schaefer, Saunders, and Ingram, 1980).

Evidence of the probable anxious attachment of an abusing parent to her own parents is consistent with the expectation of an anxious relationship between mother and child. Abusing parents have reported being abused by their own parents (Gil, 1970; Silver, Barton, and Dublin, 1967) or being severely punished in childhood (Kotelchuck, 1982). In addition, it has been argued that rejection as a child by one's parents can lead to rejection of one's own child and that this may be a less severe example of the process leading to the cross-generational transmission of abuse (Main and Goldwyn, 1984). Others have found that maltreated children show patterns of interaction with their younger siblings similar to those of their maltreating parents (Crittenden, 1984) and that abusing mothers experienced more losses and separations from their own parents in childhood (DeLozier, 1982).

Neglect. Investigations that have considered neglected children as a subgroup have reported that, as assessed in the Strange Situation, most neglected children were anxiously attached to their mothers (Crittenden, 1985a, 1985b; Egeland and Sroufe, 1981; Gaensbauer and Harmon, 1982). Moreover, like abused children, they tended to display an anxious/avoidant pattern. However, the pattern of off-modal classifications differed from that in the abuse group – neglected children who were not avoidant tended to be ambivalent. When in interaction with their mothers, neglected children tended to be passive rather than either difficult or compulsively compliant (Crittenden, 1981, 1985a).

Similarly, there is evidence that neglecting adults find it difficult to leave home and establish attachment relationships with nonfamilial partners (Crittenden, 1986). Often then the neglecting mother's own mother serves as her partner in raising the children, thus enabling the mother to avoid the primary situation in which individuals take on reciprocal, care-giving attachment relationships.

Internal conflict

Second, it is hypothesized that anxious attachments will be associated with conflicting impulses within the individual that, in extreme cases such as maltreatment, might lead to behavior that would otherwise be considered paradoxical.

Abuse. The extreme of this is, of course, the situation of the abused infant. He is genetically locked into forming an attachment to his primary caregiver and yet his experience teaches him that this attachment figure may be a source of pain and injury. There is evidence that anxiously attached children are both avoidant of and angry with the parent and also seek excessive closeness. Similarly, maltreated children would be expected to defend and protect the very parent who endangers them. Indeed, many investigations of child abuse are hampered by the child's unwillingness to implicate the perpetrating parent even when the child's protection from parental reprisal has been adequately ensured. Abused children, especially girls, have been found to care for their parents as though the parent–child roles were reversed (Flanzraich and Dunsavage, 1977; Morris and Gould, 1963; Steele and Pollock, 1974); such behavior is not dissimilar to Bowlby's concept of compulsive caregiving as both a way of maintaining closeness to an attachment figure and a means of denying pervasive anger with the person being cared for (Bowlby, 1973).

Maltreating mothers would be expected to show similar incompatible feelings toward their children although the child is particularly sought as the one person whom the mother possesses and who will love her back. In fact, the child's anger at the mother's intrusiveness may be interpreted by the mother as rejection and trigger her own rejection of him. The child's use of the avoidant response to the mother and often promiscuous seeking of affiliation with strangers may have similar effects; the mother did not want to give nurturance to her child but neither did she want a demonstration of her child's ability to get along without her or to obtain support from someone else. Finally, in spite of a desire to establish more satisfying and secure relationships, maltreated adolescents and maltreating adults would be expected to choose as partners individuals who will tend to contribute to the maintenance of distressed relationships. Many would unwittingly carry into developing relationships a wariness or suspicion of other people and excessive demands for attention from the few who were known well. When current relationships became unsatisfying, there could easily be a precipitous rush into a new and, hopefully, more rewarding attachment. However, the ambivalent ties to parents and/or previous partners would remain stressful and the individual's pattern of demandingness, distrust, and hostility would probably remain unchanged. Further, there is a reasonable likelihood that such an individual would perceive both the spouse and any children as potential sources of nurturance rather than as recipients of nurturance.

Neglect. In the case of neglect, the paradox is that individuals who desperately need the comfort and support of others rarely seek it or seem comforted by it when they receive it. Under the stress of a brief separation from the mother, neglected children respond to the need for their mothers with helplessness or random roaming around the room (Crittenden, 1985a; Gaensbauer and Harmon, 1982). Neglecting adults respond to the opportunity for relationships with withdrawal and/or a denial of feelings of loneliness and anger (Crittenden, 1988a; Polansky, Gaudin, Ammons, and Davis, 1985).

Coping with parents

Third, different types of maltreatment will be associated with different organizations of child behavior relevant to the children's interaction with the parent. Moreover, such organizations can be expected to change as a function of ontogeny and to reflect the competing desires of maltreated children. These outcomes reflect changes in the direction of development rather than an arresting of developmental processes at an infantile stage.

Abuse. When in interaction with their mothers, abused infants have been shown to be more difficult than other infants; however, the evidence suggests that this pattern of behavior is tied to the immediate interpersonal situation and not to aspects of innate infant temperament (Crittenden, 1981, 1985a). Moreover, their mothers' response to such behavior is often to avoid and/or punish the infant, thus increasing his distress. Such a mother can only feel very frustrated in her attempts to satisfy her baby. If she cannot learn to perceive and respond appropriately to her child's behavioral cues and if her child cannot learn to please her, one would expect the conflict to become increasingly severe, further endangering the infant.

In fact, there is evidence that, toward the end of the first year of life, many abused infants have learned to accommodate their mothers, first, by inhibiting signs of their anger and, later, by learning to tolerate their mothers' interference without complaint and even to comply with her desires (Crittenden, 1988c; Crittenden and DiLalla, 1988). By so doing they change the nature of the interaction from mutual anger to superficial cooperation and compliance. There is considerable evidence that many older abused children are also passive, fearful, vigilant, and compliant (Green, Gaines, and Sandgrund, 1974; Ounsted, Oppenheimer, and Lindsay, 1975).

However, not all abused children make the transition from resistant to compliant behavior. Particularly if there is no way for the child to predict what will please or anger the parent (as in abuse-and-neglect, see below), it becomes almost impossible for him or her to inhibit some behaviors and exhibit others selectively to please the mother. Thus, by the second year of life, two distinct response patterns for coping with the distress of living with an abusing parent are likely to have developed: a negative, resistant one and a compulsively compliant one.

Neglect. Parents who neglect their children would be expected to foster different patterns of child response. Like abused children, neglected children want proximity to their attachment figure when they are anxious or under stress. However, unlike abused children, they have learned that their mothers do not respond to their signals. They learn that they are ineffective at communicating their needs and obtaining maternal cooperation in meeting them. Given this experience, most children would be expected to intensify their demands. If that produced results, they would probably maintain a pattern of intense, clingy, and demanding behavior. On the other hand, if their mothers rarely responded to the intensified attachment behavior, they would be expected either to become depressed and withdrawn or to ignore their mothers entirely in their pursuit of other satisfactions. In addition, both the anxious, demanding children and the active, disorganized children could, by their efforts to draw forth a response from their environment, become a source of stress to their mothers. If their generally unresponsive mothers become frustrated and angered by their intensified demands, the children could well experience the interpersonal conditions associated with abuse-and-neglect (see below).

Coping with the environment

Fourth, it is proposed that these styles of interpersonal behavior will be related to the effectiveness of the children's exploration of their environment. Attachment theorists postulate that the attachment and exploration systems of behavior function best when balanced with each other. Thus, when there are signals of danger, the attachment system is activated, resulting in the proximity of mother and child. When child and mother feel secure, the child should feel free to explore the environment safely. Because maltreated children are neither protected adequately by proximity to the mother nor secure in the belief that she will be available, their ability to explore safely and effectively would be expected to be impaired.

Abuse. Abused children who were avoidant of their mothers could be expected to explore freely and successfully only when there were (1) no indicators of danger in the environment and (2) no indicators of maternal stress or anger. Under such conditions they could expect to be safe. When there were either environmental or maternal signals of danger, they would face approach/avoidance conflict. The studies using the Strange Situation indicate that under such conditions some abused children are able to maintain an avoidant defense strategy, whereas others are both sufficiently anxious to need close proximity to the mother and also sufficiently angry to be unable to conceal their feelings fully, displaying both avoidance and ambivalence (Crittenden, 1985a, 1985b). The avoidant children would thus be expected to benefit somewhat from exploratory behavior, whereas the more distressed abused children might be preoccupied with managing their safety and unable to explore widely. Studies by Crittenden (1985a), Dietrich et al. (1983), and Koski and Ingram (1977) support these expectations in terms of developmental quotient (DQ); abused children, as a group, have lower DQs than adequately reared children. When the DQ of the abused children is considered as a function of their tendency to use the compulsive/compliant pattern with the mother, it becomes clear that there are important within-group differences. Compliant abused children tend to have higher than normal DQs, whereas abused children who are passive/withdrawn or difficult tend to have very low DQs (Crittenden and DiLalla, 1988).

Neglect. Neglected and withdrawn children would be expected to find it difficult to separate sufficiently from their mothers to enable them to explore their environment and to establish relationships with other people; they would appear helpless and unable to exploit the learning potential of their environments. The more adventurous neglected children would have the advantage of increased experience, but at risk to their safety and without the advantage of adult support.

Niche picking

Fifth, behavior patterns of family members in attachment relationships would be expected to affect other aspects of their social ecology, such as social networks, employment, and, for the children, school experiences. The processes by which such patterns of behavior would generalize to include nonattachment relationships include the perception and interpretation of experience through internal models of reality and the tendency to repeat ingrained patterns of behavior in new situations.

Abuse. Although some abused children are compliant with adults, there is evidence that with peers many are aggressive, both in and out of school or other supervised settings (Galston, 1971; George and Main, 1979; Herrenkohl and Herrenkohl, 1981; Riedy, 1977). Their ready aggression could be motivated either by displaced anger or by increased vigilance in the context of expecting aggression *from* others. Such vigilance resulting from internal models of conflict and dominance could easily lead the abused child to misinterpret the behavior of others and to respond with aggression himself. Of course, the response of others to his aggression will only confirm his model.

The delinquent behavior of abused adolescent males and promiscuous behavior of females attest to another change in coping strategy (Silver et al., 1967). It is probable that these more mature, although equally inappropriate, patterns of behavior are associated with violence at home and reflect, for the boys, the sense of competence and control that comes from taking what one wants and, for the girls, the attempt to find security and acceptance by giving what others want.

The social networks of maltreating and adequate mothers have been found to parallel the nature of the mothers' relationships with their infants (Crittenden, 1985b). Abusing mothers appear to have the social skills to establish new friendships; however, those relationships are neither stable nor reciprocal (Crittenden, 1985b). Instead, abusing mothers perceive their help-providing friends as undependable and they in turn are perceived by their friends as being manipulative. Most abusing mothers' relationships are not only short-lived; they also end in violent quarrels and enduring bitterness (Young, 1964).

Similarly, although abusing parents find it relatively easy to obtain jobs, they are rarely able to keep them any length of time. The most common reasons for quitting their jobs are disputes with the employer or co-workers. McKinley (1964) found a negative relation between fathers' job satisfaction and harsh punishment of the children. Although this finding has been interpreted as indicating that loss of status leads to violence, it is equally possible that those men who are unable to manage personal relationships so as either to obtain satisfying jobs or to find personal satisfaction in the jobs they have are also less able to establish cooperative relationships with their children.

Neglect. Children who have been neglected tend either to be withdrawn from their schoolmates or to disorganized, active, and aggressive.

Their mothers' social relationships reflect distortions similar to those of their intrafamilial relationships. They have very few friendships outside of family; those friends they do have tend to be seen infrequently and known only briefly (Crittenden, 1985b; Gaudin and Polansky, 1986; Polansky, 1985).

Adaptation

Sixth, the children's patterns of behavior would be predicted to be adaptive to the immediate (proximate) sense of promoting their immediate survival while being maladaptive in the long-term (ultimate) sense of personal mental health and, possibly, gene survival. The maladaptation would be based in part upon the notion that defensive models imply perceptual exclusion of information and distortion of the meaning of some important perceived information.

Abuse. The adaptiveness of two patterns should be considered: compulsive compliance and overt resistance. The compulsively compliant child in interaction with his or her parent inhibits responses that the parent dislikes and substitutes others that the parent prefers. This strategy has the advantage of reducing the risk of parental violence. It is also likely to teach the child to be very sensitive to the interpersonal behavior of others; this skill may prove adaptive in many life situations. In addition, the compliant strategy may foster overachievement and/or nurturance of the parent if the parent desires and rewards such behavior. However, these outcomes are the result of the child's learning to behave in ways that do not reflect his feelings. The anger he felt in the original situations that led to inhibition may become associated with compliance, leading to a diminution of satisfaction in achievement and the association of caregiving with anger and coercion. Thus, a compulsive compliant strategy of coping with abuse may come to consist of (1) excessive social vigilance (with the attendant risk of systematic misinterpretation of others' social behavior), (2) superficial compliance in situations in which others seem threatening or powerful (with the risk of never testing the misinterpretations made regarding the possible hostility of others), and (3) inhibited anger (with the risk of possibly excluding some emotions from perception). Such a behavior pattern is often labeled manipulative and may describe the defensive response of both some abused children and many abusing parents. It is consistent with the development of representational models of others as powerful and hostile, the self as lovable only when compliant, and an emotional overtone of anxiety and repressed anger.

Abused children who remain overtly angry and resistant face different risks. They are more likely to experience continued parental anger and abuse, but less likely to deny their own feelings. Thus, their model of others may be negative, whereas their model of themselves could include justification of their own angry behavior. Therefore, overtly angry abused children may be less likely to exclude information defensively or to systematically misinterpret it. However, the costs of such a developmental pathway are both the risk of continued abuse and the possibility that anger will pervade much of the individual's behavior, thus leading to the accurate perception of rejection by others and, in the extreme, to delinquency. The balance is between retaining *open* (as opposed to defensive) models that can be consciously revised if the individual finds a more responsive substitute attachment figure and risking that the individual's anger will come to dominate all of his social interactions.

Data relevant to this rationale are scarce, but what little there are, are supportive. Adults who have been abused but do not themselves abuse their children are reported to be more open about their anger over their mistreatment and conscious in their decision not to follow their parents' model (Hunter and Kilstrom, 1979). Moreover, these parents report having supportive social relationships. Other nonabusing but formerly abused parents report having had an important supportive relationship during childhood. Such relationships could have not only the immediate advantage of helping the children through difficult experiences, but also the long-term advantage of modifying their working models to include more positive images of the self and others and an associated feeling of satisfaction. Such changes increase the likelihood that the individual will be able to form other supportive relationships in the future.

There is some limited evidence that members of abusing families do perceive or interpret experience differently from other people. Although there is no evidence that abused children are constitutionally or temperamentally different from other children (Crittenden, 1985a; Egeland and Sroufe, 1981; Kotelchuck, 1982; Starr, 1982), there is considerable evidence that their mothers perceive them to be so (Herrenkohl and Herrenkohl, 1981). Although abusing mothers have been thought to have higher expectations of their children or to attribute intentions to them inappropriately, the evidence suggests otherwise (Kravitz and Driscoll, 1983; Rosenberg and Reppucci, 1983). However, when abusing mothers have been shown videotaped behavior of children, they appear to respond more negatively and feel more angry than other mothers (Frodi and Lamb, 1980). This suggests that the problem is not with general expectations or attributions or with insufficient information about child development; instead, the problem seems to be tied to perceptions and associated emotional responses.

Turning to the situation of abused children, there is some evidence that they may be both more perceptive of the social behavior of adults (Cummings, Zahn-Waxler, and Radke-Yarrow, 1981) and less perceptive of their own or other children's behavior (Camras, Grow, and Ribordy, 1983). Furthermore, it is possible that such sensitivity is tied to IQ, with abused children who do not show IQ deficits being the more adept at interpreting emotional expressions in others (Frodi and Smetana, 1984). If abused children do adapt to their situation both by becoming hypervigiliant (Martin and Beezely, 1977, 1980) and nurturant to their parents (Cummings et al., 1981) and by denying their own emotional response, this pattern of skills and deficits would be expected. Of critical interest would be the extent to which the children retain the ability to interpret the behavior of different adults accurately (rather than assuming that all adults are similar to their abusing parent) and to recognize accurately their own emotions. There is some evidence that they respond flexibly in infancy to differences in the behavior of others (Crittenden, 1985a), but that at least some abused toddlers and preschoolers lose this resiliency (George and Main, 1979).

Neglect. For neglected children, the two primary patterns to be considered are extreme passivity (depression) and undisciplined activity. Most neglected infants find their parents too unresponsive for them to develop a secure attachment. However, as they develop mobility, they themselves become able to modify the nature of their environment. In particular, they begin to explore, seeking stimulation from all aspects of their environment. Such exploration is both adaptive and dangerous. It provides the opportunity for learning about the world as well as contingencies in it; however, because no one is watching out for the welfare of the young neglected child, there is danger of accidental harm. In addition, the child's search for stimulation is likely to be disorganized, reflecting his lack of experience with focused interaction. Current thinking about hyperactive children suggests that, rather than being overstimulated, they are understimulated to the extent that they cannot focus attention (Quay, 1985). Such a rationale would certainly fit with the unstructured behavior of some neglected children.

Other neglecting parents are able to offer little to their child beyond the physical resources to maintain life. They neither respond to their child's other needs nor encourage their child's access to a stimulating environment. Their children, therefore, neither learn strategies for engaging their parent nor for independently exploring the environment. Their passivity is a form of depression, one which results from a lack of awareness of the potential for personal effectiveness. Such children cannot be described as coping with their plight as much as being victimized by it.

Severity and abuse-with-neglect. The evidence presented suggests that the developmental impact of maltreatment differs according to type of maltreatment. However, the above presentation is distorted in two ways. First, it assumes either that all maltreatment is of similar severity or that severity is not an important factor. Second, it assumes that the conditions of abuse and neglect are mutually exclusive. Of course, neither assumption reflects the complexity of reality. The rationale was presented with these distortions for the purposes of clarity and to highlight the differential nature of the two developmental courses. On the contrary, it is necessary to grapple at least briefly with more complex situations. Data on two groups of children are relevant here: those who have been only marginally maltreated and those who have been both abused and neglected.

Children who have been marginally maltreated generally show a pattern of deficits and adaptation which is, as expected, less extreme than in maltreated children. They show mild developmental delay, general cooperativeness as infants in interaction with their parents, and mildly anxious attachment (Crittenden, 1981, 1985a, 1988a, b). Similarly, their mothers show only moderate disturbance in childrearing practices. The primary difficulty faced by these children appears not to be the maltreatment itself but rather its unpredictability. Whereas their mothers are in some ways and at some times sensitively responsive, at others they are harsh and/or unresponsive. It is difficult for the children both to determine what causes the changes in their mothers' behavior and also to develop internal models of their mothers and themselves that are consistent and useful in predicting future maternal behavior. Thus, generalized anxiety and sometimes undisciplined activity may lead these children to social and academic problems.

Abused-and-neglected children, in contrast, experience general unresponsiveness combined with bursts of harshness. Often both their exploration and their intensified demands for attention lead to parental punitiveness. The predictions of coercion and unresponsiveness that the abused and the neglected child (respectively) can make regarding their parents' behavior lead to consistent models of their parents and themselves. Although the situations offered them are distorted and unpleasant, children who experience only one type of maltreatment can often learn to cope with the predictable nature of the distortion. This is not true for the abused-and-neglected child. He experiences both types of distortions and, further, finds that his own activity endangers him. It would be expected that the coping strategies used by such children would include flagrant acting out with extreme disregard for others, extreme inhibition and withdrawal, severe psychosomatic illness, pervasive role reversal as a means of deflecting the anger of the threatening parent(s), or some combination of these (Crittenden, 1988a, b, c).

Conclusions

This chapter represents an attempt to apply the principles of attachment theory to the study of maltreatment. In the process, a number of points have been made. First, maltreatment has pervasive psychological effects; the rationale provided here applies equally well to cases with or without *physical* maltreatment. Second, the outcomes of maltreatment are developmental in nature, that is, they affect different aspects of personal functioning at different points in time. They also affect the direction of future development rather than arresting it at a problematic and immature stage. Third, although the outcomes differ at different ages, there is developmental coherence across periods (Cicchetti and Rizley, 1981, p. 49). Fourth, the developmental course selected is an outcome of individual differences as well as differences in experience. Finally, the experience of abuse is quite different from the experience of neglect with regard both to parental behavior and to the nature of child-coping strategies.

The argument offered here is not intended to focus on dyadic, attachment-related influences on maltreatment to the exclusion of organismic or societal influences. Rather, it is intended to provide a means of (1) identifying a critical variable that can explain the impact of many associated conditions and suggest why the impact of maltreatment affects so many areas of individual or family functioning and (2) identifying those individuals and families who are most vulnerable to other sources of influence and to suggest the nature of the influence. The advantage of considering anxious attachment as a critical variable is that it implies a process through which its impact can be understood, as opposed to merely identifying the correlates of risk. It is an attempt to be parsimonious without being trivial.

The predominant current theoretical approach is a transactional ecological model focusing on the environment associated with maltreatment and vulnerabilities in the child as well as on parental characteristics. As indicated above, congenital child variables do not, in well controlled studies, differentiate maltreating and nonmaltreating families. On the other hand children do differ in their ability to elicit maternal responsiveness, especially after they have experienced unsatisfying maternal behavior. Such situations are interpreted, from the perspective of attachment theory, as reflecting the nature of the relationship rather than as being a parent or a child characteristic. Thus, attachment theory is not unidirectional in its approach to causation; the focus is one how individuals' experiences with attachment figures affect what is perceived as threatening as well as what patterns of coping are shown in response.

With respect to societal influence, there is considerable evidence that the correlates of low socioeconomic status are also the correlates of maltreatment. Moreover, changes in some societal conditions have been associated with changes in rates of maltreatment – for example, increases in unemployment have been associated with increases in abuse (Justice and Duncan, 1977; Steinmetz and Straus, 1974). The nature of the association is not clear. Because not all families with an unemployed father abuse their children, it still remains to be shown why some families, and not others, are vulnerable under stress to maltreatment of their children. It is proposed here that distorted attachment relationships in the family leave family members vulnerable to the effects of crisis situations such as unemployment. The point is not that social conditions are irrelevant to the incidence of maltreatment. On the contrary, given that the quality of relationships is on a continuum, the nature of the social context may determine the point along the secure–anxious continuum at which risk for maltreatment becomes imminent. However, knowing the effect of deleterious social conditions only allows one to predict increased incidence of maltreatment. Knowing the nature of family attachment relationships and the individuals' associated representational models should enable one to specify more precisely which families and/or individuals will be the most vulnerable to external stressors.

Often the evidence needed to support this and the other hypotheses offered here is either missing or of poor quality as a result of poorly measured variables, clinical observations, etc. This is especially true in older studies and in studies of parents. In addition, very little of the evidence was initially offered in the context of testing attachment theory. This is unfortunate but does not, in and of itself, diminish the potential of attachment theory to pose integrative and testable hypotheses regarding the nature, causation, and effects of maltreatment. It is now necessary that investigators design studies (as did Kotelchuck, 1982, and Starr, 1982, to test other theoretical approaches) that test, in a single study, a range of attachment-derived hypotheses similar to those presented here. Although such an approach would not "prove" attachment theory, it would result in either finding that the theory was no more effective in explaining maltreatment than other theories or that the results were heuristically consistent and explanatory.

References

Aber, J. L., and Zigler, E. (1981). Developmental considerations in the definition of child maltreatment, *New Directions for Child Development: Developmental Perspectives on Maltreatment, 11,* 1–30.

Ainsworth, M. D. S. (1967). *Infancy in Uganda: Infant care and the growth of love.* Baltimore: Johns Hopkins University Press.

Ainsworth, M. D. S. (1980). Attachment and child abuse. In G. Gerber, C. J. Ross, and E. Zigler (Eds.), *Child abuse reconsidered: An agenda for action.* New York: Oxford University Press.

Ainsworth, M. D. S. (1985). Attachments across the life-span. *Bulletin of The New York Academy of Medicine, 61,* 792-812.

Ainsworth, M. D., Blehar, M. C., Waters, E., and Wall, S. (1978). *Patterns of attachment: A psychological study of the strange situation.* Hillsdale, NJ: Erlbaum.

Ainsworth, M. D. S., and Eichberg, C. F. (in press). Effects on infant-mother attachment of mother's unresolved loss of an attachment figure or other traumatic experience. In C. K. Parker and J. Stevenson Hinde (Eds.), *Attachment across the life cycle.*

Baldwin, J. A., and Oliver, J. E. (1975). Epidemiology and family characteristics of severely-abused children. *British Journal of Preventive Medicine, 29,* 205–221.

Belsky, J. (1980). Child maltreatment: An ecological integration. *American Psychologist, 35,* 320–335.

Belsky, J., Rovine, M., and Taylor, D. G. (1984). The Pennsylvania Infant and Family Development Project, III: The origins of individual differences in infant-mother attachment: Maternal and infant contributions. *Child Development, 55,* 718–728.

Bowlby, J. (1958). The nature of the child's tie to his mother. *International Journal of Psychoanalysis, 39,* 359–73.

Bowlby, J. (1969). *Attachment and loss, Vol. I: Attachment.* New York: Basic Books.

Bowlby, J. (1973). *Attachment and loss, Vol. II: Separation.* New York: Basic Books.

Bowlby, J. (1979). *The making and breaking of affectional bonds.* London: Tavistock Publications.

Bowlby, J. (1980). *Attachment and loss, Vol. III: Loss.* New York: Basic Books.

Bowlby, J. (1982). Violence in the family as a disorder of the attachment and caregiving systems. *American Journal of Psychoanalysis, 44,* 9–27, 29–31.

Bretherton, I. (1980). Young children in stressful situations: The supporting role of attachment figures and unfamiliar caregivers. In G. V. Coelo and P. Ahmed (Eds.), *Uprooting and development* (pp. 179–211). New York: Plenum.

Burgess, R. L., Anderson, E. S., Schellenbach, C. J., and Conger, R. D. (1981). A social interactional approach to the study of abusive families. In J. P. Vincent (Ed.), *Advances in family intervention, assessment and theory: An annual compilation of research (Vol. 2)* (pp. 1–46). Greenwich, CT: JAI Press.

Burgess, R. L., and Conger, R. D. (1978). Family interaction in abusive, neglectful, and normal families. *Child Development, 49,* 1163–1173.

Camras, L. A., Grow, J. G., and Ribordy, S. C. (1983). Recognition of emotional expression by abused children. *Journal of Clinical Child Psychology, 12,* 305–328.

Cicchetti, D., and Rizley, R. (1981). Developmental perspectives on the etiology, intergenerational transmission, and sequelae of child maltreatment. *New Directions for Child Development: Developmental Perspectives on Child Maltreatment, 11,* 31–56.

Crittenden, P. M. (1981). Abusing, neglecting, problematic, and adequate dyads: Differentiating by patterns of interaction. *Merrill-Palmer Quarterly, 27,* 1–18.

Crittenden, P. M. (1983). The effect of mandatory protective daycare on mutual attachment in maltreating mother–infant dyads. *Child Abuse and Neglect, 3,* 297–300.

Crittenden, P. M. (1984). Sibling interaction: Evidence of a generational effect in maltreating families. *Child Abuse and Neglect, 8,* 433–438.

Crittenden, P. M. (1985a). Maltreated infants: Vulnerability and resilience. *Journal of Child Psychology and Psychiatry, 26,* 85–96.

Crittenden, P. M. (1985b). Social networks, quality of child-rearing, and child development. *Child Development, 56,* 1299–1313.

Crittenden, P. M. (1986). Final Project Report. HHS Grant #90–CA–844: Differential assessment of maltreating families using interaction, attachment and family systems.

Crittenden, P. M. (1987). Non-organic failure-to-thrive: Deprivation or distortion? *Infant Mental Health Journal, 8,* 51–64.

Crittenden, P. M. (1988a). Family and dyadic patterns of functioning in maltreating families. In K. Browne, C. Davies, and P. Stratton (Eds.), *Early prediction and prevention of child abuse* (pp. 161-189). New York: Wiley.

Crittenden, P. M. (1988b). Distorted patterns of relationship in maltreating families: The role of internal representational models. *Journal of Reproductive and Infant Psychology, 6,* 183-199.

Crittenden, P. M. (1988c). Relationships at risk. In J. Belsky and T. Nezworski (Eds.), *Clinical implications of attachment* (pp. 136-174). Hillsdale, NJ: Erlbaum.

Crittenden, P. M., and Bonvillian, J. (1984). The effect of maternal risk status on maternal sensitivity to infant cues. *American Journal of Orthopsychiatry, 54,* 250–262.

Crittenden, P. M., and DiLalla, D. L. (1988). Compulsive compliance: The development of an inhibitory coping strategy in infancy. *Journal of Abnormal Child Psychology, 16,* 585-599.

Cummings, E. M., Zahn-Waxler, C., and Radke-Yarrow, M. (1981). Young children's responses to expressions of anger and affection by others in the family. *Child Development, 52,* 1274–1282.

Deitrich, K. N., Starr, R., and Weisfeld, G. E. (1983). Infant maltreatment: Caretaker–infant interaction and developmental consequences at different levels of parenting failure. *Pediatrics, 72,* 532–540.

DeLozier, P. P. (1982). Attachment theory and child abuse. In C. M. Parkes and J. Stevenson-Hinde (Eds.), *The place of attachment in human behavior* (pp. 95–117). New York: Basic Books.

Egeland, B., and Farker, E. A. (1984). Infant–mother attachment: Factors related to its development and changes over time. *Child Development, 55,* 753–771.

Egeland, E., and Sroufe, A. (1981). Developmental sequelae of maltreatment in infancy, *New Directions for Child Development: Developmental Perspectives on Child Maltreatment, 11,* 77–92.

Egeland, B., and Vaughn, B. (1981). Failure of "bond formation" as a cause of abuse, neglect, and maltreatment. *American Journal of Orthopsychiatry, 51,* 78–84.

Eichberg, C. (1986). Security of attachment in infancy: Contributions of mother's representation of her own experience and child care attitudes. Unpublished doctoral dissertation, University of Virginia, Charlottesville.

Flanzraich, M., and Dunsavage, I. (1977). Role reversal in abused/neglected families: Implications for child welfare workers. *Children Today,* 13–15.

Friedman, R. (1976). Child abuse: A review of psychosocial research. In Hefner and Company (Eds.), *Four perspectives on the status of child abuse and neglect research.* Washington, DC: National Center on Child Abuse and Neglect.

Frodi, A. M., and Lamb, M. E. (1980). Chld abusers' responses to infant smiles and cries. *Child Development, 51,* 238–241.

Frodi, A., and Smetana, J. (1984). Abused, neglected, and nonmaltreated preschoolers' ability to discriminate emotions in others: The effects of IQ. *Child Abuse and Neglect, 8,* 459–465.

Gaensbauer, T. J., and Harmon, R. J. (1982). Attachment behavior in abused/neglected and premature infants: Implications for the concept of attachment. In R. N. Emde and R. J. Harmon (Eds.), *The development of attachment and affiliative systems* (pp. 263–280). New York: Plenum.

Galston, R. (1971). Violence begins at home. *Journal American Academy of Child Psychiatry, 10,* 336–3350.

Garbarino, J. (1977). The human ecology of child maltreatment: A conceptual model for research. *Journal of Marriage and the Family, 39,* 721–727.

Gaudin, J. M., and Polansky, N. A. (1986). Social distancing of neglectful families, *Children and Youth Services Review, 8,* 1–12.

George, C., Kaplan, N., and Main, M. (1985). Adult Attachment Interview. Unpublished doctoral dissertation, University of California, Berkeley.

George, C., and Main, M. (1979). Social interactions of young abused children. *Child Development, 50,* 306–318.

Gil, D. G. (1970). *Violence against children: Physical child abuse in the United States.* Cambridge, MA: Harvard University Press.

Gray, J. D., Cutler, C. A., Dean, J. G., and Kempe, C. H. (1977). Prediction and prevention of child neglect. *Child Abuse and Neglect, 1,* 45–58.

Green, A. H. Gaines, R. W., and Sandgrund, A. (1974). Child abuse: Pathological syndrome of family interaction. *American Journal of Psychiatry, 31,* 882–886.

Grossmann, K. E., Grossmann, K., Spangler, G., Suess, G., and Unzer, L. (1985). Maternal sensitivity and newborns' orientation responses as related to quality of attachment in Northern Germany. In I. Bretherton and E. Waters (Eds.), Growing points in attachment theory. *Monographs of the Society for Research in Child Development, 50* (1–2, Serial No. 209), pp. 233–256.

Helfer, R. E. (1973). The etiology of child abuse. *Pediatrics, 51,* 777–779.

Helfer, R. E. (1976). Early identification and prevention of unusual child-rearing practices. *Pediatric Annals, 5,* 91–105.

Herrenkohl, R. C., and Herrenkohl, E. C. (1981). Some antecedents and developmental consequences of child maltreatment, *New Directions for Child Development: Developmental Perspectives on Child Maltreatment, 11,* 57–76.

Hunter, R. S., and Kilstrom, N. (1979). Breaking the cycle in abusive families. *American Journal of Psychiatry, 136,* 1320–1322.

Hurd, J. M. (1975). Assessing maternal attachment: First step toward the prevention of child abuse. *JOGN Nursing, 4,* 25–30.

Johnson, B., and Morse, H. (1968). *The battered child: A study of children with inflicted injuries.* Denver, CO: Denver Department of Welfare.

Justice, B., and Duncan, D. F. (1977). Child abuse as a work-related problem. *Journal of Behavior Technology, Methods, and Therapy, 23,* 53–55.

Kempe, C. H., Silverman, F. N., and Steele, B. F. (1962). The battered-child syndrome. *Journal of the American Medical Association, 181,* 17–24.

Koski, M. A., and Ingram, E. M. (1977). Child abuse and neglect: Effect on Bayley scores. *Journal of Abnormal Child Psychology, 5,* 79–91.

Kotelchuck, M. (1982). Child abuse and neglect: Prediction and misclassification. In R. Starr (Ed.), *Child abuse prediction: Policy implications* (pp. 67–104). Cambridge, MA: Ballinger.

Kravitz, R. I., and Driscoll, J. M. (1983). Expectations for childhood development among abusing and non-abusing parents, *American Journal of Orthopsychiatry, 53,* 336–344.

Lynch, M. A., and Roberts, J. (1977). Predicting child abuse: Signs of bonding failure in the maternity hospital. *British Medical Journal, 1,* 624–626.

Maden, M. and Wrench, D. (1977). Significant findings in child abuse research. *Victimology, 2,* 196–224.

Main, M., and Goldwyn, R. (1984). Predicting rejection of her infant from mother's representation of her own experience: Implications for the abused–abusing intergenerational cycle. *Child Abuse and Neglect, 8,* 203–217.

Main, M., and Hesse, E. (in press). Lack of resolution of mourning in adulthood and its relation to disorganization in infancy: Speculations regarding causal mechanisms. In M. Greenberg, D. Cicchetti, and M. Cummings (Eds.), *Attachment in the preschool years.* Chicago: University of Chicago Press.

Main, M., Kaplan, N., and Cassidy, J. (1985). Security in infancy, childhood, and adulthood: A move to the level of representation. In I. Bretherton and E. Waters (Eds.), Growing points in attachment theory and research. *Monographs of the Society for Child Development, 50* (1–2, Serial No. 209), pp. 66–106.

Main, M., and Solomon, J. (in press). Procedures for identifying infants as disorganized-disoriented during the Ainsworth Strange Situation. In M. Greenberg, D. Cicchetti, and M. Cummings (Eds.), *Attachment in the preschool years.* Chicago: University of Chicago Press.

Main, M., and Weston, D. R. (1981). The quality of the toddler's relationship to mother and father: Related to conflict behavior and the readiness to establish new relationships. *Child Development, 52,* 932–940.

Martin, H., and Beezley, P. (1977). Behavioral observations of abused children. *Developmental Medicine and Child Neurology.* 19, 373–387.

Martin, H., and Beezley, P. (1980). Behavioral observations of abused children. In J. V. Cook and R. T. Bowles (Eds.), *Child abuse: Commission and omission.* Toronto: Butterworth.

Marvin, R. S. (1977). An ethological–cognitive model for the attenuation of mother–child attachment behavior. In T. M. Alloway, L. Krames, and P. Pliner (Eds.), *Advances in the study of communication and affect. Vol. 3. The development of social attachments* (pp. 25–60). New York: Plenum.

Marvin, R., and Greenberg, M. (1982). Preschoolers' changing conceptions of their mothers: A social cognitive study of mother–child attachment. In D. Forbes and M. T. Greenberg (Eds.), *New directions for child development: Vol. 14. Developing plans for behavior* (pp. 47–60). San Francisco: Jossey-Bass.

Mash, E. J., Johnston, C., and Kovitz, K. (1983). A comparison of the mother–child interactions of physically abused and non-abused children during play and task situations. *Journal of Clinical Child Psychology, 12,* 337–346.

McKinley, D. G. (1964). *Social class and family life.* New York: Free Press.

Morris, M. G., and Gould, R. W. (1963). Role reversal: A necessary concept in dealing with the "battered-child syndrome." *American Journal of Orthopsychiatry, 33,* 298–299.

National Center on Child Abuse and Neglect (1978). 1977 Analysis of child abuse and neglect research (017-091-00223-1). Washington, DC: U.S. Government Printing Office.

National Institute of Mental Health (1977). *Child abuse and neglect programs: Practice and theory.* Rockville, MD: National Institute of Mental Health, DHEW.

Newberger, E. H., Newberger, C. M., and Hampton, R. L. (1983). Child abuse: The current theory base and future research needs. *Journal of the American Academy of Child Psychiatry, 22,* 262–268.

Ounsted, C., Oppenheimer, R., and Lindsay, J. (1975). The psychopathology and psychotherapy of the families: Aspects of bonding failure. In A. Franklin (Ed.), *Concerning child abuse.* Edinburgh: Churchill Livingston.

Parke, R. D., and Collmer, C. W. (1975). Child abuse: An interdisciplinary analysis. In E. M. Hetherington (Ed.), *Review of child development research,* Vol. 5. Chicago: University of Chicago Press.

Perry, M. A., Wells, E. A., and Doran, L. D. (1982). Parent characteristics in abusing and non-abusing families. *Journal of Clinical Child Psychology, 12,* 329–336.

Polansky, N. A. (1985). Determinants of loneliness among low income mothers. *Journal of Social Service Research, 8,* 1–15.

Polansky, N. A., Chalmers, M., Buttenweiser, E., and Williams, D. (1979). The isolation of the neglectful family. *American Journal of Orthopsychiatry, 49,* 149–152.

Polansky, N. A., Chalmers, M., Buttenweiser, E., and Williams, D. (1981). *Damaged parents: An anatomy of child neglect.* Chicago: University of Chicago Press.

Polansky, N. A., Gaudin, J. M., Ammons, P. W., Davis, K. B. (1985). The psychological ecology of the neglectful mother. *Journal of Child Abuse and Neglect, 9,* 265–75.

Polansky, N. A., Hally, C., and Polansky, N. F. (1976). *Profile of neglect: A survey of the state of knowledge of child neglect.* Washington, DC: U.S. Department of HEW.

Quay, H. (1985). Attention deficit disorder and the behavioral inhibition system: The relevance of the neuropsychological theory of Jeffery A. Gray for prevention. Conference on Hyperactivity as a Scientific Challenge, University of Groningen, Groningen, The Netherlands, June.

Radke-Yarrow, M., Cummings, M., Kuczynski, L., and Chapman, M. (1985). Patterns of attachment in two- and three-year olds in normal families and families with parental depression. *Child Development, 56,* 884–893.

Reidy, T. (1977). The aggressive characteristics of abused and neglected children. *Journal of Clinical Psychology, 33,* 1140–1145.

Robinson, E., and Solomon, F. (1979). Some further findings on the treatment of the mother–child dyad in child abuse. *Child Abuse and Neglect, 3,* 247–251.

Rosenberg, M., and Reppucci, N. D. (1983). Abusive mothers: Perceptions of their own and their children's behavior. *Journal of Consulting and Clinical Psychology, 51,* 674–682.

Schneider-Rosen, K., Braunwald, K. G., and Carlson, V., and Cicchetti, D. (1985). Current perspectives in attachment theory: Illustration from the study of maltreated infants. *Monographs of the Society for Research in Child Development, 50* (1–2, Serial no. 209), pp. 194–210.

Siegal, E., Bauman, K. E., Schaefer, E. S., Saunders, M. M., and Ingram, D. D. (1980). Hospital and home support during infancy: Impact on maternal attachment, child abuse and neglect, and health care utilization. *Pediatrics, 66,* 183–190.

Silver, L. B., Barton, W., and Dublin, C. C. (1967). Mandatory reporting of physical abuse of children in the District of Columbia: Community procedures and new legislation. *Medical Annals of the District of Columbia, 36,* 127–130.

Spieker, S. J., and Booth, C. L. (in press). Maternal antecedents of attachment quality: What makes social risk risky? In J. Belsky and T. Nezworsky (Eds.), *Clinical implications of attachment.* Hillsdale, NJ: Erlbaum.

Sroufe, L. A. (1985). Attachment classification from the perspective of infant–caregiver relationships and infant temperament. *Child Development, 56,* 1–14.

Sroufe, L. A., and Rutter, M. (1984). The domain of developmental psychopathology. *Child Development, 55,* 17–29.

Starr, R. (1982). A research-based approach to prediction of child abuse. In R. E. Starr, Jr. (Ed.), *Child abuse prediction: Policy implications.* Cambridge, MA: Ballinger.

Steele, B. F., and Pollock, C. B. (1974). Psychiatric study of abusive parents. In R. E. Helfer and C. H. Kempe (Eds.), *The battered child,* Chicago: University of Chicago Press.

Steinmetz, S. K., and Straus, M. A. (Eds.) (1974). *Violence in the family.* New York: Dodd, Mead.

Wasserman, G. A., Green, A., and Rhianon, A. (1983). Going beyond abuse: Maladaptive patterns of interaction in abusing mother–infant pairs. *Journal of the American Academy of Child Psychiatry, 22,* 245–252.

Wolfe, D. A. (1985). Child-abusive parents: An empirical review and analysis. *Psychological Bulletin, 97,* 462–482.

Wolock, I., and Horowitz, B. (1984). Child maltreatment as a social problem: The neglect of neglect. *American Journal of Orthopsychiatry, 54,* 530–543.

Young, L. (1964). *Wednesday's children: A study of child neglect and abuse.* New York: McGraw-Hill.

15   Patterns of maternal behavior among infants at risk for abuse: relations with infant attachment behavior and infant development at 12 months of age

Karlen Lyons-Ruth, David B. Connell, and David Zoll

Although the organization and development of mother–infant affective exchange during the first year has received a great deal of attention from developmental researchers, the majority of the work to date has focused on the development of methodologies for describing the construct of sensitive, responsive mothering (Bakeman and Brown, 1977; Belsky, Taylor, and Rovine; 1984; Kaye and Fogel, 1980; Tronick, Als, and Brazelton, 1980). However, the emphasis on assessment of the components of sensitivity has not been matched by an equally careful description of the behaviors characterizing insensitive patterns of mothering. The implicit assumption underlying most previous work has been that maternal insensitivity is adequately defined simply as the absence or opposite of maternal sensitivity. Thus, maternal sensitivity and insensitivity are regarded as quantitatively related along a single theoretical dimension. Support for this conceptualization comes not only from our natural language system regarding the usage of terms like sensitivity but also from factor-analytic studies of mother–infant interaction. These studies have shown that a strong first factor, accounting for 50 percent of the variance or more, reliably emerges and is defined by behaviors such as verbal interaction, maternal responsiveness, maternal positive affect and maternal stimulation (Belsky, Rovine and Taylor, 1984; Clarke-Stewart, 1973). This primary maternal factor is in turn

The work on which this chapter was based was supported by NIMH Grant #35122 to K. Lyons-Ruth and H. Grunebaum. Portions of these data appeared in Lyons-Ruth, K., Connell, D. G., Zoll, D., and Stahl, L. (1987), Infants at social risk: Relationships among infant maltreatment, maternal behavior, and infant attachment behavior (*Developmental Psychology, 23* [2], 223–232); copyright 1987 by the American Psychological Association. Adapted by permission of the publisher. We wish to acknowledge the dedicated work of a devoted clinical and research staff in accomplishing the aims of the project. Particular thanks go to the staff of Neighborhood Support Systems for Infants, Donna Karl, Director, for their collaborative role in the study.

464

related to positive infant affect and higher developmental scores (e.g., Clarke-Stewart, 1973). The often replicated relationship between maternal verbal responsiveness and high infant mental developmental scores has probably acted to fix attention even more strongly on this general "good mother" construct (e.g., Carew, 1980; Elardo, Bradley, and Caldwell, 1977). However, clinical observation indicates that all "sensitive" mothers and all "insensitive" mothers are not alike, and the implicit adoption of linear constructs and reliance on linear statistics may have obscured the identification of qualitatively distinct patterns of interaction that are not linearly related. Others have also called attention to the semantically and operationally complex nature of the construct of sensitive responsiveness (Belsky, Taylor, and Rovine, 1984; Stern, 1974).

In contrast to descriptive work on normal populations, high-risk studies such as the one reported in this chapter have a different mandate. In attempting to identify predictors of childhood psychopathology among populations of socially at risk infants, investigators must focus more carefully on identifying distinct patterns of early maladaptive interaction. Crittenden (1981), using a behavioral checklist approach, was able to identify patterns of maternal behavior that distinguished among abusing, neglecting, and adequate mothers of infants aged 1 to 19 months. Behaviors that distinguished abusing from nonabusing mothers were primarily instances of insensitive interference with the infants' goal-directed behavior or the display of conflicting emotional signals by the mother, usually involving covert hostility. These behaviors are listed in detail in Crittenden (1981). Behaviors characteristic of neglecting mothers were those associated with lack of interaction, including physical distance from the child, long pauses between interactive initiatives, absence of affective expression and lack of eye contact. Adequate mothers, by contrast, were distinguished by their contingent responsiveness to the infant, affectionate behavior, maternal enjoyment, and adaptation to the goals of the infant. One goal of the current study was an attempt to confirm Crittenden's findings that two distinct organizational patterns of maladaptive maternal interaction could be identified and related to risk of maltreatment.

A second aim of the present study was to examine whether the incidence of anxious infant attachment responses was related to risk of maltreatment. Attachment theory would predict that anxious infant attachment responses would be more frequent in caregiving relationships that do not function effectively as sources of comfort and security. Infants who have been maltreated would appear to be at one extreme of the continuum of caretaking casualty described by Sameroff and Chandler (1975). Therefore, anxious attachment was predicted to be more frequent among maltreated infants. Recent studies investigating the relationship between maltreatment and attachment behavior have generally concurred in finding lower incidences of secure attachment among maltreated infants (Crittenden, 1985; Egeland and Sroufe, 1981; Lamb, Gaensbauer, Malkin, and Schultz, 1985; Schneider-Rosen, Braunwald, Carlson, and Cicchetti, 1985). Investigators have not agreed, however, in their classification of the insecure behaviors observed, with some reporting a majority of anxious avoidant infants among maltreated samples (Lamb et al., 1985) and others reporting greater numbers of anxious-resistant infants (Egeland and Sroufe, 1981; Schneider-Rosen et al., 1985). Crittenden (1985) has reported that a new classification, designated "ambivalent-avoidant," was needed to account for the behavior of the largest subgroup of maltreated infants. Predating these high-risk studies, Main and Weston (1981) have also reported on a small subgroup of middle-class infants whose behavior did not fit into the traditional classification system. Thus, a secondary question that has recently emerged in the high-risk literature is how best to characterize the attachment behavior patterns of maltreated infants.

A third hypothesis of the study was that patterns of hostile interfering maternal insensitivity and patterns of insensitivity due to maternal apathy and withdrawal would impact differently on infant attachment and development. Our tentative hypothesis, on the basis of Ainsworth and colleagues' (Ainsworth, Blehar, Waters, and Wall, 1978) data, was that the intrusive pattern of maternal behavior would relate to avoidance of the mother, whereas a passive, underinvolved stance would correlate with infant resistance. Differentiated mother–infant interaction patterns characterizing avoidant and resistant infants at home had not clearly emerged from Ainsworth's original longitudinal sample of 23 mothers and infants (Ainsworth et al., 1978) because different methods of analysis yielded different results. In the first analysis, mean scores for 14 maternal home behaviors were compared across the three attachment groups. Mothers of avoidant (A) and resistant (C) infants differed in similar ways on 8 of the 14 variables from mothers of securely attached (B) infants. Different patterns of divergence from the behavior of B mothers occurred on only 2 variables. A mothers more than B mothers tended to pick up their infants in abrupt and interfering ways and C mothers more than B mothers tended to spend holding time occupied with caretaking routines.

In the second analysis, a correlational analysis relating group discriminating function scores to the same 14 maternal variables, only one of the variables was related to both avoidance and resistance, whereas 8 of the 14 related to only the A or the C discriminant function. Mothers of infants showing avoidance were more likely to pick up in abrupt and interfering ways and to be rated as insensitive, interfering, ignoring, and – especially – rejecting, than were mothers of infants who did not show avoidance. Mothers of infants showing resistance, by contrast, delayed their response to crying longer, were more likely to ignore crying altogether, and spent more holding time occupied with caretaking routines. It should be noted that these correlations reflect differences between mothers of infants with A-like and non-A-like behavior, or C-like and non-C-like behavior, rather than between mothers of A, B, and C infants, because the discriminant function scores are continuous variables without the category boundaries assigned by the classification system. Thus, B1, B2, or B4 infants may also be contributing to these effects insofar as their behavior is A-like or C-like.

Most other studies relating maternal behavior to infant attachment responses have focused on the distinction between avoidant and secure infants. Both in the original longitudinal sample and in two subsequent samples of middle-class infants, Main and colleagues have confirmed the association between infant avoidance and maternal aversion to physical contact (Ainsworth et al., 1978; Main and Weston, 1982). Main and colleagues also found that infant insecurity and, particularly, infant avoidance were strongly related to maternal anger and irritation expressed through verbal or nonverbal cues and to a restriction in emotional expression that appeared as detachment or "stiffness" rather than as bland unresponsiveness (Ainsworth et al., 1978; Main, Tomasini, and Tolan, 1979; Main and Weston, 1982). Main's hypothesis was that the stiffness was related to inhibition of expression of negative emotion. Connell (1976) found that mothers of secure infants spent more time in interaction with their infants at home than did mothers of avoidant infants, and Rosenberg (1975) found that mothers of secure infants showed greater reciprocity in a free-play laboratory situation, although not in directed play, than did mothers of avoidant infants. Maternal behavior in the resistant group was not analyzed in these studies because the numbers of 3 and 6 were considered too small.

More recently, Grossmann, Grossmann, Spangler, Suess, and Unzner (1985), studying a North German sample, found consistent differences in maternal sensitivity between mothers of secure and resistant infants over the first year and less consistent differences between mothers of secure and avoidant infants, which they attributed to cultural pressures on the mother toward early independence training. Only Belsky, Rovine, and Taylor (1984) have presented additional evidence for differential maternal correlates of avoidant and resistant infant behavior. They found that mothers of resistant infants scored lowest on measures of reciprocal interaction and maternal involvement, mothers of secure infants earned moderate scores, and mothers of avoidant infants were given the highest scores. Mothers of resistant infants were also found to be less responsive to distress and to vocalization than were mothers of secure infants. Belsky and colleagues hypothesize that avoidance may be the product of insensitive overstimulation and resistance the product of insensitive understimulation.

Overview of the sample and 12-months assessment procedures

The findings to be reported in this chapter were derived from a larger investigation of the impact of social risk indicators and the provision of preventive services on infant development in a very low income, inner city population. Half of the sample was referred to the study because area pediatric and social service providers felt the infants to be at social and psychiatric risk due to poor mother–infant relationships and economic and social stresses within the family. Eighty-nine percent of the families were supported by AFDC, 50% were single parents, and 42% had less than a high school education. Case descriptions and descriptions of the intervention services offered to the high-risk families have been presented in detail in Lyons-Ruth, Botein, and Grunebaum (1984).

This clinically referred sample was individually matched with a community comparison sample of mothers and infants drawn from the same neighborhoods who had never received social services directed at parenting skills and had never had extensive psychiatric treatment. Case and control groups were matched on family income, mother's education and race, and the child's age, sex, and birth order (firstborn, later-born). Comparisons of case and control groups, documenting differences between the groups in family histories and depressive symptoms, have been presented in Lyons-Ruth, Connell, Grunebaum, Botein, and Zoll (1984).

The 12-month sample consisted of 56 families. 28 high-risk and 28 matched controls. Thirty of the 56 infants were boys.

Infant risk status

Three levels of infant risk were identified in the sample. The lowest risk group consisted of the community comparison mothers who had never sought or received services related to parenting difficulties and had never been psychiatrically hospitalized. The second level of risk consisted of mothers referred to our home-visiting service because of service providers' concerns about their relationships with their infants. The most serious risk group consisted of the ten mothers who had been judged maltreating by the State Department of Social Services. As just described, high-risk and community mothers were matched on demographic variables. Chi-square analyses confirmed that the maltreating subgroup of the high-risk group also did not differ from the remainder of the sample on any of these variables.

Our maltreated sample was too small and heterogeneous to lend itself to a clear division between abusing and neglecting mothers. Most mothers were being followed by protective services both for providing inadequate care and for harsh or inappropriate parenting practices. Only one mother had a history of battering a previous child. In all cases the mother was considered the primary agent of abuse or neglect.

Assessment of maternal behavior at home

Naturalistic mother–infant interaction was videotaped at home for 40 minutes when the infants were 12 months of age. Mothers were told that the observer was interested in recording a typical segment of the infant's day and asked to conduct themselves as they usually would. Maternal behavior was coded in 10 four-minute intervals on 12 five-point rating scales and 1 timed variable. These included Sensitivity, Warmth, Verbal Communication, Quality and Quantity of Relational Touching (physical contact in the service of communicating affection, "touching-base," or reducing distress), Quality and Quantity of Caretaking Touching, Interfering Manipulation, Covert Hostility, Anger, Disengagement, Flatness of Affect, and Time Out of the Room, rounded to the nearest half-minute.

The Sensitivity scale was that developed by Ainsworth, Bell, and Stayton (1971) but collapsed from a 9- to a 5-point scale. The Interfering Manipulation scale rated the extent to which the mother manipulated the infant's body with abrupt movements or in ways not contigent on or responsive to the infant's current activities. The Covert Hostility scale rated the extent to which the mother's affective cues either did not match her own behavior or communicated hostility, irritation, or disgust (e.g., smiling with sharp voice tone, sweet voice with negative content). Detailed behavioral items for these two scales are available in Crittenden (1981). The Flatness of Affect scale assessed the degree to which facial and vocal tone were unchanging and expressionless. Rating scales were chosen over more detailed behavior codes because of the better long-term predictive power of ratings, as reported by Jay and Ferran (1981).

Coders were blind to all other data on the families, including risk status. Interobserver reliabilities, computed on independent ratings of 20% of the home videotapes, yielded percentages of exact agreement above 77.5% for 12 variables, with exact agreement on the thirteenth scale, Disengagement, at 68%. Mean percent exact agreement over all variables was 82.7%. Agreement within one point on the Disengagement scale was 97%, however, and agreement within one point was above 90% for all other scales, with a mean of 97.2%. Cohen's Kappa coefficients ranged from .45 to .81, all $p < .001$.

Assessment of infant attachment security and mental and motor development

Mothers and infants were assessed in the Ainsworth Strange Situation at 12 months of age, within two weeks after the home videotaped session. Before the attachment assessment, infants were administered the Bayley Scales of Infant Development by a trained staff member in a separate laboratory room. Mothers were present during the testing.

After the Bayley scales were administered, mothers and infants were videotaped in the Ainsworth Strange Situation. In this procedure, the infant is videotaped in a playroom during a series of eight structured three-minute episodes involving the baby, the mother, and a female stranger. During the observation the mother leaves and rejoins the infant twice, first leaving the infant with the female stranger, then leaving the infant alone. The procedure is designed to be mildly stressful in order to increase the intensity of activation of the infant's attachment behavior. All videotapes were coded as described by Ainsworth et al. (1978). Coders were blind to all other data on the families, including risk status. Pearson correlation coefficients for individual variables computed on independent coding of 20% of the tapes ranged from .97 to .72, with a mean of .86, all $p < .01$.

Final classification of infants as to secure, avoidant, and resistant status was accomplished according to an objective multivariate classification procedure developed by the second author using Ainsworth's original data set of 104 infants and 74 variables. The procedures and variables used in the analysis were very similar to those presented in detail in Ainsworth et al. (1978), chapter 6. A complete description is available from the second author (Connell, 1976b). The classification procedure correctly classified 97% of the 65 infants used to generate the set of discriminant functions and correctly classified 96% of the infants in the remainder of the data set used to validate the procedure. The multivariate classifier was used in preference to coder judgments because of the procedure's high reliability and because the basis for each classification decision can be explicitly specified. Much more information regarding the original classifications in the Ainsworth data set is represented in the formula used by the classifier than is available in the summary verbal descriptions provided to coders.

Both the final classifications and the reduced set of 10 behavioral variables on which the classifications were based were retained for analysis. When this study was designed, there was little data documenting the applicability of the classification system for infants from impoverished and maltreating families. Main and Weston (1981) had also reported that some patterns of infant behavior did not fit any of the three attachment classifications and questioned the wisdom of using a forced classification procedure. Thus, both the behavioral ratings and the final classification codes were examined in the data analysis. The behavioral variables were further reduced to seven by summing across the two reunion episodes or across the two stranger/baby episodes to yield single scores for avoidance, resistance, proximity-seeking and contact-maintaining to mother during reunions, a single score for resistance to the stranger, and total scores across all episodes for frequencies of crying and exploration

Table 15.1. *Principal components analysis of maternal behavior ratings*

Maternal behavior ratings	Factor 1 Maternal involvement Variance accounted for = 45%	Factor 2 Hostile intrusiveness Variance accounted for = 14%	Factor 3 Caretaking Variance accounted for = 10%	Factor 4 Flatness of affect Variance accounted for = 9%
Sensitivity	.77			
Warmth	.88			
Verbal communication	.91			
Quantity of relational touching	.78			
Quality of relational touching	.81			
Quantity of caretaking touching	.66			
Disengagement	−.91			
Anger	−.59			
Time out of room	−.51			
Covert hostility		.84		
Interfering manipulation		.71		
Quantity of caretaking touching			.61	
Quality of caretaking touching			.73	
Flatness of affect				.70

Note: Unrotated analysis, reporting all loadings > +.5 or < −.5.

Results

The organization of maternal behaviors in a high social risk sample

The 13 maternal variables were subjected to an unrotated principal components factor analysis to provide a summary description of the patterns of intercorrelation among maternal behaviors and to identify orthogonal components of variance.

Table 15.1 presents the four factors with eigenvalues greater than one that emerged from the analysis. Factor 1, Maternal involvement, accounted for 45% of the variance and replicates the sensitive-responsive first factor found in other mother–infant interaction studies (e.g., Clarke-Stewart, 1973; Belsky, Taylor, and Rovine, 1984). Maternal behaviors that loaded highly on this factor included, at the positive end, sensitivity, warmth, verbal communication, and affectionate physical contact and, at the negative end, disengagement, anger, and time out of the room. Behaviors loading positively on this factor were those identified by Crittenden as characterizing adequate mothers, and behaviors loading negatively, except for anger, were those characterizing neglecting mothers.

Factor 2, Hostile intrusiveness, which accounted for 14% of the variance, was characterized by high loadings on covert hostility and interfering manipulation, behaviors identified by Crittenden (1981) as distinguishing abusive mothers.[1]

Factor 3, Caretaking, with 10% of the variance, represented variance associated with caretaking behavior. Clarke-Stewart (1973) and Belsky and colleagues (1984) also found caretaking behavior to load on a separate factor.

Factor 4, Flatness of affect, accounting for 9% of the variance, was represented by a high loading for only one variable, flatness of affect. Lack of emotional expression was identified by Crittenden as characteristic of neglecting mothers.

Because the factoring procedure requires derived factors to be orthogonal, the actual distributions of the 13 variables along the dimensions represented by the four factors were also examined. The plot of the relationships between the variables loading highly on Factors 1 and 2 confirmed the presence of three distinct groupings of variables that corresponded well to the 3 sets of behaviors identified by Crittenden as characterizing the neglecting, abusive and adequate mothers in her sample and also confirmed the orthogonal relationship between variables indexing maternal involvement and variables indexing maternal hostile intrusiveness.

Maternal interaction and infant maltreatment

When the 13 maternal behavior ratings of mothers in the protective service group were compared with the behavior ratings of mothers in the rest of the sample, maltreating mothers scored significantly higher than nonmaltreating mothers on covert hostility, $F(1,54) = 6.25$, $p < .02$, and interfering manipulation, $F(1,54) = 4.09$, $p < .05$. As a group, they were not lower than other mothers on any of the variables composing Factor 1, the Maternal involvement factor, such as verbal communication, warmth, quality of relational touch, (direct expressions of) anger, disengagement, or time out of the room. The analysis of factor scores mirrored the findings of the separate variables, with maltreating mothers showing elevated scores only on the Hostile intrusiveness factor, $F(1,54) = 5.01$, $p < .03$.

Although the analysis of group means indicated that the maltreating mothers in our sample were rated higher than the other mothers primarily on indices of interfering behavior and covertly hostile emotional cues, the original hypothesis, following Crittenden, was that the maltreating group might be dichotomous and contain both hostile-intrusive and uninvolved mothers. Analysis of group data might obscure the presence of two quite different subgroups among the maltreatment sample.

To explore whether the dual criterion of noninvolvement *or* hostile intrusiveness would provide a more sensitive discrimination of the maltreating group, and to assess the degree to which maltreating mothers could be dis-

Table 15.2. *Proportions of mothers in each risk group exhibiting high hostile intrusiveness (Factor 2) or low involvement (Factor 1) with their infants at home*

Maternal behavior at home	n	Maltreatment group 10	High-risk group 18	Community group 28
High hostile intrusiveness (top 20% of Factor 2 scores)	11	.50(5)	.11(2)	.14(4)[a]
Low involvement (bottom 20% of Factor 1 scores)	11	.30(3)	.17(3)	.18(5)
Both	22	.80(8)	.28(5)	.32(9)
Neither	34	.20(2)	.72(13)	.68(19)[b]

[a]Maltreating mothers showed high hostile intrusiveness more frequently than did other mothers in the sample, Fisher's Exact Test $p = .001$.
[b]Maltreating mothers were significantly differentiated from all other mothers by the joint criteria of hostile intrusiveness or low involvement, Fisher's Exact Test $p = .006$.

criminated on a case-by-case basis, mothers who were either high on Hostile Intrusiveness (Factor 2) or low on Maternal Involvement (Factor 1) were compared on protective service status. Because the maltreatment group comprised roughly 20% of the sample, the most extreme 20% of scores on each factor (high scores for Factor 2, low scores for Factor 1) were compared to the remaining 80% of scores. These data are presented in Table 15.2. No mother was rated both very high on Factor 2 and very low on Factor 1.

The data in Table 15.2 confirm on a case-by-case basis that maltreating mothers were significantly more likely than other low-income mothers to receive high ratings by blind coders on hostile intrusiveness toward their infants at home. Fifty percent of maltreating mothers but only 13% of all nonmaltreating mothers (high-risk and community groups combined) were in the high scoring group, Fisher's Exact Test $p = .001$.

As shown in Table 15.2, an additional and nonoverlapping 30% of maltreating mothers were identified by low scores on Factor 1, maternal involvement. However, this figure was not significantly different from the proportion of nonmaltreating mothers who were rated low on Factor 1. Thus, for this sample, the combined criterion was not more sensitive than the Hostile Intrusiveness scores alone, Fisher's Exact Test $p = .006$, correctly identifying 80% of protective service cases and falsely identifying 30% of the remaining sample.

Table 2 also reveals the lack of discrimination afforded by maternal behavior between high-risk mothers who were not judged maltreating and other community mothers who had not been considered at high risk for parenting failures.

These findings indicate that at least two clearly discriminable and apparently mutually exclusive patterns of maternal insensitivity exist among socially at risk mothers and infants, one pattern characterized by maternal withdrawal and lack of both emotional and behavioral involvement with the infant and a second pattern characterized by maternal involvement that is insensitive to infant signals and accompanied by covert hostility.

The convergence between the current findings and Crittenden's (1981) data indicate that these patterns can be reliably identified across studies and, at least in the case of the intrusively involved pattern, reliably related to caretaking failures requiring protective services. Our inability to validate the disengaged maternal behavior pattern against protective service status is most likely a function of the small size of our protective service sample.

It is notable that mothers followed by protective services differ from other mothers not only in the relatively gross and diverse caretaking failures that result in findings of abuse or neglect (e.g., tying a child to the bed, failure to obtain medical care, battering, failure to provide adequate physical hygiene, failure to provide adequate supervision or protection against accidents), but also in subtle aspects of daily interaction with their infants. These constant aspects of mother–child interaction may be equally or more important in shaping the infant's developmental trajectory than the more discrete occurrences that typically result in the involvement of protective services.

A second notable aspect of the findings is that none of the maternal behavior scales loading highly on the Maternal Involvement factor discriminated maltreating mothers from the rest of the sample. The primary reason appears to be that some variables loading positively on this dimension, such as sensitivity, warmth, and verbal communication, are affected by both rate of interaction and appropriateness of interaction. Because the hostile-intrusive mothers were quite actively interacting with their infants, they tended to receive high scores on verbal communication and middle-range scores on other variables.

This mirrors Crittenden's (1981) findings that abusive mothers showed elevated rates of both intrusive and covertly hostile behaviors but did not differ on frequency or duration of desirable behaviors.

Infant attachment behavior and infant maltreatment

Infant attachment behaviors in the Ainsworth situation were significantly related to infant maltreatment, as can be seen in Table 15.3. Maltreated infants showed less proximity-seeking to mothers at reunion, $F(1,54) = 9.04$, $p < .004$, and greater avoidance, $F(1,54) = 4.51$, $p < .04$. Infant resistance at reunion was also marginally greater in the maltreated group, $F(1,54) = 2.98$, $p < .09$.

However, infant maltreatment was not significantly related to infant attachment classification as assigned by traditional criteria, although there

Table 15.3. *Mean infant attachment behavior scores at one year as a function of infant risk status*

Infant attachment behavior (Ainsworth coding scales)	Maltreated infants $n = 10$	Nonmaltreated high-risk infants $n = 18$	Community group infants $n = 28$
Contact maintaining at reunion (Mean rating for Reunions 1&2)	2.3[a]	2.9	2.8
Proximity seeking at reunion (Mean rating for Reunions 1&2)	2.2**	3.8	3.7
Avoidance of mother at reunion (Mean rating for Reunions 1&2)	3.6*	2.3	2.4
Resistance to mother at reunion (Mean rating for Reunions 1&2)	1.7[x]	1.4	1.2
Resistance to stranger (Mean rating for Episodes 4&7)	1.9	2.0	2.3
Total crying (Mean number of 15 second intervals/episode containing crying)	1.7	2.3	2.1
Total exploration (Mean number of 15 second intervals/episode containing locomotion and mean number of intervals/episode containing manipulation)	8.8	7.2	8.0

[a]Asterisks in this column indicate that infants in the maltreated group differed significantly from infants in the remainder of the sample.
[x]$p < .10$
*$p < .05$
**$p < .01$

was a nonsignificant trend for maltreated infants more often to be classified as avoidant – 50% as compared to 35% of the rest of the sample – and less often to be classified as secure – 40% as compared to 63% of the rest of the sample.

The discrepancy between the behavioral data and the final classification data is due to an elevated incidence of avoidant, resistant, and avoidant-resistant behavior among infants classified as securely attached by the forced classification procedure. The behavior pattern that occurred most frequently among maltreated infants classified as secure in the initial classifications was one of unstable avoidance not seen in such extreme form in previous middle-class samples. A subgroup of high-risk infants showed very marked avoidance at the first reunion but very little avoidance at the second reunion. These infants contributed to the significant relationship in Table 15.3 between behavioral avoidance and maltreatment but, in the final classifications, 83% fell into the secure category. Table 15.4 presents the frequencies for this unstable avoidant pattern in the original Ainsworth sam-

Table 15.4. *Proportion of infants in the Ainsworth, Connell, and current samples exhibiting unstable avoidant behavior in the Strange Situation*

				Change in avoidance rating from Reunion 1 to Reunion 2		
Study samples	n	Unstable avoidance [Large decrease (≥ 4 pts.)]	Small decrease (≤3 pts.)	All other patterns	Small increase (≤3 pts.)	Large increase (≥4 pts.)
Ainsworth sample[a]	104	.04 (4)[b]	.13 (13)	.71 (74)	.11 (11)	.02 (2)
Connell sample	54	.02 (1)	.09 (5)	.81 (44)	.04 (2)	.04 (2)
Current sample:						
Community group	28	0	.07 (2)	.86 (24)	0	.07 (2)
Total	186	.03 (5)	.11 (20)	.76 (142)	.07 (13)	.03 (6)
Current sample:						
High-risk group	28	.21 (6)[c,d]	.11 (3)	.61 (17)	.04 (1)	.04 (1)

[a] We appreciate the permission of M. D. S. Ainsworth to report these data.

[b] Ratings for reunions one and two for these four subjects were 5/1, 5/1, 5/1, and 6/2, and all were classified as securely attached.

[c] Ratings for reunions one and two for these six subjects were 5/1, 5/1, 5/1, 7/1, 7/1, 7/3. The first five were classified as securely attached, the last as avoidant.

[d] χ^2 comparing the high-risk group versus all others in frequency of large decreases in avoidance, large increases in avoidance and all other patterns, $\chi^2 (2, n = 214) = 17.66, p < .001$.

Table 15.5. *Proportions of infants in each of the three risk groups by attachment classification and attachment behavior*

Infant attachment behavior in the strange situation	*n*	Maltreated infants 10	Nonmaltreated high-risk infants 18	Community group infants 28	All infants 56
Attachment classifications					
Avoidant	21	.50	.28	.39	.38
Unstable avoidant[a]	5	.30	.11	0	.09
Secure	28	.10	.56	.61	.50
Resistant	2	.10	.06	0	.04
Presence of insecure behavior at reunion					
Resistance only	3	.20	.06	0	.05
Avoidance and resistance	15	.40	.28	.21	.27
Avoidance only	18	.40	.22	.36	.32
Neither	20	0[b]	.44	.43	.36

[a]Only the five infants originally classified as securely attached are included in this group. The one unstable-avoidant infant classified as avoidant is left in the avoidant category. That infant was in the maltreated group.
[b]Maltreated infants differed from nonmaltreated infants in numbers of infants showing no avoidance or resistance at reunion, Fisher's Exact Test, $p = .01$.

ples, in the middle-class sample assessed by Connell (1976a), and in the current sample.

Given the significant relationship displayed between unstable avoidance and high risk status, X^2 (2,N = 214) = 17.66 $p < .001$, and the further relationship within the current low-income sample between unstable avoidance and maltreatment status, Fisher's Exact Test $p = .01$, it is questionable whether this pattern of behavior should be included in the secure category. As Table 15.4 reveals, the behaviors of these infants differ in degree from the behaviors of infants for whom the B1 and B2 secure subcategories were originally created. If unstable avoidance, as operationally defined in Table 15.4, is classified as an insecure pattern, maltreated infants do differ significantly from the rest of the sample, Fisher's Exact Test $p = .006$. These data are shown in Table 15.5.

It is not clear from our data whether this pattern is the same as the avoidant–resistant category reported by Crittenden (1985). Two-thirds of infants in the unstable avoidance group showed no resistance at either reunion, as coded by the behavioral scale for resistance. Only one infant possibly fit the avoidant–resistant designation in that an initial high level of avoidance was replaced by a high level of resistance at the second reunion. However, Crittenden's criteria for resistance were considerably broader than the set of behaviors represented on the coding scale, and this may account for the differences in our findings.

The most important difference in attachment behavior between maltreated and nonmaltreated infants in this sample was in the proportion of infants showing no indication of ambivalence at reunion, as is also illustrated in Table 15.5. One hundred percent of maltreated infants showed some avoidance or resistance at reunion, while only 57% of nonmaltreated infants did, Fisher's Exact Test $p = .01$. In the classification subcategories described by Ainsworth and colleagues, these securely attached infants without avoidant or resistant behavior would most likely be categorized as B3, the most prototypically secure subgroup. Thus, distinctions within the groups of infants classed as secure by the traditional forced classification procedure were important in distinguishing maltreated from nonmaltreated infants in this study.

As was true of the secure classification, maltreated infants classified as avoidant also behaved somewhat differently than control infants classified as avoidant. Mixed avoidance and resistance was shown by 40% of the maltreated infants, but only 21% of community infants, as is also shown in Table 15.5. Two-thirds of avoidant and resistant infants were classified as avoidant although they differed from the traditionally described avoidant infant in the concomitant presence of resistance. Among infants classified as avoidant, 64% of the community group but only 20% of the maltreated infants showed stable avoidance without resistance as originally described by Ainsworth and colleagues (1978). This difference did not reach significance with the current small sample size, but is consistent with the report by Crittenden (1985) of elevated numbers of avoidant–resistant infants in maltreated samples.

In summary, maltreated infants showed significantly less proximity seeking and greater avoidance of their mothers at reunion in the Strange Situation, as well as a marginally reliable trend toward greater resistance. The organization of these behaviors departed somewhat from that observed in middle-class samples, resulting in nonsignificant differences between groups in the traditional forced classification procedure. However, infants showing unambivalent attachment, the B3 subgroup, were significantly absent in the maltreated sample.

Infant attachment behavior and maternal behavior at home

As with infant risk status, significant relationships between infant attachment and maternal behavior emerged from the analyses of infant reunion behaviors as assessed by the behavioral coding scales, but not from infant behavior as reflected in the final attachment classifications.

The relationships between maternal behaviors at home and infant behaviors in the Strange Situation revealed two distinct sets of mother–infant interrelationships, one centering around infant avoidant behavior on

Table 15.6. *Pearson correlation coefficients between maternal behaviors at home and infant attachment behaviors in the Strange Situation*

Maternal behaviors at home	Infant behaviors in the Strange Situation						
	CMM[a]	PSM	AVM	REM	RES	EXPL	CRY
Factor 1: Maternal involvement							
Sensitivity (+)[b]							
Warmth (+)							
Verbal communication (+)			−.27*				
Quantity of relational touching (+)							
Quality of relational touching (+)			−.20ˣ				
Disengagement (−)			.19ˣ				
Time out of room (−)			.23*				
Anger (−)						.20ˣ	
Factor 2: Hostile intrusiveness							
Covert hostility (−)	−.21ˣ	.29*			−.18ˣ	.28*	−.20ˣ
Interfering manipulation (−)							
Factor 3: Caretaking							
Quantity of caretaking touching (+)							
Quality of caretaking touching (+)							
Factor 4: Flatness of affect							
Flatness of affect (−)				.24*		−.25*	.19ˣ

[a]CMM = Contact maintaining to mother at reunion; PSM = Proximity-seeking to mother at reunion; AVM = Avoidance of mother at reunion; REM = Resistance to mother at reunion; RES = Resistance to the stranger in episodes 4 & 7; EXPL = Total exploration across all episodes; CRY = Total crying across all episodes.
[b](+) indicates positive behavior earns higher rating; (−) indicates negative behavior earns higher rating.
ˣ$p < .09$
*$p < .05$.

reunion and one around infant resistant behavior. These relationships are shown in Table 15.6.

Higher levels of infant avoidance during the two reunion episodes were related to the mother's more frequent display of covert hostility in interaction with her child. Other behaviors indicative of an avoidant attachment pattern – namely, less proximity-seeking at reunion, continued exploration of the environment, lack of overt distress, and greater acceptance of the stranger – were also marginally related to the mother's covert hostility at home. Thus, the behavioral organization of infants of covertly hostile mothers follows the pattern described by Ainsworth as characteristic of the avoidant attachment pattern.

Table 15.7. *The relationship between low maternal involvement at home and infant resistance to the mother in the Strange Situation*

		Maternal behavior	
		Low maternal involvement (bottom 20% Factor 1)	Not low maternal involvement (top 80% Factor 1)
Infant behavior	*n*	11	45
Resistance only		18%	2%
Avoidance and resistance		46%	22%
Avoidance only		9%	38%
Neither		27%	38%

Note: X^2 (2, n = 56) = 7.96, p < .025 (last two categories were collapsed for the X^2)

By contrast, infant resistance to the mother at reunion increased as mother's flatness of affect and time out of the room increased and decreased with greater verbal interaction. Resistance also tended to decrease with higher quality affectionate touching. Other behaviors consistent with the resistant attachment pattern, including increased crying and decreased exploration, were also related to flatness of affect. As can be seen in Table 15.6, the maternal behaviors associated with infant resistance were those loading on maternal Factor 1, Maternal Involvement, and Factor 3, Flatness of Affect, whereas those associated with avoidance loaded on Factor 2, Hostile Intrusiveness.

Interestingly, the more global Warmth and Sensitivity scores were not strongly related to infant attachment behaviors. Rather, specific negative behaviors of the mothers at home were related to negative responses by the infants in the Strange Situation.

The earlier analyses of attachment behavior by maltreatment status had shown that 27% of the infants displayed both avoidant and resistant behavior at reunion, as was shown in Table 15.5. From the correlational analysis relating avoidance and resistance separately to maternal behavior, it was not clear what prediction one would make regarding the behavior of the mothers whose infants showed both avoidance and resistance. Therefore, categorical analyses were also performed. As in the maltreatment analyses, infant behavior was classified as avoidant, resistant, avoidant and resistant, or neither and the maternal behavior factors were classified into two categories, the top 20% and the bottom 80% of scores. Relationships between infant behavior and maternal factor scores for Hostile Intrusiveness, Involvement, and Flatness of Affect were examined.

The relationship between low maternal involvement and infant attachment behavior is presented in Table 15.7. As can be seen, mothers who were

Table 15.8. *The relationship between maternal hostile intrusiveness at home and infant avoidance to the mother in the Strange Situation*

| | | Maternal behavior | |
| | | High hostile intrusive involvement (top 20% Factor 2) | Not high hostile intrusive involvement (Lower 80% Factor 2) |
Infant behavior	*n*	11	45
Avoidance only		82%	20%
Avoidance and resistance		18%	29%
Resistance only		0%	7%
Neither		0%	44%

Note: X^2 (2, n = 56) = 16.53, $p < .001$ (last two categories were collapsed for the X^2)

very low on involvement were more likely to have infants who responded to reunions with resistance, either alone or in combination with avoidance, than did mothers who were more interactive with their infants, Fisher's Exact Test $p = .03$. Sixty-four percent of infants with highly uninvolved mothers showed resistance, whereas only 24% of infants with more active mothers did so. Mothers who were uninvolved were particularly unlikely to have infants who responded with avoidance alone at 12 months (although see Egeland and Sroufe, 1981, for 18-months data). Analysis of the single variable, verbal communication, rather than the Factor 1 scores, yielded similar results (see Lyons-Ruth, Connell, Zoll, and Stahl, 1987). Maternal scores on Factor 3, Flatness of Affect, did not reliably relate to infant resistance on a case-by-case basis and dyads high in both Flatness of Affect and infant resistance were also high in maternal uninvolvement.

Infants whose mothers were high on the combination of hostility and intrusiveness represented by Maternal Factor 2 responded very differently to their mothers in the Strange Situation. One hundred percent of infants with mothers who were high on Factor 2 showed avoidant or avoidant–resistant behavior on reunion, while only 49% of the remaining infants did so, $X^2(2,N = 56) = 16.53$, $p < .001$, as shown in Table 15.8. Table 15.8 also reveals a more specific relationship between maternal hostile intrusiveness and avoidance unmixed with resistance, Fisher's Exact Test $p = .001$.

The relationship between the single variable, maternal Covert Hostility, and infant avoidance was also strong, $X^2(2,N = 56) = 12.17, p < .005$, with all infants of highly hostile mothers showing avoidance. The only difference was that a slightly larger proportion of infants, 33%, showed mixed avoidance and resistance when the mother's joint tendency toward interfering manipulation was not considered. Thus, the relationship with avoidance alone was slightly weaker for this variable, Fisher's Exact Test $p = .001$, than for the hostile-interfering behavior represented by the Factor 2 scores (see Lyons-Ruth, Connell, Zoll, and Stahl, 1987).

Although infant behaviors in the Strange Situation related significantly to maternal behaviors at home, the findings relating maternal behavior to the infants' final attachment classifications were much more tenuous. Only one maternal variable significantly differed by infant attachment classification. The span of time the mother was not in the same room with the infant was much greater for infants classified as resistant than for infants classified as either secure or avoidant, with means of 19 minutes, 6 minutes, and 8.5 minutes respectively. Given the small number of infants classified as resistant in this study ($n = 2$), however, this finding would be of questionable importance without confirmation from the previous analyses. In contrast to the small number of infants classified as resistant, 32% of infants in the study showed some resistance to mother on the rating scale.

The same aspects of infant behavior that reduced the relationships between attachment classification and infant maltreatment – namely, the relationships between maltreatment and unstable avoidant behavior and maltreatment and mixed avoidance and resistance – also affected the relationships between attachment classification and maternal behavior. The unstable avoidant pattern, although classified in the same group (B2) in this and previous studies (see Table 15.4), was significantly associated with high maternal Hostile Intrusiveness, Fisher's Exact Test $p = .01$. In fact, mothers of infants showing the unstable avoidant pattern received the highest Hostile Intrusiveness ratings of any classification group and were much more similar to mothers of avoidant infants than to mothers of secure infants. When these infants were classified as part of the avoidant group rather than the secure group, a significant group difference emerged between mothers of secure and avoidant infants in levels of covert hostility, $F(1,52) = 6.96$, $p < .01$. The second factor reducing the relationships between attachment classification and maternal behavior was the presence of infants showing mixed avoidance and resistance. Mixed avoidant and resistant behavior had a different set of maternal correlates than avoidant behavior alone, as previously illustrated in Tables 15.7 and 15.8 and shown in Table 15.9, yet infants with both behavior patterns were classified as avoidant.

Finally, as is also shown in Table 15.9, many infants classified as securely attached also showed some avoidant or resistant behavior. These included infants showing mild avoidance, as described for the B1 and B2 secure subgroups by Ainsworth and colleagues (1978), infants showing mild resistance or avoidance and resistance, as described for the B4 subgroup, and the unstable avoidant group, who showed more extreme forms of B2 and B4 behavior than were shown in the original middle-class samples studied by the Ainsworth group.

Table 15.9. *Relationships among infant attachment behavior: Attachment classification and maternal behavior at home*

Infant attachment classification	*n*	Infant attachment behavior	*n*	Hostile intrusive (top 20% Factor 2) 11[a]	Uninvolved (bottom 20% Factor 1) 11	Neither 34
Avoidant	21	Avoidance only	11	.36 (4)	.09 (1)	.18 (6)
		Avoidance and resistance	10	.18 (2)	.27 (3)	.15 (5)
Secure	33	Avoidance only (unstable avoidant and B1,B2)	7	.45 (5)	0	.06 (2)
		No avoidance or resistance (B3)	20	0	.27 (3)	.50 (17)
		Avoidance and resistance (unstable avoidant and B4)[1]	5	0	.18 (2)	.09 (3)
		Resistance only (B4)	1	0	.09 (1)	0
Resistant	2	Resistance only	2	0	.09 (1)	.03 (1)

Note: Numbers indicate proportions of infants in each maternal behavior grouping who exhibit a particular form of attachment behavior. All *n*'s in parenthesis.
[a]No mother was both high on hostile intrusiveness and low on involvement.

However, as shown in Table 15.9, milder forms of avoidance or resistance, consistent with a secure classification, had similar maternal correlates as the more extreme forms of avoidance and resistance that led to an insecure classification. Because of this, mothers of infants classified as securely attached by traditional criteria did not differ significantly from mothers of anxiously attached infants, with 33% and 45% of secure and anxious infants, respectively, having mothers in one of the extreme categories. Again, it was the B3 subgroup of securely attached infants who were more likely than other infants to have mothers without markedly negative behavior, $X^2(1, N = 56) = 6.19$, $p < .02$. Only 15% of B3 infants had mothers with negative behavior patterns, and all of them were mothers low on involvement, whereas 53% of infants showing avoidant or resistant behavior had mothers in one of the negative categories. Mothers of B3 infants differed reliably from both mothers of infants showing avoidance only and mothers of infants showing behavior that included resistance, Fisher's Exact Test $p = .01$, Fisher's Exact Test $p = .02$, respectively. Even *within* the group of infants classified as securely attached, infants displaying any insecure behav-

Table 15.10. *Mean infant developmental scores at one year classified by infant risk status*

Bayley Scales of Infant Development	n	Maltreated infants 10	Nonmaltreated high-risk infants 18	Community group infants 28
Mental development scores		91**[a]	101.0	104.8
Physical development scores		89**	101.6	102.1

[a]Infants in the maltreated group differed significantly from infants in the remainder of the sample.
**$p < .01$.

ior were significantly more likely to have hostile-intrusive or uninvolved mothers than were *B3* infants, Fisher's Exact Test $p = .02$. This finding is partially due to the presence within the secure classification of infants showing the unstable avoidant pattern, 80% of whom had mothers in one of the extreme categories. Other *B1, B2,* or *B4* infants were less likely than unstable avoidant infants to have mothers with extreme negative behavior. However, these infants were still more than three times as likely as *B3* infants to have mothers in one of the negative behavior categories, 50% compared to 15%.

Infant maltreatment, maternal behavior, and infant mental and motor development

Infants in the maltreatment group differed significantly in both mental and motor development scores from infants in the remainder of the sample, as shown in Table 15.10, $F(1,54) = 6.58$, $p < .01$, $F(1,54) = 8.81$, $p < .005$, respectively.

Although in previous analyses maternal Sensitivity and Warmth did not relate to security of attachment as predicted, the mother's Sensitivity, Warmth, and Verbal Communication did relate positively to infant mental development at 1 year, $r = .26$, $p < .03$, $r = .23$, $p < .04$, and $r = .25$, $p < .03$, respectively, as would be predicted from previous literature (e.g., Elardo, Bradley, and Caldwell, 1977). Verbal communication was also marginally related to motor development, $r = .21$, $p < .07$.

Only one infant behavior in the Strange Situation was related to infant developmental status at one year. Infant resistance to mother was negatively correlated with both mental, $r = -.25$, $p < .03$, and motor development, $r = -.40$, $p < .001$. By contrast, infant avoidance showed no relationship to developmental status. These relationships between infant resistance, but not

Table 15.11. *The relationship between infant resistance and infant developmental scores on the Bayley scales after controlling for maternal home behaviors*

Maternal and infant behaviors associated with infant developmental scores	% Variance accounted for in mental development indices		% Variance accounted for in physical development indices	
	Resistance entered at step one	Resistance entered at step five	Resistance entered at step one	Resistance entered at step five
Maternal behaviors associated with Bayley scores (sensitivity, warmth, verbal communication)	12%	14%	3%	8%
Infant resistance	6%	4%	16%	11%

avoidance, and lowered cognitive or verbal scores have previously been reported by Main (1983) and Connell (1976a) in middle-class samples. The negative relationship found in the present study between infant resistance and maternal verbal communication offers one explanation for the observed relationship between infant resistance and lowered mental and motor scores.

In order to evaluate the hypothesis that the association between infant resistance and infant development could be accounted for by their common relationship with maternal behavior, particularly lack of verbal communication, hierarchical multiple regression analysis was performed. Infant resistance was entered into the regression equation before and then after the three maternal variables that related to the infants' Bayley scores.

As can be seen in Table 15.11, the contribution of resistance to the prediction of mental development scores drops by only 2% when the variance shared with maternal behavior is removed. However, the 4% increment in explained variance contributed by the resistance variable is not significantly different from zero for the MDI, $F(1,51) = 2.68$, N.S. The opposite picture emerges for infant physical development. Infant resistance shares 5% of the variance in PDI with maternal behaviors. However, the unique variance contributed by infant resistance is a significant 11%, $F(1.51) = 7.22$, $p < .01$, more than three times the unique variance explained by maternal behavior.

Thus, the information contributed by infant resistance to the prediction of developmental status overlaps very little with information contributed by maternal behavior and resistance is a stronger predictor than assessed maternal behavior of physical developmental status at 12 months.

Discussion

By 1 year of age maltreated infants differed significantly from other infants in low SES families in both social and cognitive development. They were also the recipients of more covertly hostile and interfering behavior from their mothers at home. Maltreated infants scored an average of 12 points lower than other infants in both mental and motor development and were more likely to avoid their mothers at reunion after a brief separation. Resistance to the mother at reunion was also somewhat elevated in the maltreatment group. Further analyses confirmed that the tendency of maltreated infants to avoid their mothers after separation was directly related to the degree of hostile intrusiveness in the mothers' behaviors toward their infants. As would be predicted from attachment theory, infants showing no conflict in their attachment relationships with their mothers were absent from the maltreatment group.

As has also been reported by Crittenden (1985), the organization of insecure attachment behavior among maltreated infants differed from that observed in middle class samples sufficiently to cause difficulties in applying traditional classification procedures. A significant subgroup of maltreated and high-risk infants in this study showed a pattern of unstable avoidance in which very high levels of avoidance at the first reunion were replaced by little or no avoidance at the second. This pattern was more extreme than that classified as B2 in the original middle-class samples of Ainsworth et al. (1978) and was related to infant maltreatment and to highly hostile-intrusive mothering. This pattern of behavior among maltreated infants may represent a similar phenomenon to that observed by Ainsworth and colleagues (1978) when the Strange Situation was repeated with one sample of infants after an interval of only two weeks. Under the more extreme stress of a repetition of the situation, no infant classified as avoidant two weeks previously could be classified avoidant at the second assessment. Avoidance was shown by the previously avoidant infants to the extent that avoidance from session one to two was highly correlated, $r = .66$. However, the balance between approach and avoidance had shifted enough to lead the infants to approach their mothers despite their still active tendencies to avoid. The degree of stress experienced by maltreated infants from disorganized households may be such that a stable avoidant behavioral pattern is more difficult to organize and maintain by 12 months of age.

It is not clear from our data whether the unstable avoidant pattern is the same as the ambivalent–avoidant pattern noted among maltreated infants by Crittenden (1985). However, Crittenden also reports that many ambivalent–avoidant infants were initially categorized as securely attached because of the presence of approach as well as avoidance tendencies. Two-thirds of infants in the unstable avoidant group showed no coded resistance at either reunion. Only one infant possibly fit the ambivalent–avoidant designation based on the coded data in that a high level of initial avoidance was replaced by a high level of resistance at the second reunion. However, resistance as coded here included only those behaviors specified on the Ainsworth coding scale for resistance and did not include the persistent crankiness and stereotypic or maladaptive behaviors included in Crittenden's new coding system for the A/C group. The recent Disorganized/Disoriented classification developed by Main & Solomon (1986) offers the possibility of systematizing the coding of difficult to classify behaviors across studies. Whether the unstable avoidant and mixed avoidant and resistant subgroups in this study would be classified in the *D* category remains a question for future work. However, the system appears promising in that the behaviors listed by Main and colleagues were all observed among infants in the present study. In addition to the potential utility of the *D* classification, data from the current study would also strongly support the development of detailed behavioral coding scales for disorganized/disoriented behavior. Coding scales preserve more information than final category decisions and such information may be helpful in evaluating optimal placement for the category boundaries.

The relationships between maternal behavior at home and infant attachment responses in the Strange Situation were consistent with those previously reported by Ainsworth et al. (1978) and Main and colleagues (Main, Tomasini, and Tolan, 1979; Main & Weston, 1982) in middle-class groups. The repeated emphasis in these findings on the relationship between maternal anger and rejection and infant avoidance was echoed in these data. Consistent with Main's emphasis on coding subtle verbal and nonverbal signs of submerged or denied anger, the measure of covert hostility, rather than direct anger, correlated most strongly with avoidance and its associated behaviors in this sample. This probably reflects the tendency of mothers to limit direct expressions of anger in the presence of observers. Our measure of covert hostility also drew heavily on the descriptions of ambivalent behavior observed in abusing mothers by Crittenden (1981). Maltreating mothers were rated more highly on covert hostility than were nonmaltreating mothers in the current sample, confirming the chain of relationships between infant avoidance, maternal hostility, and infant maltreatment originally predicted by George and Main (1979).

The findings of Ainsworth et al. (1978) that mothers of avoidant infants also tended to be interfering and abrupt in pickups was echoed in the relationship found between maternal Factor 2, Hostile Intrusiveness, and infant avoidance. Because the single scale for interfering manipulation did not relate to avoidance per se, it would appear to be the covariance between hostility and interfering behavior expressed by the factor scores that has a particularly strong relation to infant behavior. We did not find a relationship between aspects of maternal touch and infant avoidance in these analyses. However, relationships similar to those reported by Main and Weston (1982), between quality of maternal touch at six months and infant security of attachment, are emerging in current analyses. Thus, the tender, careful quality of maternal touch earlier in the first year may be more critical to later security of attachment than touch assessed at one year.[1]

The correlates of infant resistance found by Ainsworth et al. (1978) – that is, ignoring or delay in responding to infant distress and holding primarily during caretaking – were also similar to those that emerged in the present study. Infant resistance was related to maternal unresponsiveness, as indexed by lack of verbal communication, flatness of affect, and a lack of affectionate touching, creating a similar picture of a mother who is little inclined to interact with and respond to her infant. Our measure of flatness of affect probably differs from Main's variable of lack of expression (which she related to infant avoidance) in that she emphasized the "stiffness" of the mother's demeanor and the inferred attempt to control expression of anger. Flatness of affect here refers also to a lack of variability of affect but tended to occur in our population among mothers with a more "burnt out" and depressed demeanor.

One surprising difference between our data and previous work is in the lack of findings related to maternal sensitivity and warmth. Infants classified as securely attached did not have mothers who were rated higher on sensitivity or warmth, nor did these variables relate negatively to avoidance or resistance. These variables also failed to relate to infant risk status. The most likely explanation lies in the relative absence in our sample of warmly responsive mother–infant relationships. Mothers very rarely played with their infants during the 40-minute observations and many rarely interacted with their infants even when they were in the same room. Some of the most highly interacting mothers were, in fact, the mothers rated high on hostile intrusiveness, and many of these mothers, because of their generally high rates of interaction in comparison to other mothers in the study, earned moderate scores on sensitive responsiveness. This is reminiscent of Crittenden's (1981) description of the abusive mothers in her study as trying "the hardest to create a successful interaction and yet these infants seemed the most frustrated" (p. 210). Belsky, Rovine, and Taylor's (1984) data indicating that mothers of avoidant infants were the most involved in interaction points to a similar phenomenon. Thus, it appears important in future studies to carefully disentangle rate of interaction from appropriateness and affective tone.

The overall impression gained from our data, however, is that rather than maternal sensitivity and warmth promoting security of attachment, secure attachment will develop in the absence of specific interfering maternal behaviors such as marked unresponsiveness or hostile intrusiveness. This view is consistent with the overall theoretical position of Ainsworth et al. (1978) and Bowlby (1969), which stresses that infants are preadapted to seek their primary attachment figures under stress. The evolutionary viewpoint would predict that attachment behaviors would occur under a wide range of environmental conditions and would not require especially sensitive mothering for their development. This position is also consistent with the repeated findings that middle- and lower-class mothers differ in overall levels of verbal communication and responsive interaction with their infants (Ferran and Ramey, 1980; Golden, Birns, Bridger, and Moss, 1971), yet strong class differences have not emerged in proportions of infants judged securely attached (Ainsworth et al., 1978; Egeland and Sroufe, 1981; Schneider-Rosen et al., 1985). Thus, in previous studies, the negative end of the maternal sensitivity dimension may have been more important than the positive end in accounting for variation in infant attachment. By contrast, the positive variables in this study – sensitivity, warmth, and verbal communication – do account for significant variance in infants' mental development, indicating that the aspects of sensitivity or responsiveness that are related to mental development are not necessarily the same as those related to security of attachment.

Our findings are also broadly congruent with the conclusions of Belsky, Rovine, and Taylor (1984) that mothers of avoidant and resistant infants are on opposite ends of a continuum of intensity of involvement. Both studies found that resistant infants had mothers who were less interactive than mothers of secure or avoidant infants. Belsky and colleagues reported that mothers of avoidant infants were more often stimulating their infants than mothers of secure or resistant infants. We also found that mothers of avoidant infants were highly involved in interaction, although not more so that mothers of secure infants. For example, they did not show more verbal communication or relational touching than did mothers of secure infants, and they tended to spend more time out of the room. Our data show further that the high levels of involvement of mothers of avoidant infants were accompanied by more covertly hostile emotional signals. Thus, it appears likely that our findings and Belsky and colleagues' findings are essentially congruent in emphasizing aspects of an insensitive and intrusive but active and involved mothering style. The emphasis in our data on coding the affective cues of the mother further demonstrate that a continuum of maternal affect accompanies the continuum of activity and suggests that covertly expressed hostility, in particular, plays an important role in shaping infant reactions. The importance of these affective ratings in the prediction of infant behavior supports the work of Main and colleagues (Main, Tomasini, and Tolan, 1979; Main and Weston, 1981, 1982) in indicating the usefulness of affective assessments that go beyond the commonly used discrete behavioral signs such as smiling and touching. Further work is needed to examine the relative contributions of the mothers' behavioral activity and negative emotional cues to the genesis of infant avoidance of the mother under stress.

Finally, the findings related to infant attachment point to the need in future studies for continued examination of the relationships between coded behavioral data and assignment of the final attachment classifications. The essential relationships found here between maternal behavior and infant attachment behavior emerged clearly from the behavioral codes but only faintly from the attachment classifications. Put another way, particular signs of infant insecurity in the Strange Situation were significantly and differentially related to particular signs of maladaptive mothering. However, the *balance* between approach and avoidance tendencies for the infant, on which the classifications focus, was less clearly tied to negative maternal behavior, as tendencies to maintain avoidance or resistance appeared to be overcome by the overall stressfulness of the Strange Situation or of the infant's home environment. As in the studies of Main and colleagues (Main, Tomasini, and Tolan, 1979; Main and Weston, 1981, 1982), we found that infants in the *B1, B2,* and *B4* subgroups of the secure category contributed to the obtained relationships between maternal behavior and infant avoidance and resistance, even though these infants also sought contact with the mother under stress. Because analyses that ignore classification boundaries have also produced clearer relationships between infant behavior and maternal behavior in the work reported in Main and Weston (1982) and even in the original analyses of the longitudinal sample data by Ainsworth and colleagues (1978), as noted earlier, this appears to be a general point not related to the high-risk nature of the current sample.

The findings relating infant resistance to several indicators of maternal uninvolvement provide an important clarification of the relationships that have been reported between infant attachment status and cognitive development. In Main's data (1983), Connell's data (1976a), and in the current study, infant resistance was correlated with lowered developmental or verbal scores. Although the partial correlations presented in Table 15.11 show that maternal behavior as assessed here did not account for the link between infant resistance and lowered developmental scores, mediation of this link by maternal behavior could still be occurring through several routes. The most likely possibility is that the relevant maternal behaviors were not assessed because they were not adequately represented in the coding system, because they were not present when the mothers were being observed, or because maternal behaviors characteristic of earlier periods were more influential in shaping the observed relationships than those observed at 12 months. One example fitting all these criteria would be a tendency to leave the infant for long periods in his or her crib unattended, a behavior frequently observed among mothers in our high-risk sample by their service providers. More detailed studies of the interactional patterns of maltreating mothers and their infants over the first year are needed to evaluate these possibilities. These findings also indicate that maternal behavior must be partialled out in examining the correlations reported by Connell (1976) and Waters, Vaughn, and Egeland (1980) between neonatal status and infant resistance. An impoverished intrauterine environment resulting from poor maternal nutrition, alcohol use, or drug abuse may be the correlate of a general family pattern of disorganization and maternal neglect. Multivariate analyses are needed to refine our hypotheses regarding causal relationships among infant biological status, maternal apathy, infant resistance, and infant development.

Note

1 Subsequent to the writing of this chapter, we reconsidered an early coding decision regarding the assignment of ratings for quality of comforting or caretaking touch. In this chapter, mothers who did not touch their infants during the observation period were assigned the lowest point on the scales of quality of touch. In effect, this a priori decision assumed some correlation between quantity and quality of touch. In fact, such a correlation did not occur in these data, because mothers who touched their infants only once during the observation period had means for quality of touch that were much closer to the mean of the rest of the sample than to the low scores we had arbitrarily assigned to the nontouching mothers.

These very low scores for nontouching mothers also artificially inflated the correlation between quality and quantity of touch, because the assigned low scores for quality of touch turned out to be extreme in relation to the rest of the sample. Leaving these scores blank is an even less satisfactory solution, however, because in any multivariate analysis that procedure results in the elimination of all maternal data from nontouching mothers. Therefore, in subsequent publications, a different and more conservative procedure will be used in which mothers with no touch are given the mean score for all those mothers with very low rates of touching. This avoids data loss and also results in minimal change in the correlational structure of the maternal variables. This change in coding has not altered any of the significant findings reported here.

The factor structure shifts slightly, however, in that the Hostile Instrusiveness factor also includes negative loadings for quality of comforting and caretaking touch, in replication of Main and Weston's (1981) findings regarding the covariation of poor quality of touching with suppressed maternal anger. However, the revised touch variables did *not* predict attachment behavior in themselves, apart from their common loading on Factor 2, which is consistent with the results as reported.

References

Ainsworth, M. D. S., Bell, S. M., and Stayton, D. J. (1971). Individual differences in strange situation behavior of one-year-olds. In H. R. Schaffer (Ed.), *The origins of human social relations*. New York: Academic Press.

Ainsworth, M. D. S., Blehar, M., Waters, E., and Wall, S. (1978). *Patterns of attachment*. Hillsdale, NJ: Erlbaum.

Bakeman, R., and Brown, J. V. (1977). Behavioral dialogues: An approach to the assessment of mother–infant interaction. *Child Development, 48,* 195–203.

Bayley, N., and Schaefer, E. S. (1964). Correlations of maternal and child behaviors with the development of mental abilities: Data from the Berkeley Growth Study. *Monographs of the Society for Research in Child Development, 29* (6 Serial #97).

Belsky, J., Rovine, M., and Taylor, D. (1984). The Pennsylvania Infant and Family Development Project III: The origins of individual differences in infant–mother attachment: Maternal and infant contributions. *Child Development, 55,* 718–728.

Belsky, J., Taylor, D., and Rovine, M. (1984). The Pennsylvania Infant and Family Development Project II: The development of reciprocal interaction in the mother–infant dyad. *Child Development, 55,* 706–717.

Bowlby, J. (1969). *Attachment and loss (Vol. 1): Attachment.* New York: Basic Books.

Carew, J. (1980). Experience in the development of intelligence in young children at home and in day care. *Monographs of the Society for Research in Child Development,* No. 183.

Clarke-Stewart, K. A. (1973). Interactions between mothers and their young children: Characteristics and consequences. *Monographs of the Society for Research in Child Development, 38* (6–7, Serial No. 153).

Connell, D. B. (1976a). *Individual differences in attachment: An investigation into stability, implications and relationships to structure of early language development.* Unpublished doctoral dissertation, Syracuse University.

Connell, D. B. (1976b). Multivariate classifier for the Ainsworth Strange Situation. Available from the author at ABT Associates, 66 Wheeler St., Cambridge, MA 02138.

Crittenden, P. M. (1981). Abusing, neglecting, problematic and adequate dyads: Differentiating by patterns of interaction. *Merrill-Palmer Quarterly, 27*(3), 201–218.

Crittenden, P. M. (1985). Maltreated infants: Vulnerability and resilience. *Journal of Child Psychology and Psychiatry, 26*(1), 85–96.

Egeland, B., and Sroufe, L. A. (1981). Attachment and early maltreatment. *Child Development, 52,* 44–52.

Elardo, R., Bradley, R., and Caldwell, B. (1977). Responsiveness and involvement predicts IQ: A longitudinal study of the relation of infants' home environments to language development at age three. *Child Development, 48,* 595–603.

Ferran, D., and Ramey, C. (1980). Social class differences in dyadic involvement during infancy. *Child Development, 51,* 254–257.

George, C., and Main, M. (1979). Social interactions of young abused children: Approach, avoidance and aggression. *Child Development, 50,* 306–318.

Golden, M., Birns, B., Bridger, W., and Moss, A. (1971). A social class differentiation in cognitive development among black preschool children. *Child Development, 42,* 37–45.

Grossman, K., Grossman, K. E., Spangler, G., Suess, G., and Unzer, L. (1985). Maternal sensitivity and newborn's orientation responses as related to quality of attachment in northern Germany. In I. Bretherton and E. Waters (Eds.), Growing Points in Attachment Theory and Research. *Monographs of the Society for Research in Child Development, 50* (1–2, Serial No. 209) pp. 233–256.

Jay, F., and Ferran, D. C. (1981). The relative efficacy of predicting IQ from mother–child interaction using ratings versus behavioral count measures. *Journal of Applied Developmental Psychology, 2,* 15–17.

Kaye, K., and Fogel, A. (1980). The temporal structure of face-to-face communication between mothers and infants. *Developmental Psychology, 16,* 454–464.

Lamb, M. E., Gaensbauer, T. J., Malkin, C. M., and Schultz, L. A. (1985). The effects of child maltreatment on security of infant–adult attachment. *Infant Behavior and Development, 8,* 35–45.

Lyons-Ruth, K., Botein, S., and Grunebaum, H. U. (1984). Reaching the hard to reach: Serving isolated and depressed mothers with infants in the community. In B. Cohler and J. Musick (Eds.), *Intervention with psychiatrically disabled parents and their young children.* New Directions for Mental Health Services Series, 24. San Francisco: Jossey-Bass, pp. 95–122.

Lyons-Ruth, K., Connell, D., Grunebaum, H., Botein, S., and Zoll, D. (1984). Maternal family history, maternal caretaking and infant attachment in multiproblem families. *Preventive Psychiatry, 2*(314), 403–425.

Lyons-Ruth, K., Connell, D., Zoll, D., and Stahl, J. (1987). Infants at social risk: Relationships among infant maltreatment, maternal behavior, and infant attachment behavior. *Developmental Psychology, 23*(2), 223–232.

Main, M. (1983). Exploration, play and cognitive functioning related to infant–mother attachment. *Infant Behavior and Development, 6,* 167–174.

Main, M., and Solomon, J. (1986). Discovery of an insecure-disorganized/disoriented attachment pattern: Procedure, findings, and implications for the classification of behavior. In M. Yogman and T. B. Brazelton (Eds.), *Affective development in infancy.* Norwood, NJ: Ablex.

Main, M., Tomasini, L., and Tolan, W. (1979). Differences among mothers of infants judged to differ in security of attachment. *Developmental Psychology, 15*(4), 472–473.

Main, M., and Weston, D. R. (1981). Security of attachment to mother and to father: Related to conflict behavior and the readiness to establish new relationships. *Child Development, 52,* 932–940.

Main, M., and Weston, D. R. (1982). Avoidance of the attachment figure in infancy: Descriptions and interpretations. In C. M. Parkes and J. Stevenson-Hinde (Eds.), *The place of attachment in human behavior.* New York: Basic Books, pp. 31–59.

Rosenberg, S. E. (1975). *Individual differences in infant attachment: Relationships to mother, infant, and interaction system variables.* Unpublished doctoral dissertation, Syracuse University.

Sameroff, A. J. and Chandler, M. J. (1975). Reproductive risk and the continuum of caretaking casualty. In F. D. Horowitz (Ed.), *Review of child development research* (Vol. 4). Chicago: University of Chicago Press, pp. 187–244.

Schneider-Rosen, K., Braunwald, K. G., Carlson, V., and Cicchetti, D. (1985). Current perspectives in attachment theory: Illustration from the study of maltreated infants. In I. Bretherton and E. Waters (Eds.), Growing Points in Attachment Theory and Research. *Monographs of the Society for Research in Child Development, 50* (1–2, Serial No. 209), pp. 194–210.

Stern, D. N. (1974). Mother and infant play: The dyadic interaction involving facial, vocal, and gaze behaviors. In M. Lewis and L. A. Rosenbaum (Eds.), *The effect of the infant on its caregiver.* New York: Wiley, pp. 187–213.

Tronick, E., Als, H., and Brazelton, T. B. (1980). Monadicphases: A structured descriptive analysis of infant–mother face-to-face interaction. *Merrill-Palmer Quarterly of Behavior and Development, 26,* 3–24.

Waters, E., Vaughn, B., and Egeland, B. (1980). Individual differences in infant–mother attachment relationships at age one: Antecedents in neonatal behavior in an urban, economically disadvantaged sample. *Child Development, 55,* 208–216.

16 Finding order in disorganization: lessons from research on maltreated infants' attachments to their caregivers

*Vicki Carlson, Dante Cicchetti, Douglas Barnett,
and Karen G. Braunwald*

There is more to be learnt from the study of disarray than is gained by intentionally disregarding it.[1]

Although Bowlby's original formulations on attachment emerged from observations of clinical populations (Bowlby, 1944, 1958, 1977a, 1977b; Rutter, 1979), until recently we possessed only rudimentary empirical information regarding attachment relationships in clinically disordered populations. However, during the past decade, as research in the discipline of developmental psychopathology has burgeoned (cf. Cicchetti, 1984a, 1984b; Rolf, Masten, Cicchetti, Neuchterlein, and Weintraub, in press; Rutter & Garmezy, 1983), increased attention has been paid toward understanding the organization of the attachment system in handicapped, "high-risk" and clinically disordered groups of youngsters (see, for example, Cicchetti and Serafica, 1981; Crittenden, 1988; Egeland and Sroufe, 1981a, 1981b; Radke-Yarrow, Cummings, Kuczynski, and Chapman, 1985; Sigman and Ungerer, 1984).

Proponents of attachment theory have argued that many psychopathological disorders may be brought about by deviations in the development of the attachment behavioral system or, much less commonly, by failure of its ontogenesis (Ainsworth, 1973, 1980; Bowlby, 1969/1982, 1977a, 1977b; Cic-

The writing of this chapter was supported in part by grants from the National Center on Child Abuse and Neglect (90-C-1929), the National Institute of Mental Health (R01-MH37960-01), and the Smith Richardson Foundation, Inc., to Dante Cicchetti and by a postdoctoral research training grant to Vicki Carlson (USPHMH 17104). We would like to thank the staff of the Harvard Child Maltreatment Project for their invaluable assistance in the collection of the data reported herein, especially Judy Bigelow, Ann Churchill, Carol Kottmeier, and Karen Schneider-Rosen. Moreover, we would like to extend our appreciation to J. Lawrence Aber and Mary Main for their thoughtful comments on an earlier version of this chapter. Finally, we wish to thank Victoria Gill for typing this manuscript.

chetti, 1987; Guidano and Liotti, 1983). Additionally, advocates of the attachment theory perspective have stated that strong causal relationships exist between children's experiences with their caregivers and their later capacities to develop secure affectional bonds (Bowlby, 1944, 1977a, 1977b; Sroufe and Fleeson, 1986). Because the study of risk conditions from a developmental perspective is believed to augment our understanding of normal and abnormal forms of ontogenesis (Cicchetti, in press; Cicchetti, Cummings, Greenberg, and Marvin, in press), we think that the study of attachment in maltreated infants can make significant contributions to our knowledge about relationship formation and dissolution.

Bowlby's attachment theory set out the functions and processes involved in the establishment of attachment relationships between parents and their offspring (Bowlby, 1969/1982, 1973, 1980; see Crittenden and Ainsworth, this volume, for an overview of Bowlby's attachment theory). Adequately nurturing parental care is the essence of the "environment of evolutionary adaptiveness" that, in Bowlby's theory, is the context in which the infant–caregiver attachment system evolved. In a context of adequately sensitive caregiving, the infant's attachment behavior keeps him/her "in proximity to animals that are friendly and to places that are safe and, in addition, tends to keep it away from predators and other dangers" (Bowlby, 1969/1982, p. 151). Bowlby acknowledged the existence of insensitive, even harsh, parental care and addressed its implications for theory and clinical practice – namely, how and why an offspring would form a social bond to a maltreating parent, and how the relationship to such a parent would differ from relationships formed between infants and more nurturing caretakers:

When an animal is reared in an environment other than its environment of evolutionary adaptedness, . . . *the resulting organization of behavior may be very different.* Sometimes it is *bizarre,* sometimes inimical to survival. (Bowlby, 1969/1982, p. 151, emphasis added)

In this chapter, we review theoretical and empirical work on "bizarre" infant–caregiver attachments. We describe unusual forms of attachment that have been observed in middle-class populations and in maltreated and high-risk samples. We present the results of a reanalysis of Strange Situation data from our own sample of 12-month-old maltreated and comparison infants. This reanalysis extends the basic ABC Strange Situation classification system to include Main and Solomon's (in press) disorganized/disoriented category. Finally, we consider theoretical and empirical consequences of disorganized attachment among maltreated infants and illustrate how future research with maltreated children can make important contributions to the further development and validation of this newly discovered category.

Maltreatment in attachment theory

The words "child abuse" and "maltreatment" do not appear in Bowlby's trilogy on attachment theory (Bowlby, 1969/1982, 1973, 1980). However, employing other terminology, Bowlby described conditions that would certainly fit current definitions of maltreatment. He discussed the effects of child maltreatment on the attachment system when he elaborated on two major themes in his theory. The first is the importance of *actual experience,* especially experiences of loss and separation, in shaping the quality of infant–caregiver attachment relationships, related aspects of social–emotional development, and later mental health. The second theme is the *evolutionary value* of infant–parent attachment.

The importance of real events

In contrast to Freud, who emphasized fantasy, inner dynamics, unconscious drives, and motivations unfolding through psychosexual development, Bowlby stressed the impact of caregivers' real acts, including violence, threats of abandonment, and the overall negative emotional tone of interaction.

the varied expectations of the accessibility and responsiveness of attachment figures that different individuals develop during the years of immaturity are tolerably accurate reflections of the experiences those individuals have actually had. (Bowlby, 1973, p. 202)

Bowlby (1973) gave extensive examples of how his views regarding real experience differed from Freud's. He reexamined historical documentation regarding some of Freud's most famous cases (e.g., Judge Schreber and Little Hans) and argued that the paranoid delusions Schreber experienced in his adult life could be better linked to the physically and emotionally abusive discipline practiced by Schreber's overly strict father than to inner struggles with homosexual feelings. Similarly, he argued that Little Hans's phobias might be better understood as reactions to a combination of truly frightening events, including Hans's mother's use of disciplinary threats, threats that could be seen as emotional mistreatment. In addition, Bowlby noticed that "separation" and "loss" experiences sometimes derive from situations in which the caregiver is physically present yet behaves in a distant and insensitive manner.

a mother[2] can be physically present but "emotionally" absent. What this means of course is that, although present in body, a mother may be unresponsive to her child's desire for mothering. Such unresponsiveness can be due to many conditions – depression, rejection, preoccupation with other matters – but, whatever its cause, so far as her child is concerned she is no better than half present. (Bowlby, 1973, p. 23)

In extreme cases, the negative outcomes described for literal separations and/or losses can be seen when infants experience the emotional equivalent due to caregiver unavailability, or rejection, conditions analogous to the maltreatment subcategories of physical and emotional neglect.

The evolutionary value of attachment

Bowlby used the issue of maltreatment to illustrate a second major tenet in his theory, the powerful evolutionary value of the attachment relationship between infant and caregiver. Bowlby stressed that, given the importance of the attachment bond to the offspring's survival, infants are able to form attachments to caregivers whose behaviors ranged widely across a continuum of sensitivity or nurturance. Some of the strongest evidence for this comes from animal studies. Bowlby cited detailed accounts of naturalistic and experimental animal research programs that demonstrated in numerous species the strength and resilience of the attachment bond in the face of maltreatment (see Rajecki, Lamb, and Obmascher, 1978; Reite and Caine, 1983; and Ruppenthal, Arling, Harlow, Sackett, and Suomi, 1976, for reviews).

A special but not unusual situation in which there is conflict between attachment behavior and withdrawal is when the attachment figure is also the one who elicits fear perhaps by threats or violence. In such conditions young creatures, whether human or nonhuman are likely to cling to the threatening or hostile figure rather than run away from him or her. (Bowlby, 1973, p. 91)

In Bowlby's view, had the boundaries of adequate parental performance been set too tightly, fewer offspring would have survived. Consequently, Bowlby argues that the formation of a bond can occur under conditions of maltreatment. However, questions remain concerning the *quality* of the attachment relationship that is formed and the nature of the "working models" of the self and of the self in relation to others (e.g., caregivers) that are established under such conditions.

Child studies, maltreatment, and attachment theory

In recent years, a number of well-controlled studies have been published that have confirmed Bowlby's predictions and have reinforced the findings of animal researchers (see Ainsworth, Blehar, Waters, and Wall, 1978; Sroufe and Fleeson, 1986). Studies using the Strange Situation (Ainsworth and Wittig, 1969) have demonstrated that maltreated children do form attachments to their caregivers, and that these attachments are more likely to be insecure than are those of nonmaltreated children (Crittenden, 1985, 1988; Egeland and Sroufe, 1981a, 1981b; Lamb, Gaensbauer, Malkin, and

Schulz, 1985; Schneider-Rosen, Braunwald, Carlson, and Cicchetti, 1985; Schneider-Rosen and Cicchetti, 1984).

Crittenden (1981, 1985) has gone beyond documenting that maltreatment leads to a lower proportion of secure attachments as measured by the Strange Situation. She used maltreatment samples to document specific sub-types of insensitive care correlated with different types of insecure attachments. She observed both mother–infant interactions under nonstressed conditions in the home and Strange Situation behavior in the lab to discover distinct patterns of maternal interaction style that were reliably related to particular insecure patterns of attachment in the Strange Situation. Belsky, Rovine, and Taylor (1984) and Lyons-Ruth, Connell, Zoll, and Stahl (1987) have shown relationships between particular features of maternal behavior and the development of avoidant versus resistant attachments. They have found that mothers whose interaction style was primarily intrusive and characterized by instances of covert hostility were likely to have infants who demonstrated an avoidant style of dealing with the stresses of the Strange Situation. Mothers whose interaction style was predominantly withdrawn, passive, and lacking in initiative were more likely to have babies rated as insecure/resistant–ambivalent in the Strange Situation. Crittenden (1985) demonstrated that the abusive mothers in her sample tended to show the insensitive overstimulating style, whereas neglecting mothers were insensitively understimulating.

Assessing infant attachment

Currently, the most widely used method of assessing the quality of infant–parent attachment is the Strange Situation paradigm (Ainsworth et al., 1978). This section briefly sketches the process by which the method of assessing organized attachment styles was developed. Against that background we trace the discoveries of the new, disorganized forms of attachment, including the role within that process that maltreatment research has played.

The Strange Situation: Ainsworth's original classificatory system

The Strange Situation is a 21-minute structured laboratory technique designed to produce low-level infant stress sufficient to activate the infant's attachment behavioral system. Although other nonstress methods allow observation of exploration, teaching style, and dyadic play, conditions of stress are essential to making the attachment system available for observation (see Bischof, 1975; Bretherton, 1980). Three particular stressors (introduction to a strange place, interaction with a new person, and brief separations from mother) were selected for inclusion in the Strange Situation because they are common and relatively nontraumatic, yet they provide graduations of stress that ensure activation of the attachment systems of most infants. Ainsworth devised and conducted the first "Strange Situation" procedures within the context of her prospective study of mother–child interaction in Baltimore (Ainsworth and Wittig, 1969). Twenty-three mother–infant dyads who previously had been studied in their homes were observed in a laboratory playroom, a new and "strange" situation for the babies. The 21-minute structured procedure involved an initial free play with new toys in the new room, entry and approach by a young woman the baby had not seen before, and two three-minute separations from the mother. In the first separation, the baby was left with the stranger. The baby was left alone in the room for the second separation. Observations made through a one-way mirror of the infants' behavior toward the mother, levels of play and exploration, and emotional expressions and tone were recorded by audio-taped narration. Transcripts of these observations were used to devise seven-point scales designed for rating the infant's proximity-seeking, contact maintenance, avoidance, resistance, distance-interactions, and search with mothers and strangers. Finally, qualitative categories of infant attachment were developed by sorting the transcripts into groups based on infant behavioral similarities, especially features of infant response to separation and reunion. This sorting procedure resulted in seven subgroups (A1, A2, B1, B2, B3, C1, C2), which were further grouped into three major categories. Approximately 70 percent of the infants were placed in the secure category (Type B). They responded unambivalently toward their mothers in reunions; they greeted or approached them, were readily comforted if they had been upset, then moved back to exploration and play. Twenty percent were classified as anxious/avoidant (Type A). These babies responded to reunion with a lack of either proximity-seeking or happy affect, even ignoring the mother in some cases. The 10 percent in the anxious resistant (Type C) group were distressed by separation and sought proximity, yet were not comforted by it, remaining fussy or angry, unable to return with ease to play.

The three major attachment categories were found adequate to classify an additional 83 middle-class infants who were seen in subsequent studies by Ainsworth and her colleagues (Ainsworth et al., 1978). The only addition to the classificatory system made during the process was a fourth subtype of secure attachment (B4) that described babies who were especially oriented to the mother throughout the situation, becoming quite upset during the separation episodes, yet calming eventually during reunions (Ainsworth et al., 1978).

Categories of attachment as organized strategies of behavior

Ainsworth and her colleagues examined the relationships between the mother–child interaction data from home observations made in the original study and quality of attachment as measured in the structured laboratory situation. They found that patterns of maternal caregiving behavior during the infants' early months of life were systematically related to infants' quality of attachment as measured in the Strange Situation at 1 year, a finding since replicated in American and German middle-class samples (Belsky, Rovine, and Taylor, 1984; Grossmann, Grossmann, Spangler, Suess, and Unzer, 1985) and an American lower-class sample (Egeland and Farber, 1984). What develops over the first year are caregiver-specific strategies with stressful or frightening experiences.

The attachment categories established through these home and laboratory studies are best thought of as assessments of *coherent organized strategies* for relating to the caregiver in times of stress, weariness, or illness (Sroufe and Waters, 1977). The quality of an infant's attachment relationship to his/her caregiver is believed to be a function of the history of the infant's interactions with that particular caregiver over the course of the first year of life, especially those situations in which the infant's needs are expressed (Ainsworth et al., 1978).

The securely attached infant (Type B) is characterized by a history of sensitive responsiveness in caretaking, in which the infant's expressed needs are met in a timely and appropriate fashion. In times of stress, such as in the Strange Situation, secure infants express feelings directly and rapidly seek proximity to the mother either through physical contact or through distance signals such as eye contact and vocalizations. In situations of low danger, distress is at a minimum and the infant is able to pursue play and exploration. This pattern of rapid proximity-seeking in times of stress, and easy voluntary movement away from the caregiver at other times, is called the "secure base phenomenon" (Ainsworth et al., 1978). When an infant is able to trust his or her caregiver as a secure base, he or she is able to maximize exploration and learning and minimize encounters with sources of real danger and periods of prolonged distress.

The infant who is categorized as anxious/avoidant (A) in the Strange Situation is likely to have experienced a caretaking history that was inconsistent, alternating between rejection and intrusive overinvolvement. Moreover, this pattern of interaction is out of synchrony with the infant's cues and more in tune with the caregiver's own immediate needs. The behavioral strategy developed to deal with stress in such a caregiving context seems to be one of shifting attention away from and thus reducing reactivity to fear-eliciting cues in the environment (Main and Hesse, in press). Thus, in the Strange Situation, the avoidant baby emits fewer attachment behaviors and remains more distant from the caregiver during stresses that would arouse stronger attachment responses in a securely attached baby.

The anxious/resistant or ambivalent quality of attachment (C) is the pattern shown in the Strange Situation by infants who have experienced insensitive care characterized by withdrawal and uninvolvement on the part of the caregiver. In the Strange Situation, the C infant's organized strategy is to *heighten* responsiveness to fear-eliciting cues, thus producing an increase in the expression of attachment behaviors: signalling, crying, searching during separation, and taking the initiative in seeking proximity and maintaining contact in even the early phases of the situation. With so much attention on producing attachment behavior and monitoring the whereabouts of the caregiver, these children have relatively little time for play and exploration. Their attachment behaviors increase at lower apparent levels of stress than other children.[3] A subset of C infants shows a physically more passive style. Although these infants express their distress and signal, they seem unable or unwilling to mobilize efforts to achieve contact with the caregivers. These children too have little attention focused on exploring the physical or the social world. (See Main and Hesse, in press, for descriptions of A, B, and C as organized strategies.)

New categories for the Strange Situation

Ainsworth had anticipated that there would be categorical expansion beyond the three major categories (ABC) and the eight subcategories that had been developed with the first 56 dyads in the Strange Situation.

> it seems wise to think of any classificatory system as openended. It is inconceivable that any system based on a relatively small sample could comfortably accommodate all patterns represented in the total population from which the sample is drawn. (Ainsworth et al., 1978; p. 235)

The population on which the Strange Situation was developed was a middle-class one. In recent years, the Strange Situation has been used in studies of maltreated and other high-risk infants, children drawn from populations that differ substantially from the one on which the Strange Situation was developed. Maltreated children have experienced degrees of caretaking failures much greater than those experienced by infants in the original sample. In addition, maltreated infants were more likely to be from a lower SES level than the original sample. As the Strange Situation has been employed in studies of populations other than the one on which the procedure was developed, and as reports of anomalous behavior in the situation have accrued both in normal and maltreatment samples, Ainsworth has continued to emphasize the value of adding to the system (see Crittenden and Ainsworth, this volume).

Unclassifiable Strange Situation behavior. Main and Solomon (1986, in press) have presented a chronology of reports of Strange Situation behavior that were difficult or impossible to classify using the original system. Beginning with her own dissertation research (Main 1973), Main encountered instances (5 out of a sample of 49) where Strange Situation behavior was particularly difficult to classify. For the purposes of the dissertation, all five children were "force classified" into one of the original categories. The earliest published account of hard-to-classify Strange Situation behavior was that of Sroufe and Waters (1977). In their study of 70 middle-class dyads in Minnesota they reported that 10% "could not be readily fitted" (p. 1191) into one of the ABC patterns. These cases were also force classified into ABC categories for analysis. Main and Weston (1981), in a study of 152 Strange Situations involving middle- to upper-class mothers and fathers, reported that 12.5% of the situations were unclassifiable into an A, B, or C category and they were set aside from analyses. In a subsequent study of this group, with an increased sample size, Main and her colleagues found 12.7% of 268 Strange Situations to be unclassifiable using the ABC system (Main and Solomon, in press). The majority of these unclassifiable cases, 21 of 34 or 62%, would have been force classified as secure, 15% as insecure/avoidant and 23% as insecure/ambivalent. In their review of reports of unclassifiable cases, Main and Solomon included a number of studies on maltreated or high risk children in other samples.

Investigators who have studied attachment among maltreated infants initially used the ABC classification system (Crittenden, 1985; Egeland and Sroufe, 1981a, 1981b; Gaensbauer and Harmon, 1982; Lyons-Ruth et al., 1987; Schneider-Rosen and Cicchetti, 1984; Schneider-Rosen, Braunwald, Carlson, and Cicchetti, 1985). However, upon reviewing their results, some were unsettled by the fact that there were a number of securely rated attachments among the maltreated subjects. Given the prediction of attachment theory, the outcome of a secure attachment is not expected under conditions of insensitive caregiving history such as would be expected from a maltreating caregiver (Ainsworth, 1980). Some researchers added qualifying comments to their reports of secure attachments among maltreated infants. Gaensbauer and Harmon (1982) noted that abused/neglected infants seen in their single-separation adaptation of the Strange Situation could be classified as secure, but upon more careful observation these infants' behavior appeared to be different from that of nonmaltreated secure infants. Egeland and Sroufe (1981b) chose to set some unclassifiable abuse and abuse/neglect cases aside from analyses noting that they seemed insecure but did not exhibit avoidance or resistance. Instead, they were characterized by apathy or *disorganization*. Still other investigators noticed unusual aspects of their maltreated subjects' behavior in the Strange Situation but decided to report the standard A, B, and C categories, leaving open the possibility of reanalysis at a later time (Schneider-Rosen et al., 1985).

In two laboratories, the investigators undertook the reanalysis process directly. They went back to their videotapes and carefully reviewed them, finding new types or combinations of behavior not found ordinarily among A-, B-, and C-coded infants. Two new categories were proposed as a result of that process.

The avoidant–resistant category. Spieker and Booth (1988), in a study of high-risk infants drawn from the lower-SES, encountered unclassifiable cases in the original coding process. They developed a category they labelled "A–C" to characterize the infants who had both relatively high avoidance and high resistance scores in the same reunion episodes or high avoidance in the first reunion followed by high resistance in the second reunion. They reported that the infants in this category had experienced more extreme caregiving conditions, and the mothers of these children were more depressed and had more life difficulties than mothers of infants in the A, B, and C categories.

In a case where theory provided the impetus for a new empirical formulation, Crittenden (1985, 1988) conducted an extensive reevaluation of the videotapes of maltreated securely rated infants. She had conducted Strange Situations with a population of mothers participating in a welfare-sponsored infant stimulation project. A subset of the mothers were receiving protective services for having abused or neglected their children. Forty-three tapes of children aged 11 to 24 months were coded using the ABC system. Upon examination of the data, Crittenden noticed that nine children who had experienced both abuse and neglect had been placed in the secure category. Because such a finding was almost impossible to explain theoretically, these tapes were carefully reviewed. It became apparent that the maltreated infants who had been rated as secure did not demonstrate the appropriate mixture of low avoidance and low resistance, mixed with moderate-to-high levels of proximity-seeking and contact-maintaining, which typify secure attachment relationships under conditions of stress. Instead, they displayed the unusual combination of moderate-to-high avoidance and moderate-to-high resistance. The resistance was particularly likely to be in the form of persistent crankiness and/or noncontextual aggression.[4] In addition, most of the infants displaying this blend of responses also showed some stereotypic or maladaptive behaviors, such as head cocking or huddling on the floor. Crittenden (1985) developed a coding scheme for this new category, which she labelled "A–C." In a subsequent study (Crittenden, 1988), she demonstrated that the new category could be reliably coded on a sample other than the one on which the category was devised. In this second sample, as in the first, a strong relationship was obtained between the A–C classification and a history of both abuse and neglect.

A third laboratory also discovered the need for an "A–C" category for infants who display both high avoidance and high resistance in the Strange

Situation. Radke-Yarrow et al. (1985) noted the same mix of insecure pattern in their study of the offspring of mothers with an affective disorder.

The "unstable-avoidant" category. Lyons-Ruth et al., (1987, Lyons-Ruth, Connell, and Zoll, this volume) described a second new category of attachment, also discovered in the context of an intervention project for mothers with parenting difficulties, some of whom were receiving protective services for abuse or neglect. In contrast to the theory-guided pathway to discovery illustrated in the development of the Crittenden A–C category, Lyons-Ruth and her colleagues discovered the "unstable-avoidant" pattern of attachment through analyses of unusual patterns of the 7-point interactive scale scores used in the coding of quality of attachment (e.g., proximity-seeking, avoidance, resistance, and search). They discovered that members of the high-risk sample (in particular, maltreated infants who had been coded as secure using the ABC system) exhibited patterns of scores that were extremely rare in the comparison samples. Specifically, some members of the high-risk group showed pronounced avoidance at the first reunion but minimal avoidance at the second reunion. This large difference was a drop in scale scores of 4 points or more on the 7-point avoidance scale. In Lyons-Ruth et al.'s high-risk group, 28 percent evidenced this pattern of "unstable avoidance." In order to find out if this was indeed a unique pattern, the authors reviewed the ratings from the 104 infants in Ainsworth et al. (1978). Only 4 percent of the Ainsworth et al. sample had a 4-point drop in avoidance scores from the first to the second reunion.

Development of the "disorganized/disoriented" or "D" category. Main and Solomon (1986, in press) described the process by which the D category was developed. They carefully reexamined the 34 unclassifiable video tapes that had been set aside from all 368 mother–infant and father–infant Strange Situations from the Berkeley Social Development Project. The expectation at the beginning of this review was that a number of new categories might be discovered. However, instead of finding new organizations of behavior, they were struck with the overriding impression that the Strange Situation behavior of all 34 of these infants and toddlers was *disorganized and disoriented.* What was strikingly lacking was evidence of coherent, organized strategies for dealing with the stresses inherent in the Strange Situation. Instead of new organizations, they found elements of the three major attachment patterns, combined in unusual ways. For example, they found the combination of moderate to high proximity-seeking, moderate to high avoidance and moderate to high resistance that has been labeled "A–C" (Crittenden, 1985, 1988; Radke-Yarrow et al., 1985; Spieker and Booth, 1988). In other cases, proximity-seeking was accompanied by avoidance, a combination George and Main (1979) first described in a study of physically abused toddlers. Although that study involved toddlers' behavior in a day-care center with caregivers and peers rather than with mothers, the descriptions of the behaviors of oblique approaches, detours, and approaches accomplished through backing toward the other or with head averted are very similar to the descriptions of avoidance mixed with proximity-seeking in the unclassifiable cases. Perhaps Main would have discovered this anomaly independently in her middle-class subjects had she never seen it in abused children. It is more likely that having been alerted to this form of behavior in the study of the abused children, Main was better able to recognize it in her middle-class sample.

In addition to manifesting these unusual combinations of behavior, infants with unclassifiable Strange Situations displayed other bizarre symptoms, including incomplete, undirected, and interrupted movements and expressions; asymmetrical and mistimed movements, stereotypies and anomalous postures; stilling, slow movements, freezing, and depressed affect; and direct indices of apprehension toward the parent (see Main and Solomon, in press, for elaboration).

Main and Solomon (1986, in press) drew upon data from a number of sources in their validation of the Type D attachment. First, since the Berkeley study included Strange Situations with both parents, it was possible to test the hypothesis that disorganized behavior was an expression of infant constitutional or temperamental factors rather than the result of disordered interaction histories between infants and caregivers. Only 3 of 34 infants were classified as having disorganized attachments with both parents (Main and Solomon, in press). Thus, it seems that these unusual patterns of behavior are specific to caregiver–infant interaction histories, rather than just a function of individual infant characteristics (see also Sroufe, 1985).

A second source of evidence of the uniqueness of the disorganized attachment category was the demonstration of its predictive validity. Main, Kaplan, and Cassidy (1985) reported that older children whose attachments to their mothers at 12 months had been rated as disorganized could be distinguished from children whose Strange Situation behavior had been classifiable in the A or B categories at 12 months on a number of measures, including quality of attachment on reunion with the parent, fluency of discourse, self esteem, and pictorial representation of the family, all measured at a follow-up visit when the children were 6 years old. By age 6 these children had developed an organized response to reunions with their parents. They behaved upon reunion in a *controlling* fashion, either controlling through punitive directiveness or in a caretaking style (Main and Cassidy, 1988).

Third, after establishing the D category at the behavioral coding level, Main and her colleagues turned to an examination of data from parent interviews in search of commonalities among parents whose children had been coded D in the Strange Situation. They found that the loss of a parent during childhood was a predictor of having a child with a D classification. Thirty-nine percent of the parents of disorganized/disoriented children had lost a parent prior to graduating from high school. Only eight percent of the parents of children whose Strange Situation behavior was classifiable as A, B, or C had suffered such a loss (Main and Hesse, in press). However, although loss of a caregiver's parent did serve as a significant risk factor for D attachment, Main and her colleagues were aware that not all caregivers who had lost a parent had children who were coded D in the Strange Situation. They hypothesized that the degree to which the loss had been successfully mourned would be important in differentiating parents whose behavior would or would not lead to their offspring's development of a D attachment. Main and DeMoss (cited in Main et al, 1985) developed a nine-point scale to assess the degree to which "lack of resolution of mourning" was apparent in transcripts of the Adult Attachment Interview (George, Kaplan, and Main, 1984), which was administered to the parents at a follow-up visit five years after the 12-month Strange Situation. Parents with high scores for lack of resolution of mourning lacked integrity of thought regarding the death, and showed indications of their own disorganization and disorientation in their psychological functioning. As predicted, they were also much more likely to have infants judged as disorganized/disoriented in their attachment to them than were parents who were rated as more resolved in dealing with their loss.

To summarize, the concurrent discoveries of apathetic, unstable-avoidant, avoidant–resistant, and generally unclassifiable attachment behavior have all contributed to and been integrated into the disorganized/disoriented category of attachment (although a few cases still remain unclassifiable even with the new category). We now have empirical methods to characterize those "bizarre" attachments that Bowlby indicated would develop when the caregiving context became too discrepant from the environment of evolutionary adaptiveness in which the attachment system evolved. In the following section we describe the integration of disorganized/disoriented attachment coding techniques into a reanalysis of infant–mother attachment behavior in our sample of maltreated and comparison 12-month-olds.

A reanalysis of Strange Situation data in the Harvard Child Maltreatment Project

The Harvard Child Maltreatment Project (HCMP), a longitudinal study of the developmental consequences of child abuse and neglect, is one of the research groups that has used the Strange Situation paradigm to examine attachment relationships between maltreated children and their caregivers (see Cicchetti, Carlson, Braunwald, and Aber, 1987, and Cicchetti and Todd Manly, in press, for a full description of the project). Previous reports of attachment findings from this study (Schneider-Rosen and Cicchetti, 1984; Schneider-Rosen, Braunwald, Carlson, and Cicchetti, 1985) were based on the original ABC Strange Situation system of coding. As with other maltreatment researchers (Gaensbauer and Harmon, 1982; Egeland and Sroufe, 1981a; Crittenden, 1985), coders blind to the maltreatment or comparison group status of the infants were able to classify 12-, 18-, and 24-month-old infants and toddlers into A, B, and C categories.

Following the publication of our traditionally coded Strange Situation results (Schneider-Rosen et al., 1985), we became interested in the descriptions of alternatives in coding, especially the work of Main and her colleagues on the disorganized/disoriented category of attachment. We resolved to recode the HCMP Strange Situation videotapes of 12-month-olds, this time including the D category.

We decided to employ the D classification system rather than one of the existing alternatives (e.g., "A–C") for several reasons. First, the D system had been developed after a review of Strange Situation behavior from a large and heterogeneous data set, including tapes of middle-class, lower-socioeconomic status (SES), high-risk, maltreating, and depressed mother–infant and father–infant dyads. Second, the D category seemed to encompass the essence of the proposed A–C category, as well as including additional suggested subtypes, such as "apprehensive," and "depressed." Third, use of the D system did not require redefining the Ainsworth resistance interactive scale, as is the case in the Crittenden A–C coding system. Such a redefinition may prove to be necessary, but at this point we saw merits in maintaining the behavioral coding system as it was. And fourth, the D category came with the strongest theoretical rationale and related empirical evidence (i.e., the evidence from parent histories and child follow-up data).

The sample. Forty-three mother–infant pairs, 22 from families receiving protective services for issues of child abuse and/or neglect and 21 from comparison families with no history of Protective Service involvement were included in the study.

The two groups had similar demographic characteristics (see Table 16.1). At the time of administration of the Strange Situation, the infants were an average of 12.8 months old. Ages ranged from 11.8 months to 16.1 months. Twenty-one infants were male and 22 were female; both sexes were equally represented in each group. The mothers were of an average age of 27 years with a range of 16 to 41 years. About 45 percent of the mothers in each group had received no educational degree, about half had received either a high school degree or a GED, and only one mother in each of the groups had received education beyond high school. The groups were very

Table 16.1. *Demographic characteristics of the families*

	Maltreatment $n = 22$	Comparison $n = 18$	Total	Significance level
Currently on AFDC	86%	83%	85%	ns
Mother holds the major financial responsibility	68%	65%	67%	ns
Spouse or partner in the home	36%	56%	45%	ns
Number of adults in home	1.6	2.1	1.8	$p < .05$
Number of children	3.0	1.8	2.5	$p < .01$
Adult/child ratio	.7	1.5	1.1	$p < .01$
Spouse/partner's age	34.2	30.7	32.2	ns
Mother's age	27.9	25.9	27.0	ns
Mother's highest grade	11.0	10.6	10.8	ns
Mother's occupation is housewife	91%	72%	82%	ns
Mother's religion:				
Protestant	33%	33%	33%	ns
Catholic	57%	56%	56%	
None or other	10%	11%	11%	
Race: percent caucasian	81%	100%	90%	

similar in maternal religious preference, with one third Protestant, one half Catholic, and the remainder split between "other" and "no religious preference."

All the families were from relatively low SES levels. All had received AFDC support at some point and 85 percent were currently receiving it. Thirty-six percent of the Protective Service households and 56 percent of the comparison families included a spouse or partner. Chi-Square analysis indicated this was not a significant difference. The 18 spouses/partners were an average of 32 years old, ranging from 24 to 51 years.

In addition to finding no significant differences on these separate demographic variables, we also found no difference when we employed a summary demographic measure, the Nock and Rossi (1979) household prestige score. This score combines parents' age, education, and occupational prestige rating, and number of adults and children in the household, into different formulas for two-parent, single-parent, and widowed households.

There were two areas in which the groups differed. First, all mothers in the comparison group were white, whereas the maltreatment group included two Black mothers and two of Hispanic origin. Second, there were differences in the composition of the families. The Protective Service families had significantly more children than the comparison families (an average of 3.0 per family versus 1.8 children per family; $t = 2.71$, $p = .01$), but significantly fewer adults (an average of 1.6 versus 2.1 adults per family; $t = 2.01$, $p = .05$). We checked to see if these differences operated at the individual family level by looking at the adult-to-child ratio. This variable also evidenced a significant difference ($t = -3.64$, $p = .001$). The Protective Service families had an average adult-to-child ratio of .67 and the comparison group's mean was 1.5.

Type of maltreatment. Families in the maltreatment group all had been reported to public or private protective service agencies either by a mandated or voluntary reporter or, in rare cases, through self-report. They were all assessed by the agencies to be families in need of Protective Services. This formal, legal level of definition provides a pragmatic, ecologically valid basis for characterizing a group of families as maltreating, but it lacks the kind of specificity we would like to have in developmental research. Maltreatment conditions described in official reports at the time of entry to services are not necessarily the only forms of maltreatment experienced by the children named in the report or by the siblings in the family who may not have been named. For this reason, we employed a second method of defining maltreatment. The Protective Services social worker responsible for each participating family was interviewed for details of the abuse and/or neglect experienced by all the children in the family, whether or not they had been named in a legal filing. To facilitate this process, we used a 93-item checklist developed by Giovannoni and Becerra (1979). Using the checklists, social workers indicated the specific acts and conditions of maltreatment each child had experienced during his or her lifetime. In addition, the perpetrators of each checked item were specified when that information was known. For the purpose of this study, items regarding educational neglect, moral/legal issues and substance abuse were set aside, and items relevant to four major categories of maltreatment were examined. Physical abuse included injuries ranging from cuts or bruises to major injuries. Neglect included the items characterizing medical, nutritional, or hygienic neglect and lack of adequate protection or supervision. Items in the emotional mistreatment category included rejection, psychological abuse, and emotional or psychological neglect. Sexual abuse was broadly defined as molestation by a family member or other. If any item in a category had been checked, we considered the child to have experienced that form of maltreatment.

By asking social workers to indicate the relationship of the perpetrator to the child, we were able to describe the types of maltreatment mothers had inflicted on their infants, a useful specification when looking at mother–infant interaction. According to the social workers, no mothers had physically abused their children. (However, two infants had been physically abused by their fathers.) Fifty-nine percent of the infants had experienced neglect by their mothers and 27 percent had been emotionally mistreated by them. No infants had been sexually abused. Seven children or 32 percent of the group had *no* specific checklist items indicated by the social worker. Most of these children were in family treatment plans due to prior abuse or neglect of older siblings. These infants were considered at risk for maltreatment and were being monitored by the caseworker. Eighteen percent of the infants had experienced more than one type of maltreatment from their mothers, for example, neglect and emotional mistreatment.[5]

Because we had collected checklists on all children in the families, and 19 of the 22 mothers had other children in addition to the infant seen in the Strange Situation, it was possible to characterize the mothers' perpetration of maltreatment *over their entire mothering history.* Using this definition of maltreatment, 23 percent of the mothers had physically injured one of their children, 82 percent had neglected a child, and 69 percent had emotionally mistreated a child. For only one mother was there no maltreatment item checked by the social worker. This mother had been the focus of a Protective Services report made by an obstetrical nurse at the birth of the only child in this family. The mother was destitute, had no home, and no concrete plans for caring for her child. She was referred to Protective Services and was provided with services and follow-up for at least four years. The social worker contended that, despite the impending neglect that was the basis for the filing, the services that were provided prevented neglect from actually taking place.

Coding procedures. The Strange Situation videotapes were initially coded by Carlson and Braunwald using the 1985 version of the Main and Solomon coding instructions for the D category in addition to the traditional instructions for coding ABC quality of attachment (Ainsworth et al., 1978). Interrater reliability at the ABCD level was 90 percent. Disagreements were resolved through discussions in which Cicchetti participated. We were fortunate, at this point, to have a coding review done by Mary Main, who watched and coded 17 selected tapes. The tapes were not randomly chosen, but were cases we had coded as disorganized/disoriented plus examples coded A, B, and C. The agreement between our codes and Mary Main's codes was 76 percent. Main confirmed that our coding had captured the major aspects of the D category. All the cases we had coded as D she agreed were D, but she also pointed out D features in tapes we had placed into conventional categories. For example, she pointed out facial expressions that were incongruous with other aspects of behavior, smiles that were too bright or too fast, and subtle indices of fear and wariness that took place in the context of an approach. We decided to submit the tapes to a recoding by Cicchetti and Barnett. In addition to the 1985 D coding instructions, they had feedback from the tape review process which had highlighted the more subtle features of the coding. Like the previous coders, Barnett was blind to

Table 16.2. *ABCD Codes for the Strange Situation*

	Anxious–avoidant (A)	Secure (B)	Anxious–resistant (C)	Disorganized/disoriented (D)
Maltreated group	1	3	0	18
$n = 22$	4.5%	13.7%	0%	81.8%
Comparison group	2	11	4	4
$n = 21$	9.5%	52.4%	19.1%	19.1%
Total	3	14	4	22
	6.9%	32.6%	9.3%	51.2%

the children's maltreatment status and in addition was unaware of infants' previous forced classifications. The reliability for this second round of coding was 88 percent. The two raters resolved differences through conference. The agreement between the second round of coding and Mary Main's review of the subset of these tapes was .94.

Results

The results of the Strange Situation recoding are given in Table 16.2. The majority of the infants in the Protective Service group were coded as disorganized/disoriented (81.8%). In the comparison group, the predominant rating was secure (52.4%). Given the small sample size, a significance test was conducted at the level of secure versus insecure ratings (B versus A, C, or D). The groups differed significantly from each other on the proportion of secure attachments ($X^2 = 7.35$, $p < .007$). In addition, the maltreatment group had significantly fewer secure attachments than would be expected given Ainsworth et al.'s (1978) 70% baserate ($X^2 = 30.2$, $p < .0001$). The comparison group's proportion of secure attachments was somewhat lower than the 70% baserate but was not significantly different from it ($X^2 = 3.35$, $p > .05$).

The present study's overall sample rate of 51.2% D's and the maltreatment group rate of 81.8% D's are substantially higher rates of disorganized/disoriented attachments than have been reported in any other study to date. In Main's original Berkeley middle-class sample only 13% of the Strange Situations were unclassifiable or D. A slightly higher proportion, 23%, was coded D in a subset of 60 of the Berkeley sample in a reanalysis after the D coding system was developed (Main & Solomon, in press).

In the Spieker and Booth (1988) high-risk sample, the rate of unclassifiable attachments was 18%. Only two other researchers have found a rate of unclassifiable or disorganized cases close to our rate. Crittenden's (1985) subsample of 10 abused children included 70% A–C's, and all of her subjects who were both abused and neglected were rated as A–C in this sample. O'Connor, Sigman, and Brill (1987) found that infants of mothers who had consumed a great deal of alcohol prior to, during, and following pregnancy were more likely to be insecurely attached than a comparison group of infants whose mothers were either abstinent or light drinkers during a comparable time of framework. Thirty-five percent of the entire sample of infants were classified as disorganized/disoriented. Particularly within the moderate-to-heavy drinking group, the D category was especially prevalent and a number of infants who were force classified as secure were found to be more accurately classified as disorganized/disoriented.

Forced classifications. In order to increase our knowledge about the disorganized/disoriented category, Main and Solomon recommend that whenever a D classification is assigned to a case, the coder should also rate the A, B, or C category that would have been the "forced classification" had the D category not been available. That procedure was carried out in this study. Overall, of the 22 D classifications in the sample, 55% were forced classified as A's, 27% as B's, and 18% as C's. Of the D's, 18 were from the maltreatment group, and their pattern of forced classifications were essentially the same as the aforementioned group distribution, with 50%, 33%, and 17% force coded as A, B, and C, respectively. Of the 4 D classifications in the comparison group, 3 were force classified as A and 1 as C. Thus, for the entire current sample, the avoidant category was the predominant forced classification. This finding is in contrast to Main and Solomon's (1986) Berkeley sample, where the forced classifications were predominantly secure (62% of 34 D classifications). The difference may be indicative of an overall sample difference, with the current high-risk sample simply exhibiting stronger overall avoidance reactions.

Because 35 of the children in this sample were also coded in a previous study (Schneider-Rosen et al., 1985), we thought it would be interesting to compare our recent recoding with our previous coding, substituting the current forced classifications for the children who were rated as D's. Of the 35 recodings, 10 were in disagreement with our earlier classification. Of these 10 disagreements, 8 were from the D category. This lack of ABC rating stability, found mainly in the D group, underscores the point that disorganized attachment *is* characterized by a mix of features from the three major attachment categories. Thus, we were not at all surprised to find that most of the coding disagreements with our previous classifications came primarily from infants who had disorganized/disoriented attachments. One would expect that at different times and with different raters, it would be difficult to identify one prominent style consistently. This greater lack of stability of attachment ratings in the D category further reinforces the importance of using the disorganized/disoriented classification scheme.

In addition to improving the reliability of the attachment coding system, the disorganized/disoriented category enhances the validity of the classification system. Six children in this study who were insecure Type D would have been classified as secure Type B had the new category not been available. All six of these children were from the maltreatment group. This finding is in parallel with Crittenden's (1987) and Spieker and Booth's (1988) A–C results with other maltreatment and high-risk samples. Infants given the avoidant/resistant classification in their studies were frequently rated as secure prior to the development of the new category, and they were often among the most severely maltreated in the sample or from families who had the most difficulties. By indicating limitations in the traditional tripartite scheme, these findings underscore the importance and validity of expanding the current system.

Moreover, the D category has great potential for increasing the predictive validity of the attachment system. Main et al. (1985) have already demonstrated differential sequelae at 6 years for children who were rated as insecure A and D and secure B at 12 months. Unfortunately her sample size of C's was not large enough to be included in her analyses. Still, these findings are in contrast to other studies that have not been able to distinguish sequelae of different insecure groupings. A significant criticism of the attachment paradigm has focused on the absence of specific hypotheses regarding the outcomes of the different attachment categories (Connell and Goldsmith, 1982; Lamb, 1987). The D category may help to resolve this issue. By eliminating false B's and by identifying infants who would have been force classified as A's or C's, the D category may greatly increase the predictive power of the attachment system.

Type of maltreatment. With 18 out of 22 attachments coded as D and very uneven numbers of infants who had experienced the different maltreatment types, the results of Chi-Square analyses of dichotomous variables for each type of maltreatment (neglected versus not neglected, etc.) were insignificant. However, we did informally examine the data. In particular, we wanted to know what type of maltreatment was experienced by the four infants in the maltreatment group who were *not* rated as disorganized/disoriented. Three of them were rated as securely attached and one was rated as avoidant. The three infants who were judged secure had experienced only neglect from the mother and one of these securely rated children had experienced physical abuse perpetrated by the father. The infant rated as avoidant was among the group of infants for whom social workers had indicated no experience of maltreatment.

It was surprising to find that D attachment ratings were assigned to the other six infants for whom social workers had reported no specific types of maltreatment. These children may have experienced maltreatment that went undetected even though the family was receiving protective services.

It is also possible that they experienced one or more of the other forms of interaction disruption that have been implicated in the etiology of disorganized attachment, such as maternal depression, lack of resolution of mourning of early loss, or lack of resolution of other trauma including physical or sexual abuse.

Discussion

The predominance of disorganized attachment among maltreated infants

The findings of the current study corroborate and extend the results of previous studies of attachment among maltreated infants. Maltreated infants are much more likely than comparison infants to be rated as insecurely attached to their caregivers, and are particularly likely to demonstrate a disorganized/disoriented attachment. From what we know of the caregiving environments of maltreated children, there are several reasons why this is the case.

First, the lives of maltreated infants and infants being reared in homes where parents previously have maltreated older siblings are characterized by varieties of inconsistent care (Crittenden, 1981; Egeland and Brunnquell, 1979; Garbarino and Gilliam, 1980). In the current sample, 18 percent of the infants were reported by their social workers to have experienced multiple types of maltreatment from their mothers, and the mothers of the children in the sample were reported to have perpetrated additional forms of maltreatment upon older siblings in these families. Although we do not take forms of maltreatment to be longstanding parental traits that do not change from child to child or from life circumstance to life circumstance, we do believe that infants reared in families served by Protective Services may have experienced types and degrees of maltreatment unknown to their service providers. The hidden and unreported nature of maltreatment has been well documented (USDHHS, 1981). In addition, other perpetrators (usually fathers or mothers' boyfriends) also abused and neglected some of these infants. Studies have linked insensitive overstimulation to avoidant attachment and insensitive understimulation to resistant attachment (Belsky, Rovine, and Taylor, 1984; Crittenden, 1985; Lyons-Ruth et al., 1987). Combinations of these insensitive styles could lead to combined responses such as the A–C pattern.

Second, Main and Hesse (in press) have suggested that it is the interjection of *fear* into the experience of otherwise adequate caregiving that is essential to developing a disorganized/disoriented attachment. Fear must certainly be a common experience for physically and emotionally abused children. It is also probable that there are frightening aspects to emotional and physical neglect. As Main and Hesse have described, the concurrent activation of the fear/wariness and attachment behavioral systems produces strong conflicting motivations to approach the caregiver for comfort and to retreat from him or her to safety. Proximity-seeking mixed with avoidance results as infants attempt to balance their conflicting approach and avoidance tendencies. Freezing, dazing, and stilling may be the result of overloading, when approach tendencies equal the avoidance tendencies, causing them to mutually inhibit one another (Main and Solomon, 1986). Third, in other clinical populations, infants of mothers with an affective disorder were found to be at increased risk for having avoidant/resistant attachment relationships (Radke-Yarrow et al., 1985). The mothers in our Protective Service sample had higher elevated levels of depression than our comparison mothers. Depression could have independently contributed to the development of disorganized attachment in some of the infants in our sample (cf. Gilbreath and Cicchetti, unpublished manuscript).

New categories, maltreated children, and the growth of science:
inductive and deductive approaches

The simultaneous discoveries of new patterns of attachment, disorganized/disoriented, A–C and unstable-A categories, provide diverse examples of how scientific theory and method grow. As described above, new categories evolved through both inductive and deductive processes. Main and her colleagues proceeded in a more inductive fashion: collecting anomalous cases in which the Strange Situation behavior displayed did not conform to any of the previously known attachment patterns, then carefully examining the unusual features of these behaviors in search of possible new patterns, and finally concluding that the one defining feature of the new group was the profound lack of an organized strategy for dealing with the attachment figure during stress. Lyons-Ruth and her colleagues proceeded in an analogous manner, discovering the unstable-A pattern by attending to anomalous patterns of behaviorial scale ratings, especially the ratings for avoidance. Their discovery of the group of infants with an extreme drop in avoidance ratings from the first reunion to the second, unstable avoidance, occurred *before* the investigators knew that this new pattern was overrepresented in the high-risk/maltreated group.

The development of Crittenden's A–C category exemplifies a deductive path to discovery. Her coders succeeded in applying the original A, B, and C ratings to abused and neglected children's Strange Situation behavior. Not until she reviewed her findings was she faced with a relatively large number of securely rated maltreated infants. She reexamined her Strange Situation videotapes and found anomalous behaviors that did not fit the secure, avoidant or resistant/ambivalent patterns. In both the inductive and deductive approaches, the theoretical characterization of infant attachment behavior as orderly strategies to maximize safety and learning in context-appropriate ways was central to making the new discoveries.

Common principles underlie these different pathways to discovery. First, the investigators have demonstrated that basic developmental theory and the study of abnormal populations mutually inform one another (Cicchetti, 1984b, in press, this volume; Rolf et al., in press; Rutter and Garmezy, 1983). The A–C and unstable-A categories were discovered within studies of high risk and maltreated infants. The disorganized/disoriented category was discovered in the context of basic research with low-risk families, but was validated with data from maltreatment studies. Second, investigators maintained a focus on the *organization* and *meaningfulness* of attachment strategies as they examined the infants' behavior in the Strange Situation. Thus, a lack of rationale among behaviors observed during the Strange Situation, or a lack of fit between a secure quality of attachment rating paired with a caretaking history of extreme insensitivity, was cause for reexamination of theory and method.

Future directions for the study of disorganized attachment

The value of research with maltreatment samples. Disorganized attachment patterns have only recently been disovered; therefore, additional studies are needed to complete our descriptions of them. Given the elevated levels of disorganized attachment in our own and other maltreated samples, future research conducted on these populations would ensure substantial numbers of disorganized attachments to pursue the issues outlined below.

Mapping the precursors of disorganized attachment. Ainsworth has often emphasized that a behavioral description and qualitative classification of attachment behavior at age 12 months, such as that obtained with the Strange Situation, does not provide a full understanding of a child's attachment relationship to the caregiver. Naturalistic measures of caregiving interactions over the first year are needed. Although Crittenden (1981) and Lyons-Ruth et al. (1987, this volume) have provided evidence that abusing and neglecting mothers have distinct interaction styles in the home, measured when their infants are 12 months or older, the links between the infants' disorganized Strange Situation behavior at age 1 and caregiving precursors during the first year remain to be made for the disorganized category in both middle-class and high-risk populations. Prospective studies of caregiver–infant interactions during the first year of life are required to discover which caregiver behaviors are related to disorganized attachment. Such studies are especially necessary when the Strange Situation is used with populations other than the middle-class, nonclinical samples on which the procedure was established.

Main and Solomon (in press) have called our attention to biologists' emphasis upon *history* as well as *appearance* in establishing biological classification (Mayr, 1976, cited in Main and Solomon, in press).

Prospective studies will allow us to uncover the commonalities in the developmental histories of infants with disorganized/disoriented patterns of attachment. Such commonalities are needed to confirm the categorical distinctiveness of disorganized attachment behavior, and they will provide tests of hypothesized etiologies of disorganization. Correlational studies have identified groups of infants at increased risk for disorganized attachment, including the children of depressed parents, children whose parents are characterized by unresolved mourning for the loss of their own parent, and maltreated children. Prospective studies will reveal whether these diverse groups of caregivers interact similarly with their infants during the first year of life or exhibit a variety of disorganizing interaction styles.

Predictive validity. In addition to uncovering the precursors to disorganized attachment, it is essential to document the subsequent developmental outcomes of children rated as having disorganized attachments as infants. Predictable outcomes are a part of the confirmation of the disorganized pattern as a unique category. Main, Kaplan, and Cassidy (1985) have provided the only follow-up assessment of the later development of disorganized infants. Similar studies with larger sample sizes and other populations of children with disorganized attachment, especially maltreated children, remain to be done.

In their follow-up study of 40 middle- and upper-middle-class six-year-olds, Main et al. (1985) included 12 children who had been rated as disorganized in their attachment to their mothers at 12 months of age. At the follow-up assessment, these children's reunion behavior with their mothers was characterized as controlling, either through punitiveness or through overly bright caregiving and role reversal (Main and Cassidy, in press). On other measures of mental representation of attachment, the children rated as D's in infancy appeared "depressed, disorganized and intermittently irrational in thought processes" (Main et al., 1985, p. 99). Although the controlling style seen in the reunions represents a more organized strategy than was seen when these children were in their infancy, other indicators of disordered development remain in these children's mental representations regarding attachment and in dysfluent communication with their caregivers. These preliminary findings raise a number of questions that need to be answered through future follow-up studies, both in additional nonclinical samples like the Berkeley sample, and, especially, with high-risk samples like abused and neglected children.

Do high-risk and clinical samples show five-year outcomes similar to those in the Main and Solomon sample? Given the greater instability of attachment quality over time documented in high risk samples (Schneider-Rosen et al., 1985; Vaughn, Egeland, Sroufe, and Waters, 1979), the relationships between 12-month disorganized Strange Situation behavior and 6-year-old behavior may be different among high-risk children. Is it possible that the disorganized Strange Situation behavior of some high-risk children is a result of their being *in transition* from one form of attachment to another? We have not mapped the processes by which children reformulate their attachment relationships. Longitudinal studies with special attention to disorganized features may reveal either that there are multiple pathways to a classification of disorganization, or that instability in the attachment classifications of high-risk samples is less prevalent than is currently believed. In other words, infants who have previously been reported as shifting in classification across time may have been consistently disorganized, with coders just noting different aspects of behavior as most prominent at different points in time.

Role reversal in maltreated children

The phenomenon of parent–child role reversal suggests another important link between child maltreatment and the disorganized/disoriented attachment pattern. One of the most constantly observed characteristics of abused/neglected children is that they seem to have reversed roles with their caregivers (Dean, Malik, Richards, and Stringer, 1986; Morris and Gould, 1963). In the parent–child relationships of maltreated children, the children appear to be the sensitive, nurturing members of the dyad. Hence, the role reversal of caregiving behaviors documented in 6-year-olds who were classified as Type D at 12 months (Main et al., 1985) provides a new perspective on understanding the etiology of this feature in abused and neglected children. The parentification of the maltreated child may be better understood as a specific manifestation of a more general developmental course of an underlying disorganized attachment relationship. Thus, knowledge about attachment relationships in maltreatment cases may prove to be important for prevention and intervention purposes (Cicchetti, Toth, Bush, and Gillespie, 1988). Here, again, the need for longitudinal follow-ups of children with Type D attachments is underscored.

The elaboration of subtypes of the disorganized/disoriented category

Main and Solomon (in press) have tentatively described three different subtypes within the D attachment category: depressed, apprehensive, and avoidant/resistant (A–C). Some infants show combinations of these styles.

Subtype analyses may prove to be an especially fruitful approach to studies of disorganized attachment in maltreatment and other clinical samples. Attention to different styles of disorganized attachment will add precision to studies of etiology and developmental outcome in normal and high-risk infants. We also predict that maltreatment samples will be the source of additional disorganized styles. Lyons-Ruth and colleagues (this volume) may have already discovered a new subtype of disorganization in the unstable-A category. The four-point drop in avoidance scores from the first reunion to the second is a new pattern that was exceedingly rare in the Ainsworth et al. (1978) normative sample. Egeland and Sroufe (1981b) described insecure attachments that were disorganized and *apathetic* in quality among abused and abused/neglected infants. Such attachments may be similar to the ones Main and Solomon describe as depressed, or they may be a separate subcategory. If reliable behavioral coding systems for subtypes can be developed, the prospective studies and longitudinal follow-up studies can help resolve the question regarding the existence of subtypes.

In the HCMP 12-month sample we saw novel patterns of behavior that may be the basis for a separate subtype. Unlike most anxious/avoidant youngsters, who tend to be affiliative to strangers, there were some disorganized/disoriented infants, force classified as Type A, who tended to withdraw from the strangers as well as from their caregivers. This turning inward, avoiding other possible sources of adult interaction, suggests that infants with Type D attachments may have a worse prognosis than anxious avoidant babies. In addition, several of the Type D infants in our sample seemed to show more animation and interest in play and less fearfulness when left alone at the second separation than at any other time during the Strange Situation.

One new category or several? Ainsworth's three original patterns of attachment have been empirically documented as distinct categories. They have been shown to have coding reliability, distinct caregiving precursors, and predictable developmental outcomes. At this point it is unclear whether A–C and unstable-avoidant patterns should be included as subtypes under the disorganized/disoriented classification or should be viewed as independent categories. Validation studies of the precursors and later developmental outcomes related to disorganized attachment ultimately will provide information relevant to these decisions. Currently, there is some evidence for including A–C in the disorganized category as a subtype. In a re-classification study, all of the infants Spieker and Booth (1988) had classified as A–C's were successfully reclassified as D's using the Main and Solomon system (Main and Spieker, unpublished manuscript, cited in Main and Solomon, in press). Even if Crittenden's A–C's could also be reliably coded as D's, there may still be reason to maintain the Crittenden A–C as a separate category. At issue is whether the avoidant–resistant pattern describes a coherent alternative strategy of behaving toward the caregiver in the stress of the Strange Situation, or whether A–C behavior is better characterized as disorganized and lacking in a coherent strategy. Crittenden has argued (1985; Crittenden and Ainsworth, this volume) that the avoidant–resistant form of attachment does indeed represent a meaningful strategy *for children reared in the context of abuse and neglect.*

The behavior of maltreated children in the Crittenden samples seems better described as organized around resolving the conflict between the child's needs for proximity to the mother and his expectations of his mother's reactions to his behavior. That is, the maltreated child needs proximity and contact with his mother following separation as much as other children do. In fact, his experiences of previous maltreatment heighten his distress during the brief separation of the Strange Situation making the need for contact more imperative. However, the maltreated child also has learned to expect that his bids for contact will be ignored, rebuffed, or possibly punished. The ability of such children to maintain avoidance at all following the stress of separation together with their ability to limit their resistance to noncontextual aggression directed away from the mother and their use of distal and circumspect means of achieving proximity would suggest a highly controlled, or organized pattern of behavior. (Crittenden and Ainsworth, this volume)

In addition to exploring this question at the theoretical level, additional studies would be useful. Prospective studies of infant–caregiver interaction across the first year of life may yield different correlates of Crittenden's A–C's and the A–C's that are subtypes within the D category. Follow-up studies may yield different outcomes for the A–C's versus the other D's. It is possible that such a distinction would only appear within maltreated samples. This may be an example of an extreme sample requiring the use of an adapted coding system to capture important aspects of behavior that do not appear in less extreme populations.

Remaining questions to resolve

Can a maltreated child develop a secure attachment to a maltreating caregiver? In both our original report on the quality of attachment in maltreated 12-month-olds (Schneider-Rosen et al., 1985) and in this reanalysis of those data implementing the Main and Solomon (1986) disorganized/disoriented category of attachment we have reported a few maltreated children who were rated as securely attached. Even after reanalysis of the data in which unclassifiable cases were set aside, Egeland and Sroufe (1981b) reported secure attachments in from one quarter to one half of their various subgroups of maltreated 12-month-olds. Lamb, Gaensbauer, Malkin, and Schultz (1985) reported one secure infant out of eleven infants seen in the Strange Situation with mothers who had maltreated them. Crittenden (1988), in a study that implemented the A–C category, reported 5 percent, 10 percent, and 13 percent of abused, neglected, and abused/neglected 11-

to 48-month-olds as having been rated secure in the Strange Situation. There are strong arguments for why this should not be the case. These findings would be difficult to resolve if our work were guided by a linear, "main-effects" model of development and if we did not take into consideration the limitations of our current methods of classifying the quality of attachment relationships and of assessing maltreatment. However, when viewed within the context of a transactional–developmental perspective (Sameroff and Chandler, 1975), these secure attachments in maltreated children are not necessarily an anomalous result.

The recent coding expansions that investigators have made on the original Ainsworth classification system have increased the precision of statistical findings. Infants who would have been force classified as securely attached are now being appropriately assessed as insecure. Nonetheless, although progress has been made in this area, it would be naive to assume that no further refinements will occur in the current coding system or that additional paradigms for assessing the quality of attachment will not be developed. Because it is conceivable that the current procedures employed to assess the quality of attachment may not be sensitive enough to classify all dyads properly, it is possible that an undetermined percentage of maltreated children are still being inappropriately force classified as securely attached. And, even with the addition of the D category, there are still some unclassifiable cases.

In addition to the potential shortcomings in the current attachment measures and coding schemes, there are also limitations to our present methods for operationalizing child maltreatment. Because of the heterogeneity of maltreatment phenomena and the absence of an established reliable and valid nosology for diagnosing child maltreatment (Cicchetti and Rizley, 1981), to date we have been constrained to making relatively gross comparisons of maltreated versus nonmaltreated children in our statistical analyses. As pointed out by Mineka and Rush (1978) in reference to animal studies of maltreatment, variations in the manifestations and timing of maltreatment are important variables to consider when studying the sequelae of maltreatment. Variables such as the age at which maltreatment occurred during the life cycle as well as the severity and chronicity of the maltreatment are likely to be of value when trying to understand variations in child outcome (cf. Cicchetti and Rizley, 1981). There are practical as well as ethical constraints on our ability to classify and quantify child maltreatment. At the same time, extended efforts toward developing a reliable and valid nosology of child maltreatment should be implemented.

Although work still needs to be done to increase the sensitivity of our procedures for assessing attachment and maltreatment, theoreticians and researchers have made progress in developing more sophisticated models for understanding the pathways toward competent or maladaptive developmental outcomes (e.g., Sameroff and Chandler, 1975). Drawing upon earlier descriptive studies of the etiology of maltreatment (reviewed in Cicchetti, Taraldson, and Egeland, 1978), Cicchetti and his colleagues (Cicchetti and Rizley, 1981; Schneider-Rosen et al., 1985) have proposed that the characteristics of the parent, child, and environment transact in a dynamic, mutually influencing system that is essential for interpreting the complex interplay of risk factors that operate in determining the quality of parent–child relationships and family functioning more broadly. This three dimensional, transactional model of developmental processes takes into account risk and protective factors while making temporal distinctions between enduring and transient aspects of both the risk and protective components in the model (Cicchetti and Rizley, 1981).

Implicit in the transactional model of compensatory and potentiating factors is the idea that there are multiple pathways to adaptive and maladaptive outcomes. Moreover, there may be qualitative differences underlying phenotypically similar outcomes. Hence, it is necessary to take into account long-term "vulnerabilities" (such as poor parenting skills and difficult temperament in the child) along with enduring protective factors (such as sensitive responsivity of the caregiver and resiliency to stress in the infant). At the same time, it is important to assess short-term challengers (such as physical illness) and buffers (such as the availability of daycare facilities). This model may be applied toward understanding diverse pathways toward developmental outcomes (see Cicchetti, this volume, for an elaboration of this model).

Following this perspective, an insecure attachment may not always result from maltreatment by the attachment figure. For example, if maltreatment results from the influence of short-term stress, which occurs in the broader context of more durable compensatory factors present in the parent and/or child, then an already established secure attachment might prevail. Of course, this is but one simplified example of the numerous and complex pathways and processes through which secure and anxious attachments may eventuate. Consequently, the discovery of a small number of infants who appear to be securely attached to their maltreating caregiver is not necessarily a discrepant finding. In-depth analyses focusing on the context of maltreatment and on resilient children should prove to be a fruitful avenue toward further refining the current systems for conceptualizing the quality of attachment in maltreated children as well as an initial step toward testing the transactional model of short- and long-term risk and protective factors in the parent–child–environment system.

Is lack of resolution of mourning or trauma a mechanism in the intergenerational transmission of maltreatment? If a parent's unresolved mourning regarding loss is capable of causing the interjection of disorganizing influences into later caregiving, unresolved feelings about other early attachment-related trauma, such as maltreatment, may also intrude into caregiving in a similar manner (Main and Hesse, in press). There are some data regarding the intergenerational transmission of child abuse that are consistent with lack of resolution of trauma as the mechanism. Hunter, Kilstrom, Kraybill, and Loda (1978) in a prospective study of 282 premature and ill infants (a group known to be at increased risk for child abuse and neglect) described 13 risk factors, including parent, child, and environmental characteristics, that differentiated between the families in which maltreatment was or was not reported in the first year of the child's life. One of the characteristics was a history of child maltreatment on the part of the parent. The majority of the 49 parents with a history of maltreatment did not maltreat their high-risk child, but nine (18 percent) did. In most cases, the maltreatment was in the form of neglect. Hunter (1980) commented on features that discriminated between the group of previously maltreated parents who repeated the cycle with their children and those who did not. In an extensive interview with parents about their own upbringing, maltreated parents who did *not* abuse or neglect their premature or ill infant were characterized by more resolution of their past maltreatment experiences. "Just as the non-repeaters were more open with their feelings during the nursery crisis, they were also much more detailed and emotional in discussing their own childhoods. They seemed to be actively reworking their experiences with their parents" (Hunter, 1980, p. 4). One could interpret this description as an indicator that nonrepeaters had better resolved ill feelings regarding their maltreatment, some of which may have included mourning of the adequate parenting they never had, to be able to parent their own high-risk children more effectively, just as Main and Hesse (in press) found that parents who had successfully mourned their loss of a parent tended not to have infants with D attachments.

How general and comprehensive is our understanding of the relationship between maltreatment and the formation of attachment to the caregiver? Theoretically, attachment and maltreatment have been considered from the broad perspective of evolution and across a wide range of hypothetical conditions. In empirical studies we have seen but small slices of the full picture. Animal studies have been conducted across a range of maltreatment conditions, but generalizations are limited to the few species that have been tested (Reite and Caine, 1983). The experimental animal studies that have explored maltreatment most fully have been conducted under conditions least like the natural environments in which the animals live. The findings help us examine theoretical hypotheses, but they do not provide us with generalizable knowledge of the maltreatment–attachment relationship in real life. Attention to ethological field studies could help us broaden our understanding at this point.

Research on human attachments formed under maltreatment conditions cessarily even more restricted than experimental animal studies have ῀n. Our experiments are "experiments of nature" due to ethical necessity. ɹ addition, the maltreated children we have studied have been drawn almost exclusively from lower levels of socioeconomic status. They have been most available to those of us who have depended upon protective service agencies as sources of research subjects. If we are to examine the effects of risk and protective factors on development under conditions of maltreatment, we need to broaden our sample bases to include more middle- and upper-class families.

The levels of stress under which we examine the quality of attachment in the Strange Situation paradigm are again ethically restricted to very limited levels of stress. Are the characterizations of attachment that have now become standard generalizable to more extreme conditions of stress? Only by continuing to explore actively the adjustment of maltreated children and by expanding our efforts to understand the details of their circumstances will we know how well our current theories fit the extremes.

Notes

1 Scrivens, 1961 cited in A. Kaplan (1963). *The Conduct of Inquiry.*
2 Bowlby uses the term "mother" but notes that it refers to the person who provides care for the child and to whom he becomes attached. This does not have to be the natural mother.
3 Bretherton (1980, 1985) has correctly pointed out that the attachment behavioral system does not turn on and off as with a switch; it operates continuously, monitoring signs of danger, fatigue, well-being, and proximity of the caregiver. At times no attachment signals are being emitted, the exploratory behavioral system or some other system is what is obvious and it may seem that the attachment system has shut off. Bretherton argues it is better to view the attachment system as still monitoring the availability of the caregiver and, when warranted, producing a reading of low need for attachment behaviors given an accessible attachment figure.
4 Rating general crankiness and undirected aggressiveness as "resistance" is an extension of the Ainsworth definition of resistance.
5 We believe that this percentage is lower than previous publications reported on the Harvard Child Maltreatment Project (Cicchetti, Carlson, Braunwald, and Aber, 1987) because 12-month-olds may be too young to experience some of the subtypes of maltreatment described in the literature (e.g., sexual abuse) and because it may be more difficult to document the presence of some of these subtypes at such an early age (e.g., emotional mistreatment) using conventional protective services' documentation procedures.

References

Ainsworth, M. (1973). The development of infant–mother attachment. In B. Caldwell and H. Ricciutti (Eds.), *Review of child development research,* Volume 3. Chicago: University of Chicago Press.
Ainsworth, M. D. S. (1980). Attachment and child abuse. In G. Gerbner, C. Ross, and E. Zigler (Eds.), *Child abuse: An agenda for action.* New York: Oxford University Press.

Ainsworth, M. D. S., Blehar, M., Waters, E., and Wall, S. (1978). *Patterns of attachment: A psychological study of the Strange Situation.* Hillsdale, NJ: Erlbaum.

Ainsworth, M., and Wittig, B. (1969). Attachment and exploratory behavior of one-year-olds in a Strange Situation. In B. M. Foss (Ed.), *Determinants of infant behavior* (pp. 111–136). Vol. 4. London: Methuen.

Belsky, J., Rovine, M., and Taylor, D. G. (1984). The Pennsylvania Infant and Family Development Project, III: The origins of individual differences in infant–mother attachment: Maternal and infant contributions. *Child Development, 55* (3), 718–728.

Bischof, N. (1975). A systems approach towards the functional connections of fear and attachment. *Child Development, 46,* 801–817.

Bretherton, I. (1980). Young children in stressful situations: The supporting role of attachment figures and unfamiliar caregivers. In G. V. Coelho and P. Ahmed (Eds.), *Uprooting and development* (pp. 179–210). New York: Plenum.

Bretherton, I. (1985). Attachment Theory: Retrospect and prospect. In I. Bretherton and E. Waters (Eds.), Growing Points of Attachment Theory and Research. *Monographs of the Society for Research in Child Development,* Vol. 50 (1 and 2) (pp. 3–35). Serial No. 209.

Bretherton, I. (1987). New perspectives on attachment relations: Security, communication, and internal working models. In J. Osofsky (Ed.), *Handbook of infant development* (Second Edition) (pp. 1061–1100). New York: John Wiley and Sons.

Bowlby, J. (1944). Forty-four juvenile thieves: Their characters and home life. *International Journal of Psychoanalysis, 25,* 19–52, and 107–27.

Bowlby, J. (1958). The nature of the child's tie to his mother. *International Journal of Psychoanalysis, 39,* 350–73.

Bowlby, J. (1969/1982). *Attachment and loss, Vol. I: Attachment.* (2nd ed.). New York: Basic Books.

Bowlby, J, (1973). *Attachment and loss, Vol. II: Separation.* New York: Basic Books.

Bowlby, J. (1977a). The making and breaking of affectional bonds. *British Journal of Psychiatry, 130,* 201–10.

Bowlby, J. (1977b). The making and breaking of affectional bonds. *British Journal of Psychiatry, 130,* 421–31.

Bowlby, J. (1980). *Attachment and loss, Vol. III: Loss.* New York: Basic Books.

Cicchetti, D. (Ed.), (1984a). *Developmental psychopathology.* Chicago: University of Chicago Press.

Cicchetti, D. (1984b). The emergence of developmental psychopathology. *Child Development, 55,* 1–7.

Cicchetti, D. (1987). Developmental psychopathology in infancy: Illustration from the study of maltreated youngsters. *Journal of Consulting and Clinical Psychology, 55,* 837–845.

Cicchetti, D. (in press). An historical perspective on the discipline of developmental psychopathology. In J. Rolf, A. Masten, D. Cicchetti, K. Neuchterlein, and S. Weintraub (Eds.), *Risk and protective factors in the development of psychopathology.* New York: Cambridge University Press.

Cicchetti, D., Carlson, V., Braunwald, K. G., and Aber, J. L. (1987). The sequelae of child maltreatment. In R. Gelles and J. Lancaster, (Eds.), *Child abuse and neglect: Biosocial dimensions* (pp. 277–298). New York: Aldine Gruyter.

Cicchetti, D., Cummings, E. M., Greenberg, M., and Marvin, R. (in press). Attachment beyond infancy. In M. Greenberg, D. Cicchetti and E. M. Cummings (Eds.), *Attachment during the preschool years.* Chicago: University of Chicago Press.

Cicchetti, D., and Rizley, R. (1981). Developmental perspectives on the etiology, intergenerational transmission, and sequelae of child maltreatment. In R. Rizley and D. Cicchetti (Eds.), *Developmental Perspectives on Child Maltreatment: New Directions for Child Development* (pp. 31–55). No. 11, San Francisco: Jossey-Bass.

Cicchetti, D. and Serafica, F. (1981). The interplay among behavioral systems: Illustrations from the study of attachment, affiliation and wariness in young Down's syndrome children. *Developmental Psychology, 17,* 36–49.

Cicchetti, D., Taraldson, B., and Egeland, B. (1978). Perspectives in the treatment and understanding of child abuse. In A. Goldstein (Ed.), *Prescriptions for child mental health and education.* New York: Pergamon.

Cicchetti, D., and Todd-Manly, J. (in press). A personal perspective on conducting research with maltreating families: Problems and solutions. In E. Brody and I. Sigel (Eds.), *Family research: Vol. 2, Families at risk.* New York: Academic Press.

Cicchetti, D., Toth, S., Bush, M., and Gillespie, J. (1988). Stage-salient issues: A transactional model of intervention. *New Directions for Child Development, 39,* 123–145.

Connell, J. P. and Goldsmith, H. H. (1982). A structural modeling approach to the study of attachment and strange situation behaviors. In R. Emde and R. Harmon (Eds.), *The development of attachment and affiliative systems* (pp. 213–243). New York: Plenum Press.

Crittenden, P. M. (1981). Abusing, neglecting, problematic and adequate dyads: Differentiating by patterns of interaction. *Merrill-Palmer Quarterly, 27,* 210–218.

Crittenden, P. M. (1985). Maltreated infants: Vulnerability and resilience. *Journal of Child Psychology and Psychiatry and Allied Disciplines, 26* (1), 85–96.

Crittenden, P. M. (1988). Relationships at risk. In J. Belsky and T. Nezworski (Eds.), *Clinical implications of attachment theory* (pp. 136–174). Hillsdale, NJ: Erlbaum.

Dean, A. L., Malik, M. M., Richards, W., and Stringer, S. A. (1986). Effects of parental maltreatment on children's conceptions of interpersonal relationships. *Developmental Psychology, 22,* 617–626.

Deutsch, H. (1942). Some forms of emotional disturbance and their relationship to schizophrenia. *Psychoanalytic Quarterly, 11,* 201–321.

Egeland, B., and Brunnquell, D. (1979). An at-risk approach to the study of child abuse: Some preliminary findings. *Journal of the American Academy of Child Psychiatry, 18,* 219–235.

Egeland, B., and Farber, E. A. (1984). Infant–mother attachment: Factors related to its development and changes over time. *Child Development, 55,* 753–771.

Egeland, B., and Sroufe, L. A. (1981a). Attachment and early maltreatment. *Child Development, 52,* 44–52.

Egeland, B., and Sroufe, L. A. (1981b). Developmental sequelae of maltreatment in infancy. In R. Rizley and D. Cicchetti (Eds.), *Developmental perspectives in child maltreatment, 11* (pp. 77–92). San Francisco: Jossey-Bass.

Gaensbauer, T. J., and Harmon, R. J. (1982). Attachment behavior in abused/neglected and premature infants: Implications for the concept of attachment. In R. N. Emde and R. J. Harmon (Eds.), *Attachment and affiliative systems* (pp. 245–279). New York: Plenum.

Garbarino, J., and Gilliam, G. (1980). *Understanding abusive families.* Lexington, MA: Lexington Press.

George, C., Kaplan, N., and Main, M. (1984). *Attachment interview for adults.* Unpublished manuscript, University of California, Berkeley.

George, C., and Main, M. (1979). Social interactions of young abused children: Approach, avoidance, and aggression. *Child Development, 50,* 306–318.

Gilbreath, B., and Cicchetti, D. (unpublished manuscript). Psychopathology in maltreating mothers.

Giovannoni, J., and Becerra, R. (1979). *Defining child abuse.* New York: Free Press.

Grossmann, K., Grossmann, K. E., Spangler, G., Suess, G., and Unzer, L. (1985). Maternal sensitivity and newborns' orientation responses as related to quality of attachment in Northern Germany. In I. Bretherton and E. Waters (Eds.), Growing points of attachment theory and research. *Monographs of the Society for Research in Child Development,* Vol. 50 (1 and 2) (pp. 233–256). Serial No. 209.

Guidano, V. F., and Liotti, G., (1983). *Cognitive processes and emotional disorders: A structural approach to psychotherapy.* New York: The Guilford Press.

Hunter, R. S., (1980). Parents who break with an abusive past: Lessons for prevention. *Caring, 6*(4), Chicago: The National Committee for Prevention of Child Abuse.

Hunter, R. S., Kilstrom, N., Kraybill, E. N., and Loda, F. (1978). Antecedents of child abuse and neglect in premature infants: A prospective study in a newborn intensive care unit. *Pediatrics, 61*(4), 629–635.

Kaplan, A. (1963). *The conduct of inquiry*. San Francisco: Chandler.

Lamb, M. E. (1987). Predictive implications of individual differences in attachment. *Journal of Consulting and Clinical Psychology, 55,* 817–824.

Lamb, M. E., Gaensbauer, T. J., Malkin, C. M., and Schultz, L. A. (1985). The effects of child maltreatment on security of infant–adult attachment. *Infant Behavior and Development, 8,* 35–45.

Lyons-Ruth, K., Connell, D., Zoll, D., and Stahl, J. (1987). Infants at social risk: Relationships among infant maltreatment, maternal behavior, and infant attachment behavior. *Developmental Psychology, 23*(2), 223–232.

Main, M. (1973). *Play, exploration and competence as related to child–adult attachment.* Unpublished doctoral dissertation, Johns Hopkins University.

Main, M., and Cassidy, J. (1988). Categories of response to reunion with the parent at age six: Predictable from infant classification and stable over a one month period. *Developmental Psychology, 24,* 415–426.

Main, M., and Hesse (in press). Lack of resolution of mourning in adulthood and its relationship to infant disorganization: Some speculations regarding causal mechanisms. In M. Greenberg, D. Cicchetti, and M. Cummings (Eds.), *Attachment during the preschool years.* Chicago: University of Chicago Press.

Main, M., Kaplan, N., and Cassidy, J. (1985). Security in infancy, childhood and adulthood: A move to the level of representation. In I. Bretherton and E. Waters (Eds.), Growing points in attachment theory and research. *Monographs of the Society for Research in Child Development,* Vol. 50 (1 and 2) (pp. 66–104). Serial No. 209.

Main, M., and Solomon, J. (1986). Discovery of a disorganized disoriented attachment pattern. In T. B. Brazelton and M. W. Yogman (Eds.), *Affective development in infancy* (pp. 95–124). Norwood, NJ: Ablex.

Main, M., and Solomon, J. (in press). Procedures for identifying infants as disorganized/disoriented during the Ainsworth Strange Situation. In M. Greenberg, D. Cicchetti, and M. Cummings (Eds.), *Attachment during the preschool years.* Chicago: University of Chicago Press.

Main, M., and Weston, D. (1981). The quality of the toddler's relationship to mother and father. *Child Development, 52,* 932–940.

Mineka, S., and Rush, D. (1978). Commentary on Rajecki, Lamb and Obsmascher: Toward a general theory of infantile attachment: A comparative review of aspects of the social bond. *Behavioral and Brain Sciences, 1,* 453–454.

Morris, M. G., and Gould, R. W. (1963). Role reversal: A necessary concept in dealing with the battered-child syndrome. *American Journal of Orthopsychiatry, 33,* 298–299.

Nock, L., and Rossi, P. (1979). Household types and social standing. *Social Forces, 57,* 1325–1345.

O'Connor, M. J., Sigman, M., and Brill, N. (1987). Disorganization of attachment in relation to maternal alcohol consumption. *Journal of Consulting and Clinical Psychology, 55,* 831–836.

Radke-Yarrow, M., Cummings, E. M., Kuczynski, L., and Chapman, M. (1985). Patterns of attachment in two- and three-year-olds in normal families and families with parental depression. *Child Development, 56,* 884–893.

Rajecki, D. W., Lamb, M. E., and Obmascher, P. (1978). Toward a general theory of infantile attachment: A comparative review of aspects of the social bond. *Behavioral and Brain Sciences, 1,* 417–464.

Reite, M., and Caine, N. G. (Eds.) (1983). *Child abuse: The non-human primate data.* New York: Liss.

Rolf, J., Masten, A., Cicchetti, D., Neuchterlein, K., and Weintraub, S. (Eds.) (in press). *Risk and protective factors in the development of psychopathology.* New York: Cambridge University Press.

Ruppenthal, G. C., Arling, G. L., Harlow, H. F., Sackett, G. P. and Suomi, S. J. (1976). A 10-year perspective of motherless mother monkey behavior. *Journal of Abnormal Psychology, 85,* 341–349.

Rutter, M. (1979). Maternal deprivation, 1972–1978; New findings, new concepts, new approaches. *Child Development, 50,* 283–305.

Rutter, M., and Garmezy, N. (1983). Developmental psychopathology. In P. Mussen (Ed.), *Handbook of child psychology.* Vol. IV (pp. 775–911). New York: Wiley and Sons.

Sameroff, A., and Chandler, M. (1975). Reproductive risk and the continuum of caretaking casualty. In F. Horowitz (Ed.), *Review of child development research* (Vol. 4, pp. 187–244). Chicago: University of Chicago Press.

Schneider-Rosen, K., Braunwald, K. G., Carlson, V., and Cicchetti, D. (1985). Current perspectives in attachment theory: Illustration from the study of maltreated infants. In I. Bretherton and E. Waters (Eds.), Growing points of attachment theory and research. *Monographs of the Society for Research in Child Development,* Vol. 50 (1 and 2) (pp. 194–210). Serial No. 209.

Schneider-Rosen, K., and Cicchetti, D. (1984). The relationship between affect and cognition in maltreated infants: Quality of attachment and the development of visual self-recognition. *Child Development, 55,* 648–658.

Sigman, M., and Ungerer, J. A. (1984). Attachment behaviors in autistic children. *Journal of Autism and Developmental Disorders, 14,* 231–244.

Spieker, S., and Booth, C. (1988). Maternal antecedents of attachment quality. In J. Belsky and T. Nezworski (Eds.), *Clinical implications of attachment* (pp. 95–135). Hillsdale, NJ: Erlbaum.

Sroufe, L. A. (1985). Attachment classification from the perspective of infant–caregiver relationships and infant temperament. *Child Development, 56,* 1–14.

Sroufe, L. A., and Fleeson, J. (1986). Attachment and the construction of relationships. In W. Hartup and Z. Rubin (Eds.), *Relationships and development* (pp. 51–71). Hillsdale, NJ: Erlbaum.

Sroufe, L. A., and Waters, E. (1977). Attachment as an organizational construct. *Child Development, 48,* 1184–1199.

U.S. Department of Health and Human Services. (1981). *Study findings: National study of incidence and severity of child abuse and neglect.* DHHS Pub. No. (DHDS) 81–30325, Washington, DC.

Vaughn, B., Egeland, B., Sroufe, L. A., and Waters, E. (1979). Individual differences in infant–mother attachment at 12 and 18 months: Stability and change in families under stress. *Child Development, 50,* 971–975.

17   Peer relations in maltreated children

Edward Mueller and Nancy Silverman

Recent years have witnessed an increase in attention to the development of
children who have experienced parental maltreatment. Although early studies focused mainly on documenting physical injury and cognitive impairment in maltreated children, investigators have recently begun to pay
increasing attention to the social and emotional sequelae of abuse and
neglect. As a result of this trend, a handful of studies has emerged that examine maltreated children's functioning in an important area of social and
emotional development: interaction with age-mates and the formation of
peer relationships.

Increased understanding of the relationship between maltreatment and
peer relations is important for several reasons. First, establishing successful
relations with peers is recognized to be a central task of childhood. Peer
relations may contribute uniquely to the growth of social and emotional
competence, to the acquisition of social skills and values, and to the development of the capacity to form relationships with others (Hartup, 1983;
Youniss, 1980). Furthermore, investigators have found that the quality of a
child's peer relations is significantly associated with the quality of functioning in other realms, both during childhood and in later years. In particular,
childhood peer relations have been identified as one of the most powerful
predictors of concurrent and future mental health problems, including the
development of psychiatric disorders (Cowen, Pederson, Babigian, Izzo, and
Trost, 1973; Roff, Sells, and Golden, 1972; Sundby and Kreyberg, 1968).
Maltreated children – by virtue of their placement on the extreme end of
the "continuum of caretaking casualty" (Sameroff and Chandler, 1975) –
can be hypothesized to be "at risk" for a variety of difficulties. Thus, an
increased understanding of the quality of their childhood peer relations, and

We are grateful to Drs. Vicki Carlson, Dante Cicchetti, Carolee Howes, Joseph Jacobson, and Mary Main for their helpful comments on earlier drafts of this paper.

the specific ways in which they may be disturbed, can have important implications for predicting, preventing, and ameliorating concurrent and later mental health problems in this population.

A second reason for undertaking the study of maltreated children's peer relations is that it can add to our understanding of normal developmental processes. As noted by Cicchetti and Braunwald (1984), the study of atypical populations can enhance our theory of normal development "primarily by affirming it, challenging it, and requiring a more fully integrated theory that can account for both normal and psychopathological processes" (p. 174). Studying maltreated children's peer relations allows one to address a particularly important issue in developmental psychology – the relationship between early parent–child interactions and later social relationships. Developmental theorists differ in regard to the degree to which they support a relationship between the two social realms of the family and the peer world. Additionally, they differ in regard to the emphasis placed on affective and cognitive factors in mediating such a relationship, and in terms of theories employed to explain it (Carlson and Cicchetti, this volume; Crittenden and Ainsworth, this volume; Lewis and Schaeffer, 1981; Schneider-Rosen, Braunwald, Carlson, and Cicchetti, 1985). Because maltreated children can be said to have experienced a clear disturbance in normal parent–child relations, an examination of the quality of their functioning with peers can shed light on the questions of the relative dependence/independence and nature of the relationship between the family and peer worlds.

Finally, the study of how maltreated children cope with the world of peer relationships can have important clinical applications. Specifically, it can enhance intervention strategies with at-risk and emotionally disordered children. Clinical understanding can be increased by studying both maltreated children who are having difficulties with peers and those who seem to be coping successfully despite having experienced environmental adversity. To guide intervention efforts, it is as important to identify the factors that protect or buffer a child against maladaptation as it is to uncover the negative sequelae of maltreatment. Cicchetti and Rizley (1981) note that the "identification of the competent maltreated child may suggest diagnostic and treatment interventions designed to ameliorate specific disabilities in maltreated children" (pp. 46–47). Such interventions might involve the teaching of competencies that act to reduce a more vulnerable child's risk for maladaptation.

Thus, there are several reasons why the relationship between parental maltreatment and a child's peer relations is worthy of attention. This chapter, by examining both the available empirical literature and relevant developmental theory, attempts to enhance our understanding of this relationship. First, we provide a conceptual overview of the development of peer relations in normal, nonmaltreated children. This is followed by the discussion of whether and how early familial relationships and functioning with peers are related. In that regard, two contrasting models of social development are presented. We then review the existing research on maltreated children's peer relations and offer some explanatory hypotheses. In our conclusion, we suggest some possible directions for future research in this area.

Development of normal peer relations

In order to put the effects of maltreatment into proper context, it is necessary to have some sense of the developmental course of peer relations in nonmaltreated children. It is only against the background of a normal developmental framework that one can assess the delays, deviations, and alternative pathways that maltreated children may exhibit. Space limitations preclude an exhaustive review here of the many and complex ways in which peer relations change from infancy to adolescence (for a comprehensive review, see Hartup, 1983). Thus, the description of peer relations that follows is selective and more narrow in focus. It attempts to provide a brief, general overview of the developmental changes in specific aspects of peer relations.

One of the themes highlighted in this review is that of "peer equality." A description is offered of the changes in both the ways peer equality is manifested across childhood and how children themselves may experience it at different ages. We have chosen to highlight this aspect of peer relations for several reasons. First, although the structure and form of peer relations change dramatically over the course of development, years of research on peer relations suggest that what is special about peer relations at *every* age is their equality. In his exhaustive summary of the peer literature, Hartup (1983) stated: "The unique elements in child–child relations would appear to be the developmental equivalence of the participants and the egalitarian nature of their interactions" (p. 104).

Also, the equal status of peers is quite different from what is normally found in adult–child interactions. As such, it may present children with a unique set of challenges in terms of social and communicative competence. In adult–child interactions, one of the partners is typically much more active and capable in initiating and sustaining communicative interactions. Interactions between peers, however, require that both children contribute effectively in order for the exchange to be successful. Thus, because peer relations require that the child draw on whatever social and communicative competencies are available to him or her, they may provide an important "window" through which these developing abilities can be viewed. Finally, the special set of challenges presented by peer relations has been hypothesized to contribute uniquely to the development of cooperation, morality, interpersonal sensitivity, and mutuality in relationships (Piaget, 1932/1965; Sullivan, 1953).

Although other perspectives on peer relations (e.g., the "social psychological" one; see Oden, Herzberger, Mangione, and Wheeler, 1984) recognize peer equality as important, it is often seen as just one process among others, such as peer competition or mastering social skills. The perspective offered here differs in elevating equality to the status of *the special goal and ideal endpoint of peer relations at all stages of child development.* Equality is not something that some children achieve at age 5 and others at age 10. Rather, the development of peer relations can be characterized as a progression of ever more sophisticated and coordinated "equalities." Thus, at any given point in development, the question is not "What is the function of peer relations?" but rather "What new forms of equality are manifested in children's peer relations at this developmental stage?" "Forms of equality" encompass such simple social coordinations as reciprocal visual gaze in infancy as well as such complex ones as sustained intimate relations between adolescents. In the following section, we cite recent research in an attempt to spell out the newly achieved equalities in peer contacts at each point across child development.

The following description presents eight hypothesized stages in the development of peer relations. The given chronological ages associated with each stage probably tend to vary according to other important factors, such as peer experience and temperament. Although the validity of these stages has not been tested, the model is consistent with much of the existing empirical research. It attempts to organize the disparate peer literature around the functional ideal of equality and the conscious experiences of sharing, play, and friendship.

Stage 1. Absence of peer relations: 0–5 months

During these early months, age-mates cannot relate with one another. Mueller and Vandell (1979) note that weak neck musculature prevents neonates from even seeing each other very well. Although parents can adjust posture and baby position so as to bring their faces to the optimal nine-inch distance that the newborn appears to prefer, very young infants are far from capable of making these adjustments themselves. Despite a lack of skill, young infants do display interest in their peers. Toward the end of this period, the infant's social interest in other babies is evidenced by reaching and touching (see Hartup, 1983).

Stage 2. Joint visual attention and simple elicited responses: 6–9 months

Peer communication appears to develop in relation to the control of visual attention. Thus, the control of vision appears to be a crucial motor system in early peer relations. Stern (1974) considers it to be the first of all the motor systems to become functionally mature. For this reason, it seems reasonable to consider the act of "looking at" to be the first volitional behavior towards age-mates and a necessary one for peer relations to be possible.

Visual attention appears to be the chief means humans have of expressing to potential social partners both communicative intent (Mueller, 1972) and the readiness to interact. In other words, it seems possible to conceive of mutual gaze as a sort of temporal "picture frame" identifying certain time units as high in social potential. In infant peer contacts, joint visual attention may have another important function. It may also give infants an early opportunity to "read" a peer's affective signals, a skill that may play a central role in later interactions.

The repertoire of infants' interactive skills appears to unfold in a universal sequence (Hartup, 1983). Looking is followed by touching and reaching; then, in the second half of the first year, coordinated social acts begin to appear. In a study of peer interaction at 6½, 9½, and 12½ months, Vandell, Wilson, and Buchanan (1980) found that almost half of the infants' exchanges involved such coordinated social acts. The most common sequence involved an infant's exhibiting a social behavior (e.g., vocalizing or pointing) while looking at another baby, and the other baby's responding in kind. Although most of these exchanges were short, two-unit sequences, it does seem that coordinated social interaction with peers occurs at this age. Moreover, it seems that social behavior begets social response from the very beginning of peer relations.

Two other findings from the Vandell et al. study deserve to be highlighted. First, the most common social acts at this age involved vocalizing, followed in frequency by smiling, touching, and motor gestures. At this age, crying, agonistic acts and object-related activities are rare in peer interaction. Second, the authors note that, even in these early months, infants show considerable individual variability; some infants repeatedly directed social acts toward peers, whereas others almost never did. Although these differences may be due to temperament and exposure to older siblings, it is also possible that they are related to differences in parent–infant interaction. This point will be returned to later in the chapter.

Such results support the idea that joint attention and simple social exchanges constitute the earliest "equality" in peer relations. This is an "achieved" equality only in the sense that these actions mature through exercise. It is not initially an "analyzed" or "reflective" equality; it exists in interaction before it is understood by the mind as having communicative value. Only then is it proper to speak of "meaningful joint attention," a phenomenon that characterizes the behavior of children who already know they can interact, which, as such, seems to be more characteristic of the second year.

On the contrary, this period seems to be better characterized as one of "contingent control interactions." This means that the baby is quite busy just producing a coordinated social act (see Musatti and Mueller, 1985) and cannot concern itself too much with reproducing the other's action in an imitative theme. At the same time, without a shared theme, there is nothing to sustain the interaction and it ends with the first response.

Stage 3. Shared place and shared activity on things: 10–15 months

Somewhere around the first birthday, children's peer contacts become much more purposive. They also become much more centered around toys. Often, when they come together, children struggle over toys. Yet, 1-year-olds are just as likely to imitate another baby's actions with a toy as they are to engage in a struggle over it. Imitation of other infants' actions may be due to the fact that an age-mate, capable of similar actions with a toy, provides an ideal model of what to do with it.

This can be hypothesized to be the true beginning of parallel play, a time when coming together is object-focused. It is not a sharing of direct social play so much as a sharing of activity and place. However, although this sharing may be unintended, its "sharedness" is an actual event experienced by the children themselves. In other words, we suggest that parallel play is not merely an expression of a cognitive limitation on peer relations. Instead, it is hypothesized to be the second major equality among peers: a sharing of activity with physical objects that is gradually understood by the participants as such.

Empirical support for the intensely toy-centered quality of peer contacts at this stage can be found in a study by Mueller and Brenner (1977). These investigators found that object-centered contacts in toddler free play increased from 12 to 18 months, but showed no change over the following six months. Contacts involving toys constituted 92 percent of all social interactions among toddlers at 12 months; by 23 months, it was 48 percent.

In examining these data, one tends to focus on the sharing of an activity; however, in coming together, toddlers also find themselves to be sharing a *place*, that is "the place where access to a given toy activity is possible." Although there is no research as yet on play field understanding among 1-year-olds (as there is among preschoolers; Shugar and Bokus, 1986), it is hypothesized that it is precisely at this time that children are coming to understand that they have dominion over both an activity and a place, both of which can be either shared with a peer or possessed by the self. Indeed, Brownell (1985) suggests the emergence of a personal possession rule by age 18 months.

To summarize, peer relations, which began in such a direct and vocal way, seem to take a detour through object play during the toddler period. Toddlers, it seems, come together to do things. In this sense, the toy is both a "barrier" and a "glue." It brings children together, but it also focuses peer relations outward on activities rather than inward on the social relation itself. Normally, there will be no peer intimacy for many years to come.

Stage 4. Shared meaning or topic: 18 months–3 years

Up to this point, we have described three types of equality in peer relations: shared gaze, shared place, and shared activity. Curiously, all this has occurred without any "real communication" among toddlers. This is because communication is a rather complex business, requiring both a topic (for children of this age, usually an object) and social agreement about communication. Until now, toddlers have understood the topic of "action on object" but have not reached a level of social understanding to turn that activity into a social game. They have played in parallel by doing the same things with toys, but have not yet subordinated the toy to a direct discourse with each other.

The emergence of actual communication with shared topic has been documented by Brenner and Mueller (1982). Studying boy toddlers, they found a significant increase in shared meaning games between 12 and 18 months, but no further increase thereafter. In addition, they found that the occurrence of shared meaning had the power to make social interactions significantly longer. The three most frequent shared meanings identified were "object possession struggle," "motor copy," and "object exchange." All three involve object/toy mediation, again confirming the central role of objects in the foundation of peer communication.

If shared attention and place are prerequisites for early communication, then communication of a topic is the "sufficient condition" that turns mere contingent control interaction into social communication. Moreover, it seems to be only with the beginning of shared meaning that toddler exchanges take on the playful and happy quality that leads one to relabel them as "games." Ross (1981) presents evidence that such games do not derive exclusively from adult–child interactions. She used adult tutors to provide toddlers with training sessions in potential peer games. In immediately subsequent peer sessions, unacquainted toddlers almost universally attempted play with the peer. Yet their overtures were based largely on new actions or roles and not on those just rehearsed with adults. It appears that adult training may be ineffective in training peer-relevant themes.

Stage 5. Shared pretense: 3–6 years

In the prior phase, shared meanings in children's interactions centered on the possession and use of objects, and on such simple social games as peeka-boo and run–chase. Yet around nursery school age, children's interests move beyond how objects work and embrace the complexities of how people or society works. The peer-play expression of this interest is in the form of social pretend play. Nursery school children play "family," "cops and robbers," and many other games that center on social relationships. The nature of this play – its form, rule-boundedness, and linguistic structure – has been well described (e.g., Garvey, 1977). In terms of mastery processes, what is new in this phase is the shared mastery of social roles and discourse rules.

Children's interactions during this stage are marked by other developments as well. As noted above, this period is characterized by an increase in interactive pretense play; this is accompanied by a decline in solitary pretense play (see Rubin, Fein, and Vandenberg, 1983). Also, children seem to give increasing amounts of attention to peers; they talk more with them and, in the nursery school setting, begin to direct more of their social initiations to their age-mates than to adults (Hartup, 1983). Finally, although aggressive exchanges with peers increase from age 2 to age 4, there is an overall decrease in the proportion of aggressive to friendly interactions during this period. The frequency of aggressive exchanges begins to decline after age four, and physical aggression is increasingly replaced by verbal expressions of assertiveness and anger (Hartup, 1983).

Phase 6. Play friendship (peer admiration): 6–10 years

During the elementary school years, a higher proportion of time is spent with age-mates than in early childhood. Bronfenbrenner (1970) noted that, both in the United States and in the Soviet Union, at around age 9 or 10, peers replace from parents as the primary agents of child socialization. Children also become more selective in terms of preferred play partners.

At first glance, social interactions do not seem different from the activity-focused play of the prior two stages. Indeed, this remains a phase where children base their friendships on admiration for what their partners can *do* rather than on emotional bonds based on shared feelings of loyalty. Youniss and Volpe (1978) have shown that 6- and 7-year-olds describe friends as those with whom one shares goods and physical activities. Thus, the shared activity component, described in stage 5, is not dramatically altered. What *has* changed, at this stage, is the child's ability to articulate the belief that sharing is at the heart of friendship. For the first time, the developing equality in peer relations becomes a "self-conscious" process around the idea of shared activities and exchanged possessions. The trading of objects and "doing things together" has meaning for the relationship itself.

Also, at this stage, the very goal of forming friends seems to involve a search for a new kind of equality with peers – one centered not just on shared mastery (i.e., on something performable with more or less any peer) but rather on special relationships with preferred peers. Herein could be the central feature of peer friendship. At first in small, but ever-growing, ways children at this age find sources of emotional support from peers that can reduce their dependence on parental support. Youniss and Volpe (1978) find that, by age 9 or 10, children speak of frieds as comforting and helping each other and as supporting one another when in trouble. These are functions that previously were exclusively relegated to family relationships. Across these years, friendship has moved from shared activity to shared caring.

Phase 7. Loyal friendship: 11–15 years

In the prior phase, friendships retain what might be called an "instrumental quality." The child admires her friend for what she can do, rather than for who she is. Now the "shared caring" among friends takes on deeper emotional significance.

Bigelow (1977), like Youniss and Volpe, studied children's understanding of friendship. He confirmed that early friendships are mostly a matter of shared activity. However, when he interviewed 12-year-olds, he found that older children conceived of friendship in terms of loyalty, commitment, genuineness, and the potential for intimacy.

Until this stage, emotional intimacy was largely restricted to the family orbit. However, at this time, children are beginning to conceive of peer relations as the primary system for emotional gratification and support and the family is being supplanted in this role. In terms of equality, what is new here is an equality not only of respect regarding what the partner can do, but also of what they can offer back in terms of emotional caring and intimacy.

Phase 8: Peer intimacy: 16 years and above

Despite biological maturity around age 12 or 13, Stage 7 peer relations retain a notably same-sex character, at least in most technological cultures. The growing equalities of peer relations in terms of both activity and true friendships is largely a within-sex development. Thus, a remaining task to be dealt with in peer relations is cross-sex peer equality and sexual intimacy.

From a psychoanalytic perspective, the intensity of cross-sex parent–child relations during the Oedipal phase may "color" the adolescent's attempts to form sexually intimate relations. Given the inherent asymmetry of these early intense ties, it may be difficult for adolescents and young adults to view cross-sex peer relations objectively. Instead, drawing on models of the cross-sex parent based in early childhood, they may attribute too much perfection or power to peers of the opposite sex.

Thus, a final challenge in the development of peer equality may be that of replacing an early model of cross-sex relations based on one's relation to the opposite-sex parent with one derived from the peer intimacy that began in Stage 7. In the current stage, the physical intimacy of sexual relations may entail a level of peer trust as intense as that previously given only to one's parents, or to no one at all.

Summary

Although we recognize that there are many possible approaches to this topic, we have chosen to highlight three features of the development of peer relations. First, we described the unfolding of peer relations in terms of progressively complex and coordinated equalities that are shared between peers. Second, we noted that this sense of equality increasingly becomes the felt experience of the child; moreover, it may ultimately be an important yardstick by which the satisfactions of friendships are measured. Finally, we suggested that the development of peer relations from childhood to adolescence involves a gradual transfer of function from parents to peers. Contemporaries increasingly seek one another as the primary sources of support, security, and intimacy.

We hypothesize that a history of maltreatment will have important implications for the development of egalitarian and intimate peer relationships. After we have examined the data on maltreated children's peer relations, these implications will be explored further.

Two models of the relationship between the family and peer worlds

The preceding section offered a description of the development of peer relations in normal, nonmaltreated children. However, for human infants, social development begins not with peers but within the family, especially in early parent–infant interactions. Given the temporal precedence of parent–child relations, it seems essential to address the question of what the relationship might be between the two realms of the family and the peer world.

Most of the research on the quality of maltreated children's peer relations has been undertaken or interpreted in the context of particular models of social development, each of which offers a different view of this relationship. Thus, each model also offers a different hypothesized mechanism for how child maltreatment might affect the ability to form relationships with peers.

In this section, an attachment model and a social network model of development are presented. Although other theories are relevant to this issue (e.g., social learning/modelling; Bandura, 1977), we have chosen to focus on these two models because they have been the most widely used and articulated views in research on maltreated children's social development. Additionally, they represent quite different views on the relationship between family and peer relations.

Attachment theory

Attachment theory and research (Bowlby, 1969, 1973, 1980; Bretherton, 1985; Sroufe, 1979, 1983) proposes a direct and lawful relationship between the quality of an infant's early experiences with the caregiver and later functioning with peers. It is not suggested that this relationship is a simple or invariant one. However, given a certain degree of environmental consistency, a child who has experienced a secure attachment in infancy is thought to bring quite different qualities and predispositions to the peer world than one whose attachment was insecure.

The prediction of a positive relationship between security of attachment in infancy and competence with peers has received considerable empirical support. In several separate samples, toddlers and preschoolers who were previously classified as securely attached when infants have been found to have more positively-toned and successful interactions with age-mates than those with a history of insecure attachment (Jacobson and Wille, 1986; LaFreniere and Sroufe, 1985; Lieberman, 1977; Pastor, 1981; Sroufe, 1983; Waters, Wippman, and Sroufe, 1979). There is also evidence to suggest that different types of insecure relationships in infancy are related to particular patterns of difficulty with peers. Children with a history of an insecure–avoidant relationship (thought to be related to rejection by the caregiver; Ainsworth, Blehar, Waters, and Wall, 1978; Main, 1977) have been observed to exhibit more hostility, distance, and negative behavior with peers and are more frequently found to be rejected by them (LaFreniere and Sroufe, 1985; Sroufe, 1983). On the other hand, children with a history of an insecure–ambivalent attachment (correlated with caregiver inconsistency; Ainsworth et al., 1978) have been more often observed to be passive, inept, and neglected by their age-mates (LaFreniere and Sroufe, 1985; Sroufe, 1983).

There seem to be several ways of understanding the relationship between security of attachment and later competence with peers. They all stem from the notion that a secure attachment is, at least in large part, a reflection of caregiver sensitivity and responsiveness to the infant's needs and signals (Ainsworth et al., 1978). One important result of caregiver responsiveness is that it enables the infant to utilize the parent as a "secure base" from which it can explore the environment. This, in turn, allows it to increase its experience with and mastery over both social and inanimate objects. Thus, one important implication of the secure base phenomenon for the development of social relationships outside the family is that an infant who has been able to explore more freely in the caregiver's presence will have gained experiences and skills that are relevant for competently interacting and forming relationships with age-mates later on.

The second way caregiver responsiveness and a secure attachment relationship are thought to promote competence in peer relations is through their effect on a child's "internal working models" of self, other, and relationships (Bowlby, 1969, 1973, 1980; Bretherton, 1985; Main, Kaplan, and Cassidy, 1985; Sroufe and Fleeson, 1986). Specifically, an infant who experiences a secure attachment relationship is thought to internalize a sense of others as available and of the self as worthy of attention and care. The implication of a positively toned internal working model of self and attachment figures for peer relations is that a child can then enter the peer world with more confident expectations that others will be responsive and that interactions will be pleasurable. It has been suggested that a positive affective stance (e.g., confidence, enthusiasm) is a central component of social competence in childhood because it tends to invite, organize, and perpetuate positive interactions among peers (Sroufe, Schork, Motti, Lawroski, and LaFreniere, 1984).

Finally, it can be hypothesized that the quality of early parent–child interactions may have implications for the progressive development of equality with peers that was highlighted above. Although the function of attachment is generally spoken of in terms of "protection" and "felt security" (Bischof, 1975; Bowlby, 1969), one attachment theorist has suggested that the attachment figure may also play an important role as an early playmate (Bretherton, 1985). In addition, Bowlby's description of the development of attachment behavior culminates in what he calls the "goal-corrected partnership," a phase in which the child increasingly begins to take the attachment figure's own motives and plans into account (Bowlby, 1969). The attachment relationship between infant and parent may, in this way, contribute to a decline in egocentrism, a cognitive change in early childhood that has been identified as an important component in the growth of role-taking and cooperative play with peers (Brownell, 1986). Similarly, it may provide the initial context for the growth of perspective-taking abilities and interpersonal understanding (Selman, 1980). Finally, the experience of accessibility, warmth, and contingent responsiveness (those qualities in the caregiver which promote secure attachment) may also afford the infant an initial model of reciprocity and sharing; these are the very features that seem so important in the development of positive relations with peers.

Thus, the attachment model, on both theoretical and empirical grounds, proposes a high degree of continuity between the quality of early familial relationships and functioning in the peer world. For two additional reasons, the attachment model appears to have direct relevance for studying the effects of maltreatment on peer relations. First, in two longitudinal studies, an association was found between maltreatment of the infant and insecurity of attachment (Egeland and Sroufe, 1981a, 1981b; Schneider-Rosen et al., 1985). Because the literature on normal children strongly suggests a relationship between insecurity of attachment and difficulty with peers, one could reasonably expect a similar correlation between these two phenomena in maltreated samples. Second, the results of the literature on normal subjects should also be generalizable to a maltreated population if one views maltreatment as being on the same continuum as nonabusive parenting (Egeland and Sroufe, 1981a; Main and Goldwyn, 1984). Thus, behaviors such as physical abuse and neglect may be seen as extreme forms of rejection or inconsistency of care, parental behaviors that are often found to be related to insecurity of attachment in nonmaltreating families.

Social network theory

A social network model, in contrast, proposes relative independence between parent–child and child–peer relationships. As described by Lewis (e.g., Lewis and Schaeffer, 1981), the social network model suggests that, although the quality of peer relationships may be affected by parent–child relations, it is not determined by them in an epigenetic sense. That is, unlike the attachment model, the social network perspective does not require that a child first form a bond to its primary caregivers before being able to bond to other children. Also, it does not suggest that the particular quality of the parent–child bond will in and of itself determine the nature of later peer relationships.

The social network model instead proposes two alternate ways in which the parent–child relationship may affect subsequent functioning with peers. The first is through the availability of peer contact. The model proposes that if a parent does not facilitate early contact with peers, poor peer relationships might result because of a lack of relevant experience and the failure to develop interaction skills. Moreover, it is suggested that parents who are inadequate in terms of facilitating secure attachments in their infants may also be those who fail to provide their children with peer experience. There is some evidence that security of attachment and parent provision of peer contact are, in fact, positively related (Lieberman, 1977). Thus, problems in attachment and problems with peers may co-occur. However, the causal variable is presumed to lay outside of the parent–child relationship, namely, in the degree of the parent's facilitation of peer contact.

The second way parent–child and peer relationships could be related is through "generalized fear." Thus, if attachment difficulties result in a general fearfulness, which in turn leads the child, itself, to shy away from peer interactions, this could also lead to the development of poor peer relations. Again, it would be a lack of contact caused by fearfulness, rather than anything inherent in the parent–child relationship that affects the ability to form relationships with other children. Although the concept of generalized fear does refer to a state of mind, it differs from the concept of internal working model described above. Generalized fear does not seem to refer to a particular set of expectations, beliefs, and understanding of roles that are used to organize and interpret new interpersonal experiences. Moreover, unlike Bowlby's notion, there is no suggestion that the beliefs formed in the context of early parent–infant interactions may be the most influential and difficult to modify (Bowlby, 1980).

One well-established finding makes it likely that this model is relevant to the issue of maltreatment and later social development. It has frequently been found that maltreating parents themselves tend to be quite socially isolated from their communities and extended family resources (Parke and Collmer, 1975). One could hypothesize that these parents' greater social isolation would extend to their children as well, either because they actively restrict their children's contact with others or because it is simply less available.

Research on maltreated children's peer relations

An overview of both the development of peer relations and its hypothesized associations with early parent–child interactions has been presented. Using this as an essential background, we turn now to the central question of this chapter: What is the relationship between a history of maltreatment and a child's functioning with peers?

In this section, we will review the existing literature on the peer relations of maltreated children. The studies are divided into two types: clinical studies and comparison group studies. Only research that involved direct behavioral observations of maltreated children's interactions with their peers is included. Thus, studies that focused on aspects of socioemotional or personality development that are relevant for social behavior (e.g., the development of empathy) but did not involve actual assessments of behavior with peers are not discussed.

Clinical studies

Clinical studies of maltreated children are those that do not employ comparison groups. The use of appropriate comparison groups is particularly important in the study of the sequelae of maltreatment because abuse and neglect are frequently accompanied by other factors that can have a negative impact on a child's development, such as poverty, family disorganization, and highly stressful life circumstances. Thus, the conclusions about the effects of maltreatment per se that can be drawn from clinical studies are limited. Nonetheless, they often provide rich descriptions of maltreated children in clinical and naturalistic settings and suggest hypotheses that can then be tested in a more controlled fashion.

Most clinical descriptions of maltreated children's interactions with their peers suggest that they behave toward them in one of two ways: either excessively aggressive and provocative, or exhibiting excessive withdrawal and avoidance of other children (Galdston, 1971; Green, 1978; Martin, 1980; Martin and Beezley, 1977). Galdston, for example, made daily observations of 42 maltreated infants, toddlers, and preschoolers in a childcare facility. He reported that the abused children initially appeared listless, apathetic, and uninterested in toys, adults, or other children. When they began to respond to their environment, the abused children engaged in play with toys and adults far more than with their peers. Even after several months in the facility, they showed little awareness of one another, and Galdston describes their attitude toward other children as one of seemingly active denial, the maltreated boys exhibiting unpredictable and apparently purposeless violent behavior that appeared to be aimed at obtaining adult attention and recognition, the maltreated girls exhibiting mostly isolated or clinging behaviors.

The authors of the various clinical studies mentioned above offer several interpretations of the interactional styles observed in maltreated children. They suggest that heightened aggressiveness may represent an identification with the abusive parent as an attempt to ward off feelings of anxiety and helplessness (Green, 1978). They also suggest that it may represent a means of seeking recognition and attention from adults, a preoccupation maltreated children may have because their needs for adult responsiveness were not sufficiently met in their own families (Galdston, 1971). This last notion has recently received empirical support. Aber, Allen, Carlson, and Cicchetti (this volume) found that maltreated school-age children exhibited more attention- and approval-seeking and were more dependent on social reinforcement from novel adults than middle-class, nonmaltreated children.

Comparison group studies

Several researchers have employed control groups in their studies of maltreated children's relations with their peers. As mentioned above, the use of a comparison group allows one to control for important variables relevant to the study of the sequelae of maltreatment, such as socioeconomic status (SES), age, gender, previous peer experience, and family composition. The studies described below all involve behavioral observations of maltreated children's peer relations. They vary in the degree to which they have successfully met the many methodological challenges involved in the study of maltreatment and the degree to which they have employed theoretically derived, stage-salient measures of peer functioning (cf. Aber and Cicchetti, 1984).

George and Main

One of the first published studies to employ behavioral observations of maltreated children's interactions with their peers and to compare them with a control group was conducted by George and Main (1979). This study compared the social interactions of 10 physically abused toddlers (sexually abused and neglected children were excluded from the sample) with 10 control children. The two groups were well matched on important demographic variables and were reported to have roughly equivalent amounts of prior peer experience. The abused subjects were obtained from two daycare centers that specifically served maltreated children. The comparison children were recruited from two other daycare centers serving "families under stress." The authors state that the presence and absence of abuse was verified in the maltreated and comparison samples, respectively. Unfortunately, the observers in the study were not blind to the children's maltreatment status.

The study was undertaken in the context of research on parent–child attachment in nonmaltreating families. It aimed to test the hypothesis that physically abused children would resemble insecurely attached infants in normal samples who had experienced maternal rejection. Previous studies had shown that maternal rejection of normal infants was correlated with the infant's increased avoidance of and aggression towards the mother and increased avoidance of other adults (Main, 1977). The authors hypothesized that physically abused children would similarly display heightened levels of aggression, avoidance, and approach–avoidance conflict behavior with peers and daycare teachers.

The results of the study confirmed the hypothesis that physically abused toddlers would show more disturbed patterns of social interaction than an equivalent group of nonmaltreated children. Although the majority of the differences observed concerned the nature of interaction with the daycare teachers, important and significant differences were also observed in how the abused and comparison children interacted with their peers. The abused children were more likely to exhibit aggressiveness and avoidance toward other children, and to display approach–avoidance conflict behaviors, particularly following a friendly overture by another child. When abused children did respond to another's affiliative action, they were more likely to do so indirectly (e.g., by approaching from the side or from behind).

Recently, the authors extended their analysis of these data (Main and

George, 1985). Based on narrative records of the social interactions of the abused and nonabused toddlers in their daycare settings, a blind judge coded the responses of the subjects during instances where distress was exhibited by another child in the facility. The authors report that the abused and nonabused children responded to other children's distress in very different ways. In general, the nonabused toddlers tended to exhibit interest, empathy, sadness, or concern; these are the behaviors frequently described in the literature on the development of prosocial behavior in nonabused, middle-class children (e.g., Zahn-Waxler, Radke-Yarrow, and King, 1979). The abused toddlers, however, responded very differently. They were often observed to respond to a peer's distress with fear, threats, and angry behavior (including active physical attack). Moreover, in some of the abused toddlers, comforting and attacking behaviors were intermingled (e.g., gentle patting that became vigorous hitting). The authors remark that, for the abused toddlers, caregiving and aggressive behaviors seemed to stimulate one another in a striking way.

The George and Main studies provide important information about maltreated children's social development. First, they provide evidence that maltreatment can indeed impair a child's ability to meet a central task of early childhood – namely, the exploration and engagement of the social environment. The heightened aggressiveness, avoidance, and aberrant responses to both friendliness and distress in other children exhibited by these toddlers suggest that they do not enter the peer world with a readiness to engage in positive ways. Rather, it appears that the opportunity to interact with agemates is somehow stressful for these children; moreover, they manage this stress in ways that may decrease the likelihood of further interaction and the fostering of relationships.

We are particularly struck by the finding that situations of mutual attention (e.g., an approach by a peer) seem to be threatening for abused children, and that these toddlers avoided their peers more than they sought interaction with them. Drawing upon ethological theory, the authors suggest that avoidance may be a way of maintaining behavioral organization (George and Main, 1979). They suggest that maltreated infants, because of their experience of violent interactions with adults, may find situations of mutual attention disorganizing, because they arouse feelings of fear, distress, and anger. We would add that such avoidance of mutual attention and interaction is contrary to the sharing of activity, place, and meaning with peers that was highlighted in the stage model presented above. Thus, although it may allow for the maintenance of behavioral organization, the child may do so at the expense of experiencing a sense of sharing and equality with peers that was proposed to be a central aspect of social development.

Second, the George and Main studies also have relevance for the issue of the intergenerational transmission of maltreatment. The authors note that the difficulties in social interaction exhibited by maltreated children bear resemblance to those shown by their parents (i.e., heightened aggressiveness, avoidance/isolation, and an angry reaction to distress in others; Frodi and Lamb, 1980; Parke and Collmer, 1975). Although their research does not answer the question of *how* these behaviors might be transmitted, it does offer striking evidence that abused children can develop "abusive" behavior patterns quite early in life.

Finally, their study suggests that maltreatment can be viewed, at least in some respects, as being on the same continuum as nonabusive parent–child relations. The authors observed behaviors in their maltreated sample that are similar to those seen in rejected, but nonabused, infants and toddlers.

The George and Main studies have certain methodological limitations – in particular, the small numbers of children studied and the fact that some of the observations were made by individuals who were not blind to the children's maltreatment status. Additionally, the toddlers in this study were seen in groups of either all maltreated or all nonmaltreated children. There is some evidence (Jacobson and Wille, 1986; Pastor, 1981) that suggests that the nature of the peer partner (e.g., whether she or he has a history of a secure or insecure attachment relationship), in and of itself, influences the quality of the interaction. This raises a question about the generalizability of these results, that is, whether maltreated toddlers would behave similarly if they were interacting in a group that included nonabused as well as abused children.

However, we feel that this research has significant strengths. In particular, the authors utilized measures derived from prior research on normal development; specifically, they chose to examine behaviors that had been found to reflect disturbances in parent–child attachment. We believe that this enabled them to detect differences in behavior that are subtle and that would not have been predicted on intuitive grounds alone (i.e., it is not immediately obvious why a maltreated child would respond with aggressiveness or avoidance to distress or friendliness in other children). Moreover, their use of theoretically derived, stage-salient measures allows one to integrate their data with what is known about normal development, thereby increasing understanding of both the meaning of the behaviors they describe and the mechanisms that may possibly account for them (cf. Aber and Cicchetti, 1984).

Herrenkohl and Herrenkohl

As part of a larger study, Herrenkohl and Herrenkohl (1981) observed the social behavior of maltreated and nonmaltreated children in a preschool setting. The authors believed that an environment marked by maltreatment could interfere with the attainment of social competencies, such as negotiation and conflict-resolution strategies and impulse control.

Four groups of families participated in their study: families with one or more maltreated children ($n = 72$), nonmaltreating, Protective Service families ($n = 74$), non-child-welfare families in a Head Start program ($n = 50$), and non-child-welfare families served by daycare programs ($n = 50$). It is unclear exactly how many children participated in the study, although the numbers of families suggest it was very large. Also unclear is exactly what is encompassed by "maltreatment" in this sample (e.g., physical abuse, emotional mistreatment, gross neglect).

The children, who ranged in age from 3 to 5 years, were observed in free play situations in their preschools for two 30-minute observation periods. The authors did not mention whether the observers were blind to the children's maltreatment status or to the hypotheses of the study. The children were rated on such behaviors as aggression or withdrawal in the face of frustration, leadership of others, withdrawal from others, and task-oriented behavior.

The children were chiefly found to differ in terms of aggression. The maltreated children behaved more aggressively, especially in response to frustrating situations, such as a difficult task or interfering behavior by others. This difference was found while controlling for important demographic variables and characteristics of the classroom and the child.

The results of this study seem useful in two respects. First, the finding of heightened aggressiveness in maltreated children's peer interactions is in accord with other investigations, thereby increasing one's confidence in the validity of this phenomenon. Second, the author's attention to the context in which aggression occurred (e.g., following a frustrating experience) provides a more specific picture of the ways in which the social interactions of maltreated children may be negatively affected. Maltreated preschoolers may not be prone to behave aggressively in all situations; rather, they may have a particularly low threshold for the arousal of aggressive responses when they are faced with frustration. The additional finding by the Herrenkohls (1981), that maltreating parents are themselves less able to cope with frustration without resorting to aggressive solutions, suggests that one causal variable may be lack of a parental model of alternate means of containing aggressive impulses.

The tendency to respond aggressively to frustrations (in both social and task-related contexts) may prove to be an important target for interventions with maltreated children. Certainly, learning to cope successfully with frustrating experiences seems to be an essential aspect of social development. Successful conflict resolution has been observed to be an important skill in the development of friendships in nursery-school-age children (Rubin, 1980). Additionally, aggressive behavior is a frequent correlate of rejection by peers during the elementary school years (Coie and Kupersmidt, 1983; Dodge, 1983). Moreover, the amelioration of aggressive responses to frustration in maltreated children may have implications for preventing the intergenerational transmission of abuse and neglect, given the resemblance in this regard between maltreated children and maltreating parents that this study suggests.

Lewis and Schaeffer

Lewis and Schaeffer (1981) also investigated the social interactions of young maltreated children in comparison to their nonmaltreated counterparts. These authors were particularly interested in investigating the relationship between the quality of mother–child attachment and functioning with peers in light of the two models of social development described above – attachment theory and social network theory. By concurrently assessing the quality of both mother–child and child–child interactions, they hoped to answer the question of the relative independence/dependence of these two social realms.

A total of 26 children (ages 8–32 months) participated in the study. All of the children were attending a full-day daycare center. Of these children, 12 had been verified as abused/neglected; 14 had no history of maltreatment. The authors report that the children were equivalent in regard to SES, presence of the father in the home, number of siblings, and birth order. Each child was observed for 12 five-minute periods during both free- and structured-play sessions in the daycare center. The authors did not mention whether the observers were blind to the children's maltreatment status; nor did they mention whether the children were equivalent in terms of prior peer experience and familiarity with one another.

Behavior ratings consisted of frequency counts of various peer-directed behaviors. The authors report that an overall MANOVA found no difference between the maltreated and nonmaltreated children on these variables. The only significant difference that did emerge involved a variable labeled "positive play," a composite of several discrete behaviors (offer, share, show, accept, throw, and follow). Maltreated children were found to exhibit fewer positive-play behaviors than the comparison children; however, the authors noted inconsistency within this variable in that the maltreated children scored higher on some of the discrete, composite behaviors, whereas the comparison children scored higher on others.

Observations of mother–child interactions did reveal significant differences between the maltreated and nonmaltreated subjects. In general, maltreating mothers were described as more negative in their orientation to their children; the maltreated children were described as exhibiting behaviors toward their mothers that were reminiscent of those seen in insecurely attached children.

Lewis and Schaeffer interpret their results as being in support of the social network model of social development. They conclude that poor parent-child relations do not necessarily lead to disturbances in peer interactions. Moreover, they hypothesize that the maltreated children were found to be functioning adequately with peers mainly because the experience of maltreatment had not decreased their opportunity for peer interaction and experience. As stated by the authors: "Thus, poor maternal relationship will lead to a subsequently poor peer relationship only if the poor maternal relationship leads to early peer isolation" (1981, p. 219).

The Lewis and Schaeffer study, however, has several methodological limitations that prevent an unequivocal acceptance of this conclusion. First, the sample size employed in this study was not only small, but it also encompassed quite a large and developmentally significant age range. The period from 8 to 32 months involves important changes in all domains of development, including a child's behavior and approach to age-mates (Jacobson and Wille, 1986; Kagan, 1984). Thus, a sample of 12 maltreated children consisting of infants as well as toddlers and neglected as well as abused children seems overly heterogeneous and, in and of itself, could have introduced variability that obscured group differences.

Second, the authors assert that maltreatment did not deleteriously affect the children's peer relations, because daycare provided them with an opportunity to be with peers. It is possible, however, that the daycare experience provided more than just an opportunity for peer interaction; it may also have functioned as a therapeutic intervention that prevented or ameliorated impairments in social functioning. Even if the program was not designed to be therapeutic per se, research suggests that variations in the quality of day care (e.g., adequacy of materials, quality of program organization, quantity of verbal interaction between staff and children) are significantly and positively associated with measures of social competence in children; this has been found for both maltreated (Bradley, Caldwell, Fitzgerald, Morgan, and Rock, 1986) and nonclinical samples (McCartney, Scarr, Phillips, and Grajek, 1985). Because the authors do not provide information regarding the nature of the daycare experience, it is not possible at this point to accept the conclusion that the provision of an adequate social network was the sole cause of the comparability they observed across groups.

Third, the subjects in this study are described by the authors as "abused/ neglected." It is not clear from their description what subtype(s) of maltreatment these children experienced. As will be discussed in more detail below, however, physical abuse and neglect appear to have very different effects on social and emotional development, including behavior with peers. If the sample in this study included a mixture of abused and neglected children, as well as children who had experienced both subtypes of maltreatment, this could have introduced a degree of variability that would effectively mask differences in social behavior between the maltreated and comparison children.

Finally, the assessment of peer behavior in this study consisted mostly of frequency counts of discrete behaviors. Although such a method can provide useful descriptions of a child's interactional style, it often fails to capture the psychological meaning of a child's behavior and, indeed, may not truly measure the construct of interest, namely, competence with age-mates (cf. Waters and Sroufe, 1983). For example, merely counting the number of times a child approaches peers may reveal very little about the actual quality of that child's social interactions. Although high frequency of approaches may reflect one preschooler's sense of enthusiasm and ability to engage smoothly in social exchanges, it may have a quite different meaning for another child (e.g., high dependency, an inability to read other children's cues, a lack of social skill; see, e.g., Putallaz and Gottman, 1981).

Thus, it does not seem possible to draw conclusions about social competence without paying some attention to the meaning of behaviors, both in terms of their psychological significance and in regard to the broader context in which they occur. Because Lewis and Schaeffer relied so extensively on frequency counts of discrete behaviors, one is left with the question of whether their measures were in fact sensitive enough to detect relevant differences between the maltreated and the comparison children, if they were present. An acceptance of the null hypothesis of no difference between these two groups does not seem warranted while the construct validity of the measures used in this study is so open to question.

Although we have methodological concerns about this study that prevent us from accepting its results as definitive, we feel that the attempt to assess mother–child and child–peer interactions concurrently represents an important step in research on maltreatment and social development. The examination of the relationship between the family and peer worlds requires the assessment of behavior in both contexts. This point will be more fully elaborated in a later section of this chapter.

Jacobson and Straker

Jacobson and Straker (1982) compared the social interaction styles of physically abused, school-age children with those of their nonabused peers. They were particularly interested in investigating abused children's styles of interacting on dimensions they felt were associated with the behavior of abusing parents, such as withdrawal from social interaction and heightened aggressiveness.

Nineteen 5- to 10-year-old abused children were studied. All children had been injured to the extent that a hospital admission was warranted; other specific criteria were also employed to ensure verification of maltreatment. Additionally, cases of sexual abuse, neglect, and children with evidence of organic impairment were excluded from the sample. The abused children were compared with 38 control children, who were matched on developmental and demographic variables. The control children were recruited from the maltreated subjects' classrooms. The authors do not mention whether nonabuse was verified in the control sample.

The children were observed in groups of three during a free-play session in a laboratory setting. Each triad consisted of one abused child and two control children from their classroom, thus ensuring that, in each triad, the children were equally familiar to one another. Five minutes of videotaped free play were then rated by independent raters who were blind to the children's maltreatment status.

The children were rated on several dimensions that described both affect and behavior with peers. All of the ratings were then subjected to a principal components analysis and two components were derived: "social interaction" (reflecting willingness and enjoyment of interaction and relating creatively in a sustained fashion) and "hostility" (reflecting aggressiveness and lack of warmth). The children were compared on the two components using separate ANOVAs. They were found to differ significantly on the social interaction component, with abused children interacting less, with less enjoyment, and in a less sustained and imaginative fashion. No difference was found between the two groups of children on the hostility component.

Based on these results, Jacobson and Straker suggest that abused children resemble abusing adults in that they appear socially withdrawn and isolated. They note that the fact that they found no difference between abused and comparison children in terms of hostility conflicts with the results found by others. The authors suggest that their definition of aggressiveness may have been too global; they propose that a difference on this variable might have emerged if attention was paid to the context in which aggression occurred, to the target of the aggressive behavior, and to its relation to other variables such as anxiety and fear.

The failure to detect significant differences between the maltreated and comparison children on the measure of aggressiveness brings up an important issue in research on the sequelae of maltreatment. As noted by Aber and Zigler (1981), measures of psychological constructs in maltreated children must be operationalized in ways that are age- and stage-appropriate. Because the expression of these constructs changes over the course of development, one must be particularly sensitive as to how a given construct is manifested by children of different ages. In terms of measuring aggression, Aber and Zigler note that lawful developmental changes have been documented in the causes, type, and dominant mode of expressing aggression from infancy through the school-age years. This raises a question as to whether the assessment of aggression in the Jacobson and Straker study was developmentally appropriate for the 5- to 10-year-olds in their sample. For example, in accord with developmental changes, did they distinguish between instrumental and hostile aggression? Similarly, did they assess fantasy and verbal aggression in addition to aggression expressed primarily in a physical mode? Because the authors do not list the specific behaviors that constituted their measure of aggression, it is not possible to determine whether their measure was in fact sensitive to these developmental changes. However, we would be surprised if a measure used to assess aggressiveness in a toddler or preschooler would do so with equal success for older children without being specifically adjusted for developmental differences.

Another possible explanation for the failure to detect differences in aggressiveness is that the children interacted for too short a period of time for aggressive responses to occur in a laboratory setting. Although the authors offer justifications for limiting their data coding to five minutes of free play, it is possible that this does not constitute an ecologically valid and representative sample of school-age children's interactions. Also, one can imagine that school-age children could be quite sensitive to the effects of a laboratory setting and the presence of a video camera, and that these factors might further have inhibited the expression of any aggressive behavior.

Finally, the children in this study may have been more severely abused than those in the other studies reported here. The authors state that "only those cases of abuse which had been severe enough to warrant a hospital referral were included in the sample" (Jacobson and Straker, 1982, p. 322). It is possible that severity of abuse may be related to behavior with peers, and to the expression of aggressiveness, in unexpected ways. For example, the association between severity of abuse and child aggressiveness may resemble an inverted-U function rather than a linear relationship. Thus, it is possible that the most severely abused children do not behave aggressively in middle childhood. This notion could be tested empirically. It suggests, however, that it is necessary to have a taxonomy of maltreatment that includes not only subtypes of abuse and neglect but also variables like severity and chronicity.

Hoffman-Plotkin and Twentyman

Hoffman-Plotkin and Twentyman (1984) undertook a multimodal assessment of social and cognitive functioning in physically abused, neglected, and nonmaltreated preschoolers. Their goal was to extend the findings of previous research by including behavioral observations and multiple sources of information, employing a matched control group.

Forty-two 3- to 6-year-old children participated in the study. The sample consisted of abused, neglected, and nonmaltreated children (14 per group); presence or absence of maltreatment was confirmed through a social service agency. The children were reported to be roughly equivalent on the length of time elapsed since the last reported instance of maltreatment, and the three groups were matched on relevant demographic variables and the amount of time spent in day care.

Data were obtained from several sources, including cognitive assessments, parent and teacher ratings, and behavior ratings made by blind raters during classroom free play. Of the rated behaviors most relevant to peer interaction, maltreated children were found to differ from control children in the following ways: The physically abused children were observed to exhibit more aggressive behavior than the other two groups; the neglected children appeared to be more generally withdrawn from social interaction; both groups of maltreated children were found to exhibit less prosocial behavior than the control subjects; and, finally, the abused children were observed to be more generally disruptive in the classroom and were disciplined more frequently by teachers.

The results of this study not only suggest that maltreatment can deleteriously effect a child's social interactions, but they also provide important information on the differential consequences of abuse and neglect. It is not surprising that differing parental styles would have different sequelae for children. Therefore, it is likely that investigators who treat maltreatment as a homogeneous variable will be obscuring important differences between abused and neglected children (for an elaboration of this notion, see Cicchetti and Rizley, 1981). Additionally, these findings could have important clinical implications in terms of the type of intervention required by children exposed to different subtypes of maltreatment. For example, an abused, aggressive child may require a period of individual therapy with an adult who represents a less aggressive object of identification; a withdrawn, neglected child may be ready immediately for interventions with peers (Mueller and Cohen, 1986).

Hoffman-Plotkin and Twentyman interpret the behavioral differences between abused and neglected children as reflecting the process of social learning/modelling. They propose that the abused children had learned to be aggressive because their parents modelled aggressive behavior at home; similarly they speculate that the neglected children avoided interaction because they had observed socially withdrawn behavior in their parents. Although this notion may be valid, it is also possible that the differences in abused and neglected children's behavior are not as straightforward as they seem. For instance, do neglected children also experience feelings of anger, but just not express them in most contexts? To answer this question, it might be useful to assess variables like aggression not just on the level of overt behavior but with less direct means, such as a measure of fantasy aggression. In general, before concluding that neglected children are simply more withdrawn than others, and that this is a result of behavioral modelling, it would be useful to have a fuller understanding of their subjective experiences in social contexts (i.e., are they fearful of interaction? anxious about being rebuffed? depressed and therefore lacking in motivation/ energy?).

Howes and colleagues

Howes and colleagues (Howes, 1984; Howes and Eldredge, 1985; Howes and Espinosa, 1985) conducted three separate studies of maltreated children, each of which involved behavioral observations in naturalistic settings. As the most recent research of which we are aware, these studies are of interest for several reasons. First, they try to reconcile some of the contradictory findings that emerged from prior studies by examining maltreated children in more than one type of peer situation. Also, they explore the effects of an intervention program that was specifically aimed at ameliorating difficulties in peer relations. Although the studies do not include a "no treatment" control group of maltreated children, they do provide preliminary evidence about the possibilities of preventing and treating maladaptive behavior in maltreated children.

In *Study 1* (Howes, 1984), Howes compared 12 maltreated infants and toddlers to 23 of their nonmaltreated peers. Maltreated subjects were recruited through social service agencies and were all court-verified cases of abuse and/or neglect (Howes, personal communication, 1985). It is not clear exactly which subtypes of maltreatment these children had experienced, although five of them are specifically described as "physically abused." Howes does not describe how the comparison sample was recruited into the study and does not mention whether and how the absence of maltreatment was verified in these subjects. The children in the two groups ranged in age from 8 to 28 months and are described as being all of lower socioeconomic status and mostly from single-parent homes.

All of the children were attending a full-time therapeutic daycare facility. The intervention program for the maltreated children was focused on the facilitation of peer relationships; the intervention also included therapy for the maltreating parents (Howes, 1984; Howes, personal communication, 1985). Observations were made during free-play sessions when the maltreated and nonmaltreated children had an opportunity to interact with one another. The free-play sessions constituted half of the children's scheduled time in the program; during the other half, children were in their "home-rooms," which consisted of either all maltreated or all nonmaltreated peers.

Raters, who were blind to the children's maltreatment status, coded peer interactions along two dimensions: (1) whether children met specified criteria for having formed a friendship with a peer, and (2) the content and complexity of interactions (e.g., success at initiating interactions, the degree of reciprocity in play, frequency of aggressive or prosocial exchanges). Coding of behavior involved a mixture of both quantitative and qualitative elements. For instance, although some ratings involved recording the mere occurrence of a behavior (e.g., number of interactions), others were aimed at capturing the quality of exchanges (e.g., whether they involved "positive affective sharing" or "shared meaning"; see Waters et al., 1979, and Brenner and Mueller, 1982, respectively, for an elaboration of these concepts).

When interacting with children from their own homeroom, the maltreated and comparison subjects were found to be similar in the degree to which they engaged in interactions and had established friendships with other children. For both groups, the relationships were more positive and the interactions more complex when the children were from the same homeroom. In general, neither group of children appeared to have established friendships with children from outside of their homeroom. Additionally, on some dimensions, the maltreated children were found to be more socially competent than the comparison children (e.g., they had a higher proportion of contacts that involved sustained, complementary, and reciprocal play). Thus, the intervention program appears to have been effective in that it did foster positive peer relations among the maltreated children who were in the same homeroom. It is important to note, however, that both groups of subjects were found to exhibit a lower proportion of friendships than children who were neither maltreated nor of lower socioeconomic status (Howes, 1984).

Although maltreated children appeared to function similarly to the comparison children when they interacted with a familiar peer, differences emerged when their interactions with toddlers from different homerooms were examined. During free play, the nonmaltreated children tended to ignore their unfamiliar peers. The maltreated children, in contrast, tended to become involved in physically aggressive exchanges with them.

In *Study 2* (Howes and Espinosa, 1985), the peer relations of abused and neglected children were again compared to those of their nonmaltreated counterparts. In this study, however, a second comparison group was included: nonmaltreated children who had been referred to an outpatient clinic for psychiatric treatment. Besides comparing the children in terms of their diagnostic status (physically abused, neglected, clinic-referred, and normal), the children were assessed in terms of whether they were members of well-established intervention groups (similar to the groups in Study 1) or were seen in groups that were newly formed for the purpose of the study. Finally, in this study, a larger sample and wider age range was included.

All observations took place during free-play sessions. The total sample, which ranged in age from 14 to 61 months, consisted of 26 physically abused children, 4 neglected children, 21 clinic-referred children, and 26 normal children. Blind raters coded peer interactions on the following dimensions: frequency of expression of positive and negative emotions, frequency of positive and negative behaviors directed towards peers, the number of interactions a child initiated, and the complexity of play (ranging from parallel to complementary and reciprocal play).

Similar to Study 1, the central finding that emerged here was that the physically abused children's behavior differed according to context (i.e., whether they were seen in the newly formed or the well-established group). In the established, intervention group, the abused children's peer interactions and ability to form friendships closely resembled those of normal, nonmaltreated children (who functioned similarly regardless of which group they were seen in). In the newly formed group, however, the physically abused children appeared less socially competent. In that context, they exhibited fewer positive emotions, directed less behavior toward peers (positive or negative), initiated fewer interactions, and engaged in less complex play. Additionally, when the data from the newly formed group were analyzed for the effects of age, abused children were found to display less positive affect with increasing age, whereas the opposite held true for the normal children.

The neglected children (who were assessed only in an established group) showed a different pattern. For these children, the intervention program did not appear to increase social competence and participation. Rather, they were found to resemble the abused and clinic children in the newly formed group in that they exhibited less affect (positive or negative) in peer encounters, directed fewer positive behaviors toward peers, initiated fewer interactions, and engaged in less complex play. These results must be taken as tentative, given the very small number of children in this subsample ($n = 4$). However, they lend further support to the notion that physical abuse and neglect have different developmental sequelae. Also, they raise intriguing questions about whether different types of intervention are best suited for children with different maltreatment histories. The intervention program in this study is not described in enough detail to permit specific hypotheses about why it was less successful for the neglected children than for the physically abused children. It may be that neglected children, similar to socially withdrawn children in one nonmaltreated sample, would do better in an intervention that involved one-to-one interactions with a younger child rather than being treated in a group of same-age or older peers (Furman, Rahe, and Hartup, 1979).

In *Study 3* (Howes and Eldredge, 1985), the goal was to elaborate the behavioral context in which maladaptive behavior occurred. Specifically, the authors were interested in whether maltreated and comparison children responded differently to their peers when those children were exhibiting specific behaviors.

Eighteen children participated in the study: 5 physically abused children, 4 neglected children, and 9 nonmaltreated children. All of the subjects were attending a daycare center; it is not clear whether this was the same therapeutic program as the one discussed above. The children were observed in both free-play and structured-play settings. The structured setting involved 20 minutes of play with one other child in a smaller room; an adult was present but was instructed to not interact with the toddlers and to redirect all bids for contact to the peer.

Blind raters coded both the free-play and the structured-play sessions for the following types of social behaviors: friendly behaviors, prosocial responses to the distress of the partner, aggressive behaviors, resistance of social offers, and resistance of attempts to take a toy. The data were then analyzed to see whether abused, neglected, and nonmaltreated children responded differently to specific behaviors in a peer partner (the child they were engaged with at the time).

During the free-play session, the abused and neglected children were as likely as the nonmaltreated children to respond to a peer's friendly behavior in a positive way. During the structured-play session, however, the abused and neglected children were more likely to resist their partner's friendly offers than were the nonmaltreated subjects. In response to aggression by a peer partner, the nonmaltreated children tended to respond with distress or resistance. Although the maltreated children tended to respond similarly during free play (although with more resistance), they were more likely than the nonmaltreated children to behave aggressively in response to a peer's aggression when it occurred during the structured dyadic interaction. Finally, the abused children responded quite differently to the appearance of distress in a peer partner than did the nonmaltreated children. Although the nonmaltreated children tended to respond to distress with prosocial behavior, the physically abused children tended to respond aggressively in both the free-play and the structured-play settings. This last finding replicates the results reported by Main and George (1985).

The authors note that the types of responses they observed in the maltreated children not only differed from those of their comparison subjects, but also diverge from what has been observed in developmental research with other nonmaltreated samples. For example, it is not uncommon for a toddler to respond with prosocial behavior (rather than aggression) in response to distress in another child (Howes and Farver, 1984). Similarly, even very young children have been found capable of employing nonaggressive strategies to resolve conflicts with other children (Hay and Ross, 1982).

Although the Howes research has certain methodological weaknesses (e.g., the age-appropriateness of the measures given the large age range studied), we feel that it provides interesting data that are worthy of further exploration. The central theme of the findings seems to be that the effect of maltreatment on children's social functioning is not necessarily a global phenomenon that manifests itself uniformly in all contexts. Instead, these studies suggest that several variables may be important in determining whether maltreatment will result in maladaptive behavior with peers. Similarly to Main and George, Howes found that certain behaviors in another child seem to be especially provocative for children with a history of maltreatment. In particular, the appearance of distress in an age-mate seems to stimulate aggressive behavior that might not otherwise occur. Other contextual variables this research suggests are important are the degree of familiarity of the peers and the interactional setting and whether the situation involves free play or is structured so that the child cannot avoid one-to-one interaction with another child. In regard to the latter point, it is interesting to note that in nonmaltreated samples, more mature and complex play tends to occur among toddlers in dyadic as opposed to larger group settings (Vandell and Mueller, 1977). Finally, the research suggests that therapeutic interventions can prevent or ameliorate maladaptive peer relations in some maltreated children. This finding must be taken as tentative given the absence of a "no treatment" control group.

Howes interprets her data as supporting early intervention for abused children and suggests that the intervention was effective because it provided the children with an enlarged social network and increased opportunities for social interaction that were not being supplied by their families. Thus, Howes interprets her data as supporting the social network model of development. However, there may be other plausible explanations for the results she obtained. First, it is possible that the intervention functioned as more than just an enlargement of the children's social networks. The stated aim of the program was the fostering of peer relationships. Because Howes does not specify what was involved in the intervention, it is difficult to specify exactly how it affected the children's peer interactions. However, there is much evidence to suggest that the mere provision of peer contact does not necessarily lead to improved social functioning. This body of evidence includes the majority of studies reviewed here (many of which involved observations in daycare settings) as well as the aforementioned research on the relationship between the particular quality of a daycare setting and social competence in children.

Also, we believe that one could offer an explanation of these differences based on attachment theory. One of the results of an insecure attachment is that it can impair a child's ability to explore in a new environment. Because the experience of maltreatment is correlated with a heightened incidence of insecure attachments (Egeland and Sroufe, 1981a, 1981b; Schneider-Rosen et al., 1985), it is possible that the less socially competent behavior of Howes's maltreated subjects in the newly formed groups was due in some manner to earlier attachment difficulties that had reduced environmental engagement and interfered with the attainment of social competence. Also, because a newly formed group may constitute a more stressful experience for a child than an ongoing group, the more vulnerable maltreated children may have found it particularly difficult to maintain the sense of "felt security" (Sroufe and Waters, 1977) that could have facilitated successful engagement of peers in that context.

Discussion

Summarization of the findings

As should be clear from this review, only a handful of published studies on the peer relations of maltreated children exists at this time. Moreover, the nature of the data base imposes limitations on the degree to which one can generalize about the nature of maltreated children's social functioning. These limitations stem from several sources. First, the studies vary widely in terms of the ages of children studied. Given the dramatic changes that occur over the course of development, it is difficult to assess the degree of comparability of a behavioral characteristic when it appears in a toddler as compared with a preschooler or a latency-aged child. Second, the studies differ in how they treat the variable of maltreatment. Some combine physically abused and neglected children into a single group; others examine children according to maltreatment subtype. Treating maltreatment as a homogeneous variable can obscure differences between abused and neglected children. It also limits the degree to which one can draw conclusions about the differential effects of abuse and neglect at this time. Third, although this group of studies demonstrates the vast improvement that has been made in terms of scientific rigor in research on maltreatment, some of the studies still fail to attend sufficiently to basic methodological necessities. These include the use of appropriate comparison groups, verification by an independent source of the presence/absence of maltreatment, and the employment of experimenters and raters who are blind to the children's maltreatment status. Fourth, the studies vary in the aspects of behavior they examine. Moreover, even when they address the same characteristic (e.g., aggression), they vary in their definition of the variable and the measure employed to assess it. The lack of standardization of measures across studies, although not surprising given the nascent state of this area of research, adds to the difficulty one has in making generalizations from the data. Finally, some of the studies suffer from a certain behavioral superficiality. As discussed above, frequency counts of discrete behaviors are limited in that they often fail to capture the psychological significance of a behavior and its connotation in a particular context.

Despite these limitations, the data from both clinical and comparison studies concur to a substantial extent in their descriptions of the social functioning of maltreated children. One theme that emerges rather clearly from the existing data is the heightened aggressiveness seen in maltreated – especially physically abused – children in their interactions with their peers. This finding emerged in all but two of the studies described, and in those two, aggressiveness appears to have been inadequately measured. Heightened aggressiveness, however, does not appear to be a global, across-the-board phenomenon in maltreated children. Rather, the studies strongly suggest that context can be quite important in determining whether a child will behave aggessively. In that regard, the degree to which peers and the interactional setting are familiar seems to be an important variable. Additionally, there is evidence to suggest that heightened aggressiveness and other difficulties with peers can be prevented or ameliorated when children receive treatment specifically aimed at this issue. Moreover, two of the studies concur in their observation that this heightened aggressiveness at times appears in a surprising context, namely, following the occurrence of distress in another child. We feel this is an intriguing finding, and it will be discussed in more detail below.

A second characteristic frequently described in maltreated children is an excessive degree of withdrawal and avoidance of interaction with peers. Although some of the studies suggest that this is more prevalent in neglected children, others report this for more than a single type of maltreated child. Additionally, two of the studies suggest that this withdrawal does not consist of merely being passive around other children; both the George and Main and the Howes studies suggest that maltreated children may actively avoid or resist the friendly overtures of other children.

Finally, the Howes studies and the Hoffman-Plotkin and Twentyman study offer beginning support to the notion that physical abuse and neglect have quite different effects on a child's social development. Whereas physically abused children are more often described as behaving aggressively or actively avoiding interaction, neglected children are more frequently depicted as withdrawn and restricted in affective expression.

The two models of social development

We turn now to the question of what the studies can contribute in terms of assessing the relevance of the two models of social development described earlier in this chapter. In general, the data are not conclusive enough to allow one to accept one model over the other as being sufficient to account for the relationship between maltreatment and peer relations. Moreover, we believe that both models have some relevance for understanding the impact of maltreatment on a child's ability to form relationships with peers. This belief stems from a recognition that child maltreatment is a complex and multifaceted phenomenon. It appears linked to several etiological factors and manifests itself on many levels of a child's developmental ecology (cf. Belsky, 1980). We would not expect the sequelae of maltreatment to arise out of only one aspect of this phenomenon. Rather, we believe that a child's social development will be affected both by the particular quality of the parent–child relation (e.g., the quality of attachment) and by a family's intercourse with the broader social system in which it is embedded (e.g., relative isolation). Additionally, other factors will be important (e.g., the presence/ absence of other supportive adults) insofar as they buffer or potentiate the effects of maltreatment. It does not seem fruitful for investigators to attempt to document that the sequelae of maltreatment are attributable to a single feature of a child's ecology. Instead, we propose that researchers attempt to study the variety of ways in which the experience of maltreatment may affect a child's functioning with peers.

In addition, it is possible that the nature of a child's social network and the quality of his or her attachment to parents are not independent but, instead, are themselves related. For example, Lieberman (1977), in an investigation of attachment and peer relations, found that mothers of secure preschoolers facilitated more peer contacts for their children than did those of insecure ones. Thus, her data suggest that the quality of attachment and of social contacts with peers may be linked via parent behavior (although these two factors may affect different aspects of behavior with age-mates).

Other conceptions of the relationship between attachment and social network quality are also possible. For instance, the nature of a parent's social network may affect his or her level of stress or depression (e.g., Levitt, Weber, and Clark, 1986), factors that have been found to be associated with child attachment quality and other developmental tasks (Radke-Yarrow, Cummings, Kuczynski, and Chapman, 1985). Another way in which the quality of attachment and of the social network may be linked is through the parent's own conceptions and expectations of relationships. Crittenden (1985), for example, found that the nature of a mother's social network (e.g., length of friendships, frequency of contact, level of satisfaction with support received) was associated with the quality of her child's attachment to her. In her discussion of these data, Crittenden suggests that the link between network variables and infant attachment quality may be mediated by the mother's mental representations of relationships. Thus, a mother who expects support and satisfaction from relationships may facilitate the establishment of stable and positive relations with her own peers and family and a secure relationship with her infant. Relatedly, the infant of such a parent may be more prone to create a supportive and satisfying social network as he or she enters the world of age-mates. Thus, our understanding of the relationship between parental maltreatment and children's peer relations may be enhanced by attending not only to the factors present in a child's developmental ecology on an individual basis, but also to the complex interrelationships among those factors.

However, although both models seem relevant for understanding the peer relations of maltreated children, the social network model, as defined by Lewis and Schaeffer (1981), seems less adequate than the attachment approach. First, we feel that the social network explanation is too narrow. Although social isolation is certainly an important feature of many maltreating families, this concept alone is inadequate to describe what goes on in abusing and neglecting families. "Abuse" and "neglect" suggest to us particular kinds of parent–child relationships. Given that research on nonmaltreating families has shown lawful relationships between particular styles of parenting and child development (e.g., Ainsworth et al., 1978; Baumrind, 1967, 1971; Belsky, Rovine, and Taylor, 1984; Block and Block, 1980; Grossmann, Grossmann, Spangler, Suess, and Unzner, 1985; Sears, Maccoby, and Levin, 1957), we would expect the same to hold true for maltreating families. This seems especially likely given that in these families childrearing is characterized by such dramatic and, indeed, traumatic features.

Additionally, the social network model does not fit much of the existing data on maltreated children's social and emotional development. For instance, it cannot explain the fact that maltreatment results in maladaptive peer relations even in situations where availability of peer contact is not of central concern. For example, the children in the Jacobson and Straker study were equally familiar to one another; they were also of an age where, by virtue of school attendance, children are no longer dependent on parents to expose them to peers. Yet, the maltreated children in this sample were found to differ in significant ways from their nonmaltreated classmates. The social network model also cannot explain other features of maltreated children's social behavior that emerged in these studies. For example, why would abuse and neglect have different effects on peer relations, if deprivation of peer contact is the only relevant factor? Also, although early lack of peer contact might reasonably be expected to result in shyness and withdrawal around age-mates, it is more difficult to understand how it alone would account for heightened aggressiveness and aggressive responses to distress in others. Finally, the social network model cannot account for findings that emerged from other studies on the socioemotional sequelae of maltreatment that were not focused specifically on peer relations. For example, how would it explain that maltreated children show more dependency on social reinforcement from novel adults (Aber et al., this volume)? Similarly, how would it account for the finding that maltreated youngsters have been found to consider children responsible and blameworthy when they are treated unkindly by adults (Dean, Malik, Richards, and Stringer, 1986)?

We believe that these problems encountered by the social network model in trying to explain the sequelae of maltreatment are due to three features of that approach: an exclusive focus on only one aspect of maltreatment (i.e., social isolation), a failure to recognize that behavioral continuity does not necessarily imply behavioral isomorphism, and a lack of attention to the mediating variables between the experience of maltreatment and a child's observed behavior (specifically, the internal working models of self, other, and relationships). In contrast, the attachment model (or, more broadly, a "relational" approach) does not suffer from these limitations. Although the relationship between quality of attachment and later peer relations in maltreated children has not yet been investigated empirically, an attachment/relational approach offers several concepts that seem useful not only for accounting for much of the data on maltreated children's peer relations, but also for generating hypotheses about the causal mechanisms underlying this behavior. These hypotheses are described in the following discussion.

An interpretation of the data on maltreated children's peer relations

The authors of the studies discussed above offered a variety of explanations for the behavior they observed. Examples include inadequate learning of conflict-resolution strategies, modelling of abusive parenting, and employment of defenses, such as displacement. In this section, we present some of our speculations about how a history of maltreatment leads to the kinds of behavior maltreated children were found to exhibit with peers. In particular, we speculate about the mechanisms underlying the heightened aggressiveness observed in abused children. These speculations draw upon the ideas of attachment, self, and object relations theorists.

Both object relations theorists (see Greenberg and Mitchell, 1983) and attachment theorists (e.g., Sroufe and Fleeson, 1986) suggest that the construction of the self begins in the early parent–infant dyad. They suggest that features of this dyadic relationship are ultimately internalized by the child to form the initial core of personality. Moreover, they suggest that the type of self that has formed will be reflected in the types of relationships that the child later seeks out and creates. Expectations and beliefs about self and other that emerge from the primary relationship will, thus, be carried forward to new interpersonal situations.

Furthermore, in internalizing this relationship, the child is said to learn not one, but both sides of the relationship (Sroufe and Fleeson, 1986). Thus, in recreating this early relationship in new interpersonal situations, the child can draw upon both her own and her parents' role. In this light, a maltreated child can be said to have learned the roles of both the abuser and the abused. We believe that this notion can be used to explain the heightened aggressiveness described in maltreated children's interactions with peers. From the theory of relationships just presented, we surmise that these children are, in fact, reenacting what they experienced earlier, with one important difference: they are now in the more powerful role of the aggressor rather than the one receiving the aggression.

What might be the motivating force that leads to this aggressive behavior? We hypothesize that the underlying process is basically a defensive one; it is aimed at decreasing anxiety and maintaining organization in the face of distressing feelings (Freud, 1926/1977; A. Freud, 1937/1966). Thus, in part, it may represent an identification with the aggressor, such that the child "transforms himself from the person threatened into the person who makes the threat" (A. Freud, 1937/1966, p. 113) and, in this way, manages to avoid the feelings of helplessness and trauma associated with being abused. A child who has experienced hostility, rejection, or coercion from caregivers may enter the peer world with expectations of similar treatment by age-mates. By adopting the role of the aggressor, a maltreated child may, thus, be seeking the "comfort" of predictable, albeit harsh, encounters. This notion is reminiscent of Bowlby's description of adults who, as children, had caregivers who were rejecting or unavailable. Bowlby suggests that, for such individuals, "the world is seen as comfortless and unpredictable; and they respond by shrinking from it or by doing battle with it" (1973, p. 208). Although such interactions are probably far from pleasant or satisfactory, their predictability and familiarity may mitigate the psychological pain associated with seeking support and, instead, receiving a rejecting or abusive response.

The aggressiveness observed in maltreated children's peer interactions may function as a defense in another way. It may represent an attempt on the child's part to hold onto a positive sense of self and other, and to keep conscious experience of the reality of an abusive relationship at bay. In his discussion of internal working models, Bowlby (1973, 1980) suggested that individuals sometimes have more than one model of the self and the attachment figure. Further, he suggested that such multiple models can, at times, become defensively dissociated in an attempt to avoid the more painful ones, such as those associated with having been rejected or abused by a parent. In this regard, a maltreated child might construct a conscious image of the self as valued and of the attachment figure as available and caring, even though this stands in contrast to what was actually experienced. The dissociated models, however, are thought to continue to be capable of guiding behavior, although they may operate outside of conscious awareness. We suggest that such a process (an attempt to hold onto a positive view of self and other while repressing a more negative one) may also underlie the heightened aggressiveness seen in maltreated children. In particular, it may help to explain the reported finding that abused children frequently strike out at a peer who is exhibiting distress.

We suggest that such hitting is not an elicited response to crying, but is instead related to the particular *meaning* that a peer's distress has for a maltreated child. Such an explanation might run as follows: Like all children, the maltreated child is trying to construct a positive view of self and other, because all children's objective dependency on adults requires that they try to be loved and valued by others (Fairbairn, 1950). Only if they are successful in making others value them can they see themselves as worthy and confident children (Horner, 1984). The maltreated child enters the peer situation with doubts about the value of self and other based on the actual experience of abuse and rejection. It appears that few children are so cognitively disabled by maltreatment, however, as to be unable to perceive peers objectively, that is, as different from adults. Most appear to retain their ability to perceive the physical and behavioral similarities between themselves and peers. Some experience of interest in the age-mate and of felt equality between self and peer seems unavoidable, although the child may feel wary and avoidant. It is precisely for these reasons that the social network point of view is correct in stressing peer interest and imitation in all children, regardless of the quality of the parent–child relationship. A healthy parent–child relation may not be prerequisite for some expression of peer interest.

However, precisely because the age-mate is perceived as similar to the self, a peer's distress may be quite anxiety-provoking for a previously maltreated child. The display of distress and strong attachment behavior in someone so like the self may function as a powerful symbol. Specifically, it may serve to evoke mental images and memories of instances when he or she was similarly in distress but attachment needs were rejected or unmet. For a child who is attempting to keep conscious awareness of such experiences at bay, a peer's distress may be intolerable. Moreover, he or she may know that it is essential to stop such a display because of its symbolic power to reelicit intolerable aspects of the self and of the relationship to the parent. Such a need may be experienced with urgency or desperation and lead the child to the most direct means: striking out at the peer. It is not that such a child is somehow untaught or unskilled in comforting, as a "social skills" argument might suggest. Just because a child is abused does not mean that she is unfamiliar with being comforted. Rather, the striking out reflects the urgency of her own need not to be reminded of the distress, helplessness, and attendant anger in her own personality.

The behavioral descriptions of abused toddlers witnessing the distress of age-mates provided by Main and George (1985) offer some support to this notion. The vignettes included in their report suggest that these toddlers were experiencing strong stress and urgency as they struck out at the distressed peer. For example, one abused toddler was described as loudly saying "Cut it out! Cut it out!" as he progressed from patting to hitting a crying child (p. 410). Although such behavior may represent feelings of anger and/

or modelling of maltreating parents' responses to infant distress (see Frodi and Lamb, 1980), the extreme emotional reactions described in these children suggest that another process may be involved as well: an urgent need to bring the display of distress to an end.

In summary, we are suggesting that maltreated children, like all children, enter the peer world with a relationship history that organizes their thoughts, feelings, and behavior in interpersonal contexts. Encounters with peers are not approached de novo. Rather, they are strongly influenced by the models of self and other that have been formed and by the child's need to avoid intolerable amounts of distress and anxiety. For maltreated children, this may result in a somewhat paradoxical situation: their need to avoid experiencing an overwhelming amount of negative affect does not lead them to create positive relationships but, instead, to create ones marked by aggressiveness and avoidance. It may be, however, that the most pressing need is for a familiar, predictable, and consistent experience of the self and of relationships with others. We speculate that this may be particularly true for maltreated children who have experienced traumatic encounters over which they had no control whatsoever.

The implications of a history of maltreatment for the development of peer relations

In our description of the development of peer relations, we gave a central role to the notions of sharing and equality. We suggested that the very heart of peer relations, a felt equality between partners, involved developing a working model of relationships that was based on sharing, equality, and nonexploitation. The experiences of abuse and neglect seem antithetical to developing such a model. The theoretical reason why peer relations may be so difficult for the maltreated child is that it is extremely hard to develop a model of equality and trust when one's formative experiences have involved exploitation, submission, and the violation of trust.

The difficulties in establishing and maintaining a sense of felt equality might be most apparent if the friendships of school-age and adolescent maltreated children were examined. It is during those stages that equality – in the forms of reciprocity, genuineness, and intimacy – seems to become the aspect of friendship that children themselves experience as most important. However, the available data on maltreated children's peer relations deals mostly with much younger children and focuses more on the quality of interactions than on the quality of relationships. Nonetheless, the research reviewed above does suggest that the development of egalitarian and trusting relations between peers may be negatively affected in several ways by a history of maltreatment.

As noted in the discussion of the George and Main and the Howes studies, it seems that the experience of abuse can interfere with the expression of simple equalities, such as the sharing of activity and place. We would speculate that it is also likely to interfere with the development of more complex equalities, such as shared meanings and interactive pretend play. In part, this may be because situations of mutual attention and interaction cannot be sustained. It may also be, however, that play, as a spontaneous expression of the self, is too threatening for the maltreated child. Play, particularly in its less rule-bound and structured forms, may be inherently frightening to the child who is trying to keep certain aspects of the self from being expressed.

Maltreatment may interfere with the development of sharing and equality in another way. Maltreated children may tend to create relationships with their peers that are so dominated by the difficulties they experienced with parents that they cannot deal with a peer in his or her own right. This is evidenced in maltreated children's heightened aggressiveness. In that instance, the need to re-create an abuser–abused relationship seems to override the development of relations based on equality and nonexploitation. It is as if the child were "stuck" or "fixed" in the conflictual relationship with the abusive parent, and only that relationship is meaningful to the child for "playing out" in peer relations.

Maltreatment may also interfere with another aspect of the development of peer relations – the gradual transfer of the functions of support, security, and intimacy from parents to peers. Difficulty with this task may occur, in part, because maltreating relationships do not afford a very good model of trust and intimacy. We also wonder, however, whether the experience of maltreatment and rejection could lead a child to turn to peers prematurely, in the hope that other children might fulfill the needs that are being unmet at home. Thus, the gradual transfer of function may become accelerated and, in certain instances, distorted. Although such peer relations might occur most frequently in middle childhood and adolescence, presumably even very young children may reach out to the peer world hoping to find the emotional support lacking at home.

An example of such a process in very young children can be found in a study by Jacobson and colleagues of the peer interactions of normal, non-maltreated toddlers (Jacobson, Tianen, Wille, and Aytch, 1986). These authors found that children with a history of an insecure–ambivalent attachment relationship displayed greater sociability and eagerness, although not more success, in their interactions with their peers than did those with a history of a secure attachment. Jacobson et al. note that an insecure–ambivalent relationship has been found to be related to inconsistent responsiveness on the part of the caregiver (Ainsworth et al., 1978). They speculate that uncertainty regarding maternal responsiveness may have made these toddlers anxious concerning the responsiveness of others and, thus, overly eager to receive a response from a playmate. Although we are not aware of any research that describes in depth the quality of friendships that maltreated children form with their peers, we hypothesize that some of them may be similarly characterized by an attempt to use peers to compensate for what is lacking in the parent–child relationship.

Conclusions and future directions

We began this chapter by presenting what we felt were three compelling reasons for the study of peer relations of maltreated children. We suggested that (1) it would allow us to specify maltreated children's difficulties in an important area of development, (2) it could enhance our understanding of normal developmental processes, and (3) it might add to our knowledge about how to prevent or treat social maladaptation in abused and neglected children. These three reasons can also be viewed as three important challenges or questions facing investigators in this area. With these in mind, we can then ask: To what extent have these questions been answered by the available literature? Further, what avenues should future investigators pursue in order to answer them more fully?

The first controlled, observational study of maltreated children's peer relations appeared not even a decade ago. Despite the nascent state of this research, however, we feel that progress toward answering these three questions has been made. First, we feel that we can conclude that a history of maltreatment can indeed impair a child's functioning with peers in significant ways. Earlier, we reviewed the specific difficulties that maltreated children have been found to exhibit. Our confidence in this conclusion is enhanced by the fact that we examined the data on maltreated children's peer relations in the context of a normal developmental framework. For example, the knowledge that normal development entails an increasing ability to interact with peers in nonaggressive ways allowed us to identify this as a particularly vulnerable area for abused children.

These studies also afforded an examination of how well two different models of normal social development could account for the behavior of maltreated children with their peers. Although we concluded that neither model alone was sufficient to explain the data, we felt that a central claim of the social network model was unsupported. It seems that, for maltreated children, and perhaps for all children, it is necessary to go beyond the concept of "availability of peer contact" to account for the relationship between family interactions and a child's functioning with peers.

Finally, throughout our discussion of the studies, we tried to highlight the implications of the data for interventions with maltreated children who are having difficulty with peers. Although the data do offer some preliminary guidelines for preventive and therapeutic efforts, the existence of only one study focusing directly on this issue makes it a particularly important area for future research.

Overall, then, the studies reviewed here provide important information about the relationship between a history of maltreatment and a child's social functioning. However, although they allow us to conclude that maltreatment can deleteriously affect peer relations, we feel that our understanding of this is still quite global. Therefore, we hope that future investigations can build upon this foundation by elaborating the sequelae of maltreatment in greater depth and increasing our understanding of the underlying developmental processes. Based on our review of the existing literature and with these goals in mind, we offer the following suggestions for future research in this area.

> 1. *Investigators should choose measures for studying the effects of maltreatment on peer relations in light of theory and research on normal development.*

When studying the effects of maltreatment on development, measures should be chosen and results interpreted in light of what is known about the normal developmental course of the behavior of interest. For instance, as noted above, there are age- and stage-specific changes in the manifestation of aggression. Thus, in studying whether maltreated children are more aggressive toward age-mates, it would be important to assess this construct in a developmentally sensitive way. Relatedly, it would be significant if maltreated children were found not only to exhibit more aggression than their peers, but also to be doing so in less developmentally mature ways.

A concern about developmental salience and appropriateness should also guide investigators in their initial choices of what behaviors to assess. Instead of merely recording whatever behavior occurs, investigators need to ask themselves what features normally characterize the interactions of children at different ages. Additionally, they need to ask which areas of functioning are most likely to be impaired by the experience of abuse or neglect. Choosing developmentally salient measures should lead to both an increase in sensitivity to group differences and to greater understanding of the import of the results obtained (as they can be interpreted in light of their courses and correlates in normal samples). Moreover, the measures chosen should be capable of detecting subtle or covert vulnerabilities (Aber and Cicchetti, 1984).

A second point is that investigators of maltreated children's peer relations have yet to make use of the growing literature on normal children's peer relations, including the body of research focused on peer status and the correlates of acceptance, rejection, and neglect by peers (e.g., Schneider, Rubin, and Ledingham, 1985). This body of research, however, offers assessment strategies and methodological guidelines that could advance our understanding of the difficulties exhibited by maltreated children. For instance, the literature on peer status has moved toward a refinement of the construct of "social competence" such that the dimensions of healthy and impaired functioning with peers are becoming increasingly clear. Asher (1983), for example, describes three qualitative dimensions of competent social interactions, including the relevance of social initiations (the ability to interpret a social situation and adapt behavior accordingly), responsiveness to the initiations of other children, and children's own ideas and theories concerning the best way to engage a peer in interaction. What all of these dimensions have in common is that they cannot be assessed with simple, behavioral frequency counts (e.g., rate of interaction). Although this body of research suggests that the assessment of social competence is a complex and challenging task, it does offer suggestions and strategies that investigators of maltreatment might fruitfully apply to research on abused and neglected children.

Another point that emerges from the body of developmental research on normal children's peer relations is that there are several contextual variables that can influence peer interactions. For instance, a child's behavior can vary according to whether she is interacting with a peer with a history of a secure or an insecure attachment (Jacobson and Wille, 1986; Pastor, 1981). Moreover, children behave differently with peers in different environments; for example, popular children have been found to make more social initiations than socially rejected children on the playground; the opposite occurs in the classroom. Similarly, certain behavioral measures (e.g., social participation) are quite sensitive to variations in the ecology of observations, such as class size and the proportion of disturbed children (LaFreniere and Sroufe, 1985). Thus, there are several variables that can effect the nature of children's social behavior and the validity of measures of social competence. Unless researchers are aware of them, however, they can confound results and lead to erroneous conclusions.

Finally, we propose that future investigations attempt to study the peer relations of maltreated children in greater depth. In a recent volume on peer relations in normal children, Hartup (1985) noted that researchers in that area have begun to move beyond the study of friendliness to the investigation of friendships. We advocate a similiar effort on the part of those who study maltreatment. Studying maltreated children's relationships in greater depth may reveal areas of both vulnerability and coping not evident in their interactions with acquaintances and unfamiliar peers. Furthermore, the study of friendships would allow an examination of the hypothesis that maltreated children's relationships can entail a reenactment of or an attempt to compensate for what they experienced at home.

> 2. *Researchers should attempt to assess children's internal working models of self, others, and relationships in addition to measuring overt behavior.*

We believe that children's internal working models (their expectations, beliefs, and conceptions) are the variables that mediate between a history of maltreatment and behavior with peers. Although difficult to assess, we believe that knowledge of these models will both significantly increase understanding of the observational data and help to resolve apparently discrepant results (e.g., why children behave aggressively in some circumstances and not in others). An example of how the interpretation of maltreated children's behavior can be expanded by a move to the level of mental representation was offered earlier in regard to abused children's responses to distress in a peer partner. Although this discussion was speculative, we believe that certain methods already exist in both the normal and maltreatment literature that provide avenues for exploring the mental representations of maltreated children.

Previous studies on the socioemotional development of maltreated children have employed self-report and projective measures from which one can draw a preliminary sketch of the internal life of maltreated children. Although these results have not been integrated into a coherent picture, maltreated children have been found to have more negative self-concepts (Kinard, 1980), higher levels of fantasy aggression (Reidy, 1977), and a greater tendency toward negative self-attributions (Dean et al., 1986) than comparison samples of nonmaltreated children. One could hypothesize that these thoughts and feelings have important relationships to maltreated children's overt behavior. For example, it is possible that aggressiveness is related not only to excessive anger but also to low self-esteem. However, these beliefs about the self and feelings about others are not necessarily evident when one looks only on the behavioral level.

Relatedly, research on normal samples has shown that children's self-conceptions are not synonymous with their status among peers or with their interactional styles. For example, withdrawn children have been found to perceive themselves as unpopular and socially incompetent, although they are not actually disliked by peers and appear to have adequate social problem-solving skills (Rubin, 1985). Negative self-concepts, however, may prove to be quite significant in that they may place a child at risk for later difficulties involving depression or low self-esteem. However, the negative self-concept of withdrawn children is not apparent from either measures of behavioral frequencies (i.e., the fact that they interact less) or single indices of social functioning (e.g., sociometric status).

Thus, we suggest that research on maltreated children's social competence would be enhanced by including assessments of these children's concepts of themselves and others. Ideally, this research would involve a multimodal scheme in that it would include information from several sources (e.g., adult observers, peers, the child him- or herself) and more than one observational level (e.g., overt behavior, self-report, projective techniques). We are aware of the challenges involved in the assessment of internal models, yet we believe that significant advances have already been made such that reliable, valid, and creative methods are beginning to be available (Hymel and Franke, 1985; Main et al., 1985). As noted above, we believe that a move to the level of representation will be an important component of fleshing out the global descriptions of maltreated children as "aggressive" and "withdrawn" with their peers.

> 3. *Researchers should attmept to assess directly the relationship between the quality of parent–child and child–peer relations.*

At the beginning of this chapter, we suggested that one of the central reasons for undertaking the study of maltreated children's peer relations was that it could then contribute to our understanding of normal developmental processes. In particular, we felt it could illuminate the nature of the relationship between the family and peer worlds. The authors of the studies we reviewed have certainly been concerned with this issue and, throughout this review, we have described their various hypotheses concerning the developmental origins of the behaviors they observed in maltreated children's peer interactions. However, due to the nature of the studies, few conclusions could be drawn as to the relative validity of these different explanations. This is largely because all of the studies were cross-sectional in nature and, with the exception of the Lewis and Schaeffer study, most assessed behavior in only one context and only with peers.

We hope, however, that future investigations can employ an approach that is longitudinal in nature and begins with assessments of parent–infant interactions or, if cross-sectional, involves concurrent assessments of behavior in more than one context (i.e., with family members as well as peers). We feel that such assessments could add to our understanding of maltreatment and peer relations in two ways. First, assessments of parent–child interactions in maltreating families could provide a more elaborated picture of what actually is encompassed by the rather global descriptors "abuse" and "neglect." The advantage of a more richly elaborated understanding of the subtypes of maltreatment can be seen in a study by Egeland and Sroufe (1981b). In that study, the authors included qualitative aspects of parenting such as "psychological unavailability" in their typology of different maltreating behaviors. These qualitative distinctions proved quite important as the children of psychologically unavailable mothers were found to evidence the most severe sequelae of maltreatment in the entire sample. Such qualitative aspects of a child's experience with parents is often not captured by the report of a social service agency stating that the child has been abused or neglected. Although confirmed reports of maltreatment by social agencies are certainly important in these studies, they cannot provide the depth and richness obtained in actual observations of family interactions.

A second reason to conduct observations in more than one context is that children behave differently according to context. Thus, it is not possible to understand fully the effects of familial factors on peer relations by only assessing interactions with age-mates. The relationship between childrearing history and later peer relations may not be characterized by behavioral isomorphism. Thus, in nonmaltreated samples, children who are aggressive with peers are not necessarily found to come from homes that are characterized primarily by aggressiveness; rather, aggressiveness with peers has been found to be related to a mother–child relationship that is lacking in warmth and, depending on the child's age, is characterized by either permissiveness or control and hostility (Hinde and Stevenson-Hinde, 1986). This suggests that although the relationship between different social realms may be lawful, it is not necessarily characterized by homotypic continuity; thus, it cannot be inferred from data from only a single context.

As a result of the efforts of the investigators whose studies were reviewed here, we now have a far better description of maltreated children's behavior with peers than was available less than a decade ago. Moreover, the results of the studies strongly suggest that maltreatment can deleteriously affect children's development in an important sphere: interacting and forming relationships with peers. Although much remains to be understood about this process, the research discussed clearly supports the importance of this topic for future investigations and provides a solid foundation upon which they can build.

References

Aber, J. L., and Cicchetti, D. (1984). The socio-emotional development of maltreated children: An empirical and theoretical analysis. In H. Fitzgerald, B. Lester, and M. Yogman (eds.), *Theory and research in behavioral pediatrics, Vol. 2.* New York: Plenum.

Aber, J. L., and Zigler, E. (1981). Developmental considerations in the definition of child maltreatment. In R. Rizley and D. Cicchetti (Eds.), *Developmental perspectives on child maltreatment.* San Francisco: Jossey-Bass.

Ainsworth, M., Blehar, M., Waters, E., and Wall, S. (1978). *Patterns of attachment.* Hillsdale, NJ: Erlbaum.

Asher, S. R. (1983). Social competence and peer status; Recent advances and future directions. *Child Development, 54,* 1427–1433.

Bandura, A. (1977). *Social learning theory.* Englewood Cliffs, NJ: Prentice Hall.

Baumrind, D. (1967). Child care practices anteceding 3 patterns of preschool behavior. *Genetic Psychology Monographs, 75,* 43–88.

Baumrind, D. (1971). Current patterns of parental authority. *Developmental psychology monograph, 4* (1), 1–103.

Belsky, J. (1980). Child maltreatment: An ecological integration. *American Psychologist, 35,* 320–335.

Belsky, J., Rovine, M., and Taylor, D. G. (1984). The Pennsylvania Infant and Family Development Project, 3: The origins of individual differences in infant–mother attachment: Maternal and infant contributions. *Child Development, 55,* 718–728.

Bigelow, B. J. (1977). Children's friendship expectations: A cognitive developmental study. *Child Development, 48,* 246–53.

Bischof, N. (1975). A systems approach toward the functional connections of attachment and fear. *Child Development, 45,* 801–817.

Block, J. H., and Block, J (1980). The role of ego-control and ego-resiliency in the organization of behavior. In A. Collins (Ed.), *Minnesota symposium of child psychology* (Vol. 13). Hillsdale, NJ: Erlbaum.

Bowlby, J. (1969). *Attachment and loss, (Vol. 1): Attachment.* New York: Basic Books.

Bowlby, J. (1973). *Attachment and loss, (Vol. 2): Separation.* New York: Basic Books.

Bowlby, J. (1980). *Attachment and loss, (Vol. 3): Loss, sadness and depression.* New York: Basic Books.

Bradley, R. H., Caldwell, B. M., Fitzgerald, J. A., Morgan, A. G., and Rock, S. L. (1986). Experiences in day care and social competence among maltreated children. *Child Abuse and Neglect, 10,* 181–189.

Brenner, J., and Mueller, E. (1982). Shared meaning in boy toddler's peer relations. *Child Development, 53,* 380–391.

Bretherton, I. (1985). Attachment theory: Retrospect and prospect. In I. Bretherton and E. Waters (Eds.), *Growing Points in Attachment Theory and Research: Monographs of the Society for Research in Child Development,* Vol. 50 (1 and 2), Serial No. 209. Chicago: University of Chicago Press.

Bronfenbrenner, U. (1970). *Two worlds of childhood: U.S. and U.S.S.R.* New York: Russell Sage.

Brownell, C. A. (1985). Toddler peer interactions in relation to cognitive development. Paper delivered at the biennial meetings of the Society for Research in Child Development, Toronto, April.

Brownell, C. A. (1986). Convergent developments: Cognitive–developmental correlates of growth in infant–toddler peer skills. *Child Development, 57,* 275–286.

Cicchetti, D., and Braunwald, K. G. (1984). An organizational approach to the study of emotional development in maltreated infants. *Infant Mental Health Journal, 5* (3), 172–183.

Cicchetti, D., and Rizley, R. (1981). Developmental perspectives on the etiology, intergenerational transmission, and sequelae of child maltreatment. In R. Rizley and D. Cicchetti (Eds.), *Developmental perspectives on child maltreatment.* San Francisco: Jossey-Bass.

Coie, J. D., and Kupersmidt, J. (1983). A behavioral analysis of emerging social status in boys' groups. *Child Development, 54,* 1400–1416.

Cowen, E. L., Pederson, A., Babigian, H., Izzo, L. D., and Trost, M. (1973). Long-term follow-up of early detected vulnerable children. *Journal of Consulting and Clinical Psychology, 41* (3), 438–446.

Crittenden, P. M. (1985). Social networks, quality of child rearing, and child development. *Child Development, 56,* 1299–1313.

Dean, A. L., Malik, M. M., Richards, W. and Stringer, S. (1986). Effects of parental maltreatment on children's conceptions of interpersonal relationships. *Developmental Psychology, 22* (5), 617–626.

Dodge, K. A. (1983). Behavioral antecedents of peer social status. *Child Development, 54,* 1386–1399.

Dodge, K. A. (1985). Facets of social interaction and the assessment of social competence in children. In B. H. Schneider, K. H. Rubin, and J. E. Ledingham (Eds.), *Children's peer relations: Issues in assessment and intervention.* New York: Springer-Verlag.

Egeland, B., and Sroufe, L. A. (1981a). Attachment and early maltreatment. *Child Development, 52,* 44–52.

Egeland, B., and Sroufe, L. A. (1981b). Developmental sequelae of maltreatment in infancy. In R. Rizley and D. Cicchetti (Eds.), *Developmental perspectives on child maltreatment.* San Francisco: Jossey-Bass.

Fairbairn, W. R. D. (1950). *An object relations theory of personality.* New York: Basic Books.

Freud, A. (1937/1966). *The ego and the mechanisms of defense.* New York: International Universities Press.

Freud, S. (1926/1977). *Inhibitions, symptoms and anxiety.* New York: Norton.

Frodi, A. M., and Lamb, M. E. (1980). Child abuser's responses to infant smiles and cries. *Child Development, 51,* 238–241.

Furman, W., Rahe, D. F., and Hartup, W. W. (1979). Rehabilitation of socially withdrawn preschool children through mixed-age and same-age socialization. *Child Development, 50,* 915–922.

Garvey, C. (1977). *Play.* Cambridge, MA: Harvard University Press.

Galdston, R. (1971). Violence begins at home: The parents center for the study and prevention of child abuse. *Journal of the American Academy of Child Psychiatry, 10,* 336–350.

George, C., and Main, M. (1979). Social interactions of young abused children: Approach, avoidance, and aggression. *Child Development, 50,* 306–318.

Green, A. H. (1978). Psychopathology of abused children. *Journal of the American Academy of Child Psychiatry, 17,* 92–103.

Greenberg, J. R., and Mitchell, S. A. (1983). *Object relations in psychoanalytic theory.* Cambridge, MA: Harvard University Press.

Grossmann, K., Grossmann, K. E., Spangler, G., Suess, G., and Unzner, L. (1985). Maternal sensitivity and newborn's orientation responses as related to quality of attachment in Northern Germany. In I. Bretherton and E. Waters (Eds.), *Growing Points in Attachment Theory and Research: Monographs of the Society for Research in Child Development,* Vol. 50 (1 and 2), Serial No. 209. Chicago: University of Chicago Press.

Hartup, W. W. (1983). Peer relations. In E. M. Hetherington (Ed.), P. H. Mussen (Series Ed.), *Handbook of child psychology,* Vol. 4, *Socialization, personality and social development.* New York: Wiley.

Hartup, W. W. (1985). Foreword. In B. H. Schneider, K. H. Rubin, and J. E. Ledingham (Eds.), *Children's peer relations: Issues in assessment and intervention.* New York: Springer-Verlag.

Hay, D., and Ross, H. (1982). The social nature of early conflict. *Child Development, 53,* 105–113.

Herrenkohl, R. C., and Herrenkohl, E. C. (1981). Some antecedents and developmental consequences of child maltreatment. In R. Rizley and D. Cicchetti (Eds.), *Developmental perspectives on child maltreatment.* San Francisco: Jossey-Bass.

Hinde, R. A., and Stevenson-Hinde, J. (1986). Relating childhood relationships to individual characteristics. In W. W. Hartup and Z. Rubin (Eds.), *Relationships and development.* Hillsdale, NJ: Erlbaum.

Hoffman-Plotkin, D., and Twentyman, C. (1984). A multimodal assessment of behavioral and cognitive deficits in abused and neglected preschoolers. *Child Development, 55,* 794–802.

Horner, A. J. (1984). *Object relations and the developing ego in therapy.* New York: Aronson.

Howes, C. (1984). Social interactions and patterns of friendships in normal and emotionally disturbed children. In T. Field, J. Roopnarine, and M. Segal (Eds.), *Friendships in normal and handicapped children.* Norwood, NJ: Ablex.

Howes, C., and Eldredge, R. (1985). Responses of abused, neglected, and non-maltreated children to the behaviors of their peers. *Journal of Applied Developmental Psychology, 6,* 261–270.

Howes, C., and Espinosa, M. P. (1985). The consequences of child abuse for the formation of relationships with peers. *Child Abuse and Neglect, 9,* 397–404.

Howes, C., and Farver, J. (1984). Toddler responses to the distress of their peers. Paper presented at the International Conference on Infant Studies, New York.

Hymel, S., and Franke, S. (1985). Children's peer relations: Assessing self-perceptions. In B. H. Schneider, K. H. Rubin, and J. E. Ledingham (Eds.), *Children's peer relations: Issues in assessment and intervention.* New York: Springer-Verlag.

Jacobson, J. L., Tianen, R. L., Wille, D. E., and Aytch, D. M. (1986). Infant–mother attachment and early peer relations: The assessment of behavior in an interactive context. In E. C. Mueller and C. R. Cooper (Eds.), *Process and outcome in peer relations,* New York: Academic.

Jacobson, J. L., and Wille, D. E. (1986). The influence of attachment pattern on developmental changes in peer interaction from the toddler to the preschool period. *Child Development, 57,* 338–347.

Jacobson, R. S., and Straker, G. (1982). Peer group interaction of physically abused children. *Child Abuse and Neglect, 6,* 321–327.

Kagan J. (1984). *The nature of the child.* New York: Basic Books.

Kinard, E. M. (1980). Emotional development in physically abused children. *American Journal of Orthopsychiatry, 50,* 686–696.

LaFreniere, P. J., and Sroufe, L. A. (1985). Profiles of peer competence in the preschool: Interrelations between measures, influence of social ecology, and relation to attachment history. *Developmental Psychology, 21,* 56–69.

Levitt, M. J., Weber, R. A., and Clark, M. C. (1986). Social network relationships as sources of maternal support and well-being. *Developmental Psychology, 22,* 310–316.

Lewis, M. L., and Schaeffer, S. (1981). Peer behavior and mother–infant interaction. In M. L. Lewis and S. Schaeffer (Eds.), *The uncommon child.* New York: Plenum.

Lieberman, A. F. (1977). Preschoolers' competence with a peer: Relations with attachment and peer experience. *Child Development, 48,* 1277–1287.

Main, M. (1977). Analysis of a peculiar form of reunion behavior seen in some daycare children: Its history and sequelae in children who are home-reared. In R. Webb (Ed.), *Social development in childhood: Daycare programs and research.* Baltimore: Johns Hopkins University Press.

Main, M., and George, C. (1985). Responses of abused and disadvantaged toddlers to distress in agemates: A study in the day care setting. *Developmental Psychology, 21* (3), 407–412.

Main, M., and Goldwyn, R. (1984). Predicting rejection of her infant from mother's representation of her own experience: Implications for the abused–abusing intergenerational cycle. *Child Abuse and Neglect, 8,* 203–217.

Main, M., Kaplan, N., and Cassidy, J. (1985). Security in infancy, childhood and adulthood: A move to the level of representation. In I. Bretherton and E. Waters (Eds.), *Growing Points in Attachment Theory and Research: Monographs of the Society for Research in Child Development,* Vol. 50 (1 and 2), Serial No. 209. Chicago: University of Chicago Press.

Martin, H. P. (1980). The consequences of being abused and neglected: How the child fares. In C. H. Kempe and R. E. Helfer (Eds.), *The battered child* (3rd ed.). Chicago: University of Chicago Press.

Martin, H. P., and Beezley, P. (1977). Behavioral observations of abused children. *Developmental Medicine and Child Neurology, 19,* 373–387.

McCartney, K., Scarr, S., Phillips, D., and Grajek, S. (1985). Day care as intervention: Comparisons of varying quality programs. *Journal of Applied Developmental Psychology, 6,* 247–260.

Mueller, E. (1972). The maintenance of verbal exchanges between young children. *Child Development, 49,* 930–938.

Mueller, E., and Brenner, J. (1977). The origins of social skills and interaction among playgroup toddlers. *Child Development, 48,* 854–861.

Mueller, E., and Cohen, D. (1986). Peer therapies and the little latency: a clinical perspective.

In E. C. Mueller and C. R. Cooper (Eds.), *Process and outcome in peer relationships.* New York: Academic.

Mueller, E., and Vandell, D. H. (1979). Infant–infant interaction: a review of research and concepts. In J. Osofsky (Ed.), *Handbook of infant development.* New York: Wiley Interscience.

Musatti, T., and Mueller, E. (1985). Expressions of representational growth in toddlers' peer communication. *Social Cognition, 3,* 383–399.

Oden, S., Herzberger, S. D., Mangione, P. L., and Wheeler, V. A. (1984). Children's peer relationships: an examination of social processes. In J. C. Masters and K. Yarkin-Levin (Eds.), *Boundary areas in social and developmental psychology.* New York: Academic.

Parke, R. D., and Collmer, C. W. (1975). Child abuse: An interdisciplinary analysis. In E. M. Hetherington (Ed.), *Review of child development research* (Vol. 5). Chicago: University of Chicago Press.

Pastor, D. L. (1981). The quality of mother–infant attachment and its relationship to toddlers' initial sociability with peers. *Developmental Psychology, 17* (3), 326–335.

Piaget, J. (1932/1965). *The moral judgment of the child.* New York: Free Press.

Putallaz, M., and Gottman, J. M. (1981). An interactional model of children's entry into peer groups. *Child Development, 52,* 986–994.

Radke-Yarrow, M., Cummings, E. M., Kuczynski, L., and Chapman, M. (1985). Patterns of attachment in two- and three-year-olds in normal families and families with parental depression. *Child Development, 56,* 884–893.

Reidy, T. J. (1977). The aggressive characteristics of abused and neglected children. *Journal of Clinical Psychology, 33,* 1140–1145.

Roff, M., Sells, S. B., and Golden, M. M. (1972). *Social adjustment and personality development in children.* Minneapolis: University of Minnesota Press.

Ross, H. S. (1981). The establishment of social games amongst toddlers. Paper delivered at the biennial meetings of the Society for Research in Child Development, Boston, April.

Rubin, K. H. (1985). Socially withdrawn children: An "at risk" population? In B. H. Schneider, K. H. Rubin, and J. E. Ledingham (Eds.), *Children's peer relations: Issues in assessment and intervention.* New York: Springer-Verlag.

Rubin, K. H., Fein, G. G., and Vandenberg, B. (1983). Play. In E. M. Hetherington (Ed.), P. H. Mussen (Series Ed.), *Handbook of child psychology,* Vol. 4, *Socialization, personality and social development.* New York: Wiley.

Rubin, Z. (1980). *Children's friendships.* Cambridge, MA: Harvard University Press.

Sameroff, A., and Chandler, M. (1975). Reproductive risk and the continuum of caretaking casualty. In F. Horowitz (Ed.), *Review of child development research* (Vol. 4). Chicago: University of Chicago Press.

Schneider, B. H., Rubin, K. H., and Ledingham, J. E. (Eds.) (1985). *Children's peer relations; Issues in assessment and intervention.* New York: Springer-Verlag.

Schneider-Rosen, K., Braunwald, K., Carlson, V., and Cicchetti, D. (1985). Current perspectives in attachment theory: Illustration from the study of maltreated infants. In I. Brethertin and E. Waters (Eds.), *Growing Points in Attachment Theory and Research: Monographs of the Society for Research in Child Development,* Vol. 50 (1 and 2), Serial No. 209. Chicago: University of Chicago Press.

Sears, R. R., Maccoby, E., and Levin, H. (1957). *Patterns of child rearing.* Evanston, IL: Row, Peterson.

Selman, R. (1980). *The growth of interpersonal understanding.* New York: Academic Press.

Shugar, G. W., and Bokus, B. (1986). Children's discourse and children's activity in the peer situation. In E. C. Mueller and C. R. Cooper (Eds.), *Process and outcome in peer relationships.* New York: Academic Press.

Sroufe, L. A. (1979). The coherence of individual development: Early care, attachment and subsequent developmental issues. *American Psychologist, 34,* 834–841.

Sroufe, L. A. (1983). Infant–caregiver attachment and patterns of adaptation in preschool: The roots of maladaptation and competence. In M. Perlmutter (Ed.), *Minnesota Symposia on Child Development* (Vol. 16, pp. 41–83). Hillsdale, NJ: Erlbaum.

Sroufe, L. A., and Fleeson, J. (1986). Attachment and the construction of relationships. In W. H. Hartup and Z. Rubin (Eds.), *Relationships and development*. Hillsdale, NJ: Erlbaum.

Sroufe, L. A., Schork, E., Motti, F., Lawroski, N., and LaFreniere, P. (1984). The role of affect in social competence. In C. E. Izard, J. Kagan, and R. B. Zajonc (Eds.), *Emotions, cognition, and behavior*. New York: Cambridge University Press.

Sroufe, L. A., and Waters, E. (1977). Attachment as an organizational construct. *Child Development, 48*, 1184–1199.

Stern, D. N. (1974). Mother and infant at play: The dyadic interaction involving facial, vocal and gaze behaviors. In M. Lewis and L. A. Rosenblum (Eds.), *The effect of the infant on its caregiver*. New York: Wiley.

Sullivan, H. S. (1953). *The interpersonal theory of psychiatry*. New York: Norton.

Sundby, H. S., and Kreyberg, P. C. (1968). *Prognosis in child psychiatry*. Baltimore: Williams and Wilkins.

Vandell, D. L., and Mueller, E. C. (1977). The effects of group size on toddler's social interactions with peers. Paper presented at the meeting of the Society for Research in Child Development, New Orleans, March.

Vandell, D. L., Wilson, K. S., and Buchanan, N. R. (1980). Peer interaction in the first year of life: An examination of its structure, content, and sensitivity to toys. *Child Development, 51*, 481–488.

Waters, E., and Sroufe, L. A. (1983). Social competence as a developmental construct. *Developmental Review, 3*, 79–97.

Waters, E., Wippman, J., and Sroufe, L. A. (1979). Attachment, positive affect, and competence in the peer group: Two studies in construct validation. *Child Development, 50*, 821–829.

Youniss, J. (1980). *Parents and peers in social development*. Chicago: The University of Chicago Press.

Youniss, J., and Volpe, J. (1978). A relationship analysis of children's friendship. In W. Damon (Ed.), *Social cognition* (New Directions for Child Development, No. 1). San Francisco: Jossey-Bass.

Zahn-Waxler, C., Radke-Yarrow, M., and King, R. A. (1979). Child rearing and children's prosocial initiations towards victims of distress. *Child Development, 50*, 319–330.

18 The effects of maltreatment on development during early childhood: recent studies and their theoretical, clinical, and policy implications

J. Lawrence Aber, Joseph P. Allen, Vicki Carlson, and Dante Cicchetti

Introduction

In several recent reports, we have presented initial results of studies of the socioemotional development and behavioral symptomatology of maltreated preschool and early school-age children (Aber and Allen, 1987; Aber, Allen, and Cicchetti, 1988; Aber, Trickett, Carlson, and Cicchetti, 1989; Cicchetti, Carlson, Braunwald, and Aber, 1987). The purposes of this chapter are to summarize the results of these studies and to discuss their implications for a variety of unresolved scientific, clinical, and policy issues. In order to accomplish these purposes, it is first necessary to briefly describe the theoretical, clinical, and policy contexts in which these studies were designed and conducted.

Contexts for the research

Scientific theoretical context

As we have noted elsewhere (Aber and Allen, 1987; Aber and Cicchetti, 1984; Cicchetti et al., 1987), until very recently, the few scientific studies of the effects of maltreatment were largely atheoretical. In our opinion, atheo-

The studies reported in this chapter were supported by grants from the National Center on Child Abuse and Neglect (90–C–1929) to Dante Cicchetti and from the National Institute of Mental Health (1–R01–MH37960–01) to Dante Cicchetti (Principal Investigator) and Lawrence Aber and Vicki Carlson (Co-Investigators). Preparation of this report was made possible by a Spencer Fellowship from the National Academy of Education to Lawrence Aber.

Study 1 (pp. 588–95) is reprinted by permission from J. L. Aber and J. P. Allen, The effects of maltreatment on young children's socio-emotional development: An attachment theory perspective, *Developmental Psychology, 23* (1987), 406–414; copyright 1987 by the American Psychological Association.

retical research in child maltreatment is only slightly better than no research at all. This is because no single study or set of studies will provide us with all the knowledge necessary to guide our clinical and policy efforts on behalf of maltreated children. Rather, it is by developing accurate, comprehensive theories of the etiologies of child maltreatment and the development of maltreated children that cumulative knowledge may serve as the basis for effective actions.

Thus, a central issue at the very start of our studies was the selection of the general and specific theoretical frameworks within which we could conduct our studies. Although rarely commented upon, the *selection* of theoretical frameworks within a scientific world of multiple and competing paradigms is a critical stage of scientific research.

Our overall theoretical approach was based upon both a careful review of the extant research literature on the developmental sequelae of child maltreatment (Aber and Cicchetti, 1984) and upon emerging theories in the fields of developmental psychopathology and risk research (Cicchetti and Rizley, 1981; Cicchetti et al., 1987). Described more fully elsewhere, we nonetheless wish to reemphasize several of our key theoretical premises:

1. Studies of the development of maltreated children, like studies of other populations of high-risk children, should begin by focusing on children's competencies and incompetencies in broad domains of adaptive functioning. Both theory and research on normal development can serve as initial guides to the identification of crucial domains of adaptive functioning.
2. The crucial domains of adaptive functioning to be investigated should both be stage-salient and bear a clear theoretical relationship to the nature of the risk to which the child is exposed and to relevant findings and/or concepts of the children's prior and future functioning.
3. Maltreatment is a complex and heterogeneous phenomenon that probably involves complex and heterogeneous etiologies and developmental outcomes. Hence, we should not assume single, discrete causes or outcomes; instead, we should examine a range of causes and effects of maltreatment, both direct and indirect.

With these premises in mind, we decided to base our studies on no single theory of behavior and development, but rather on a constellation of theories, notably attachment theory, social-cognitive developmental theory, developmental-structural theory (Ainsworth, Blehar, Waters, and Wall, 1978; Kohlberg, Ricks, and Snarey, 1983; Sroufe and Rutter, 1984) and ecological theory (Belsky, 1980; Bronfenbrenner, 1979; Garbarino, 1982). These subtheories were further ordered and integrated using principles from Werner's organismic-developmental theory (Werner and Kaplan, 1963) as recently reinterpreted by Sroufe, Cicchetti, and others (Cicchetti, 1984). For example, these subtheories were used to generate testable hypotheses about the development of maltreated children. From attachment theory, we generated the hypothesis that maltreated children would demonstrate a higher proportion of insecure attachments to their primary caretakers than would a demographically matched sample of nonmaltreated children. Based upon social-cognitive developmental theory, we proposed that a history of maltreatment would disrupt the optimal development of the self-system. From ecological theory, we proposed that the family ecologies of maltreated children would be characterized by more authoritarian control and less access to community resources. And from developmental-structural theory, we hypothesized that impairments in developmental-adaptational traits with a cognitive-structural base associated with a history of maltreatment would also be associated with elevated levels of behavioral symptomatology. After initial studies of components of our comprehensive theory, we intend to draw upon "organizational" principles to describe the relationship between attachment, the self-system and emergent psychopathology in maltreated children as adaptations to certain types of childrearing environments.

Our research with infants and toddlers has essentially supported the first two of these hypotheses regarding the effects of maltreatment on security of attachment and the development of the self-system (Carlson, Cicchetti, Barnett, and Braunwald, this volume; Schneider-Rosen and Cicchetti, 1984; Schneider-Rosen, Braunwald, Carlson, and Cicchetti, 1985). Just as these hypotheses were tested in infancy and toddlerhood, we wished to test similar (but not identical) hypotheses concerning the effects of maltreatment during the preschool and early school-age years.

Unfortunately, one cannot always immediately direct new research to the most important or reasonable theoretical question; one must also take into account the status of measurement and description of the key constructs that make up the theory one wishes to test. Hence, when we began constructing the studies of the effects of maltreatment on development in the preschool and early school-age years, we wished to pursue similar questions to those we had proposed in infancy and toddlerhood; namely, how a history of maltreatment affected both attachment and the self-system. But attachment theory and research had not yet developed to the point of generating measures of key constructs in the preschool or school-age years (although recently that problem has been addressed by Main (Main and Cassidy, 1988; Main, Kaplan, and Cassidy, 1985) and others (Greenberg, Cicchetti, and Cummings, in press). Even if a measure of "security of attachment" per se were available for older children, it is not immediately apparent that it would be the best measure to employ. Although attachment to the primary caregiver continues to be important beyond toddlerhood, perhaps another stage-specific aspect of the attachment system (such as the ability to establish positive relationships with novel adults) would be a better measure of the quality of adaptive functioning in the attachment domain for preschool and early school-age maltreated children. In any case, for both methodological and theoretical reasons, in designing studies of maltreated preschool and early school-age children, we were guided by the same set of premises and the same general set of questions, but had to adapt specific questions and methods in light of the state of the research tools available at the time.

In this respect, we were fortunate to have the advice of Edward Zigler of Yale University in the design of our initial studies. Although the effects of maltreatment on preschoolers' attachment relationships and self-system had not been directly investigated per se, Zigler alerted us to a related line of his own research on the effects of social deprivation on the development of pre-schoolers' social relationships (especially with novel adults) and effectance motivation. According to attachment theory, these constructs should be systematically related to the quality of attachment with the primary caregiver (Sroufe, 1983; Sroufe, Fox, and Pancake, 1983).

As we have argued elsewhere (Aber and Allen, 1987; Cicchetti et al., 1987), we believed that these concepts and measures from social deprivation theory could be used in studies of the effects of maltreatment on preschool and early school-age development that would parallel in essential features the infant/toddler studies. The specific rationale, methods, and results of these studies are described below. But first, we wanted to make a point by briefly describing the general theoretical premises and the history of interpretations and adaptations of theoretical frameworks and measurement strategies employed in these studies. Studies of the development of maltreated children must be theoretically grounded to be valuable; but creating the theoretical framework, especially an integrative framework that permits the study of key developmental constructs across developmental epochs, will not be a simple, straightforward endeavor.

Clinical context

When we started our study, in 1979, both the state we lived in (Massachusetts) and the nation as a whole were still in the midst of a child abuse report explosion of unprecedented proportions. Although the increased number of reports of child maltreatment and the creation both of criteria for reports and of response systems are largely policy issues (Aber, 1980), they also influence the clinical context of services to maltreated children and their families. This context influenced our research.

Most child protective service workers have not received adequate training compared to many other human service professionals, yet they must handle some of the most serious and difficult cases possible. It was our judgment at the time we began our studies that child protective service workers in particular (and, to be fair, children's service professsionals in general, including professionals from the fields of health, mental health, day- and child-care, education, and welfare) were severely hampered in their abilities to provide clinical services to maltreated children and their families by our lack of knowledge of the development of maltreated children, especially their social–emotional, behavioral, and cognitive development. Although workers could identify physical injuries and obvious problems in physical development (e.g., severe malnutrition), little guidance could be provided on the psychological development of maltreated children.

At the time, maltreated children were being described in the clinical literature in confusing and sometimes contradictory ways; for example, as both hyperaggressive and as withdrawn, as overly dependent and as isolated (see Aber and Cicchetti, 1984, for a review). If left unchanged, the contradictory and unordered clinical picture of the psychological development of maltreated children would surely limit the accurate identification of new cases of child maltreatment (especially emotional maltreatment and neglect) and in addition hinder the targeting of limited services available on the children in most need and on those key impairments with the greatest impact on the children's long-term health and development.

In short, we hoped that our work in describing the socioemotional, cognitive, and behavioral development of maltreated children would produce clinically useful knowledge. Our greatest hope was to provide empirical evidence in support of a unifying theory that would help bring order to the prevailing chaotic picture.

Policy context

The last twenty years are filled with a variety of examples of the complex relationship between behavioral and social science research (e.g., in child development) and the construction of social policies (e.g., child welfare policy). Our studies commenced at a particular point in that history, when data from one of the few rigorously conducted scientific studies of the long-term effects of child maltreatment appeared to call into serious question whether maltreatment had a negative effect on child development over and above the effects of poverty and welfare dependency (Elmer, 1977). Definition and design limitations of this study call this conclusion itself into question (see Aber and Cicchetti, 1984). Curiously, this bit of scientific evidence seemed to support current trends among libertarian policymakers and analysts who wished to reduce the amount of unnecessary state intervention into private family life as well as conservative policymakers and analysts who wished to construct rationales for reducing human service budgets at both the federal and state levels.

Our approach to this complex set of issues was orthodoxly (perhaps hopelessly) scientific (as opposed to policy-oriented). For reasons detailed elsewhere, we strongly questioned the inferences drawn from Elmer's work, due largely to limitations in the design of her study (Aber and Cicchetti, 1984);

yet, like Elmer, we wished to use an empirical, scientifically based approach to help develop policy-relevant data on the effects of maltreatment. We hoped to reorient the debate on the wisdom of expanding the protective service system by focusing more on what we can know about the development of maltreated children. We hoped that our research eventually could help distinguish maltreated children who were not suffering serious effects from those who were and use this information to guide decisions both on initial intervention and on service delivery to the children at highest risk. Yet we suspected that this "targeting" of intervention and service guided by knowledge of development could not be accomplished through such popular devices as the construction of simple risk profiles for use by hospital personnel and the like (Cicchetti and Aber, 1980). Instead, in this highly complex arena, we believed careful, textured judgments (not recipes for decisions) would always be required; and that such judgments would likely be improved by a more accurate and refined picture of the development of maltreated children.

Summary

Thus, our major goal was (and is) to construct an empirically supported theory of the development of maltreated children. This comprehensive theory would need to be informed by a variety of specific theories and would need to be consistent with what we were learning about maltreated children at various stages of development. We hoped and believed that such a theory could prove useful to both clinical- and policy-decision making on behalf of maltreated children, although we were certainly aware of some of the dangers in the minefield that lay between scientific knowledge and its application in social action.

Research questions

With these general theoretical, clinical, and policy contexts as background, we now turn to the specific theoretical rationales for and research questions of our first set of studies.

As we have described above, we designed these studies first and foremost to contribute to theory because we believe Lewin's old adage that there is nothing so practical as a good theory. Guided by organismic-developmental theory, we decided to focus on four broad domains of adaptive functioning that seemed especially important during the preschool and early school-age years and that previous theory and/or research suggested may be affected by a history of maltreatment. Each of these four domains are briefly introduced below and discussed more fully elsewhere (Aber and Allen, 1987; Aber, Allen, and Cicchetti, 1988).

Relations with novel adults

As young children move out from their family systems to spend an increasing amount of time in the child care and/or school systems, their relationship with unfamiliar adults, especially new teachers, becomes increasingly important.

Attachment theory suggests that children's expectancies of adult availability and responsiveness are generalizations developed during infancy and toddlerhood through interactions with their primary attachment figure(s). These expectancies concerning adult availability and responsiveness are carried forward via internal representational models of self-in-relationships. These cognitive-affective models influence both the construction of new relationships and the ability to explore and cope with the demands of new and stressful situations later in development (Bowlby, 1980; Main and Weston, 1981; Sroufe and Fleeson, 1986).

Previous research suggests that histories of social deprivation and/or insecurity of attachment to the primary caregiver may distort young children's relationships with unfamiliar adults outside the home, leading, for example, to excessive dependency and possibly excessive wariness and imitation as well (Balla and Zigler, 1975; Sroufe, 1983; Sroufe, Fox and Pancake, 1983; Yando, Seitz, and Zigler, 1978; Zigler and Balla, 1982).

Effectance motivation

Conceptualized as the child's motive to deal competently with his or her environment for the intrinsic pleasure of mastery (White, 1959), effectance motivation also has been found to be negatively associated with both insecurity of infant attachment and with a child's history of social deprivation (Arend, Grove, and Sroufe, 1979; Harter, 1978; Harter and Zigler, 1974). Effectance motivation may figure prominently in the young child's successful adaptation to the problem-solving orientation and task demands of most American classrooms.

Cognitive maturity

Poor performance on measures of cognitive maturity (e.g., mental age as measured by standard intelligence tests) has been associated with a history of maltreatment (Barahal, Waterman, and Martin, 1981; Hoffman-Plotkin and Twentyman, 1984; Rohrbeck and Twentyman, 1986). Other research provides support for the notion that such deficits may result from interpersonal expectancies that impair performance. For instance, research on the motivational factors that increase the competence–performance gap in the symbolic play of insecurely attached children (Belsky, Garduque, and

Hrncir, 1984), on family socialization and motivational factors that lower the performance of disadvantaged children on IQ-like tests (Moore, 1986; Zigler, Abelson, and Seitz, 1973; Zigler, Abelson, Trickett, and Seitz, 1982) and on the link between maltreatment and on externally oriented social-cognition style (Barahal et al., 1981) all are consistent with the concept of an interpersonal expectancy component as a mediating factor in the poor cognitive performance of maltreated children.

Behavioral symptomatology

This fourth domain of young children's adaptive functioning that may be affected by a history of maltreatment has been investigated for the longest period of time and has progressed from initial clinical descriptions, through uncontrolled empirical studies, to well controlled studies employing reliable, valid measures (see Aber and Cicchetti, 1984, and Aber, Allen, and Cicchetti, 1988, for reviews). Surprisingly, although most clinical reports of maltreated children describe them as much more symptomatic than nonmaltreated children, the empirical literature is inconclusive. Until certain problematic features in the designs of previous studies are overcome, it will remain unclear whether and when maltreated children are more symptomatic than demographically well-matched comparison children. Another key issue is whether maltreatment leads to an increase in externalizing symptoms (e.g., aggression), internalizing symptoms (e.g., depression), or both.

As noted above in our discussion of the theoretical context for these studies, theories like attachment theory, self-system theory, and social deprivation theory were used to generate first-level, specific hypotheses about young maltreated chidlren, which we wished to test. Thus, on the basis of the rationales presented above, we predicted that, *as a group,* maltreated preschool and school-age children would exhibit more dependency and wariness toward novel adults, less effectance motivation, lower cognitive maturity, and higher levels of behavioral symptomatology than a well-matched sample of nonmaltreated children. Indeed, we viewed the tests of these first-level hypotheses as key to evaluating Elmer's (1977) assertion that maltreatment appeared to have no additional effect on children's development over and above the effect attributable to the family chaos associated with poverty and welfare dependency (Elmer, 1977).

But we also noted that, in addition to the simple, first-order hypotheses about group differences (maltreated versus comparison children) in single domains of development, we wished to employ: (1) organismic-developmental (Werner and Kaplan, 1963), developmental-structural (Greenspan and Porges, 1984), and organizational theories (Sroufe and Rutter, 1984; Cicchetti, 1984) to help formulate and test hypotheses about relations among domains of development, and (2) ecological theory to help formulate and test hypotheses about within-group differences.

In our initial studies, we twice examined sets of relations among domains of development. First, guided by the organizational concept of the dynamic relationship between the attachment and exploratory systems of behavior in infancy and toddlerhood, we wished to examine the connection between relations with novel adults and effectance motivation in the preschool and early school-age years. Just as insensitive (noncontingent, rejecting, unpredictable) parenting in infancy led to both insecurity of attachment and to impaired exploration, so too, we reasoned, a history of maltreatment would lead to a connection between excessive dependency concerns and reduced effectance motivation in the preschool years (Aber and Allen, 1987). Second, guided by the developmental–structural and organizational theories of Kohlberg, Greenspan, Sroufe, and Cicchetti, we hypothesized a relationship between lags in socioemotional development (especially those areas built upon what Kohlberg calls a "cognitive-structural base") and behavioral symptomatology (Aber, Allen, and Cicchetti, 1988). In both of these instances, we wished to extend our analyses of the impact of maltreatment beyond its effects on single domains of development to its effects on the relationships between domains of development.

Finally, our initial studies, although pointing to important between-group differences in the development of poor maltreated and nonmaltreated children, also increased our awareness of the considerable within-group differences. Our initial premise that maltreatment has a wide range of effects led to the hypothesis that these within-group differences could be accounted for in part by important environmental characteristics like authoritarian child-rearing practice and lack of access to community and other resources at (respectively) the micro- and meso-system levels of the ecology of human development (Belsky, 1980). In addition, we wished to explore whether certain parenting and family ecology variables mediate the relation between a history of maltreatment and children's socioemotional, cognitive, and behavioral development.

In summary, our first series of studies were designed to address three major issues: (1) Does maltreatment have an effect on socio-emotional development over and above the effects attributable to the family chaos associated with lower-class status and welfare dependency? Specifically, are maltreated preschool and early school-age children impaired in their relations with novel adults (e.g., more dependent and wary), less motivated by effectance, less cognitively mature (Study 1), and more behaviorally symptomatic (Study 2) than a well-matched sample of nonmaltreated children? (2) Is there evidence of an "organizational" effect of maltreatment on development; does maltreatment affect children across several interrelated domains of development (Studies 1 and 2)? (3) Are within-group differences in child development variables attributable to within-group differences in the family ecologies of maltreated children at the microsystem (parent–child relations) and mesosystem (access to community resources) levels (Study 3)?

We have completed studies that address the first two of these issues (Studies 1 and 2) and preliminary analyses that address the third (Study 3). In the next sections, we will summarize both the methods and the results of our studies. (Detailed methods and results are available in Aber and Allen, 1987; Aber, Allen, and Cicchetti, 1988; and Aber, Trickett, Carlson and Cicchetti, 1989.)

Study 1

Methods

Design. In order to enhance the generalizability of the findings of this study and thus narrow the gap between basic and applied research on the sequelae of child maltreatment, Study 1 focused upon a sample of maltreated children representative of the preschool and early school-age children in the caseloads of public and private social service agencies (Aber, 1982). Most families of these maltreated children (93 percent) were receiving or recently had been receiving Aid to Families with Dependent Children (AFDC). This investigation employed a two-comparison group strategy, comparing maltreated children both to children whose families are on AFDC and share other important sociodemographic characteristics and to nonmaltreated children from middle-class families, allowing the developmental status of the maltreated children to be compared to that of a "normative" sample of middle-class children and to a "high-risk" sample of lower-class children. This enabled us to begin to distinguish those aspects of socioemotional developmental status unique to the maltreated children from those aspects shared with the high-risk sample by virtue of their lower-class status (Aber and Cicchetti, 1984; Elmer, 1977).

Subjects. The children in this study comprised a cohort of 190 preschool and early school-age children from a short-term longitudinal study of the development of maltreated children (Cicchetti et al., 1987; Cicchetti and Rizley, 1981). Three samples of children between the ages of 4.0 and 8.1 years old were recruited for the study. The mean age for the children in each of the three samples was 5.7 or 5.8 years old.

The *children from maltreating families* (n = 93, 52 boys and 41 girls) were referred to the study by social workers from public and private protective

Table 18.1. *Demographic characteristics for maltreated, AFDC, middle-class children and their families*

	Group					
	Maltreated (n = 93)		AFDC (n = 67)		Middle Class (n = 30)	
Demographic characteristics	M	SD	M	SD	M	SD
Child's age (years)	5 .7	1.2	5.7	1.3	5.8	1.2
Child's race (% minority)	11%		15%		17%	
Household prestige score (1–100 scale)	47.4	5.3	49.2	5.9	60.6	7.7
Annual family income (in thousands of dollars, 1981–1984)	$9.0	$6.8	$7.7	$6.1	$28.4	$14.3
Ratio of adults to children in the home	.69	.53	.74	.43	.81	.46
Mother's age (years)	30.1	5.1	30.5	5.1	34.3	4.8
Mother's highest grade	11.1	2.0	11.7	2..1	14.6	2.3
Spouse/partner in home (% yes)	40%		28%		73%	

service agencies in urban and suburban communities in a New England state. Each child in this group either (1) was reported to the state as a maltreated child (n = 87), or (2) had a sibling reported to the state as maltreated and the child himself or herself was named in the treatment plan as in need of protective services (n = 6). In either case, the initial report of maltreatment was investigated by the state and confirmed. As reported by their case workers, the children suffered from multiple and overlapping types of maltreatment, most commonly physical neglect (71%), emotional mistreatment (41%), and physical injury (40%). (See Carlson, Cicchetti, Barnett, and Braunwald, this volume, for a fuller description of our methods for measuring types of maltreatment.)

The *children from AFDC families* (n = 67, 34 boys and 33 girls) were recruited through advertisements placed in welfare offices, in housing projects, neighborhood stores, and laundromats near welfare offices, and in newspapers with heavy readership in poor communities. Each child in this group lived in a family presently receiving welfare stipends.

The *children from middle-class families* (n = 30, 13 boys and 17 girls) were recruited by advertisements asking for volunteers to participate in studies of family life and child development. Each child in this group lived in a family that had at least one working parent and was not receiving welfare stipends. Before participation in the study began, a parent of each nonmaltreated (AFDC and middle-class) child was interviewed to ensure that the child had not been reported to the state for child abuse or neglect.

Table 18.1 presents data on family and child demographic characteristics

Table 18.2. *Measures of socioemotional development*

Domain	Construct	Measure
Relationships with novel adults	Dependency	Marble-in-the-hole
	Wariness	Marble-in-the-hole
	Interpersonal distance	Felt board game
	Verbal attention-seeking	Sticker game
	Imitation	Sticker game
	Approval-seeking smiles	Puzzle preference task
Effectance motivation	Pictorial curiosity	Cardboard houses task
	Variability-seeking	Box maze task
	Level of aspiration	Puzzle preference task
Cognitive maturity	IQ-equivalent	Peabody picture vocabulary test

for each of the three groups of children. The household prestige scores presented are based upon Mueller and Parcel's (1981) suggested use of Nock and Rossi's (1979) measures of family socioeconomic status, which account for differences between one- and two-parent families. Appropriate one-way analyses of variance were performed on group means for each continuous variable and chi-square analyses were performed for each categorical variable. As anticipated, there were no significant differences between AFDC and maltreating families on any demographic measures. There were consistent differences between these two groups and the middle-class group on all demographic characteristics except for the controlled variables of age, gender, and the ratio of adults to children in the home.

Measures. Study 1 focused on the socioemotional development of maltreated children in three domains of development: (a) relations with novel adults, (b) effectance motivation, and (c) cognitive maturity. Table 18.2 presents a summary of the domains of development, the constructs within each domain, and the measures of each construct used in Study 1. (A complete description of each construct and measure is available in Aber and Allen, 1987.)

Procedures. Family participation in the study was solicited either during initial recruitment interviews with parents at each child's home or by phone. Family and parent demographic data were collected during a subsequent interview. Child measures were collected in the first hour of each of two two-hour laboratory visits. In each visit, child and mother were greeted by a research assistant who described the measures and procedures and obtained informed consent. Then the research assistant escorted the child to an experimental room (which was furnished much like a big family playroom) and introduced the child to an experimenter whom the child had never met before.

The marble-in-the-hole game and the sticker game were administered in fixed order in visit 1. The felt board game, curiosity task, box maze task, puzzle preference task, and Peabody picture vocabulary test were administered in fixed order in visit 2. At the end of each visit, all families were paid $15.00 for their participation that day.

Different experimenters conducted visits 1 and 2. Experimenter's sex was assigned randomly and remained constant across visits for each child. Experimenters were drawn from a pool of approximately one dozen male and female experimenters who received extensive training and ongoing supervision in the administration of the measures. All experimenters were blind to children's group status (maltreated versus AFDC versus middle-class) as well as other salient family characteristics like parent education, occupation, income, and marital status.

Results

Analyses of the results of this study occurred in two stages. First, the psychometric characteristics and interrelationship of the 10 dependent measures described above were explored, with a factor analysis used to guide the construction of summary developmental outcome variables. These developmental outcome variables were then used in examining differences among maltreated, AFDC, and middle-class children in socioemotional development.

Summary developmental outcome variables. Scores on three of the measures (dependency, verbal attention-seeking, and imitation) were skewed in their distribution. Thus, they were subjected to natural log transformations and transformed scores were used in all subsequent analyses. Following this, the interrelationship of the 10 dependent measures was explored. Table 18.3 presents the intercorrelations of these variables for this sample. A principal factors analysis, varimax rotation, using squared multiple correlations for initial communality estimates was used to explore the factor structure underlying these 10 constructs.

The results are presented in Table 18.4. Two factors accounted for 100 percent of the variance in the reduced correlation matrix. Children who score high on Factor 1 are high in pictorial curiosity, variability-seeking, and cognitive maturity and low in dependency. This factor appears to tap children's "secure readiness to learn and to explore in the company of unfamiliar adults." Children who score high on Factor 2 are high on verbal attention-seeking, approval-seeking smiles, wariness, and imitation. This factor appears to tap children's compliant, externally-oriented style of problem

Table 18.3. *Zero-order correlations among dependent measures of development*

Developmental variables	Relationships with novel adults						Effectance motivation			IQ
	1	2	3	4	5	6	7	8	9	10
A Relationships with novel adults										
1 Dependancy (NL)										
2 Wariness	.03									
3 Interpersonal distance	.04	.02								
4 Verbal attention-seeking (NL)	−.06	.26	−.13							
5 Imitation (NL)	−.04	.07	.04	.22						
6 Approval-seeking smiles	.13	.05	−.10	.28	.20					
B Effectance motivation										
7 Pictorial curiosity	−.21	−.11	−.04	−.16	−.20	−.10				
8 Variability-seeking	−.11	−.20	.00	−.13	−.05	.04	.35			
9 Level of aspiration	−.11	.00	−.08	−.07	.04	−.07	.11	.18		
C Cognitive maturity										
10 IQ (derived)	−.16	.13	−.09	.03	−.06	.03	.28	.13	14	

Table 18.4. *Principal factors analysis of developmental variables*

Developmental variables	Factor loadings	
	Factor 1 (secure readiness)	Factor 2 (outer directedness)
A Relationships with novel adults		
Dependency[a] (NL)	−.34	
Wariness		.33
Interpersonal distance		
Verbal attention-seeking (NL)		.52
Imitation (NL)		.31
Approval-seeking smiles		.41
B Effectance motivation		
Pictorial curiosity	.57	
Variability-seeking	.47	
Level of aspiration		
C Cognitive maturity		
IQ (derived)	.45	

[a]NL denotes that variable was submitted to a natural log transformation.

Table 18.5. *Mean scores for and analyses of variance on summary developmental outcome variables*

| Summary developmental outcome variables | Group | | | | | | F (2,187) main effect for group | Post-hoc comparison of means |
| | Maltreated (n = 93) | | AFDC (n = 67) | | Middle class (n = 30) | | | |
	M	SD	M	SD	M	SD		
Secure readiness (Factor 1)	−.91	2.38	.43	2.35	1.98	2.00	19.28***	Maltx < AFDC < M.C.
Outer-directedness (Factor 2)	.21	2.42	.00	2.49	−.91	1.93	2.57^a	Maltx > M.C.

***$p < .001$
$^a p < .07$

solving, which is referred to as "outer-directedness." Factor scores for each factor were constructed by summing the unit weightings of standard scores of each variable loading above .30 on a factor.

Group differences on outcome variables. Prior to examining the main effects of Group on the secure readiness and outer-directedness factors, MANOVAs were performed to determine the main effects of child's age and gender, experimenter gender, and the interaction of each of these three variables with Group on the factors. A significant main effect of age was revealed using Wilk's criterion (F [2, 187] = 27.66; $p < .001$). Simple correlations revealed that child's age was significantly positively related to secure readiness ($r = .39$, $p < .001$) and significantly negatively related to outer-directedness ($r = .34$; $p < .001$). A significant effect for child gender was revealed (F [2, 187] = 3.48; $p < .05$) and followed with ANOVAs that revealed a significant effect of child gender on outer-directedness. Boys appeared more outer-directed than girls (means: boys = .39, girls = −.51; F [1, 188] = 6.99, $p < .01$). Given these findings, child's age and gender were covaried in further analyses involving both outer-directedness and secure readiness. No significant main effects of experimenter gender or interactions of Group with child's age or gender or with experimenter gender were found for the two factors.

A MANCOVA was next performed to test the effect of Group on the factors while covarying the effects of child's age and gender. The null hypothesis was rejected using Wilk's criterion (F [4, 368] = 11.57, $p < .001$). This analysis was followed with one-way analyses of covariance of the effects of group on children's scores for each of the two factors with a posteriori tests of differences between pairs of means conducted using the Duncan method. As Table 18.5 indicates, a significant main effect for group was found for secure readiness. Maltreated children scored lower than AFDC children, who in turn scored lower than middle-class children. Although no group differences were found in outer-directedness in a 3-group analysis, post-hoc comparisons of means indicated that both maltreated and AFDC children scored higher than middle-class children.

Discussion

These data indicate that the multiple measures of children's socioemotional functioning that we used in this study represent two theoretically meaningful underlying constructs of early childhood development: secure readiness to learn and outer directedness. Further, the data reveal that these two underlying constructs are differentially sensitive to a history of maltreatment over and above the effects of low socioeconomic status.

The Secure Readiness factor is composed of high effectance motivation (pictorial curiosity and variability seeking), high cognitive maturity, and low dependency. This factor can be interpreted tentatively as an organizational construct of competence in early childhood, because it seems to reflect the integration of cognitive, social, and emotional functioning required to meet the adaptational demands of a particular stage-salient task (Sroufe, 1979; Sroufe and Waters, 1977; Waters and Sroufe, 1983). Similar to the organizational construct of security of attachment in infancy, secure readiness to learn in early childhood also appears to represent a dynamic balance between establishing safe, secure relationships with adults and feeling free enough to venture out to explore the world in a manner that is likely to promote maturation of cognitive competencies.

As the results of the MANCOVA for the effects of Group indicated, children's secure readiness to learn showed a clear association with group status. Maltreated children demonstrated significantly less secure readiness to learn than did AFDC children, who in turn demonstrated significantly less than the middle-class children. These findings of group differences in secure readiness are consistent with previous research of the effects of maltreatment on infant and toddler development (Egeland and Sroufe, 1981; Schneider-Rosen et al., 1985). At both developmental stages, maltreatment appears to distort the balance between children's security-promoting operations and effectance-promoting operations.

The Outer Directedness factor is composed of verbal attention seeking, approval-seeking smiles, wariness, and imitation. Theoretically, outer directedness has been defined as an orientation to problem solving in which the young child relies on external cues rather than on his or her own cognitive resources. Zigler believes that this dimension also taps the extent of children's conformity to or compliance with adults, especially for children from environments where a high degree of compliance has adaptive value (Zigler and Balla, 1982).

Consistent with earlier findings (Zigler and Balla, 1982), the two more cognitively immature and socially deprived groups – maltreated children and AFDC children – scored higher on outer directedness than did the middle-class children. However, the maltreated and AFDC groups did not significantly differ from each other in their degree of outer directedness. Thus, unlike its effect on secure readiness to learn, maltreatment does not appear to have an effect on young children's outer directedness over and above the effects attributable to their lower socioeconomic status.

Study 2

Methods

Design. Study 2 addressed several limits of the existing work on the behavioral symptomatology of maltreated children (see Aber, Allen, and Cicchetti, 1988, for a discussion of the limits). It employed a research design with both sufficient power to detect moderate-sized effects and an appropriately matched comparison group to examine the effects of maltreatment on symptomatology independent of the effects of socioeconomic status. These design features also enabled us to examine differences between poor maltreated and poor nonmaltreated children by age (preschool versus school-age) and by gender. In addition, we employed a normed measure of children's behavioral symptomatology – the Child Behavior Checklist (CBCL) (Achenbach and Edelbrock, 1983). Use of the CBCL allowed us to compare the results of this study to the results from Achenbach's and Edelbrock's norming studies, and thus increase the generalizability and interpretability of the findings.

Finally, following the developmental–structural approach to child psychopathology articulated by Kohlberg and others, Study 2 examined the relationship between children's behavioral symptomatology and the two developmental variables suggested by Study 1 of the socioemotional development of maltreated preschool and school-age children (Aber and Allen, 1987): (1) children's secure readiness to learn in the company of novel adults, and (2) children's outer directed style of problem solving. Both of these constructs meet Kohlberg's criteria of a developmental–adaptational trait and have been theoretically and empirically linked to high-risk status in previous studies of maltreated and/or socially deprived children (Aber and Allen, 1987; Zigler and Balla, 1982). Thus, this study went beyond the test of group differences in behavioral symptomatology between maltreated and nonmaltreated children to an examination of several underlying developmental processes thought to be associated with symptomatology.

Subjects. The children in this study consisted of a cohort of 128 preschool and school-age children from the larger short-term longitudinal study of the development of maltreated children (Aber and Allen, 1987; Cicchetti et al., 1987). The middle-class sample included in Study 1 ($n = 30$) was dropped from Study 2 because of funding limitations and because the initial sample was too small to permit analyses by age and gender. Of the 160 remaining maltreated and lower-class comparison children, we were unable to collect symptomatology data on 20% ($n = 32$) for a variety of reasons such as the family moving to an unknown address, or parents deciding to end participation in the study. Thus, we were able to retain for this study a preschool sample (ages 4.0 to 5.9) that consisted of 40 maltreated and 28 lower-class comparison children (mean ages 4.8 and 4.9 respectively) and a school-age sample (ages 6.0 to 8.8) comprised of 29 maltreated and 31 lower-class comparison children (mean ages 6.7 and 6.9 respectively).

In addition to the samples described above, we used published norms on the child symptomatology reported by parents of clinical and nonclinical samples of children that were part of the standardization study for the CBCL (Achenbach and Edelbrock, 1983). Norms are based upon data on 400 children ages 4 to 5 and 1200 children aged 6 to 11, divided equally between genders and between a clinical sample of children referred to mental health service settings and a nonclinical sample obtained through random sampling of families in Washington, D.C., Northern Virginia, and Maryland. Both clinical and nonclinical samples were racially and socioeconomically heterogeneous, although there was a slight underrepresentation of the lowest 2 steps of Hollingshead's (1957) measure of socioeconomic status in the nonclinical sample. (See Achenbach and Edelbrock, 1983, for a more complete description of the sampling procedure.)

Measures. In addition to the measures described in Study 1, which resulted in the two composite measures of "secure readiness to learn" and "outer-directedness," Study 2 included a parent rating of the frequency of the child's symptomatic behaviors over the prior 12 months. From this Child Behavior Checklist (CBCL), we derived a measure of the child's *overall behavioral symptomatology* as well as measures of the four "narrow-band syndromes" derived from factor analysis of the CBCL (Achenbach and Edelbrock, 1983) and which were common to both boys and girls in the preschool and early school-age years. These narrow-band syndromes were: aggression (e.g., tantrums, fighting), depression (e.g., feeling guilty, feeling worthless), social withdrawal (e.g., refusing to talk), and somatic complaints (e.g., stomach problems, aches and pains). (These narrow-band syndromes and their composition are described more fully in Achenbach and Edelbrock, 1983.)

Although these syndromes are not arithmetically independent – several items load on more than one syndrome – analysis of these syndromes does permit exploration of the type of symptomatology present, which the simple total score for behavioral symptomatology does not allow. In this sample, intercorrelations between syndrome scores ranged from .14 to .62, with the strongest correlations between the aggressive, depressed, and social withdrawal syndromes. Use of common syndromes across the age and gender groupings studied allows for consideration of developmental and gender-specific effects of maltreatment upon symptomatology. Because the syndromes are constructed somewhat differently for different age-gender groupings, scores from these syndromes were standardized within each of the four age-gender groupings for analyses that combined samples across either age or gender.

Procedure. The data collection procedures for the composite variables for "secure readiness" and "outer directedness" have been described above in Study 1.

In addition, for Study 2, the CBCL was administered to each child's mother either while the child was taking part in an experimental session or during a separate home visit. The child was never present during the administration of this measure. Because of logistical difficulties, the lag-time between collection of the laboratory measures of socioemotional development and collection of the CBCL averaged 4.4 months for this study (s.d. = 9.6 months). The CBCL was collected at most 1.8 years before to 2.8 years after the lab visits.

Results

Results of the study are presented in three parts. First, the main effects of maltreatment on symptomatology and the interactions of maltreatment with age and gender are examined using the maltreating and lower-class samples in this study. Next, these two samples are briefly compared to the normal and clinical populations of children studies by Achenbach and Edelbrock (1983) in the standardization of the CBCL. This was done so as to place the results from the samples collected for this study in the context of broadly sampled normative data. Finally, correlations between reported symptomatology and developmental status and the interactions of these with maltreatment are presented to illuminate the relationship between socioemotional development and reported symptomatology in maltreated and poor nonmaltreated children.

Group symptomatology comparisons. Because the four different measures of behavioral syndromes were based upon some identical items and were nonindependent, experiment-wise protection against Type I errors was achieved by first examining the effects of maltreatment on the total level of behavior symptomatology. Only when significant differences in levels of total symptomatology were found were specific behavioral syndromes examined. This is appropriate in terms of assuring that effects with behav-

Table 18.6. *Group differences in symptomatology*

	4- to 5-year-olds			6- to 9-year-olds		
	Maltx (n = 40)	LowCl. (n = 28)	F(1,64)	Maltx (n = 29)	LowCl. (n = 31)	F(1,56)
Total behavior problems [a]	50.1 (18.2)	48.2 (22.4)	0.13	55.9 (24.6)	41.0 (21.2)	6.20*
Aggressive	16.3 (8.5)	14.3 (8.4)	0.77	19.0 (10.0)	14.9 (8.5)	3.00+
Depressed	8.3 (4.9)	9.5 (6.0)	1.20	9.6 (5.4)	6.4 (4.9)	5.52*
Social withdrawal	5.0 (3.4)	5.8 (4.9)	0.58	4.9 (2.8)	3.2 (2.7)	5.39*
Somatic complaints	4.4 (3.7)	3.8 (3.8)	1.63	2.8 (2.8)	2.6 (3.0)	0.03

Note: Syndromes at different ages are comprised of slightly different behaviors. Similarly, syndrome scores are comprised of varying numbers of items. Thus, comparisons in absolute levels of symptomatology across age or across syndromes should not be made.
[a] Because of missing data, each analysis with total behavior problems has 1 fewer degree of freedom in the error term than other analyses.
+ p < .10
* p < .05

ioral syndromes are interpreted only if they reflect significant overall differences in symptomatology (when syndromes are most likely to be clinically significant).

A 3-way analysis of variance (ANOVA) was conducted initially to determine the overall effects of maltreatment and its interactions with age (4–5 vs. 6–9) and gender groupings upon children's total level of behavioral symptomatology. This test revealed a significant main effect of maltreatment on reported symptomatology, with maltreated children exhibiting higher levels of symptomatic behaviors than lower-class comparison children (M maltreated = 52.5, M lower class = 44.4, F [2, 229] = 44.4, p < .04). It also revealed a trend toward an interaction effect of maltreatment with age of child (F [1, 119] = 2.93, p < .09), in which maltreated children exhibit substantially more symptomatology than comparison in the school-age group, but only slightly more in the preschool-age group. No interactions of gender with maltreatment or age were found. As a result of these findings, follow-up analyses with narrow-band scales of symptomatology were conducted separately for preschool and school-age children.

Table 18.6 presents data on symptomatology separately for preschool and school-age children along with the results of ANOVAs to determine whether significant differences exist between maltreated and lower-class comparison children. The results presented in Table 18.2 indicate that school-age maltreated children are reported by their mothers to display more depressed and socially withdrawn behaviors as well as a higher level of overall symptomatology than do school-age children in lower-class comparison families. A trend in this direction was also found with aggressive behaviors. No significant differences were found between groups at the preschool level. Because this study sought to explore fully the effects of within-group differences among children (e.g., gender and age), tests for interaction of child's gender with maltreatment were also conducted at this level. No significant interactions were found.

Comparisons to normative data. The second phase of analysis involved comparing the two samples collected for this study to established norms for clinical and nonclinical populations of children. Published data on the means, standard deviations and sample sizes for the symptomatology measures from Achenbach and Edelbrock's (1983, Appendix D) samples of children were used for these analyses.

One-way ANOVAs were used to examine group differences among the two normative samples and the maltreated and lower-class comparison children in this study. Significant ANOVAs were followed with Duncan *a posteriori* tests of differences between pairs of means. These results, presented in Table 18.7, show that for total behavioral symptomatology across all four age X gender groupings, maltreated children had significantly more symptomatology than Achenbach and Edelbrock's nonclinical sample and were never statistically distinct from the clinic-referred sample. In all cases, the lower class children also were rated as significantly more symptomatic than the nonclinical samples. For the school-age children, but not the preschool children, the lower-class sample was rated as significantly less symptomatic than the clinical and maltreated samples.

Examination of group differences on the specific symptom scales revealed that, for the preschool children, the nonclinical normative sample was typically significantly less symptomatic than each of the other three samples. Clinical, maltreated and lower-class children could not typically be statistically distinguished from each other at this age. For the school-age children, a similar pattern existed, except that for about half of the comparisons the lower-class comparison children were significantly less symptomatic than the clinical and maltreated samples of children. Overall, these data indicate patterns of results that were almost identical to those found with total behavioral symptomatology. In 15 of 16 possible comparisons of groups using the four behavior problem scales across the four age–gender groupings, the maltreated children were significantly more symptomatic than the Achenbach and Edelbrock nonclinical sample and were statistically indistin-

Table 18.7. *Comparisons with Achenbach and Edelbrock (1983) normative data on symptomatology: means and standard deviations*

	Maltx	LowCl	Clin	NonClin	F(3,232)	Post-hoc comparison of means
4- to 5-year-old boys						
	(n = 22)	(n = 14)	(n = 100)	(n = 100)		
Total						
behavior	48.4	47.1	59.8	24.1	41.01***	C, M, L > N
problems	(19.3)	(19.1)	(30.1)	(14.2)		& C > L
Aggressive	17.6	17.4	23.9	9.7	23.27***	C, M, L > N
	(9.4)	(6.2)	(11.7)	(6.4)		
Depressed	9.8	10.7	12.6	5.4	18.71***	C, L, M > N
Social	4.4	5.5	5.9	1.9	22.10***	C, L, M > N
withdrawal	(3.4)	(4.6)	(4.5)	(2.0)		
Somatic	2.0	1.5	2.0	0.6	11.25***	C, M > N
complaints	(1.7)	(1.2)	(2.4)	(0.9)		
4- to 5-year-old girls						
	(n = 18)	(n = 14)	(n = 100)	(n = 100)		
Total						
behavior	52.2	49.4	58.8	25.2	35.18***	C, M, L > N
problems	(16.9)	(26.0	(29.1)	(17.1)		
Aggressive	14.7	11.1	15.2	5.8	23.27***	C, M, L > N
	(7.2)	(9.4)	(10.4)	(5.2)		
Depressed	6.5	8.3	9.3	3.4	22.74***	C, L, M > N
	(2.8)	(6.2)	(6.1)	(4.1)		
Social	5.7	6.1	7.1	2.2	22.01***	C, L, M > N
withdrawal	(3.4)	(5.3)	(5.4)	(2.9)		
Somatic	7.4	6.1	7.8	3.6	19.78***	C, M, L > N
complaints	(3.4)	(4.0)	(4.8)	(3.0)		
6- to 11-year-old boys						
	(n = 13)	(n = 16)	(n = 300)	(n = 300)		
Total						
behavior	56.8	45.6	58.9	21.7	173.4***	C, M > L > N
problems	(25.0)	(20.9)	(24.0)	(15.0)		
Aggressive	19.5	16.2	19.1	7.3	119.41***	M, C, L > N
	(10.3)	(9.2)	(9.2)	(5.7)		
Depressed	8.1	6.4	10.1	3.2	90.69***	C, M, L > N
	(5.6)	(5.1)	(6.4)	(3.4)		& C > L
Social	4.0	2.9	4.8	1.7	76.02***	C, M > N
withdrawal	(2.5)	(2.0)	(3.1)	(1.8)		&C > L
Somatic	1.4	2.1	1.9	0.8	18.10***	C, L > N
complaints	(1.2)	(2.5)	(2.3)	(1.3)		
6- to 11-year-old boys						
	(n = 16)	(n = 15)	(n = 300)	(n = 300)		
Total						
behavior	55.1	36.1	58.4	19.9	168.27***	C, M > L > N
problems	(25.1)	(21.1)	(26.2)	(14.2)		

Table 18.7. *(cont.)*

	Maltx	LowCl	Clin	NonClin	F(3,232)	Post-hoc comparison of means
Aggressive	18.6	13.5	20.2	7.2	123.16***	C, M > L > N
	(10.2)	(7.7)	(10.1)	(6.0)		
Depressed	10.9	6.3	12.9	4.2	123.56***	C, M > L, N
	(5.1)	(4.9)	(7.0)	(3.7)		
Social	5.7	3.4	6.4	1.8	101.32***	C, M > L, N
withdrawal	(2.9)	(3.4)	(4.2)	(1.9)		
Somatic	4.0	3.1	4.3	1.7	34.40***	C, M > N
complaints	(3.3)	(3.5)	(3.9)	(2.0)		

Note: M = Maltreated children, L = Lower class children, C = Clinical normative group, N = Nonclinical normative group. Clinical and nonclinical groups are from Achenbach and Edelbrock (1983) normative data. Syndromes at different ages are comprised of slightly different behaviors. Thus, comparisons in absolute levels of symptomatology across age should not be made.

N's and degrees of freedom for analyses involving 4-year-old girls total symptomatology and 6-year-old girls total symptomatology are 1 less than other analyses presented for these groups due to missing data.

***$p < .001$

guishable in symptomatology from their clinical sample. Lower-class comparison children most frequently were classified similarly to maltreated children. Overall, in 11 of 16 comparisons, lower-class children were significantly more symptomatic than the nonclinical sample. Finally, in 5 of 16 comparisons, lower-class children were significantly less symptomatic than the clinic-referred children.

Relationship of symptomatology and developmental status. The final stage of analysis examined the correlations between behavioral symptomatology and developmental status to explore the relationship between development and symptomatology in groups of children-at-risk. Given the interactions of age with the effects of maltreatment on symptomatology reported previously, these analyses were conducted separately for preschool and school-age children. Initial analyses were performed to determine whether the relationship between developmental status and reported symptomatology differed across maltreatment status. These tests revealed interaction effects

Table 18.8. *Correlations of developmental status with reported symptomatology*

	Total behavior problems	Aggressive	Depressed	Social withdrawal	Somatic complaints
Preschool					
Maltx (n = 40[a])					
Secure readiness	−.37*	−.32*	−.30+	−.34*	.05
Outer-directedness	.17	.13	.10	.15	.01
Non-Maltx (n = 28)					
Secure readiness	.06	−.03	.23	−.22	−.02
Outer-directedness	.44*	.54**	.17	.47*	.27
Early school-age					
Combined Sample (n = 60)					
Secure readiness	.07	.08	.18	.06	.30*
Outer-directedness	−.02	−.07	−.04	−.00	.13

[a]Because of missing data, each analysis with total behavior problems has 1 fewer degree of freedom than other analyses.
+$p < .10$
*$p < .05$
**$p < .01$

for preschool-age children in which maltreatment status affected the relationship of total reported symptomatology to both secure readiness to learn ($F [1, 61] = 3.88; p < .04$) and outerdirectedness ($F [1, 61] = 3.49; p < .05$). No interaction effects were found for school-age children (all $ps < .25$). Thus, the correlations between reported symptomatology and measures of developmental status are reported in Table 18.8 separately by maltreatment status for younger children and for the combined sample of maltreated and nonmaltreated school-age children.

Examination of the correlations reported in Table 18.8 reveals different patterns of relationships between symptomatology and developmental status for maltreated and nonmaltreated preschool-age children. For maltreated preschoolers, low levels of secure readiness to learn are related to total reported behavioral symptomatology and to syndromes of aggressive, depressed, and socially withdrawn behavior. No such relationship between secure readiness and symptomatology was found for nonmaltreated preschoolers. However, for these children, outerdirectedness was significantly correlated with total levels of reported symptomatology and with syndromes of aggressive and socially withdrawn behavior; however, no relationship between outerdirectedness and symptomatology was found for maltreated preschoolers.

For school-age children, no significant relationships were found between either measure of developmental status and overall symptomatology. A positive correlation was found between secure readiness and somatic complaints, although its statistical and practical significance may be questioned.

Discussion

The results of Study 2 refine and extend the results of previous studies that have investigated the behavioral symptomatology of maltreated children. The pattern of group differences and the relationship between behavioral symptomatology and developmental-adaptational processes varies considerably with the children's developmental stage.

Preschool years. Direct comparisons of the levels of symptomatology between poor maltreated preschoolers and poor nonmaltreated preschoolers revealed no group differences. However, additional analyses employing norms from Achenbach's and Edelbrock's (1983) study indicated that both the poor maltreated and poor nonmaltreated preschoolers were more symptomatic than a nonclinical sample. Further, the levels of symptomatology among the maltreated and comparison children were indistinguishable from the levels of symptomatology in Achenbach's and Edelbrock's clinically referred sample. These data suggest that the lack of group differences between the poor maltreated and poor nonmaltreated preschoolers is, at least in part, a reflection of the elevated levels of symptomatology in the nonmaltreated comparison group.

Consistent with the position of such theorists as Kohlberg, Sroufe, and Greenspan, preschoolers' levels of symptomatology were associated with their scores on measures of developmental–adaptational characteristics. Interestingly, the developmental correlates of symptomatology differed for the two groups of preschoolers studied. Low secure readiness was associated with greater symptomatology for maltreated preschoolers, but high outer-directedness was not. In contrast, high outerdirectedness (but not low secure readiness) was associated with greater symptomatology for the poor non-maltreated preschoolers.

Early school-age years. In contrast to the findings for preschoolers, direct comparisons of the levels of symptomatology from poor maltreated and nonmaltreated school-age children revealed clear group differences. Maltreated school-age children were more symptomatic in general, more depressed, socially withdrawn, and marginally more aggressive in terms of behavioral syndromes. The additional analyses employing Achenbach's and Edelbrock's norms indicate that, in general, maltreated children's levels of symptomatology could not be distinguished from the levels of a clinic-referred sample. Both the maltreated and clinic-referred children scored higher in symptomatology than the poor, nonmaltreated children, who in turn scored higher than a nonclinical, normal sample.

Finally, we found no relationships between either secure readiness or outerdirectedness and total behavioral symptomatology among the school-age children. Perhaps these constructs are less sensitive measures of adaptation at this developmental stage. Or perhaps school-age children's levels of symptomatology are related to deficits in different areas of development, such as the development of intention cue detection skills (Dodge, Murphy, and Buchsbaum, 1984).

Study 3

Methods

Design. Due to our participation in a multisample study of social class differences in the sequelae of physical child abuse (Trickett, Aber, Carlson, and Cicchetti, 1989), we have recently begun to analyze data that permits us to address the question of within-group differences in the development of maltreated and lower-class comparison children. For the purposes of this preliminary study, we wished to investigate whether differences in the ecologies of children-at-risk are associated with differences in their levels of cognitive maturity (PPVT scores) and behavioral symptomatology (CBCL total symptom scores).

For analytic purposes, we wished to explore aspects of the child's ecology at the microsystem (e.g., parent–child relations) level and at the mesosystem (parent–community interactions) level. Thus, we measured: at the microsystem level, aspects of parents' childrearing values and practices thought to be related both to risk for maltreatement and to child developmental outcome, specifically parental (1) authoritarian control, (2) enjoyment of the child, and (3) encouragement of child autonomy; and, at the mesosystem level, aspects of the family environment, including (4) level of family resources (e.g., cohesion, expressiveness, and lack of conflict) and (5) access to various types of community resources (e.g., intellectual/cultural, activities/recreational, moral/religious). These measures were selected both because of their relevance to theories of key elements of the ecology of child maltreatment (Belsky, 1980; Garbarino, 1982) and because of their potential to account for some of the variance in child development outcomes usually associated with more global measures of risk or socioeconomic status.

In summary, in Study 3 we hypothesized that for both poor maltreated and poor nonmaltreated children, within group differences in parents' childrearing values and practices and family environments would be significantly associated with differences in children's behavioral symptomatology and cognitive maturity.

Subjects. Because these data were analyzed for a collaborative multisample study (Trickett et al., 1989), only those children who met the criteria for the collaborative study (who were between the ages of 4.0 and 8.0 and who had been physically abused but not sexually abused) were included in this preliminary study. Thus, 90 of the 128 children from Study 2, 37 maltreated and 53 lower-class comparison children, were subjects for Study 3. As in Studies 1 and 2, the two samples did not differ on any measured demographic features, including age and gender of child; SES, race, and education of the mother; or proportion of single-parent families.

Measures. In addition to the demographic variables and the Peabody Picture Vocabulary test (described in Study 1) and the Child Behavior Checklist (described in Study 2), two additional measures of the children's ecologies were included in Study 3. During a visit to the home, each child's mother responded to the Child Rearing Practices Q-sort (CRPQ) (Block and Block, 1980) and the Family Environment Scale (FES) (Moos and Moos, 1981). From the CRPQ, three superordinate scales were derived from a subset of the authors' 23 original scales: authoritarian control, enjoyment of the child, and encouraging autonomy. From the FES, two superordinate scales were derived from a subset of the author's 10 original scales: family resources and community resources. The precise methods of calculating these three superordinate scale scores of the child's microsystem (parent-child relations) and the two scale scores of the child's mesosystem (family ecology) are described in Trickett et al., 1989.

Results

In order to begin to examine the hypothesis that within-group differences in children's ecologies were associated with within-group differences in child developmental outcomes, two sets of Pearson correlations were computed. Families' five superordinate scale scores were correlated with children's scores on the PPVT and CBCL. These 10 correlations were computed separately for the poor maltreated and poor nonmaltreated samples. The results are presented in Table 18.9.

For the maltreated children, several different characteristics of their ecologies were related to child outcomes. Maltreated children whose parents reported enjoying them less (microsystem) and having more limited access to community resources (mesosystem) were described by their parents as

Table 18.9. *Correlations between children's ecologies and their developmental outcomes by group*

	Maltreated children		Comparison children	
Ecological variables	Total Beh. Prob.	PPVT	Total Beh. Prob.	PPVT
Microsystem:CRPQ				
Authoritarian control	.19	−.24	−.08	−.28
Enjoyment of child	−.52**	.05	−.33*	.08
Encouraging autonomy	−.06	.42*	.21	.21
Mesosystem:FES				
Family resources	−.21	.13	−.10	.25
Community resources	−.42*	.31	−.10	.01

$*p < .05$
$**p < .01$

more behaviorally symptomatic. Maltreated children whose parents reported less encouragement of autonomy (microsystem) scored lower on the PPVT, a measure of relative cognitive maturity.

In contrast, only one feature of the poor nonmaltreated children's ecologies was related to child outcome. Like the maltreated children, comparison children whose parents reported enjoying their child less were described by those parents as more behaviorally symptomatic.

Discussion

In summary, of the 10 correlations between ecology and outcome, 3 were significant for the maltreated children and 1 was significant for the nonmaltreated children. In addition, seven of the total 20 correlations ranged in absolute value between .21 and .33 and may prove significant with a larger sample size. Also, with a new and larger sample, a priori tests of the multivariate relationships between features of the children's ecologies and their development would be instructive.

Despite these limits to this preliminary study, it seems fair to conclude that for maltreated children, within-group variation in developmental outcomes is associated with theoretically meaningful within-group variation in their ecologies at the micro- and mesosystem levels. Not enjoying one's child and lack of access to community resources are strongly associated with high levels of behavioral symptomatology in maltreated children. In addition, discouraging autonomy is associated with lower cognitive maturity scores. For the poor nonmaltreated children, variation in ecology appears to be more weakly associated with variation in children's development. Two additional points are noteworthy. First, despite our predictions, authoritarian control appears less important as a source of within-group variation in the development of children-at-risk than do other features of their ecologies (but see Trickett et al., 1989). Second, different features of children's ecologies appear to predict to distinct features of children's development. The implications of these tentative findings for scientific theory, clinical, and policy concerns are discussed in the next section of this chapter.

General discussion

Theoretical/research issues

The results of Study 1 indicate that a history of maltreatment has a discernable effect on children's socioemotional development over and above the effects attributable to poverty and welfare dependency. These effects – on children's dependent relations with novel adults, effectance motivation, and cognitive maturity – are best described as "organizational." Across these three interrelated domains of adaptive functioning, poor maltreated children perform less well than an appropriately matched sample of poor nonmaltreated children. This suggests an effect on the organization of development, not just on individual, separate features of development. We have interpreted this pattern to indicate that maltreated preschool and early school-age children are less securely ready to learn in the company of novel adults.

In two other domains of socioemotional development, other patterns of group differences (between poor maltreated and poor nonmaltreated children) were observed. In Study 1, on a composite measure of children's outerdirectedness (a less mature form of cognitive problem-solving), poor maltreated children and poor nonmaltreated children both scored significantly higher than middle-class nonmaltreated children, but did not differ from each other. These data suggest that socioeconomic status, not maltreatment status, may have the determining influence on outerdirectedness. Similarly, in Study 2 on a composite measure of behavioral symptomatology, poor maltreated and poor nonmaltreated children were rated significantly higher than a middle-class nonclinical sample of children; but the maltreated children's level of symptomatology exceeded that of the comparison children only in the early school-age years (6–8 years old), not the preschool years (4–5 years old). Perhaps the poor maltreated children were rated as more symptomatic than the poor nonmaltreated children only for the older group years because symptomatology is a function of the duration of maltreatment (and older children may have been mistreated longer). Alternatively, perhaps the level of maltreated children's symptomatology becomes clearer to their parents when the children attempt to meet the adaptational demands of school and parents begin to receive negative feedback on their children via teacher reports and comparisons to peers.

We also presented evidence in Study 2 that suggests that poor maltreated children and poor nonmaltreated children may travel different developmental pathways to behavioral symptomatology in the preschool years. Specifically, for maltreated preschoolers, low secure readiness (but not outerdirectedness) was associated with increased symptomatology; conversely, for nonmaltreated preschoolers, high outerdirectedness (but not secure readiness) was associated with greater symptomatology. Although this specific finding requires replication, it nonetheless serves to illustrate the importance of a basic premise of the emerging field of developmental psychopathology: different processes may underlie the development of psychopathology for different subpopulations of children-at-risk.

The results of Study 3 indicated that within-group differences in maltreated children's developmental outcomes were associated with some within-group differences in the micro- and mesosystems levels of their developmental ecologies. Parents' enjoyment of their children and access to community resources were negatively associated with children's symptomatology; parents' encouragement of the children's autonomy was positively associated with children's cognitive maturity. Fewer and weaker associations between family ecology and child outcome were observed for the poor nonmaltreated children. (This complex set of issues concerning the interactive influence of maltreatment and socioeconomic status on family ecologies and child development is being explored more fully in a set of collaborative studies with Penelope Trickett of NIMH; see Trickett et al., 1989 and Aber et al., 1989.)

In summary, the hypotheses we derived from a variety of independent, domain-specific theories (attachment, social-cognitive, developmental–structural, and ecological theories) concerning the comparative development of poor maltreated and poor nonmaltreated children in the preschool and early school-age years were largely supported. We believe that this demonstrates the potential value of specific theories as the bases for specific hypotheses about the comparative development of maltreated children. However, these theories, and the specific hypotheses they can and do generate, do not yet constitute a unifying theory of the development of maltreated children. As we noted above, we hoped that our studies could contribute to such a unifying theory as the basis for informed, effective actions on behalf of maltreated children.

In order for a developmental theory both to be unifying and to constitute a useful basis for social action, it must effectively describe a finite set of lawful relationships between constructs. The theory will be as effective as it is able to (a) successfully summarize a large amount of complex information on relations between constructs, (b) help generate and integrate new information, (c) be used in a manner to assess the meaning of actions, and (d) provide a framework for the evaluation of success or failure of actions. In other words, for theory to guide action, it must be solidly grounded in fact and hence not as ethereal or irrefutable as "grand theories" like psychoanalysis. A useful theory must also function like a good metaphor, effectively summarizing and connoting as well as denoting. We have come to recognize and value this "metaphorical function" of theory (in general, and of the development of maltreated children in particular) through our work with clinicians, protective service workers, program planners, and policymakers. These actors clearly wish to gain more comprehensive and accurate knowledge of maltreated children on which to base their actions; but they cannot – indeed they should not have to – master the details of the very complex research literature emerging on the causes and effects of child maltreatment.

For these reasons, we wished to use superordinate principles to integrate our studies with others on the development of maltreated children and thus arrive at an initial formulation of the *central* (not the only) impact of maltreatment on early childhood development. We tentatively conclude that the central impact of maltreatment on early development is a distortion in the child's dynamic balance between security-promoting operations and competence-promoting operations. Extensive data consistent with this formulation are available from studies of the development of maltreated infants and toddlers based on attachment theory (Carlson et al., this volume; Cicchetti et al., 1987; Egeland and Sroufe, 1981; Lyons-Ruth, Connell, Zoll, and Stahl, 1987; Schneider-Rosen et al., 1985). These studies clearly demonstrate that maltreated infants and toddlers are less able to derive security and comfort from their primary caregiver and consequently are less able to competently explore the environment. Aber and Allen (1987), summarized in this chapter in Study 1, is the first study to test predictions drawn from attachment theory on the effects of maltreatment on development in the preschool and early school-age years. In our study, maltreated children exhibited increased dependence concerns, decreased effectance motivation, and an accompanying deficit in cognitive maturity. Because our data are so consistent with findings on the effects of maltreatment at earlier stages of development, we are persuaded that this imbalance in security-promoting versus competence-promoting operations will prove to be a replicable across-stage feature of the development of maltreated children.

This formulation of the central impact of maltreatment on early childhood development can form the basis for the theoretical integration of a variety of other findings. In our studies, the formulation helps provide a theoretical rationale for the process by which maltreatment results in higher levels of behavioral symptomatology. We have argued that preschoolers' "secure readiness to learn" constitutes what Kohlberg calls a "developmental-adaptational trait," a sequence in emotional development that has a cognitive–structural base. Kohlberg argues that lags in developmental–adaptational traits are the best childhood predictors of adult psychopathology. We have simply extended his argument to assert that such lags are effective predictors of childhood psychopathology as well. In short, we propose that "structuralized" preoccupation with security-promoting operations over competence-promoting operations is a causal/mediating factor that links a history of maltreatment with psychopathology in the preschool years.

Similarly, this formulation may help integrate the results of future ecological analyses of the development of maltreated children. A distortion in the dynamic balance between security-promoting and effectance-promoting operations can be viewed as the maltreated child's adaptations to characteristic features of maltreating families' childrearing environments. Although such adaptations may make short-term "sense" (for example, by reducing the probability that the child may provoke an abusive or severely rejecting response from the parent), previous theory and research from an organizational perspective suggests that such adaptations place the children at risk for adaptational failures at future key developmental tasks (Cicchetti and Aber, 1986; Sroufe and Rutter, 1984).

Finally, our formulation of the central impact of maltreatment on early childhood development suggests several key hypotheses that could be tested in future studies. The first set of hypotheses concerns the effect of maltreatment per se on development. As we have indicated, we believe that we've demonstrated that maltreatment can have an effect on development over and above the deleterious effects of the family disorganization associated with low socioeconomic status. As we become increasingly refined in specifying the developmental ecologies of maltreated children, we can use the same type of logic to ask if maltreatment has a discernable impact on development over and above certain features of the children's ecologies (for instance, over and above the parents' self-reported childrearing values and practices or their access to community resources; see Aber et al., 1989). Thus, in future studies, we wish to (1) identify several key features of the children's ecologies (e.g., parental characteristics like psychopathology and cognitive maturity and parent–child behavioral interaction styles like coerciveness in addition to childrearing values and family climate), and (2) examine the multivariate relationships among maltreatment status, socioeconomic status, and ecological variables and developmental outcome. Through such analyses, we hope to specify those features of the ecologies of maltreated children that have a causal influence on their development.

The second set of hypotheses concern the future adaptation of maltreated children. If maltreated children are less securely ready to learn, they may

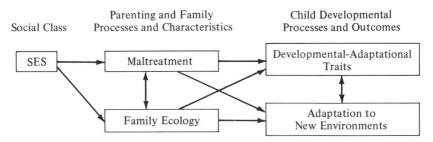

Figure 18.1. Schematic diagram of a unifying theory of the development of maltreated children.

also expereince difficulties in adapting to major demanding out-of-home environments like school and peer groups. According to organizational principles, incompetence at an earlier adaptational task (e.g., secure readiness) should predict incompetence at later tasks that make related adaptational demands. Thus, we hypothesize (a) that maltreated children will experience problems in establishing effective relationships with teachers and peers as well as problems in tasks requiring cognitive and academic competence in school, and (b) that the relationship between a history of maltreatment and these problems of adaptation to the school and peer environments will be mediated by developmental–adaptational traits such as secure readiness to learn and outerdirectedness.

In summary, the unifying theory of the development of maltreated children we are beginning to build is presented in Figure 18.1. Across the top line, we represent the general and successfully replicated findings that poverty is positively assoicated with maltreatment (Garbarino and Sherman, 1980; Gelles, 1975) and that maltreatment has a negative effect on development (Aber and Allen, 1987; Augostinos, 1987; Carlson et al., this volume; Lamphear, 1987). The lower line represents still poorly understood but important qualifications in the general set of relationships between social class, maltreatment, and developmental–adaptational traits. For example, as Studies 2 and 3 indicated, the level of impairment in maltreated children's development is associated with (a) variation in the nature of their family ecologies, and (b) variation in other outcomes such as symptomatology. More generally, our emergent unifying theory suggests that: (1) the effect of poverty on the probability of maltreatment is mediated by other features of the family's ecology; (2) similarly, the effects of maltreatment on children's development is also mediated by key features of their ecologies; and (3) the effects of maltreatment on children's adaptation to new environments (like school) is mediated by developmental–adaptational traits (like security).

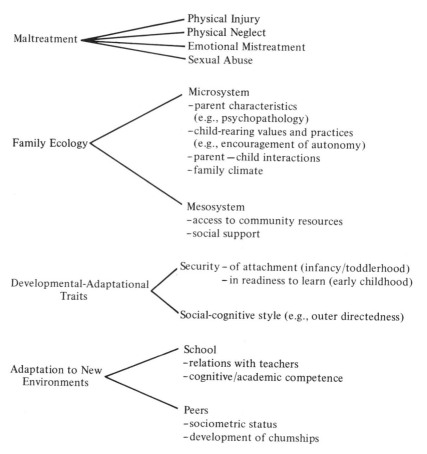

Figure 18.2. Latent variable structure for model of the effects of maltreatment on development.

Figure 18.2 presents examples of how each of these general constructs in our unifying theory could be operationalized. Indeed, the Harvard Child Maltreatment Project has collected these and other data on the children participating in these studies via home visits and follow-up studies of the children in their school environments. Thus, this emergent theory will guide our next phase of analyses of the effects of maltreatment on development during early childhood. These future analyses will employ structural equations modelling techniques to test the goodness of fit between this proposed model and the observed data. If the results confirm the heuristic value of our model, then we will be a significant step closer to a unifying theory of the development of maltreated children.

Clinical and policy implications

As we noted earlier, there are many difficulties and dangers involved in attempting to employ developmental knowledge to guide practical actions, especially in the area of child maltreatment. Clinicians who must identify, assess, treat, and follow up maltreated children and their families face terribly complex and painfully difficult decisions daily. Similarly, policymakers who must decide on which standards do and do not justify coercive state intervention and who must choose between devoting resources to this or other very pressing social problems also face complex, difficult decisions that greatly influence the lives of maltreated children and their families. In light of the prevailing conditions such as the confusion over what constitutes maltreatment, the dramatic increase in official reports of maltreated children and the severe limits in human and fiscal resources to address the problem, how can improved knowledge of the development of maltreated children possibly help the clinical and policy decisionmakers who are on the front lines?

We fear that as scientists, we ask this question too infrequently. But we have been enormously excited by the response of both protective service workers and child welfare service planners and policymakers when we do present the results of our studies to them. It appears as though our work can help them in several possible ways.

First, studies like those summarized in this chapter can help clinicians and policymakers become clearer about the "emotional damage" inflicted by maltreatment. The wisdom of using such a subjective concept as "emotional damage" to justify state intervention has come under severe criticism for its vagueness and potential race and class bias (Solnit, 1980). However, because so many citizens and professionals believe that emotional damage often is the most serious or important harm to the maltreated child, others have recommended retaining it as a basis for state intervention but limiting its potential bias by requiring that it be "evidenced by severe anxiety, depression, withdrawal or untoward aggression toward self or others" (Juvenile Justice Standards Project, 1977). Although specifying and documenting actual physical harm is relatively straightforward, it is much more difficult to specify and document emotional harms such as severe anxiety, depression, or withdrawal (Aber and Zigler, 1981). Studies such as those summarized by Carlson et al. (this volume) and by this chapter begin to sketch the parameters of how to operationalize and dimensionalize "emotional damage." In our opinion, an overconcern with dependence/security issues and an underconcern with competence/effectance issues is the most ubiquitous and may be the most sensitive, useful index of emotional damage. When clinicians view our tapes of insecure–avoidant or insecure–disorganized infants and dependent, non-competence-motivated preschoolers, they begin to *see* what emotional damage can look like. Indeed, providing clinicians with a framework to observe key features of the socioemotional development of maltreated children may be the greatest service our research can offer to them. Improving operational definitions of emotional damage through research on the socioemotional development of maltreated children can help service planners and policymakers by providing a method by which to target services on children at greatest risk for damage.

Second, a unifying theory of the development of maltreated children could provide clinicians and policymakers with a framework within which to target, design, and evaluate protective services. For instance, if future research confirms the causal relationship between family ecological variables and severity of developmental outcome for maltreated children hypothesized by our theory, perhaps preventive services should be targeted at parents who least enjoy their children, most discourage their children's autonomy, and have the least access to community resources. Similarly, perhaps scarce protective services should be targeted at the least secure maltreated children. (Although the entire issue of targeting the children most at risk strikes us as a modern Solomon's dilemma, in light of the scarcity of resources we can hardly shrink from our responsibility to provide some guidance on this pressing issue.)

Regarding the design of services, our formulation of the central impact of maltreatment on early childhood development provides a theoretical focus and rationale for clinical and program efforts. Specifically, our research in the context of contemporary attachment theory (Belsky and Nezworski, 1988; Bretherton and Waters, 1985; Greenberg, Cicchetti, and Cummings, in press) suggests that children's expectations of adult responsiveness and availability be the primary focus of services. Many of the other problems maltreated children exhibit (poor self-esteem and self-regulation; aggressive/rejecting and/or withdrawn/isolated relations with peers; lags in cognitive and academic competence; elevated levels of behavioral symptomatology) appear to us to be derivative of the central problem – an overconcern with security issues reflecting an expectation of unresponsive, unavailable, rejecting adults. We wish to emphasize that we do *not* believe that a distortion in the balance between security-promoting and effectance-promoting operations has been *proven* to be the central impact from which other problems derive. Nor do we believe that if this were the case, simply by encouraging children's expectations of adult responsiveness and availability and thereby enhancing their sense of security, other problems that may have developed (e.g., aggressive peer relations) would automatically be solved. On the contrary, we consider our formulation of the central impact of maltreatment as a working hypothesis for service providers because it has some empirical support, it makes considerable theoretical sense, and it provides some grounded guidance for how to design services for maltreated children. Likewise, our own organizational perspective suggests that early insecurity affects later adaptational tasks, failures that themselves become "structuralized" over development. Consequently, it may prove necessary to work directly on impaired peer relations even after maltreated children's expectations of adults have begun to change. In the context of our unifying theory, we are simply asserting that the relationship between children's developmental–adaptational traits and their adaptation to new environments is complex and probably overdetermined such that a positive change in the former does not guarantee a positive change in the latter.

Finally, theory and research on the development of maltreated children may eventually result in a framework within which to evaluate the efficacy of various types of preventive and protective services. With one or two very important exceptions (e.g., Olds et al., 1986), the evaluation studies of preventive and protective services for high-risk and maltreated children and their families in the last decade have been both atheoretical and prone to using very gross measures of impact (e.g., on [re]injury rate or [re]reporting of abuse). By being atheoretical, evaluation studies have failed to add to the cumulative knowledge of what works and what doesn't in the prevention of child maltreatment. By using gross measures of impact, we limit our abilities to detect meaningful, if subtle, effects of intervention. In the end, without theories of what causes maltreatment and what the causal factors are in the development of maltreated children and without sensitive measures of the impact of both maltreatment and services on development processes, it proves almost impossible to synthesize information across various evaluation studies and come to powerful conclusions about the efficacy of various treatment and prevention studies.

Although we are still quite a distance from truly adequate theories and measures to guide evaluations of service, we believe that the studies and theory reported in this chapter, when combined with the work of other investigators in this volume, have moved us significantly closer to such a theoretical and measurement framework. To provide one limited but clear example of recent progress, we believe that theory and research on infant attachment in maltreating families provide a sufficient basis for the design and conduct of a coordinated series of studies of the relative efficacy of prevention programs for high-risk parents and infants. Similarly, we believe we are just several years away from being in a similar position to provide both theory and methods for the design and conduct of comparative prevention and intervention studies in the preschool and early school-age years. These will be the studies of maltreated children with the greatest clinical and policy relevance. But they will require the active collaboration and best efforts of developmental scientists to design and conduct successfully. In short, when this present generation of studies of the "natural history" of child maltreatment are completed, we will be prepared to enter the next generation of studies. In the future generation, we are likely to learn most about the causes and consequences of maltreatment by systematically trying to change the causes and consequences, guided by the best theory and data available from the present generation of studies.

References

Aber, J. L. (1980). The involuntary child placement decision: Solomon's dilemma revisited. In G. Gerbner, C. Ross, and E. Zigler (Eds.), *Child Abuse: An Agenda for Action.* New York: Oxford University Press, 156–182.

Aber, J. L., and Allen, J. P. (1987). The effects of maltreatment on young children's socio-emotional development: An attachment theory perspective. *Developmental Psychology, 23,* 406–414.

Aber, J. L., Allen, J., and Cicchetti, D. (1988). The behavioral symptomatology of maltreated children: A developmental analysis. Unpublished manuscript.

Aber, J. L., and Cicchetti, D. (1984). The socio-emotional development of maltreated children: An empirical and theoretical analysis. In H. Fitzgerald, B. Lester, and M. Yogman (Eds.), *Theory and Research in Behavioral Pediatrics* (Vol. 2, pp. 147–205). New York: Plenum.

Aber, J. L., Trickett, P., Carlson, V., and Cicchetti, D. (1989). The relationship between family ecology and child developmental outcomes in maltreating and nonmaltreating high-risk families. Unpublished manuscript.

Aber, J. L., and Zigler, E. (1981). Developmental considerations in defining child maltreatment. In R. Rizley and D. Cicchetti (Eds.), *Developmental Perspectives on Child Maltreatment: New Directions for Child Development* (pp. 1–29). San Francisco: Jossey-Bass.

Achenbach, T. M., and Edelbrock, C. (1983). *Manual for the Child Behavior Checklist and Revised Child Behavior Profile.* Burlington, VT: Queen City Printers.

Ainsworth, M., Blehar, M., Waters, E., and Wall, S. (1978). *Patterns of Attachment.* Hillsdale, NJ: Erlbaum.

Arend, R., Gove., F. L., and Sroufe, L. A. (1979). Continuity of individual adaptation from infancy to kindergarten: A predictive study of ego-resiliency and curiosity in preschoolers. *Child Development, 50,* 950–959.

Augostinos, M. (1987). Developmental effects of child abuse: Recent findings. *Child Abuse and Neglect, 11,* 15–27.

Balla, D., and Zigler, E. (1975). Preinstitutional social deprivation and responsiveness to social reinforcement in institutionalized retarded individuals: A six-year follow-up study. *American Journal of Mental Deficiency, 80M,* 228–230.

Barahal, R. M., Waterman, J., and Martin, H. P., (1981). The social cognitive development of abused children. *Journal of Consulting and Clinical Psychology, 49,* 508–516.

Belsky, J. (1980). Child maltreatment: An ecological integration. *American Psychologist, 35,* 320–335.

Belsky, J., Garduque, L, and Hrncir, E. (1984). Assessing performance competence and executive capacity in infant play: Relations to home environment and security of attachment. *Developmental Psychology, 20,* 406–417.

Belsky, J., and Nezworski, T. (1988). *Clinical Implications of Attachment.* Hillsdale, NJ: Erlbaum.

Block, J. H., and Block, J. (1980). The role of ego control and ego resiliency in the organization of behavior. In W. A. Collins (Ed.), *Minnesota Symposium on Child Psychology* (Vol. 13, pp. 39–101). Hillsdale, NJ: Erlbaum

Bowlby, J. (1980). *Attachment and Loss: Vol. 3. Loss.* New York: Basic.

Bretherton, I., and Waters, E. (Eds.) (1985). *Growing points of attachment theory and research.*

Monographs of the Society for Research in Child Development, Vol 50 (1 and 2) Serial No. 209.

Bronfenbrenner, U. (1979). *The Ecology of Human Development: Experiments by Nature and Design.* Cambridge, MA: Harvard University Press.

Carlson, V., Cicchetti, D., Barnett, D. and Braunwald, K. (this volume). The contribution of child maltreatment research to attachment theory and method.

Cicchetti, D. (1984). The emergence of developmental psychopathology. *Child Development, 55* (1), 1–7.

Cicchetti, D., and Aber, J. L. (1980). Abused children – abusive parents: An overstated case? *Harvard Educational Review, 50,* 244–255.

Cicchetti, D., and Aber, J. L. (1986). Early precursors to later depression: An organizational perspective. In L. P. Lipsitt (Ed.), *Advances in Infancy Research* (Vol. 3). Norwood, NJ: Ablex, 1986, 87–137.

Cicchetti, D., Carlson, V., Braunwald, K., and Aber, J. L. (1987). The sequelae of child maltreatment. In R. J. Gelles and J. B. Lancaster (Eds.), *Child Abuse and Neglect: Biosocial Dimensions,* Hawthorne, NY: Aldine, 277–298.

Cicchetti, D., and Rizley, R. (1981). Developmental perspectives on the etiology, intergenerational transmission and sequelae of child maltreatment. In R. Rizley and D. Cicchetti (Eds.), *Developmental Perspectives on Child Maltreatment* (pp. 31–55). San Francisco: Jossey-Bass.

Dodge, K., Murphy, R., and Buchsbaum, K. (1984). The assessment of intention–cue detection skills in children: Implications for developmental psychopathology. *Child Development, 55,* 163–173.

Egeland, B., and Sroufe, L. A. (1981). Developmental sequelae of maltreatment in infancy. In R. Rizley and D. Cicchetti (Eds.), *Developmental Perspectives on Child Maltreatment* (pp. 77–92). San Francisco: Jossey-Bass.

Elmer, E. (1977). A follow-up study of traumatized children. *Pediatrics, 59,* 273–279.

Garbarino, J. (1982). *Children and Families in the Social Environment.* Hawthorne, NY: Aldine.

Garbarino, J., and Sherman, D. (1980). High-risk neighborhoods and high-risk families: The human ecology of child maltreatment. *Child Development, 51,* 188–198.

Gelles, R. (1975). The social construction of child abuse. *American Journal of Orthopsychiatry, 45,* 363–371.

Giovannoni, J., and Becerra, R. (1979). *Defining Child Abuse.* New York: Free Press.

Greenberg, M., Cicchetti, D., and Cummings, M. (in press). *Attachment in the Preschool Years.* Chicago: University of Chicago Press.

Greenspan, S., and Porges, S. (1984). Psychopathology in infancy and early childhood: Clinical perspectives on the organization of sensory and affective-thematic experience. *Child Development, 55,* 49–70.

Harter, S. (1978). Effectance motivation reconsidered: Toward a developmental model. *Human Development, 21,* 34–64

Harter, S., and Zigler, E. (1974). The assessment of effectance motivation in normal and retarded children. *Developmental Psychology, 10,* 169–180.

Hoffman-Plotkin, D., and Twentyman, C. (1984). A multimodal assessment of behavioral and cognitive deficits in abused and neglected preschoolers. *Child Development, 52,* 13–30.

Juvenile Justice Standards Project (1977). *Standards Relating to Abuse and Neglect.* Cambridge, MA: Ballinger.

Kohlberg, L., Ricks, D., and Snarey, J. (1983). Childhood development as a predictor of adaptation in adulthood. In L. Kohlberg (Ed.), *Developmental Psychology and Early Education.* New York: Longman.

Kohlberg, L., LaCrosse, J., and Ricks, D. (1972). The predictability of adult mental behavior from childhood behavior. In B. Wolman (Ed.), *Manual of Child Psychopathology.* New York: McGraw-Hill.

Lamphear, S. (1987). The impact of maltreatment on children's psychosocial adjustment: A review of the research. *Child Abuse and Neglect, 9,* 251–263.

Lyons-Ruth, K., Connell, D., Zoll, D., and Stahl, J. (1987). Infants at social risk: Relationships among infant maltreatment, maternal behavior, and infant attachment behavior. *Developmental Psychology, 23*(2), 223–232.

Main, M., and Cassidy, J. (1988). Categories of response to reunion with the parent at age 6: Predictable from infant attachment classifications and stable over a 1-month period. *Developmental Psychology, 24,* 415–426.

Main, M., Kaplan, N., and Cassidy, J. (1985). Security in infancy, childhood and adulthood. A move to the level of representation. In I. Bretherton and E. Waters (Eds.), *Growing points in attachment theory and research. Monographs of the Society of Research in Child Development* (pp. 66–104). Chicago: University of Chicago Press.

Main, M., and Weston, D. (1981). The quality of toddler's relationship to mother and father. Related to conflict behavior and the readiness to establish a new relationship. *Child Development, 52,* 932–940.

Moore, E. G. (1986). Family socialization and the IQ test performance of traditionally and transracially adopted black children. *Developmental Psychology, 22,* 317–326.

Moos, R. H., and Moos, B. S. (1981). *Family Environment Scale Manual.* Palo Alto, CA: Consulting Psychologists Press.

Mueller, C., and Parcel, T. (1981). Measures of socioeconomic status: Alternatives and recommendations. *Child Development, 52,* 13–30.

Nock, S. L., and Rossi, P. H. (1979). Household types and social standing. *Social Forces, 57,* 1325–1345.

Olds, D. S., et al. (1986). Preventing child abuse and neglect: A trial of nurse home visitation. *Pediatrics, 78,* 65.

Rohrbeck, C., and Twentyman, C. (1986). Multimodal assessment of implusiveness in abusing, neglecting and nonmaltreating mothers and their preschool children. *Journal of Consulting and Clinical Psychology, 54,* 231–236.

Schneider-Rosen, K., Braunwald, K., Carlson, V., and Cicchetti, D. (1985). Current perspectives in attachment theory: Illustration from the study of maltreated infants. In I. Bretherton and E. Waters (Eds.), *Growing points in attachment theory and research: Monographs of the Social of Research in Child Development* (pp. 194–210). Chicago: University of Chicago Press.

Schneider-Rosen, K., and Cicchetti, D. (1984). The relationship between affect and cognition in maltreated infants: Quality of attachment and the development of visual self-recognition. *Child Development, 55,* 648–658.

Solnit, A. (1980). Too much reporting, too little service: Roots and prevention of child abuse. In G. Gerbner, C. Ross, and E. Zigler (Eds.), *Child Abuse: An Agenda for Action.* New York: Oxford University Press.

Sroufe, L. A. (1979). The coherence of individual development: Early care, attachment and subsequent developmental issues. *American Psychologist, 34,* 834–841.

Sroufe, L. A. (1983). Infant–caregiver attachment and patterns of adaptation in the preschool: The roots of maladaptation and competence. In M. Perlmutter (Ed.,), *Minnesota Symposium in Child Psychology, 16,* 41–83.

Sroufe, L. A., and Fleeson, J. (1986). Attachment and the construction of relationships. In W. Hartup and Z. Rubin (Eds.), *Relationships and Development* (pp. 51–71). New York: Cambridge University Press.

Sroufe, L. A., Fox, N., and Pancake, V. (1983). Attachment and dependency in developmental perspective. *Child Development, 54,* 1615–1627.

Sroufe, L. A., and Rutter, M. (1984). The domain of developmental psychopathology. *Child Development, 55,* 17–29.

Sroufe, L. A., and Waters E. (1977). Attachment as an organizational construct. *Child Development, 48,* 1184–1199.

Trickett, P., Aber, J. L., Carlson, V., and Cicchetti, D. (1989). The influence of socioeconomic status on the etiology and developmental sequelae of physical child abuse. Manuscript submitted for publication.

Waters, E., and Sroufe, L. A. (1983). Social competence as a developmental construct. *Developmental Review, 3*, 79–97.

Werner, H., & Kaplan, B. (1963). *Symbol Formation: An Organismic-Developmental Approach to Language and the Expression of Thought.* New York: Wiley.

White, R. W. (1959). Motivation reconsidered: The concept of competence. *Psychological Review, 66,* 297–323.

Yando, R., Seitz, V., and Zigler, E. (1978). *Imitation: A Developmental Perspective.* Hillsdale, NJ: Erlbaum.

Zigler, E., Abelson, W. D., and Seitz, V. (1973). Motivational factors in the performance of economically disadvantaged children on the Peabody Picture Vocabulary Test. *Child Development, 44,* 293–303.

Zigler, E., Abelson, W., Trickett, P., and Seitz, V. (1982). Is an intervention program necessary in order to improve economically disadvantaged children's IQ scores? *Child Development, 53,* 340–348.

Zigler, E., and Balla, D. (1982). Atypical development: Personality determinants in the behavior of the retarded. In E. Zigler, M. Lamb, and I. Child (Eds.), *Socialization and Personality Development* (pp. 238–245). New York: Oxford University Press.

19   Social cognition in maltreated children

Judith G. Smetana and Mario Kelly

There is increasing interest in the psychological consequences of child mal-treatment, as evidenced by the recent attention and journal space given to the topic. Most of this research has focused on behavioral effects – such as heightened aggression – or socioemotional effects – such as deficits in the development of empathy. Although research on the development of social cognition in normal children has been burgeoning over the past 15 years, research on the effects of maltreatment on social-cognitive development has been virtually ignored.

In this chapter, we contend that studying the social cognition of mal-treated children is important for several reasons. First, it is important to determine how children who have experienced extended social interactions in environments that are abusive or neglectful construct, interpret, and structure their social world. We do not know, for instance, whether and in what ways maltreated children's developing understanding of others' emo-tions, attributions for others' behavior, justifications for their own behavior, or moral judgments differ from nonmaltreated children. These represent important but unanswered questions that fall within the social-cognitive realm. Knowledge of normative social-cognitive development can be used to identify deficits or delays in development that are related to experiences of maltreatment.

Second, knowledge of social-cognitive development in maltreated chil-dren can compliment and enrich our knowledge by offering unique oppor-tunities to test hypotheses about normative development. Most theories of social-cognitive development are based upon the Piagetian premise of an active child structuring his or her social world through social interactions. Therefore, studying the social reasoning of children who have experienced deviant social interactions offers an opportunity to test a number of inter-esting hypotheses about the role of such interactions in development and about developmental processes more generally.

Finally, studying social cognition in maltreated children offers the potential for establishing links between social cognition and social behavior. This has been considered an important goal of research on normal children (Shantz, 1983), and it may be a particularly relevant issue for maltreated children, as aspects of their social behavior have been found to be problematic. For instance, research indicates that maltreated children are either more withdrawn or more aggressive, especially in response to frustration, than normal children (Burgess and Conger, 1978; George and Main, 1979; Reidy, 1977; Straker and Jacobson, 1981). An understanding of maltreated children's judgments about aggressive situations may ultimately lead to new, more successful methods for remediation than would be obtained by focusing on behavior alone. Further, relationships between judgments and actions have been extensively studied in normal children, and the extent and nature of the judgment–action relationship has been subject to much debate (see Blasi, 1980; Turiel and Smetana, 1984). Describing such relationships in atypical populations could potentially contribute to our understanding of the judgment–action relationship in normal as well as in maltreated children.

The primary objectives of this chapter are to review the existing literature on the effects of child abuse and neglect on social-cognitive development and to provide an example, through our own research, of how research on social cognition in abused and neglected children can illuminate basic issues in developmental psychology, as well as define some consequences of maltreatment for children's social-cognitive development. In addition, because so little has been done, we will comment on the most obvious gaps in our knowledge of the social-cognitive consequences of maltreatment. We will begin by defining social cognition as it is used here and the types of research that have been included under this rubric.

The development of social knowledge

Historically, interest in social-cognitive development can be directly traced to Piaget's theorizing and research on cognitive development. Although it was not until the 1960s that interest grew in applying this approach to social development, the assumptions guiding Piaget's work on cognitive development have formed the theoretical basis of much of the research on social cognition. Thus, a good deal of research has been aimed at identifying the principles of organization that underlie children's social knowledge and the patterns of age-related qualitative changes, or restructuring, of knowledge.

Our definition of social cognition also takes into consideration another often overlooked but equally salient aspect of Piaget's theorizing (Piaget, 1967): his concern with classifying systems of knowledge. We define social-cognitive development here in terms of three broad aspects of children's developing social knowledge: their understanding of persons as psychological systems (psychological knowledge), social relations (morality), and social systems (societal knowledge). Although there may be instances of overlap or intersection between the domains, they are proposed to form separate, self-regulating developmental systems.

Much of what often has been referred to as social cognition (cf. Shantz, 1975, 1983) can be classified as aspects of children's understanding of persons as psychological systems. This domain pertains to children's concepts about how people relate to others in systematic ways, including inferences about others' thoughts, feelings, and intentions, and knowledge of personality, self, and identity. A great deal of research, usually described in terms of discrete topics such as person perception, causal attributions, self-concepts, role-taking, and so forth, has been conducted on aspects of children's psychological knowledge (see Shantz, 1983, for a review).

Not all social interactions pertain to children's attempts to understand persons as psychological systems, however. From their social interactions, children may also develop theories of social relations. That is, from their experiences as victims or observers to transgressions, children develop abstract notions of right and wrong, good and bad, that form the basis of their moral understanding. The moral domain can be defined as a prescriptive system, based upon an underlying conceptualization of justice, that is concerned with how individuals ought to behave toward one another. Moral judgments concern such issues as others' welfare, trust, responsibility, and the fair distribution of resources.

Children also construct an understanding of culture and social organization that is distinct from their understanding of morality. We refer here to this form of knowledge as the societal domain. It includes children's concepts of groups, authority, social roles, social structure, and social conventions (see Table 19.1).

These different types of social knowledge are organized systems that are constructed out of interactions, that is, the child's actions upon and interactions with the environment. However, social interactions are not of one type; children engage in different types of interactions with fundamentally different types of objects and events. Because conceptual knowledge is constructed through an interactive process, different types of individual–environment interactions should lead to the construction of different types of social knowledge (Smetana, 1983; Turiel, 1983).

For example, consider the following events, which we observed in interactions among twelve 36-month-old toddlers in a daycare center:

> *Event A:* Lisa, Michael, and David are all rocking in a rocking boat. Jenny, who has been waiting nearby for a turn, finally approaches. As the rocking slows down, she bites Lisa in the arm. Lisa screams and then cries.

Table 19.1. *Domains of social knowledge*

Moral knowledge	
Defined as	Prescriptive judgments of right and wrong
Structured by	Concepts of justice
Pertaining to	Issues of welfare, rights, fairness, trust
Criteria	Generalizability, independence from rules and authority sanctions, obligatoriness, universalizability, unalterability
Societal knowledge	
Defined as	Judgments regarding systems of social relations
Structured by	Concepts of social organization
Pertaining to	Social conventions, social roles, authority
Criteria	Rule contingency, alterability, contextualism, relativity, authority jurisdiction
Psychological knowledge	
Defined as	Understanding the self and others as psychological systems
Structured by	Concepts of the person
Pertaining to	Self, identity, personality, personal issues, inferences and attributions regarding the causes of self's and others' behavior
Criteria	Personal jurisdiction, independence from societal regulation and moral concern

> *Event B:* It is snack time, and the teachers instruct the children to sit in their seats. Cindy is kneeling in her chair. The teacher tells her, "Cindy, bottoms have to be on the chair before children can have their snacks." Cindy sits down; the other children pay no attention.

From the child's perspective, both of these events share similar features: both are wrong, and both are prohibited by adults. Yet, they also differ in important ways. Consider Event A. A salient aspect of the event is the pain inflicted on Lisa (or Jenny's apparent perception of unfairness). Children who observe (or are the victims of) experiences with harm or the perceived violation of rights generate prescriptions regarding such events through their abstractions from their experiences. The child need not be told that the act is a rule violation or that it is wrong; she will construct this knowledge from her experience of the event. Children's attempts to understand their social experiences thus result in judgments about what is fair, right, or good (and correspondingly, what is unfair, wrong, or bad). Thus, awareness of the effects of actions on others' rights and welfare results in the development of prescriptive (moral) judgments about how individuals ought to behave toward one another.

Now consider Event B. There is no intrinsic basis for knowing that children must be seated before a snack is served; this knowledge is based upon understanding of the social regulations of the school. In other daycare centers, families, or even cultures, snacks might always be eaten while standing up! Thus, such interactions differ from moral interactions and are likely to produce a different type of social knowledge. This knowledge has been referred to as social-conventional. Social conventions are one aspect of the societal domain and refer to the arbitrary, consensually agreed-upon behavioral uniformities that structure social interactions within social systems (Turiel, 1975, 1983). Social-conventional knowledge is generated through an understanding of the prohibitions regarding acts rather than from the acts themselves.

It has been proposed that from early childhood on, children distinguish between morality and social convention (Smetana, 1983; Turiel, 1975, 1983). For instance, in one study (Smetana, 1981), 2½- to 5-year-old children in daycare centers were presented with familiar transgressions representing prototypical moral (for instance, hitting, not sharing) and conventional (not putting toys away in the correct place, not sitting appropriately during snack time) events. Children were asked to judge the acts' seriousness, amount of deserved punishment, contingency on rules, and contextual relativity. All preschool children judged moral transgressions to be more serious and deserve greater punishment than conventional transgressions. Further, the wrongness of moral transgressions was judged to be generalizable across social contexts and independent of rules, whereas the wrongness of conventions was judged to be contingent on the presence of rules.

These findings have been replicated and extended in other studies. Indeed, research indicates that across a wide age range, children judge moral concepts to be unalterable, generalizable, and independent of rules and authority jurisdiction, whereas they judge conventional concepts to be contextually relative, alterable, contingent on rules, and subject to subordinate jurisdiction (Davidson, Turiel, and Black, 1983; Nucci, 1981; Smetana, 1981, 1985; Turiel, 1978). Children's understanding of these distinctions appears to be present very early in development; although these criteria may be applied to a broader range of issues with age, they are not reorganized or changed qualitatively with development. (This is in contrast to others, for example, Kohlberg, 1971; Piaget, 1932/1948, who have proposed that morality develops from a global confusion of moral and nonmoral judgments. According to these theorists, the process of development is seen to entail the progressive differentiation of principled moral judgments from a morality comprised of the habitual, customary, or conventional.)

Other age-related changes occur within these three social–cognitive domains that also do not entail qualitative transformations in social knowledge. Within the psychological domain, for instance, children have also been found to develop skills or methods for gathering information about the social world that, through experience, may improve quantitatively in accuracy or scope. These methods include such activities as communication, observation, imitation, and symbolically taking the perspective of another (role-taking). Although these methods of information are constrained by children's development within a conceptual domain, they are analytically separable from the development of knowledge within the psychological domain.[1]

Finally, children's psychological, moral, and societal concepts each appear to change qualitatively with age and increasing social experience. It would be beyond the scope of this chapter to describe all of the developmental research supporting this proposition. Nevertheless, research examining developmental changes within these domains supports the notion that concepts within each of these domains form interrelated groups that follow the same age-related sequential transformations, yet differ across domains (although there may be coordinations or intersections). For instance, in a study focused on concepts of distributive justice in children 6 to 10 years of age, Damon (1977) found that children developed an increasing understanding of concepts of equality and reciprocity. In contrast, in research on children's concepts of social convention, Turiel (1975, 1983) reports that children's social-conventional understanding develops through a sequence of alternating affirmations and then negations of the importance of conventions in regulating social life. Children develop an increasing understanding of the functions of conventions in coordinating social interactions. In the remaining category, the psychological domain, there have been several studies examining age-related developmental patterns. The results of studies on concepts of self or personal identity (Broughton, 1978; Lemke, 1973; Nucci, 1977), understanding other persons (Pratt, 1975), and the causes of behavior generally indicate that young children rely on situational or behavioral characteristics in making psychological judgments and do not have concepts of stable, internal, psychological processes; these concepts appear to develop between the ages of 7 and 12.

Social–cognitive development in maltreated children

As the previous discussion suggests, social-cognitive development encompasses a wide range of social concepts and, correspondingly, should provide a rich source of hypotheses regarding the role of maltreatment in development. Surprisingly, few studies have addressed these issues. In the following sections, we consider the available research on the effects of maltreatment on children's knowledge of psychological topics, morality, and concepts of society.

Several criteria were used in our selection of studies. We originally intended only to survey studies that had control groups of nonmaltreated children, so that developmental differences between maltreated and nonmaltreated children could be compared. Happily, we found that the few available studies of the social-cognitive consequences of maltreatment all employed control groups, unlike more clinical studies, which dominated the research on the psychological consequences of maltreatment until the early 1970s (Aber and Cicchetti, 1984). Second, although the development of empathy is sometimes included under the rubric of social cognition, research on empathy in maltreated children is not reviewed here, as it is more properly considered within a discussion of socioemotional development. Finally, in keeping with our definition of social cognition as children's concepts of persons qua persons, social relations, and social systems, we did not include studies of behavior, emotional adjustment, or personality characteristics. The remaining studies concern three aspects of psychological concepts – understanding of others' behavior (in particular, the abusing parent), understanding of others' emotions, and role-taking ability, as well as moral judgments and social role concepts. These studies are summarized in Table 19.2.

Several characteristics of the remaining studies are worth noting. First, research on maltreated children's social–cognitive concepts has been conducted almost exclusively on physically abused children. Neglected children have rarely been studied and, further, types of physical abuse have not been differentiated. Also, despite increasing interest in follow-up and longitudinal prospective studies on the effects of maltreatment, no such research designs have been implemented to study social-cognitive development among maltreated samples.

Psychological knowledge

Psychological knowledge encompasses a broad range of topics that have been well-studied in normal children. The effects of maltreatment on children's knowledge in this domain would appear to be both a natural extension of this research and extremely relevant to an understanding of maltreatment. Yet, few studies have been conducted. Typically, the results of normative research on the quantitative dimensions of children's psychological knowledge have been used as indices on which to compare normal and maltreated children. As the following studies illustrate, maltreated children have been hypothesized to experience delays or deficits along different dimensions of social-cognitive development.

One comparative study examined a range of psychological characteristics thought to differentiate abused from nonmaltreated children (Herzberger, Potts, and Dillon, 1981). Of interest here are their findings regarding children's attributions for others' (e.g., the abusing parents') behavior. These authors predicted a range of deficits among abused as compared to normal children, although they did not specifically define the deficits in terms of the developmental processes by which children form attributions.

Table 19.2. *Studies of social cognition in maltreated children*

Study	Topic	Subjects	Tasks	Major Findings
Barahal, Waterman, and Martin (1981)	Social sensitivity	17 physically abused and 16 matched controls, age range = 6–8 years, $\bar{X}$ = 7.5	Rothenberg's Social Sensitivity Task	Controls > abused, ns with IQ controlled
	Social roles		Watson and Fischer's Social Role task	Controls > abused in comprehension and imitation; spontaneous production ns
	Role-taking		Flavell, Botkin, Fry, Wright, and Jarvis's 1968 Boy–Dog–Tree Test	ns
	Moral judgment		Piaget's heteronomy task	ns
Herzberger, Potts, and Dillon (1981)	Causes of (parental) behavior	14 physically abused males and 10 matched control males, age range = 8–14 years, $\bar{X}$ = 10.79	Interview regarding attributions for parental behavior	Mother-abused males, compared to controls, saw behavior as undeserved
Frodi and Smetana (1984)	Social sensitivity	8 physically abused, 12 neglected, 21 matched controls, and 19 high income, high IQ comparisons, age range = 3–5 years, $\bar{X}$ = 4.40	Rothenberg's Social Sensitivity Scale	High IQ comparison group > abused, neglected, and matched controls; abused, neglected, and matched control ns

In this study, father-abused, mother-abused, and a comparison group of nonabused males' perceptions of parental treatment and attributions for their parents' behavior were compared. The results indicated that almost all children took responsibility for parental spankings and felt that such punishment was in response to their bad behavior. Such attributions did not preclude additional attributions to their parents' personalities, however. Subjects who had been abused by their fathers were significantly more likely than nonabused controls to feel that their punishment was due to their father's mean character; a similar though nonsignificant trend was found among mother-abused males. Children were also asked whether they deserved to be treated in that way; father-abused and nonabused children did not difffer in their responses. About half of the father-abused and control males felt that their parental treatment was deserved. Children who were abused by their mothers, in contrast, were much less likely than control males to feel that their parental treatment was undeserved. Abusive mothers were perceived to feel less bad about hitting their sons than nonabusive mothers. Finally, when questioned about their perceptions of the amount of hitting in their families as compared to other families, abused and non-abused children alike did not differ in their perceptions of other families. However, nonabused children viewed the frequency of hitting in their families as comparable to other families, whereas abused children saw themselves as being hit significantly more frequently than in other families. Thus, the results of this study suggest that abused children perceived themselves as being uniquely punished.

Interestingly, the finding that all children take responsibility for incurring parental punishment and that maltreated children differed from nonmaltreated children only in their attributions regarding their parents' behavior seems to contradict the hypothesis that abused children suffer social-cognitive deficits; rather, abused children appear to make accurate attributions regarding the causes of their mistreatment. Unfortunately, however, because no developmental measures were obtained, little can be said about whether either the process or the developmental rate of forming causal attributions differs in abused and nonabused children.

Based on observations that abusive parents are often insensitive to others' needs and emotions, Barahal, Waterman, and Martin (1981) proposed that abused children's social-cognitive style would differ from nonmaltreated children. More specifically, they proposed that their ability to role-take and to label the emotional states of others would be less developed than non-abused children. To test this hypothesis, abused children between 6 and 8 years of age were compared with matched nonabused children on a measure of social sensitivity developed by Rothenberg (1970) and on a test of per-spective-taking ability developed by Flavell, Botkin, Fry, Wright, and Jarvis (1968)[2] (other social-cognitive measures used by these investigators are discussed in the following section). These investigators found that abused children were less able to identify appropriate feelings, were less advanced in describing the social and interpersonal causes of the specific emotions, and were poorer in role-taking ability than were nonabused children. The strength of these findings was reduced (and most group differences became nonsignificant), however, when differences in IQ between the two groups were controlled. The authors intriguingly suggest that perhaps differences in maltreated children's social-cognitive abilities lead to a reduction in their performance on IQ tests rather than that their lower IQ scores account for the social-cognitive differences obtained. That is, children who are underachievers and dependent on external cues in evaluating their own performance may suffer on standardized examinations, where intrinsic motivation and self-feedback are required.

Developmental acceleration due to experiences of maltreatment has also been predicted. Frodi and Smetana (1984) predicted that the development of social sensitivity would be enhanced in abused and neglected as compared to nonmaltreated children. This hypothesis was based on the observation that children of abusive parents adaptively learn to monitor the behavior of adults (A. Freud, 1952; Ounsted, Oppenheimer, and Lindsay, 1974) and that young children who are constantly exposed to naturally occurring parental anger are more socially sensitive than other young children who experience little or no parental anger (Cummings, Zahn-Waxler, and Radke-Yarrow, 1981). Subjects in this study were 3- to 5-year-old neglected, physically abused, and nonmaltreated children who were divided into two comparison groups. One group was carefully matched to the maltreated children on a number of variables, including IQ. The second comparison group was composed of middle-class children with higher IQ's; they were included to separate the effects of IQ from those of maltreatment, as maltreated children often have been reported to have low IQ's. (Unfortunately, however, social class and IQ remained confounded.) As in the previous study, the Rothenberg scale was used to measure social sensitivity. Abused and neglected children were not found to differ significantly from the matched control group. However, all three groups differed significantly from the higher IQ comparison group. Thus, the results of this study, as well as those of the Barahal et al. study, point to the importance of unconfounding the effects of IQ and socioeconomic status in examining the social–cognitive development of maltreated children. We cannot conclude from these findings that there are developmental deficits among maltreated children because of the uncontrolled differences in IQ.

Moral and societal knowledge

The effects of maltreatment on children's moral and societal knowledge have received little attention. The Barahal et al. (1981) study is the only research, other than our own, to explore the consequences of maltreatment for children's social knowledge in these domains. Their research examined two aspects of children's moral and societal concepts: social role concepts (based on work by Watson, 1977), and moral judgment (based on Piaget's 1932 theory of moral judgment). Barahal et al. proposed that abused children may be deficient in their understanding of social roles, based on the observation that abusive adults are often confused about appropriate role responsibilities. They also proposed that abused children would be more likely to make moral judgments based on external sanctioning of behavior than on intentionality, based on the observation that abusive adults are more likely to prefer physical than psychological modes of discipline that emphasize the child's behavioral intentions. With the effects of IQ controlled, they found that nonabused children were more effective in comprehending and imitating increasingly complex social roles than were abused children, although there were no differences in abused and control children's ability to spontaneously produce social role concepts. They found no differences between abused and control children's use of intentionality – nearly half the children in both groups were found to make moral judgments on the basis of external rewards and sanctions. This was not surprising, however, because the children were at an age (between 6 and 8) when this transition to intentional moral judgments would be expected to occur. This measure might have been more discriminating had the research subjects been older.

A study conducted by Smetana, Kelly, and Twentyman (1984) examined whether, based upon their experiences of abuse and neglect, maltreated children use the same criteria to evaluate moral conduct as nonmaltreated children, and whether abused and neglected children judge events that affect others' welfare and rights as prescriptively wrong, as do normal children. We began with the rather obvious observation that, compared to normal children, abused children have had aberrant experiences regarding welfare and rights. As victims of physical abuse, for instance, abused children have continually experienced situations in which the abusing parent has seemingly violated moral principles regarding welfare. In addition, observational studies on the effects of maltreatment have consistently found that maltreated children are more aggressive, particularly in response to frustration, than nonabused children (Burgess and Conger, 1978; George and Main, 1979; Herrenkohl and Herrenkohl, 1981; Hoffman-Plotkin and Twentyman, 1984; Reidy, 1977). At present, the link between moral judgments and aggression has not been examined, but we viewed them as potentially related (see Turiel, 1987; Turiel and Smetana, 1984). Therefore, we speculated that maltreated children's moral judgments, particularly those pertaining to welfare, might differ from nonmaltreated children's.

From an internalization perspective, these observations might suggest that children who have been maltreated may develop different standards of moral behavior. For instance, the findings on maltreated children's aggressive behavior might be seen as suggesting that, through processes of imitation and observational learning, abused children come to consider physical or psychological harm to be more permissible than do nonabused children. Similarly, as victims of gross neglect who have been deprived access to physical and emotional resources, neglected children come to consider psychological distress or the unfair distribution of resources to be more justifiable than do nonmaltreated children.

Our predictions differed. Because moral judgments are hypothesized to develop from the intrinsic effects of actions on others, such as harm, injury, or the perceived violation of rights, it is also possible that children who have experienced extended interactions in social environments that are abusive or neglectful might be more sensitive to the justice or welfare issues intrinsic to the effects of moral events. This would lead to a different prediction: that maltreated children treat moral transgressions as less permissible than normal children.

These contrasting predictions were tested in a sample of abused, neglected, and nonmaltreated preschool children. This study also provided a way of elucidating the role of social experience in normal social-cognitive development. The methods for this investigation were drawn from research on the criteria normal children use to evaluate moral and conventional rules and transgressions. Because we hypothesized that maltreatment might affect children's prescriptive moral judgments, we examined the extent to which children applied criteria of generalizability and rule contingency (the permissibility of actions in the absence of rules) to familiar nursery school moral and conventional transgressions. In addition, we examined children's judgments of seriousness and deserved punishment regarding these transgressions. These judgments were chosen in part because normative data are available for preschool children (Smetana, 1981, 1985). We also distinguished between types of maltreatment: Our sample included both children who had suffered physical abuse and children who had experienced neglect. We hypothesized that different types of maltreatment might be differentially related to children's judgments. In addition, judgments regarding different types of moral transgressions, including physical harm, psychological distress, and unfair resource distribution, were examined. Finally, we examined children's judgments as they pertained either to themselves or to others. This was done to test the hypothesis that, compared to normal children, abused and neglected children judge moral transgressions to be more permissible when committed by themselves than by others.

Subjects were 44 preschool children divided between 12 abused, 16 neglected, and 16 nonmaltreated children between the ages of 38 to 68 months ($\overline{X} = 52.84$). The abused and neglected children were drawn from a daycare center serving abused and neglected children who had been referred from the local Department of Social Services Child Protective Division. As maltreated children are more likely to be classified as neglected rather than abused due to stringent legal requirements regarding physical evidence of abuse, classifications of abuse and neglect were based upon ratings of four therapists who had extensive ongoing contact with the children's families. Although there was some overlap between the abuse and neglect categories, for the most part, children could be clearly categorized within a single category. The comparison group was matched as closely as possible on parental income, IQ (using the Peabody Picture Vocabulary Test), maternal education, age, and race. The sample was racially mixed, lower SES, and somewhat lower than average IQ ($\overline{X}$ = 87.73); mothers of subjects had, on the average, less than a high school education.

Using standard and reliable methods that had been developed previously (Smetana, 1981), subjects were shown pictures of children committing 11 familiar nursery school transgressions. There were three each pertaining to physical harm (hitting, kicking, and biting), psychological distress (making another child cry, teasing, and being mean to another child) and social conventions (not listening to the teacher during story time, not keeping quiet during nap time, and leaving the classroom without permission). Two transgressions pertained to unfair resource distribution (taking away another child's snack and not taking turns with a toy). Children were asked to make four judgments: (1) whether the event would be permissible if there were no rule about it in the preschool, indicating the rule contingency of the event, (2) whether the transgression would be permissible at home or in another school, indicating the generalizability of the transgression, (3) the seriousness of the transgression (on a three-point scale) and (4) the degree of deserved punishment (also on a three-point scale; for a more detailed description of the methods, see Smetana, Kelly, and Twentyman, 1984). For half of the children in each maltreatment (or nonmaltreated) group, children were asked to make judgments in terms of themselves as the transgressor (the "self"condition); for the other half, children were asked to make judgments in terms of a hypothetical transgressor (the "other" condition).

As expected, maltreated and normal children alike applied the same criteria to their evaluation of moral and conventional transgressions. That is, all children treated moral transgressions as more serious, more punishable, more wrong in the absence of rules, and more generalizably wrong than conventional transgressions. Further, all children were found to judge all transgressions as more permissible when committed by the self than by others; they judged transgressions as more serious, more punishable, and more wrong in the absence of rules when committed by others than by the self (means are presented in Table 19.3). Thus, regardless of maltreatment status, all children were egocentric when making judgments for themselves versus others.

Table 19.3. *Mean responses to questions concerning the seriousness, rule contingency, rule relativity, and punishment due moral and social-conventional transgressions*

	Seriousness[a]				Rule contingency "OK if no rule"[b]				Rule relativity "OK in different context"[b]				Amount of punishment[c]			
	M^1	M^2	M^3	S-C	M^1	M^2	M^3	S-C	M^1	M^2	M^3	S-C	M^1	M^2	M^3	S-C
Abused																
Self(6)	2.87	2.53	2.20	1.67	.40	.27	.60	.60	.27	.20	.50	.33	1.33	1.40	1.20	1.27
Other(6)	2.83	2.67	2.58	2.44	0	.11	.17	.39	.06	.11	.17	.56	2.67	2.50	2.42	2.50
Neglected																
Self(8)	2.83	2.38	2.19	1.71	.11	.37	.44	.85	.11	.22	.06	.37	2.04	1.67	1.81	1.79
Other(8)	2.83	2.54	2.44	2.04	.14	.48	.43	.52	.14	.48	.43	.43	2.04	1.88	2.00	1.50
Control																
Self(8)	2.83	2.33	2.06	1.71	.29	.50	.44	.67	.29	.42	.44	.50	1.50	1.33	1.50	1.50
Other(8)	2.88	2.54	2.38	1.67	.08	.29	.31	.67	.13	.33	.25	.63	2.58	2.42	2.19	2.08

[a] Responses reflect a 3-point scale where 1 = OK, 2 = Bad, and 3 = Very, very bad
[b] Responses were scored as 0 = No, 1 = Yes
[c] Responses were scored as 1 = No punishment, 2 = A little punishment, 3 = A lot of punishment

[1] Physical harm
[2] Psychological distress
[3] Resource distribution

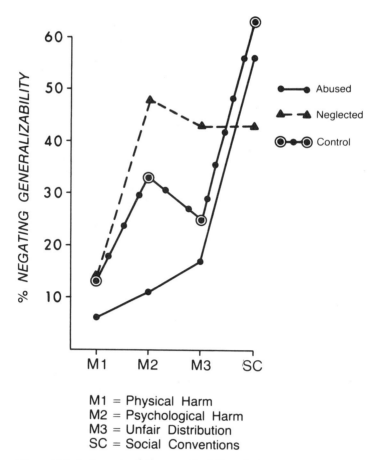

M1 = Physical Harm
M2 = Psychological Harm
M3 = Unfair Distribution
SC = Social Conventions

Figure 19.1. Judgments of the generalizability of transgressions for others.

The expected interactions between maltreated status and types of transgressions were not found. There was, however, a significant interaction between maltreatment status, transgression type, and judgments of self versus others for judgments of generalizability that was consistent with our predictions. That is, abused subjects were found to consider transgressions that cause psychological distress to be more universally wrong when committed by others than did neglected subjects. In contrast, neglected subjects considered transgressions regarding unfair resource distribution to be more generalizably wrong when committed by the self than did abused subjects (see Figures 19.1 and 19.2). It can be hypothesized that both abused and neglected children experience psychological distress as a consequence of their maltreatment and, thus, it is not clear why these differences were found. The findings of abused children are consistent, however, with those

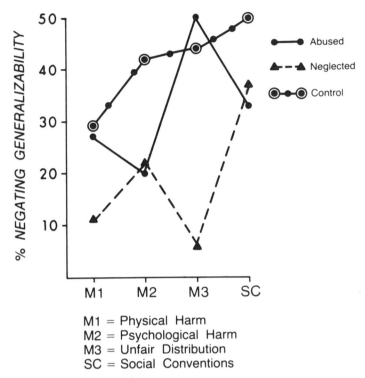

M1 = Physical Harm
M2 = Psychological Harm
M3 = Unfair Distribution
SC = Social Conventions

Figure 19.2. Judgments of the generalizability of transgressions for self.

of Herzberger, Potts, and Dillon (1981), who found that abusing mothers are perceived as more emotionally neglecting than nonabusing mothers. (Remember, however, that the Herzberger et al. study did not include a comparison sample of neglected children.) No differences according to maltreatment status in judgments regarding physical harm were found, probably because there was a ceiling effect for these judgments. All children treated transgressions causing physical harm as extremely serious (mean = 2.85 on a three-point scale); 83 percent of all children judged the wrongness of causing physical harm as not contingent on rules, and 84 percent judged causing physical harm as generalizably wrong. Finally, it is also not clear why the findings regarding psychological harm occurred in judgments for others, whereas the findings regarding distributive justice occurred in judgments for the self.

In addition, there were group differences in children's judgments of deserved punishment for self versus others. Abused and comparison children evaluated all transgressions as deserving significantly less punishment for themselves than for others, whereas neglected children made no distinction between the amount of punishment the self versus others deserved.

Thus, consistent with the aforementioned finding, neglected children seem to view themselves as culpable and more deserving of punishment than other children.

Three aspects of these findings deserve comment. First, they indicate that abused and neglected children's moral evaluations differ only in judgments that may be seen as most closely related to experiences of maltreatment. Chronic experiences with social interactions entailing physical or psychological harm or injury appear to result in increased rather than decreased sensitivity to the intrinsic wrongness of such moral offenses. The findings are also consistent with the assertion that children's social judgments are actively constructed from social experience (Smetana, 1983; Turiel, 1983). Thus, the findings further our understanding of both normal development and the social-cognitive consequences of maltreatment. Second, the results indicate that, in most respects, abused and neglected children's moral evaluations are similar to those of normal children when background variables such as IQ and social class are taken into account. Therefore, this study demonstrates that research on normal social-cognitive development can be generalized beyond the previously studied relatively homogeneous samples of middle-class "normal" children (e.g., Smetana, 1981, 1985). Finally, the results indicate the importance of distinguishing between abuse and neglect, despite the conceptual confusion and pragmatic difficulties of doing so, as the group differences found in this study were between abused and neglected rather than between maltreated and normal children.

The results of this study also raise an intriguing issue. They indicate that children who have been maltreated do not internalize different standards of behavior. Rather, as predicted, maltreated children appear to be more sensitive to the intrinsic wrongness of transgressions most closely related to their experiences of abuse or neglect. Yet, we began by observing that both abused and neglected children are more aggressive than their nonmaltreated counterparts. Thus, the findings point to an apparent discrepancy between maltreated children's moral evaluations and their aggressive behavior. Rather than concluding that they are not related, it is necessary to examine the links between children's abstract moral judgments and judgments in actual situations (see Turiel and Smetana, 1984, for a discussion of this issue). Thus, the next step in the research was to determine whether abused, neglected, and nonmaltreated children's interpretations of the situations that elicit aggressive behavior differ. The following section describes the results of research, conducted by the second author in his doctoral dissertation, that examined this issue.

Moral judgments and actions in maltreated children

The subjects in this study were 10 abused, 10 neglected, and 20 nonmaltreated preschool children, 10 each in two comparison groups, who were drawn from the same two daycare centers as in Smetana, et al. (1984). Children in the maltreated groups were racially mixed, lower-class SES, and had lower than average IQs, as assessed by the Peabody Picture Vocabulary Test ($\overline{X}$ = 88.15, SD = 8.95). Children in one comparison group were matched to the maltreated children on SES, race, IQ, mother's education, and age; the mean age in these three groups was 49.17 months (SD = 5.17). Children in the additional comparison group were middle-class, so that the effects of social class on judgments and actions could be examined. Unfortunately, however, social class and IQ were confounded, as these children also had somewhat higher than average IQs ($\overline{X}$ = 113.70, SD = 6.76).

Several procedures were used in this study. First, children were asked to make judgments about hypothetical transgressions. The study was more narrowly focused than that of Smetana et al. (1984) on specific moral behaviors; the hypothetical transgressions pertained to intentional harm (that is, aggression (hitting) and unfair resource distribution (not sharing a toy). Children were asked to judge the acts' permissibility and their permissibility at two levels of harm ("a little" or "a lot"). They were also asked to rate on a three-point scale the amount of harm (for aggressive acts) or sadness (for unfair acts) they perceived the acts to cause and to reason about, or justify, the acts' wrongness.

To obtain judgments regarding actual behaviors, observations were conducted during free-play sessions at the daycare centers. An observer waited for a naturally occurring aggressive or unfair act, and then the perpetrator of the act was immediately interviewed. The child was first asked why he or she committed the act. She was then asked to judge the permissibility of her behavior, rate on a three-point scale the amount of harm or sadness she perceived her behavior to cause, and reason, or provide justifications, for engaging in the act. Observations were continued until each subject had been interviewed about both types of transgressions.

Children's justifications for the wrongness (or permissibility) of hypothetical acts and actual behaviors and their reasons for their own behavior were coded into justification categories – presented in Table 19.4 – that were based upon previous research (Davidson, Turiel, and Black, 1983; Smetana, 1985) and a content analysis of a subset of protocols.

The findings revealed some interesting differences in children's reasoning and evaluations of the permissibility of hypothetical versus real-life transgressions. Regardless of maltreatment status, children were more likely to judge hypothetical than actual transgressions as wrong (96% versus 49%, respectively). This finding is not too surprising, as the perpetrators, not the victims, were judging the permissibility of the actual transgressions. Further, all children rated victims as more harmed in the hypothetical than in real-life situations (see Table 19.5).

Regardless of maltreatment status, children also reasoned somewhat differently about hypothetical versus actual situations. They were more likely

Table 19.4. *Justification categories*

Category	Description
Harm	Reference to physical or psychological harm ("It's wrong because it hurt her"; "It's OK because he pushed me into the wall")
Fairness	Reference to unfairness or injustice ("She took my little people [toys]"; "I had it first and she took it")
Egocentric goal	Reference to personal wants, desires, or needs
Achievement	("Because I wanted it")
Interpersonal incompatibility	Reference to personal dislike ("Because I hate him")
Rule violation	Appeal to rules, standards, or authority dictates ("Because the teacher says so")
Punishment	Reference to sanctions expected from authority ("Because your mama'll beat your butt")
Undifferentiated	Global, undifferentiated reasons for act's wrongness ("It's bad"; "It's not a nice thing to do"; "It's just not nice")
Don't know	

Table 19.5. *Proportion of subjects judging acts as wrong*

	Hypothetical transgressions			Actual transgressions
	No consequences	Low harm	High harm	Actual
Abused	85	65	85	35
Neglected	100	85	95	20
Low SES control	100	95	95	45
High SES control	100	100	100	95

to justify actual than hypothetical situations in terms of egocentric goal achievement (7% versus 0% for actual versus hypothetical transgressions), fairness (e.g., restoring a balance of rights; 27% versus 5%, respectively), and interpersonal incompatibility (10% versus 0%), whereas they were more likely to justify hypothetical than actual situations in terms of punishment avoidance (24% versus 5% for hypothetical versus actual transgressions, respectively) and global evaluations of wrongness (33% versus 14%, respectively). Children acted aggressively primarily in retribution for the victim's perceived harmful behavior, whereas they acted unfairly in retribution for their victim's perceived violation of their rights or to achieve egocentric personal goals.

Differences according to maltreatment status were found when children were asked to judge the permissibility of transgressions described with varying levels of hypothetical harm. Across the two levels of harm, children in both high and low SES comparison groups were more likely to judge hypothetical behavior as not permissible (100% and 95%, respectively) than those abused (75%), but they did not differ from neglected (90%) children. In other words, although virtually all abused children, like other children, judged hypothetical moral transgressions to be wrong, some abused children judged the same events to be permissible when the harmful consequences of those acts were included in descriptions of the transgressions!

The actual level of harm did not influence these judgments; merely the mention of consequences, whether mild or severe, served to differentiate abused children's judgments from those of other children. Further, level of depicted harm differentially affected abused children's (but not other children's) judgments. Although not quite statistically significant, acts that were described as causing high levels ("a lot") of harm were seen as more permissible by abused children than all other children, whereas acts that were described as causing low levels of harm ("a little") were seen as less permissible by high SES than by all other children. Abused children did not differ from other children, however, in their perceptions of the amount of harm actual or hypothetical transgressions caused.

Group differences were also found in judgments of the permissibility of actual transgressions. High SES comparison children were significantly more likely than low SES comparison, abused, and neglected children to judge actual transgressions as wrong (95%, 45%, 35%, and 20%, respectively). Further, in both hypothetical and actual situations, high SES comparison children were more likely than all other children to justify the wrongness of acts by referring to rules. Maltreated and nonmaltreated children did not differ, however, in their justifications for their own behavior.

Thus, the methods of this study provide some important insights into the interrelationships between maltreated (and normal) children's hypothetical moral judgments and judgments in real-life situations. Presented hypothetically and without mention of consequences, maltreated children, like other children, judged aggression and unfair resource distribution to be wrong. Further, they reasoned about the wrongness of these acts using justifications that have been associated with morality in previous studies (Davidson, Turiel, and Black, 1983; Smetana, 1985). These findings are consistent with those of Smetana et al. (1984) in suggesting that maltreated children do not differ from nonmaltreated children in their hypothetical judgments of right and wrong.

When reasoning about actual transgressions or when the consequences of hypothetical acts are made salient, however, abused children are more likely than other children to view transgressions that violate others' rights or welfare to be permissible, especially when the acts were described as causing high levels of harm. How can these two sets of findings be reconciled? Two explanations seem plausible. The first clue comes from children's justifications. The results suggest that, to some extent, all children see their actual behavior as *morally* justified – that is, as exacting retribution for another's misbehavior. Thus, all children are acting on a (perhaps immature) moral code in which unfairness and aggression are seen as just rewards for behavior in kind. In addition, both abused and neglected children were somewhat more likely than other children to justify their actual behavior on the basis of egocentric goals and interpersonal incompatibility. Although all children are more egocentric in making hypothetical judgments for the self than others (Smetana et al., 1984), abused children may be less able than other children to inhibit their egocentrism in actual behavior. Finally, the results also suggest that abused children may develop different thresholds for pain and evaluate acts that cause pain as less serious and more permissible than do other children. Thus, abused children may, paradoxically, be both *more* sensitive to the intrinsic effects of acts for hypothetical others' rights and welfare and *less* sensitive to the intrinsic effects of acts for real-life others' rights and welfare than other children.

These findings, as well as those of others (Barahal et al., 1984; Frodi and Smetana, 1984) also raised questions about the effects of social class on children's judgments, as middle-class children's judgments differed from both maltreated and nonmaltreated lower class children's judgments. First, high SES children were found to be more likely than other children to judge their actual behavior as wrong. This may be partially accounted for by the finding that all children considered actual situations to be only mildly harmful and that high SES children were found to be somewhat more likely than other children to consider mildly harmful (hypothetical) transgressions wrong. However, it is not clear why high SES children were more sensitive than all other children to the mildly harmful consequences of acts for others' welfare, nor is it clear whether this difference is due primarily to differences in social class, IQ, or both. As high SES children were also more likely than other children to justify hypothetical and actual transgressions by appealing to rules, it is possible that middle-class preschool children are more likely than other children to attend to regulations, even when the transgressions are not seen as particularly harmful or unfair. It is also possible that middle-class children were more aware of the socially desirable responses. This question, as well as others raised by these findings, await further research.

Directions for future research

There are many questions regarding the development of maltreated children's psychological, moral, and societal knowledge that remain to be addressed. Particularly lacking are studies that draw upon normative developmental research to examine qualitative changes in maltreated children's social knowledge. Given its relevance to understanding the social-cognitive effects of maltreatment, the psychological domain has been understudied. For instance, there have been no social-cognitive studies of maltreated children's conceptions of self, although it can be hypothesized that this aspect of children's psychological knowledge might be particularly susceptible to the effects of maltreatment. Such an approach to self knowledge might entail an investigation of how children's conceptions of self are qualitatively restructured through development, including a determination of whether maltreated children develop at the same rates, and in the same ways, as normal children. Researchers have described qualitative changes in normal children's understanding of the social, physical, active, and psychological selves (e.g., Damon and Hart, 1982). Developmental delays in self-knowledge among maltreated children may be global, or they may be restricted to particular aspects of self that are most closely related to experiences of maltreatment. For example, the development of conceptions of the physical self may be more susceptible to developmental delays among physically abused as compared to normal or neglected children. To our knowledge, no such investigations have been conducted. (Although there has been a great deal of interest in maltreated children's self-concept or self-esteem, this more personality-oriented dimension of the self-system is distinguishable from children's conceptions of self as described here. See Harter, 1983, for discussion of this issue.)

Similarly, there have been no comparisons of qualitative changes with age in normal and maltreated children's causal attributions; these need to be assessed broadly, as we do not know whether maltreatment results in generalizably different patterns of attributions or whether differences are restricted to the abusing parent.

The value of a developmental approach is not limited to this type of study. Knowledge of normative development can also be used to predict interactions between maltreatment status and development. For instance, Herzberger et al.'s (1981) findings raise intriguing questions when considered in light of the available developmental data regarding children's conceptions of persons. Research on the development of person perception (Livesley & Bromley, 1973; Peevers and Secord, 1973) indicates that the ability to make attributions regarding dispositional characteristics (e.g., a "mean character") develops with age. Although it is not clear whether maltreated children would suffer general developmental delays in their ability to make causal attributions (although, again, this hypothesis would need to be investigated), developmental changes in children's causal attributions and understanding of persons and psychological characteristics may interact with maltreatment status to produce deficits only at particular points in development. For instance, maltreated children's perceptions of the abusing parent may not differ from normal children's until they develop the ability to make dispositional attributions. This type of question can only be addressed by research informed by an understanding of normal development.

There are many other quantitative changes with age in children's psychological knowledge and skills that bear investigation in relation to maltreatment. The Barahal et al. (1981) study is unique in its focus on the quantitative dimensions of psychological development, but there is further need for careful studies of maltreated children's perspective-taking and communicative abilities. We issue one caveat for such research, however. Too often, such research is engaged in without adequate attention to and understanding of the developmental phenomenon under investigation, resulting in inappropriate hypotheses and conclusions. For example, Barahal et al.'s hypotheses were based upon the perceived social-cognitive deficits of adult abusers. It is highly unlikely, however, that the kinds of age-related changes in role-taking and social sensitivity that the Flavell et al. (1968) and Rothenberg (1970) measures, respectively, were designed to assess can be equated with these deficits, especially because virtually all children achieve a ceiling on these measures by middle childhood or early adolescence. In this context, how can group differences be interpreted? Lower scores in middle childhood do not necessarily point to arrested development, and may have no bearing at all on outcomes in adulthood. Therefore, hypotheses need to be thoughtfully generated, measures must be carefully chosen to be age-appropriate, and findings must be interpreted with caution.

In the moral and societal domains, there are many important developmental issues that remain to be addressed, each having serious implications for treatment and intervention. For instance, it is surprising that no studies have been conducted to determine whether children who have been abused or neglected are less developmentally mature moral reasoners compared to a nonmaltreated sample. The measurement of moral maturity represents an ongoing problem that has stymied researchers (we cannot recommend using Kohlberg's measures [see Colby and Kohlberg, 1987], because we believe the scoring entails confusions of moral and societal concerns and that these domains need to be conceptually and epistemologically distinguished), but other conceptually clear measures of young children's reasoning are available (e.g., Damon, 1977). We also do not know how maltreated children's concepts of parental authority or familial conventions, both aspects of the societal domain, differ as a consequence of suffering maltreatment, nor whether these vary as a function of type of maltreatment. A developmental approach to these questions must be based upon an understanding of the qualitative aspects of normative development.

Research on the criteria and justifications children use to distinguish among domains of social knowledge also offers some intriguing directions for further research. Research (Nucci and Herman, 1982) has indicated that, as compared to normal children, behaviorally disordered children do not treat moral actions of hitting and hurting as wrong independent of rules; they also appear to have a less developed sense of personal jurisdiction than normal children. It is possible that abused and neglected children also may differ in their construction of the parameters of the moral domain – that is, in what constitutes a moral problem – in subtle ways that were not captured by the two studies described here (Kelly, 1986; Smetana et al., 1984). More speculatively, it is possible that such differences in childhood may lead to and underlie abusing and neglecting parents' behavior. The distinct domain perspective offers a rich source of hypotheses regarding maltreated children's social-cognitive development.

Such investigations would further our understanding of the effects of maltreatment on social-cognitive development, as well as enrich our understanding of normal development. Although more research in this area is clearly needed, we offer two more caveats for future research. First, in most previous research, maltreatment has been defined in terms of physical abuse. In future research, maltreatment must be more broadly defined, and careful distinctions among types of maltreatment (physical, psychological, and sexual abuse and neglect) must be carefully made. The consideration of only one type of maltreatment may obscure differences that emerge between types of maltreatment, as well as between maltreated and normal children. This was illustrated by the findings of Smetana, Kelly, and Twentyman (1984), where significant differences occurred primarily between abused and neglected children.

Second, appropriate comparison groups, carefully matched on relevant characteristics, must be employed. The research discussed in this chapter points to the importance of unconfounding IQ and social-cognitive variables (Barahal et al., 1981; Frodi and Smetana, 1984; Kelly, 1986). Further, if IQ is found to have an effect on social-cognitive performance, Barahal et al.'s (1981) intriguing proposal that social-cognitive deficits among maltreated children leads to lower performance on IQ tests, rather than the reverse, must be seriously considered. Thus, in future research, the effects of social class and IQ need to be more carefully separated, so that the social experiences that lead to deficits in social judgments can be identified.

Finally, we believe that, to understand maltreated children's social behavior, it is necessary to examine the interrelationships between hypothetical social-cognitive judgments and judgments in actual social situations, as was done in the study by Kelly (1986) described here. Using methods informed by an understanding of social-cognitive domain distinctions (Turiel and Smetana, 1984), this study suggested that maltreated children's social behavior is related to their interpretation of aggressive and unfair situations. Although these findings need to be replicated and expanded, they further underscore the importance of considering maltreated children's interpretations and structuring of their social world.

Notes

1 This view is consistent with the large body of empirical research on role-taking, which indicates that children's ability to take another's perspective varies according to the type of role-
taking task used (see Ford, 1979, for a review of the role-taking research and Turiel, 1983,
for a further elaboration of this argument).
2 The Rothenberg scale assesses the accuracy of children's labeling of specific affects and of the
underlying motives for the affects, whereas the test of perspective-taking ability, the so-called
Boy–Dog–Tree test, assesses the degree to which children are able to tell a story that is missing essential elements and keep the story free of contamination from these stimuli.

References

Aber, J. L., and Cicchetti, D. (1984). The socio-emotional development of maltreated children:
An empirical and theoretical analysis. In Fitzgerald, H. E., Lester, B. M., and Yogman, M.
W. (Eds.), *Theory and Research in Behavioral Pediatrics: Vol. 2* (pp. 147–205). New York:
Plenum.
Barahal, R., Waterman, J., and Martin, A. P. (1981). The social–cognitive development of
abused children. *Journal of Consulting and Clinical Psychology, 49,* 508–516.
Blasi, A. (1980). Bridging moral cognition and moral action: A critical review of the literature.
Psychological Bulletin, 88, 1–45.
Broughton, J. (1978) Development of concepts of self, mind, reality, and knowledge. In W.
Damon (Ed.), *New directions for child development. Vol. 1: Social cognition.* San Francisco:
Jossey-Bass.
Burgess, R. L., and Conger, R. D. (1978). Family interaction in abusive, neglectful, and normal
families. *Child Development, 49,* 1163–1173.
Colby, A., and Kohlberg, L. (1987). *The measure of moral judgment: Vol. 2.* Cambridge: Cam-
bridge University Press.
Cummings, E. M., Zahn-Waxler, C., and Radke-Yarrow, M. (1981). Young children's responses
to expressions of anger and affection by others in the family. *Child Development, 52,* 1274–
1282.
Damon, W. (1977). *The social world of the child.* San Francisco: Jossey-Bass.
Damon, W., and Hart, D. (1982). The development of self-understanding from infancy through
adolescence. *Child Development, 53,* 841–864.
Davidson, P., Turiel, E., and Black, A. (1983). The effect of stimulus familiarity on the use of
criteria and justifications in children's social reasoning. *British Journal of Developmental
Psychology, 1,* 49–65.
Flavell, Botkin, Fry, Wright, and Jarvis (1968). *The development of role-taking and communi-
cation skills in children.* New York: Wiley.
Ford, M. E. (1979). The construct validity of egocentrism. *Psychological Bulletin, 86,* 1169–
1188.
Freud, A. (1952). The role of bodily illness in the mental life of children. *Psychoanalytic Study
of the Child, 7,* 69–81.
Frodi, A., and Smetana, J. (1984). Abused, neglected, and normal preschoolers' ability to dis-
criminate emotions in others: The effects of IQ. *Child Abuse and Neglect, 8,* 459–465.
George, C., and Main, M. (1979). Social interactions of young abused children: Approach,
avoidance, and aggression. *Child Development, 50,* 306–318.
Harter, S. (1983). Developmental perspectives on the self system. In E. M. Hetherington (Ed.),
Handbook of child psychology: Socialization, personality, and social development (pp. 275–
386). New York: Wiley.
Herrenkohl, R. C., and Herrenkohl, E. C. (1981). Some antecedents and developmental con-
sequences of child maltreatment. In R. Rizley and D. Cicchetti (Eds.), *New directions for*

child development: Developmental perspectives on child maltreatment. San Francisco: Jossey-Bass.

Herzberger, S. D., Potts, D. A., and Dillon, M. (1981). Abusive and nonabusive parental treatment from the child's perspective. *Journal of Consulting and Clinical Psychology, 49,* 81–90.

Hoffman-Plotkin, D. L., and Twentyman, C. T. (1984). Cognitive and behavioral characteristics of abused and neglected children. *Child Development, 55,* 794–802.

Kelly, M. A. (1986). Relations between moral judgment and moral actions in abused, neglected, and nonmaltreated children. Unpublished doctoral dissertation, University of Rochester.

Kinard, E. M. (1980). Emotional development in physically abused children. *American Journal of Orthopsychiatry, 50,* 686–696.

Kohlberg, L. (1971). From is to ought: How to commit the naturalistic fallacy and get away with it in the study of moral development. In T. Mischel (Ed.), *Cognitive development and epistemology* (pp. 151–232). New York: Academic Press.

Lemke, S. (1973). Identity and conservation: The child's developing conceptions of social and physical transformations. Unpublished doctoral dissertation, University of California, Berkeley.

Livesley, W. J., and Bromley, D. B. (1973). *Person perception in childhood and adolescence.* London: Wiley.

Nucci, L. (1977). Social development: Personal, conventional, and moral concepts. Unpublished doctoral dissertation, University of California, Santa Cruz.

Nucci, L. (1981). The development of personal concepts: A domain distinct from moral or societal concepts. *Child Development, 52,* 114–121.

Nucci, L., and Herman, S. (1982). Behavioral disordered children's conceptions of moral, conventional, and personal issues. *Journal of Abnormal Child Psychology, 10,* 411–426.

Ounsted, C., Oppenheimer, R., and Lindsay, J. (1974). Aspects of bonding failure: Treatment of families of battered children. *Developmental Medicine and Child Neurology, 16,* 447–445.

Peevers, B. H., and Secord, P. F. (1973). Developmental changes in the attribution of descriptive concepts to persons. *Journal of Personality and Social Psychology, 27,* 120–128.

Piaget, J. (1932/1948). *The moral judgment of the child.* Glencoe, IL: Free Press.

Piaget, J. (1967). *Six psychological studies.* New York: Random House.

Pratt, M. A. (1975). A developmental study of person perception and attributions of causality: Learning the what and why of others. Unpublished Ph.D. dissertation, Harvard University.

Reidy, T. J. (1977). The aggressive characteristics of abused and neglected children. *Journal of Clinical Psychology, 33,* 1140–1145.

Rothenberg, B. (1970). Children's social sensitivity and the relationship to interpersonal competence, intrapersonal comfort, and intellectual level. *Developmental Psychology, 2,* 335–350.

Shantz, C. U. (1975). The development of social cognition. In E. M. Hetherington (Ed.), *Review of child development research.* (Vol. 5). Chicago: University of Chicago Press.

Shantz, C. U. (1983). Social cognition. In J. H. Flavell and E. M. Markman (Eds.), *Handbook of child psychology: Cognitive development* (pp. 495–555). New York: Wiley.

Smetana, J. (1981). Preschool children's conceptions of moral and social rules. *Child Development, 52,* 1333–1336.

Smetana, J. (1983). Social–cognitive development: Domain distinctions and coordinations. *Developmental Review, 3,* 131–147.

Smetana, J. (1984). Toddlers' social interactions regarding moral and conventional transgressions. *Child Development, 55,* 1167–1176.

Smetana, J. (1985). Preschool children's conceptions of transgressions: The effects of varying moral and conventional domain-related attributes. *Developmental Psychology, 21,* 18–29.

Smetana, J. G., Kelly, M., and Twentyman, C. T. (1984). Abused, neglected, and nonmaltreated children's conceptions of moral and conventional transgressions. *Child Development, 55,* 277–287.

Straker, G., and Jacobson, R. S. (1981). Aggression, emotional maladjustment and empathy in the abused child. *Developmental Psychology, 17,* 762–765.

Turiel, E. (1975). The development of social concepts: Mores, customs, and conventions. In D. J. DePalma and J. M. Foley (Eds.), *Moral development: Current theory and research.* Hillsdale, NJ: Erlbaum.

Turiel, E. (1978). Social regulations and domains of social concepts. In W. Damon (Ed.), *New directions for child development: Vol. I: Social cognition* (pp. 45–74). San Francisco: Jossey-Bass.

Turiel, E. (1979). Distinct conceptual and developmental domains: Social convention and morality. In C. B. Keasey (Ed.), *1978 Nebraska symposium on motivation.* Lincoln: University of Nebraska Press.

Turiel, E. (1983). *The development of social knowledge: Morality and convention.* Cambridge: Cambridge University Press.

Turiel, E. (1987). Potential relations between the development of social reasoning and prevention of childhood aggression. In D. Crowell, I. Evans, and C. R. O'Donnel (Eds.), *Childhood aggression: Sources of influence, prevention, and control.* New York: Plenum.

Turiel, E., and Smetana, J. (1984). Social knowledge and action: The coordination of domains. In W. M. Kurtines and J. L. Gewirtz (Eds.), *Morality, moral behavior, and moral development.* New York: Wiley.

Twentyman, C. T., Bousha, D. M., and Hoffman-Plotkin, D. L. (1981). *Behavioral interactions in abusive, neglectful, and comparison children.* Paper presented at the Third International Congress on Child Abuse and Neglect, Amsterdam.

Watson, M. (1977). A developmental sequence of role playing, Paper presented at the meeting of the American Psychological Association, San Francisco.

20   The effects of maltreatment on the development of young children

Martha Farrell Erickson, Byron Egeland,
and Robert Pianta

> Her school performance is extremely erratic. One day she does fine and the
> next day she can't seem to do anything. Then she usually becomes frus-
> trated and ends up tearing up the work she did the day before. Her behavior
> is an enormous problem for everyone in the school. One minute she is sweet
> and loving, holding my hand, and the next minute she is screaming and
> throwing things. I have never seen such anger! She is a bomb ready to
> explode!
>
> *– Teacher's description of a 6-year-old victim of maltreatment*

Although harsh treatment and inadequate care of children has a long history, widespread recognition of child maltreatment as a social problem, and
particularly recognition of the lasting psychological consequences of maltreatment, is a relatively recent phenomenon. Parenting practices that today
are recognized as abusive actually were accepted as standard practice and,
in fact, were recommended by childrearing "experts" as recently as the late
1930s. Historians of childrearing trends (e.g., DeMause, 1974; Newson and
Newson, 1974) describe open advocacy of child beating into the eighteenth
century and continued recommendation of harsh, swift discipline well into
this century. Not only was physical punishment advocated, but parents were
counseled to behave in ways that today would be considered neglectful of
the child's basic psychological and physical needs. For example, in 1928
Watson warned mothers against "mawkish, sentimental" handling of their
babies. If a baby cried she or he should not be picked up; crying did not hurt
the baby, but only hurt the parent to listen. An infant was expected to be
quiet, obedient, and to submit early on to firm parental control (Newson
and Newson, 1974). From the early childhood education movement and

This research was supported by a grant from the Maternal and Child Health Service
to the Department of Health, Education and Welfare (MC–R–270416–01.–0). This
research is currently supported by a grant from the Office of Special Education,
Department of Education, Washington, DC (G008300029) and the Wm. T. Grant
Foundation, New York City.

647

from psychoanalysis came ideas and observations that challenged these attitudes. In the late 1920s and 1930s, extensive observations of children in
their natural environments (e.g., Isaacs, 1930; Piaget, 1952) led to a new
understanding of the complexities of human development and an appreciation of the importance of play, exploration, and self-assertion to the young
child's development. And from psychoanalysts such as Spitz (1945) and
Bowlby (1951) came dramatic evidence attesting to the importance of warm,
affectionate care to the child's healthy development. The lack of such care
was shown to result in serious social and emotional problems, if not physical
illness or even death. Further support for this view came from ethologists
and zoologists (e.g., Harlow, 1961; Lorenz, 1952).

Improved understanding of child development and a new awareness of
the importance of loving care for infants and children helped to pave the
way for public recognition of maltreatment and its impact on a child's
development. However, it was not until Kempe's landmark paper in 1962
that abuse actually was recognized as a major social problem. (Interestingly,
Margaret Lynch, 1985, cites a paper written almost 100 years ago that is
strikingly similar to Kempe's; however, that paper apparently was ignored
– perhaps, as Lynch contends, because society was not yet ready to recognize
the problem.)

And although Kempe's paper stirred public response to the problem of
overt, intentional physical abuse of children, public recognition of other
forms of maltreatment (e.g., physical and emotional neglect) lagged behind.
In 1973 Newberger wrote, "We are coming to see that the essential element
in child abuse is not the intention to destroy a child but rather the inability
of a parent to nurture his offspring" (p. 15). Eleven years later, Wolock and
Horowitz (1984) still observed that, although neglect is more prevalent and
has been shown to have consequences as serious for the child as abuse, it
continues to receive far less attention both publicly and professionally.

Early awareness of the consequences of both abuse and neglect focused on
observable physical effects and only recently has attention turned to the psychological consequences of maltreatment. Yet, as Garbarino and Vondra
(1987) contend, it is the psychological consequences that are the unifying
factor in all types of maltreatment. Regardless of the occurrence of physical
trauma or injury, the legacy of maltreatment in its various forms is damage
to the child's sense of self and the consequent impairment of social, emotional, and cognitive functioning.

Empirical findings on psychological outcomes for maltreated children

Much of the evidence attesting to the psychological consequences of abuse
comes from clinical descriptions and uncontrolled studies. Disproportionate numbers of abused children have been found to perform below the aver-

age range on IQ tests (e.g., Martin, Beezley, Conway, and Kempe, 1974; Morse, Sahler and Friedman, 1970; Sandgrund, Gaines, and Green, 1974). Abused children also have been described as presenting multiple and varied social and emotional problems, including aggression, hostility, passivity, apathy, and withdrawn behavior (e.g., Galdston, 1971; Kempe and Kempe, 1978; Martin and Beezley, 1977). Steele (1977), looking not only at physically abused, but also at neglected, emotionally deprived, and sexually abused children, called attention to the learning problems and low self-esteem among children who were maltreated early in life, and noted a high incidence of juvenile delinquency among these children in subsequent years.

A few studies have used control groups to examine more systematically the behavior of abused children. For example, George and Main (1979) found that abused toddlers were more aggressive and avoided peers more than nonabused toddlers. These children also failed to show empathy in response to the distress of their age-mates, and, in fact, responded with fear, anger, or even physical aggression toward the distressed peer (Main and George, unpublished manuscript, as cited in Main and Goldwyn, 1984). Kinard (1980) compared the performance of abused and nonabused school-age children on a battery of psychological tests and reported that abused children's responses suggested more aggression, lower self-concept, and problems in social relationships with both peers and adults. A number of other carefully controlled studies now are underway, as discussed later in this chapter and elsewhere in this volume (e.g., Crittenden and Ainsworth; Aber et al.).

Subtypes of maltreatment

In addition to comparing abused children to a control group of nonabused children, some researchers also have found significant differences when comparing physically abused children with children who were neglected. For example, Reidy (1977) reported that both abused and neglected school-age children displayed more aggressive behavior in school than nonabused children, but that abused children expressed more aggression in fantasy and free play than the neglected children. In a recent study of preschoolers, Hoffman-Plotkin and Twentyman (1984) found that abused children were more aggressive than either neglected or nonmaltreated children. The neglected children in their study interacted less frequently with peers than either abused or control group children. Likewise, Crittenden (1985b; Crittenden and Ainsworth, this volume) traced different patterns of developmental consequences among groups of abused and neglected infants. Abused children in her study were described as temperamentally difficult, angry when stressed, and showing mild developmental delay. In contrast, neglected children were passive, somewhat helpless when stressed, and exhibited significant developmental delays.

The reported differences between neglected and abused children in the studies cited above highlight the importance of separating the various forms of maltreatment when investigating the consequences for children. Failure to do so may obscure important differences between maltreated and nonmaltreated children. Furthermore, identifying the consequences of particular patterns of maltreatment can have important implications for detecting maltreatment, intervening with maltreated children and/or their families, and for legal and social policy decisions relevant to child maltreatment. However, as Aber and Cicchetti (1984) discussed in their review of maltreatment research, there is no hard, clear line separating subtypes of maltreatment. Many children experience more than one form of maltreatment. Thus, subtype groups are bound to overlap, a fact researchers should not deny by attempting to force cases into one group or another. Research also might address the question of whether different combinations of types of maltreatment lead to different consequences for children. (The Harvard Child Maltreatment Project [Cicchetti & Rizley, 1981; see also Cicchetti, this volume; Cicchetti, Barnett, and Braunwald, this volume; Carlson, this volume] and our own Mother–Child Project, discussed subsequently, are attempting to address those issues and questions.)

Child neglect has more than one form; there are subtypes within the broader category. Some children are victims of physical neglect in that their basic physical needs (food, clothing, health, hygiene) are not met. Others are well fed and appropriately clothed, but are emotionally neglected. The most extreme consequences of emotional neglect are described as nonorganic failure to thrive syndrome, failure to grow (and sometimes even failure to survive) despite adequate nutrition (e.g., Gardner, 1972; MacCarthy, 1979; Patton and Gardner, 1962). The psychological consequences of emotional neglect persist even after diagnosis and intervention. In a clinical follow-up of medically diagnosed failure-to-thrive infants, MacCarthy (1979) described attention-seeking behavior and superficial displays of affection among these children following out-of-home placement. Later in childhood, these children were observed to be selfish and spiteful and to engage in stealing. Similarly, Polansky, Chalmers, Buttenweiser, and Williams (1981) described the hostile, defiant behavior of 11- to 12-year-old children who had earlier been diagnosed as failure-to-thrive infants. And Hufton and Oates (1977) found that failure-to-thrive children presented a variety of academic and behavior problems in early elementary school.

Even in less serious cases of emotional neglect the long-term consequences of this form of maltreatment are profound. As discussed later in this chapter, our own assessments of emotionally neglected children (children whose mothers are what we have called "psychologically unavailable") reveal increasingly severe problems in cognitive and socioemotional functioning from infancy through the preschool years (Egeland and Erickson, 1987; Egeland, Sroufe, and Erickson, 1983).

Another subtype of maltreatment that typically has been the subject of a separate body of literature is sexual abuse – perhaps the most difficult pattern of maltreatment to study. To date there is a notable lack of published research comparing sexually abused children either to nonmaltreated children or to children experiencing other forms of maltreatment, but such comparisons are being undertaken as part of the Minnesota Mother–Child Interaction Project, as described in a subsequent section of this chapter. Although the research on sexual maltreatment that has been published so far is scant and methodologically limited, it does suggest some of the possible psychological consequences for children who are sexually abused. A number of studies have shown an extremely high incidence of prior sexual abuse among drug abusers (e.g., Benward and Densen-Gerber, 1973) and prostitutes (James and Meyerding, 1977). Clinical symptoms of women who were sexually abused in childhood include isolation, depression, guilt, poor self-concept, sexual problems, and difficulty in social relationships (e.g., Herman and Hirschman, 1981; Meiselman, 1980; Tsai and Wagner, 1978). Although studies have concentrated largely on female victims of sexual abuse, Tyler (1983) noted that a large proportion of adult males who perpetrate sexual abuse were themselves victims of sexual abuse as children. Retrospective studies such as these, however, look only at victims who present clear-cut problems and tell us nothing about the coping strategies or developmental outcomes for other victims of child sexual abuse.

Furthermore, consequences for the sexually maltreated child might be expected to vary depending on the type of sexual activity engaged in, the use of force, the age of the child, the age of the perpetrator, and the relationship of the perpetrator to the child. In one of the few studies to consider those variables, Finkelhor (1979) found the severity of psychological consequences of sexual abuse to be related to the degree of force used, the age difference between the victim and the perpetrator, and the closeness of the relationship between the child and the perpetrator. On the basis of clinical experience with sexually abused children, Summit and Kryso (1978) hypothesized that psychological consequences of sexual abuse are mediated by the environmental response to the act; particularly, that children suffer psychological damage if they are aware of the inappropriateness or the exploitive quality of the act – an awareness that would vary with age and cognitive ability. This question has not been explored systematically.

Separating the effects of maltreatment from the effects of other environmental influences

Many researchers and clinicians have noted that maltreated children often live in poverty and/or in families with multiple problems. Therefore, an important question to address is to what extent a child's subsequent problems are due to the maltreatment per se or to other aspects of the environment in which the child is being reared. In an often-cited study, Elmer (1977) compared abused and nonabused children from homes of low socio-economic status and found very few differences. Instead, she reported extensive problems in cognitive functioning, language, and social–emotional behavior among all of her subjects, leading her to conclude that consequences of poverty and its many environmental correlates may override the effects of abuse. Although this was an important study and called much-needed attention to the risks of poverty, Elmer's conclusion should be viewed somewhat cautiously. To a certain extent, her findings may be an artifact of the procedure by which she identified her groups. Specifically, the two nonabused comparison groups were (1) children who were hospitalized for accidental injury, and (2) children who were not victims of trauma (either accident or abuse) but were matched for history of hospitalization (i.e., for acute illnesses). As Aber and Cicchetti (1984) note, by matching her control group and maltreatment group not only on SES but also on history of hospitalization, Elmer may have skewed the representativeness of her control group. A more accurate conclusion of her study might "be that those socio-demographic features of a family that lead to infant hospitalization may have an impact on child development that appears as strong as the impact of a history of maltreatment" (p. 175).

More recent research that we and our colleagues have conducted (described in a subsequent section of this chapter) indicates that maltreatment does have consequences above and beyond the effects of poverty and its correlates. Comparing maltreated children with nonmaltreated children from the same low SES, high-risk population, we have found maltreated children to function more poorly in the cognitive and social-emotional domains from infancy through the early school years (Egeland and Erickson, 1987; Egeland and Sroufe, 1981; Egeland, Sroufe, and Erickson, 1983).

Although one can control for poverty and other sociodemographic characteristics, it is more difficult (if not impossible) to tease out the effects of abuse from the effects of other aspects of family interaction and home environment. For example, several researchers (e.g., Giaretto, 1976; Rosenfeld, 1977; Herman and Hirschman, 1977) have noted that the occurrence of sexual abuse (whether perpetrated directly by a family member or allowed to happen within the home) suggests general family dysfunction, and they contend that it is this dysfunction rather than the abuse per se that accounts for psychological outcomes for the child. (The same might be said in regard to other forms of maltreatment.) Indeed, a close examination of abusing and neglecting families usually reveals that maltreatment is not an isolated event within an otherwise normally functioning family. In our own research we have found that maltreatment usually represents a pervasive, persistent pattern of interaction within home environments that in many ways fail to foster the child's healthy development (see, for example, Egeland and Erickson, 1987; Egeland and Sroufe, 1981; Egeland, Sroufe, and Erickson, 1983; Pianta, Egeland, and Erickson, this volume). Perhaps the issue of separating "maltreatment" from "family dysfunction" is more a semantic issue than a real one if one adopts a broad view of maltreatment as "inability of the parent to nurture his offspring" (Newberger, 1973).

Developmental considerations in examining consequences of maltreatment

Many of the early studies of maltreatment described negative consequences for groups of children of widely varying ages. Yet, given what is known about the rapid and dramatic changes children undergo over time, it is reasonable to expect that the consequences of maltreatment would be manifest differently at different developmental periods. More recent cross-sectional studies have looked at children within a specific age range and longitudinal studies have begun to follow children over time, through different stages of development. Importantly, a number of researchers are using measures sensitive to the particular demands and issues at each stage of development. To date, most of these developmental assessments of the consequences of maltreatment have focused on infancy and early childhood. For example, Gaensbauer, Mrazek, and Harmon (1980) described ways in which maltreated infants deviated from normal development of emotional expression and affective communications with their caregivers. The authors classified infants into one of four categories of affective expression and hypothesized as to the caretaking history that may have led to the particular pattern observed. A pattern of developmental and affective retardation was thought to be the outcome of extreme neglect and deprivation. Children who appeared depressed, but were able to perform at age level on developmental tasks, were thought to have experienced initial adequate care followed by separation from the caregiver or psychological separation due to maternal depression. Alternating periods of adequate care and maltreatment were hypothesized to lead to an ambivalent, affectively labile pattern of communication. And infants who were angry and destructive were thought to be victims of frequent, harsh punishment.

Much of the recent research on the development of maltreated infants has been facilitated by attachment theory (Bowlby, 1969, 1973, 1980) and the Strange Situation paradigm (Ainsworth, Blehar, Waters, and Wall, 1978), which has been demonstrated to be a theoretically sound and empirically valid means of assessing the quality of the infant's adaptation within the context of the infant–caregiver relationship. One of the major studies of maltreated children currently underway is the Harvard Child Maltreatment Project (Cicchetti and Rizley, 1981). Early results from that project found

maltreated children to be more likely than nonmaltreated infants to be insecurely attached (Schneider-Rosen, Braunwald, Carlson and Cicchetti, 1985;
Schneider-Rosen and Cicchetti, 1984). These researchers also noted a
marked increase from 12 to 24 months in the percentage of maltreated
infants who presented an anxious–avoidant pattern of attachment. (See
Carlson, et al., this volume, for a detailed discussion of the findings.)

Using a modification of the Strange Situation procedure, Lamb, Gaensbauer, Malkin, and Schultz (1985) found that children who were abused or
neglected by their primary caregiver were more likely than nonmaltreated
children to demonstrate insecure attachments with their biological mothers
and, to a lesser extent, with foster mothers. For children abused by someone
else this was not true. Crittenden (1985b) also reported a high incidence of
insecure attachment among abused and neglected children. And she found
that abused children were angry until their second year of life, at which time
they were observed to inhibit that anger with their mother. Neglected children showed no such change in strategy in the second year, and the author
suggests that the inhibition of the anger reflects the abused children's new
cognitive ability to form expectancies about the mother's behavior (Crittenden, 1985a).

Developmental studies of maltreated children converge with studies of
the development of nonmaltreated children to help us understand the
impact of the early infant–caregiver relationship on various aspects of the
child's development. A number of studies have shown secure mother–infant
attachment to lead to subsequent competence and anxious attachment to
relate to later problems in cognitive and socioemotional functioning (e.g.,
Arend, Gove, and Sroufe, 1979; Erickson, Sroufe, and Egeland, 1985; Matas,
Arend, and Sroufe, 1978; Sroufe, Fox, and Pancake, 1983; Waters, Wippman, and Sroufe, 1979). Studies conducted by Main and her colleagues illustrate the similarity of outcomes for abused infants and nonabused infants
whose caregivers reject their attachment behavior. As noted earlier, these
researchers found abused toddlers to be aggressive, avoidant, and nonempathic (George and Main, 1979). As Main and Goldwyn (1984) discuss, they
and other researchers have observed behaviors similar in kind, but not
degree, in children whose mothers rejected their attachment behavior (e.g.,
Ainsworth, Blehar, Waters, and Wall, 1978; Blanchard and Main, 1979;
Main and Weston, 1981; Sroufe, 1983). These children typically are
avoidant of their mothers in the Strange Situation, and in other situations
they are aggressive, nonempathic, and avoidant of both peers and adults.

In our own research we also have found a high incidence of insecure
attachment among children experiencing various forms of maltreatment
and, as discussed in following pages, we have chronicled the difficulties these
children exhibit in developmentally appropriate situations at subsequent

stages. Aber and Cicchetti (1984) lauded the increasing sophistication of research tracing the early development of maltreated infants and children and they called for the development of broad-band measures to assess the quality of adaptation of children at later stages of development. Cicchetti and colleagues on the Harvard Project are now engaged in such efforts. Such work is also underway as part of our project as we continue to assess the children from our sample in early elementary school, at home, and in the laboratory. Early results of those assessments are presented in this chapter.

New directions in maltreatment research

In summary, in the years since Kempe and his colleagues first called attention to the plight of physically abused children, researchers and clinicians have documented the harmful consequences of maltreatment in its many forms. Although early evidence came from uncontrolled studies or clinical descriptions, recent studies have shown increasing refinement and rigor in attempting to build the body of knowledge about the ways in which various forms of maltreatment affect children. Early focus on overt physical harm has given way to recognition of psychological consequences, and emphasis on the most blatant forms of abuse and neglect has broadened to include more subtle forms of maltreatment that may have equally damaging effects. Separate subtypes of maltreatment have been identified and the different consequences related to these subtypes are beginning to be explored. Important questions have been raised about the effects of maltreatment above and beyond the effects of other environmental influences, particularly those associated with poverty, and a few controlled studies have begun to address those questions. And recently researchers have examined the sequelae of maltreatment within a developmental framework, beginning to identify the ways in which the effects of maltreatment are manifest during different stages of development.

The Minnesota Mother–Child Interaction Project, initiated in 1975, was one of the first investigations to address systematically many of these major questions about the developmental consequences of different patterns of maltreatment. In the remainder of this chapter we will discuss findings from this ongoing longitudinal, prospective study and will consider how it has added to our understanding of maltreatment and its effects. We will review briefly the studies, presented in detail elsewhere, that follow our subjects from infancy through preschool. We then will present a recent examination of maltreated children from our sample as they enter school, including for the first time a group of children identified as having been sexually abused. Finally, we will consider the implications of these findings for future research and practice.

The Minnesota Mother–Child Interaction Project

The Minnesota Mother–Child Project is a prospective longitudinal study designed to follow the development of a sample of children born to first-time mothers identified as being at risk for caretaking problems due to poverty, youth, lack of support, low education, and generally unstable life circumstances. As part of this investigation, we have studied the various factors that influence the quality of care the child receives, particularly the antecedents of abuse and neglect, and we have examined the effects of various forms of maltreatment on the development of these children from birth through the early school years. (A brief overview of the Minnesota Mother–Child Project is presented in a chapter by Pianta, Egeland, and Erickson in this volume and will not be repeated here.)

Maltreatment groups at two years

Although the Mother–Child Project has examined the entire qualitative range of caregiving, the detailed and comprehensive data we have collected allow us to focus on the consequences of maltreatment, addressing the question of whether specific patterns of maltreatment result in specific developmental outcomes. From among the original sample of 267 mothers, four maltreatment groups were identified when the children were 2 years of age, based on data collected from birth: physically abusive ($n = 24$), hostile/verbally abusive ($n = 19$), neglectful ($n = 24$), and psychologically unavailable ($n = 19$). (There is considerable overlap among these maltreatment groups. See Pianta, Egeland, and Erickson, this volume, for details.) Behaviors of physically abusive mothers in this sample range from frequent, intense spanking when disciplining their children to unprovoked outbursts of anger resulting in serious injuries. Mothers in the hostile/verbally abusive group engaged in constant harassment and berating of their children, chronically finding fault and criticizing them in a harsh manner. Neglectful mothers, either through incompetence or irresponsibility, failed to provide necessary health or physical care and protection for their children. Although these mothers sometimes expressed interest in their children's well-being, their efforts to care for their children were inconsistent and inadequate. Mothers in the psychologically unavailable group were emotionally unresponsive to their children. These mothers appeared detached, interacting with their children only when necessary, and gave no indication that they experienced joy or satisfaction in their relationship with them. (A detailed description of the procedures and criteria for identifying these maltreatment groups is presented in Pianta, Egeland, and Erickson, this volume.) A control group of 85 nonmaltreated children also was selected from the original high-risk sample, allowing us to distinguish the consequences of maltreatment from the influences of poverty and other environmental factors. If there was some doubt as to whether a child was being maltreated, the case was not included in the control group or any of the maltreatment groups.

Outcomes measures: infancy through preschool

Our assessments were designed to capture the overall quality of the child's adaptation, the way in which the child handled salient developmental tasks at each age period. Three months postpartum, mother and infant were observed in a feeding situation, and at 6 months mother and infant were observed in two feeding and one play situations. Following the observations, the observer rated a variety of mother, infant, and interactional behaviors. Separate factor analyses of the feeding and play situations yielded three-factor solutions, with one of the factors for each being a baby factor. The 3- and 6-month baby feeding factor loaded on baby's responsiveness to mother's interaction, baby's disposition, and social behavior. The baby play factor loaded on baby's activity level, baby's coordination, baby's satisfaction, and baby's attention. In order to have an index of the infant's cognitive and motor development, the Bayley Scales of Infant Development (BSID, 1969) were administered at 9 and 24 months.

Quality of the mother–infant attachment was assessed at 12 and 18 months using the Ainsworth, Blehar, Waters, and Wall (1978) Strange Situation procedure. (See appendixes for a description of this procedure and criteria for group classification.) At 24 months of age, measures of independent engagement of tasks, emerging autonomy, and resources for coping with frustration reflect the salient developmental task. Thus, we videotaped the 24-month-old children with their mothers in a series of tool-using problem-solving tasks designed to capture those behaviors. The first two problems were simple and were not included in the scoring. The last two problems, however, were too difficult for a 2-year-old to solve without the help of an adult: putting two sticks together, end to end, in order to get a prize from a long plexiglass tube; weighting down the end of a lever with a block to raise a prize through a hole in a plexiglass box. Mothers were told to let the child work on the problem alone and then to "give any help you think the child needs." Observers, blind to the child's family history or maltreatment classification, rated the children on five- to seven-point scales on the following dimensions: enthusiasm, dependency, noncompliance, anger, frustration toward the mother, coping, and persistence.

When the children were 42 months of age, they were videotaped alone in the Barrier Box task and with their mothers in a series of four teaching tasks. The Barrier Box was designed to assess the child's reaction to frustration, whereas the teaching tasks provided an opportunity to observe how the mother and child worked together on a series of age-appropriate learning tasks. In the Barrier Box situation the child was allowed to play with a variety of attractive toys on the floor while the project assistant worked at a table nearby. In the center of the room was a large plexiglass box containing a set of toys identical to those on the floor. The box was latched in a way that a young child could not open it. After one minute the project assistant removed the toys the child was playing with, telling the child they belonged in another room. She then left the child with a few unattractive toys and told the child she or he could play with those or with the toys in the box. For ten minutes the child was allowed to try to open the box, play with the few available toys, or wander around the room. Activities available to the child were limited in order to encourage the child's continued efforts to open the Barrier Box. At the end of the session the project assistant opened the box for the child and allowed him or her to play for several minutes with the toys. During the session the child was videotaped and then was rated on three- to seven-point scales on the following variables: self esteem, ego control (how well the child controls impulses and modulates responses), apathy/withdrawal, flexibility, creativity, agency (the child's confidence and assertiveness in approaching the task), hyperactivity/distractibility, dependency on the project assistant for help or support, directness and intensity of help-seeking, and positive and negative affect. In addition to these rating scales, the child's persistence was assessed by computing the portion of time he or she spent on the task.

In the 42-month teaching tasks, we videotaped mother and child in a series of tasks difficult enough to require that the mother use some teaching strategies to enable the child to complete the tasks. In the first task, the child was told to construct copies of a large wooden block, using smaller blocks of various shapes. Task 2 was a verbal problem in which the mother asked the child to name as many things with wheels as he or she could think of. In Task 3 the child was asked to place objects on a matrix, matching stimuli on dimensions of shape and color. In the final task, the child used an Etch-a-Sketch to trace a maze drawn on the screen of the toy. Children were rated on their persistence, enthusiasm for the tasks, anger/negativity (directed at the mother or the environment in general), compliance with mother's directions and suggestions, reliance on mother for help and support, affection for mother, avoidance of mother, and the general quality of their experience in the session. Ratings of the children in the Barrier Box situation were done independent of the ratings of the mothers and children in the teaching tasks, and again raters were blind to family history or maltreatment classifications.

At approximately 4½ to 5 years of age, 96 children from our total sample were observed extensively in their preschool or daycare settings. Forty of the children attended a special laboratory preschool at the University of Minnesota. Others attended a variety of preschools and daycare centers throughout the metropolitan area. Using seven-point rating scales, observers assessed the children on the following dimensions: agency, ego control, dependency on teachers for support and nurturance, social skills in the peer group, positive affect, negative emotional tone, and compliance with teacher's directions and suggestions. In addition, a childcare provider or preschool teacher completed the Preschool Behavior Questionnaire (Behar and Stringfield, 1974), which consists of 31 items often associated with social or emotional problems in young children. Teachers also completed the Behavior Problem Scale (Erickson and Egeland, 1981), similar in format to the Preschool Behavior Questionnaire, and consisting of an additional 30 behaviors considered indicative of adjustment problems in preschool children.

Adaptation of maltreated children: infancy through preschool

To determine the effects of maltreatment, each maltreatment group was compared to the control group on the child outcome variables described above. Because physical abuse often accompanies other forms of maltreatment, a second set of analyses also was done, in which physically abused children were subtracted from each maltreatment group and each of those subgroups (e.g., neglected without physical abuse; psychologically unavailable without physical abuse) was then compared to the control group. These earlier findings from the Mother–Child Project demonstrate that the consequences for children from each maltreatment group were varied and severe. Maltreated children were functioning much more poorly in many areas of social and emotional behavior at each stage of development than were children from similar backgrounds who did not have a history of maltreatment. These earlier findings, which have been recorded in detail elsewhere (cf. Egeland and Sroufe, 1981; Egeland, Sroufe, and Erickson, 1983) are summarized here in Table 20.1 through Table 20.3. (Note that the data analysis procedures used here are consistent with those used in the 1983 article. However, a slightly different procedure was used in the 1981 article; thus there are a few discrepancies from the figures reported there.)

Physically abused children. No significant differences were found between physically abused and nonmaltreated children in this sample through the age of 12 months (Tables 20.1, 20.2). However, by 18 months, physically abused children were more likely to present an anxious pattern of attachment in the Strange Situation (Table 20.3). Fifty percent of these children were anxiously attached (32% A's, 18% C's), compared to 29% in the control group who were anxiously attached. At 24 months of age, in the tool-using tasks, physically abused children differed from the control group on several measures (Table 20.1). They were angry, frustrated with their mothers, and noncompliant, and they exhibited less enthusiasm for the task than did the

Table 20.1. *Comparisons between controls and early maltreatment groups on outcome measures from infancy through preschool*

	Control group versus					
Variables	Physical abuse	Neglect	Neglect without physical abuse	Psychologically unavailable	Psychologically unavailable without physical abuse	Verbal[a] abuse
3-month feeding						
Baby social behavior				U > C*	U > C*	
6-month feeding						
Baby social behavior		C > N*	C > N*			
6-month play						
baby social behavior						
BSID (9 months)						
BSID (24 months)	C > P**	C > N**	C > N**	C > U**	C > U**	C > V**
24-month tool-using tasks						
Dependency						
Noncompliance	P > C**	N > C**	N > C*	U > C**	U > C**	V > C**
Frustration	P > C**	N > C**		U > C**	U > C**	V > C**
Persistence						
Coping	C > P*	C > N**	C > N**	C > U*		
Enthusiasm		C > N**	C > N*	C > U*	C > U**	
Anger	P > C**	N > C**		U > C**	U > C**	V > C**
Positive affect		C > N**			C > U*	C > V*
Negative affect	C > P**	N > C**	C > N**	C > U**		V > C**

42-month barrier box task:

Self-esteem	C > P**	C > N**	C > N**		C > V**
Ego control	C > P**	C > N**	C > N*		C > V**
Apathy/withdrawal		N > C*	N > C*		
Flexibility		C > N**	C > N**		
Creativity	C > P*	C > N**	C > N*	C > U*	
Agency	C > P*	C > N**	C > N**		
Hyperactivity/distractibility	P > C**	N > C**	N > C**		
Dependency					
Directness of help-seeking					
Intensity of help-seeking					
Positive affect	P > C*	C > N*	C > N**		
Negative affect		N > C**	N > C**		V > C*
Persistence (proportion of time on task)					

42-month teaching tasks:

Persistence	C > P**	C > N**	C > N**	C > U**	C > V**
Enthusiasm	C > P**	C > N**	C > N**	C > U**	C > V**
Negativity	P > C**	N > C**	N > C**	U > C**	V > C**
Compliance	C > P**	C > N**	C > N*	C > U**	C > V**
Quality of experience	C > P**	C > N**	C > N**	C > U**	C > V**
Reliance		N > C**			
Affection for mother	C > P**	C > N**	C > N**	C > U**	C > V**
Avoidance of mother	P > C**	N > C**		U > C**	V > C**

Preschool variables:

Preschool data available for too few subjects to allow analysis.

Preschool behavior questionnaire	P > C*	N > C*		U > C**	

Table 20.1. (*cont.*)

Variables	Control group versus					
	Physical abuse	Neglect	Neglect without physical abuse	Psychologically unavailable	Psychologically unavailable without physical abuse	Verbal[a] abuse
Behavior problem scale				U > C**		
Agency						
Ego control	C > P**	C > N**	C > N**	C > U**	C > U*	
Dependency		N > C**	N > C**	U > C*	U > C**	
Social skills						
Positive affect						
Negative emotion	P > C*			U > C*		
Compliance	C > P**			C > U**		

*p < .05
**p < .01
[a]Because there were only four subjects in the verbal without physical abuse group, that group was not included in this table.

Table 20.2. *Distribution of 12-month attachment classes among early maltreatment groups*

Row # Row %	A Anxious/avoidant	B Secure	C Anxious/resistant	Total
Control group	15	57	13	85
(nonmaltreated)	18%	67%	15%	
Physically abused	6	13	4	23
	26%	57%	17%	
Hostile/verbal abuse	4	12*	2	18
	22%	67%	11%	
Hostile/verbal without	0	3*	0	3
physical abuse	0%	100%	0%	
Neglect	7	7	7	21
	33%	33%	33%	
Neglect without physical	2	3	4	9
abuse	22%	33%	45%	
Psychologically unavailable	7	8	3	18
	39%	44%	17%	
Psychologically unavailable	3	4	0	7
without physical abuse	43%	57%	0%	

Table 20.3. *Distribution of 18-month attachment classes among early maltreatment groups*

Row # Row %	A Anxious/avoidant	B Secure	C Anxious/resistant	Total
Control group	13	60	11	84
(nonmaltreated)	16%	71%	13%	
Physically abused	7	11	4	22
	32%	50%	18%	
Hostile/verbal abuse	2	11*	4	17
	12%	65%	23%	
Hostile without physical	0	3*	1	4
abuse	0%	75%	25%	
Neglect	7	11	2	20
	35%	55%	10%	
Neglect without physical	3	6	0	9
abuse	33%	67%	0%	
Psychologically unavailable	11	5	1	17
	65%	29%	6%	
Psychologically unavailable	6	1*	0	7
without physical abuse	86%	14%	0%	

*Several of these children do not present a pattern of secure attachment, nor do they show clearcut avoidance or resistance. In the earlier report of these data a D classification was used for these children who are difficult to classify.

control group. On the Bayley Scales of Infant Development, also given at 24 months, physically abused children earned significantly lower scores ($\overline{X} = 89$) than children in the control group ($\overline{X} = 107$).

In the Barrier Box task alone when they were 42 months old, physically abused children were hyperactive and distractible, lacked self control, expressed much negative affect, and showed little creativity in their approach to the problem. They were judged to lack agency (confident assertiveness) and to be low in self esteem compared to nonmaltreated children. Also at 42 months when observed with their mothers in a series of age-appropriate teaching tasks, physically abused children again were noncompliant and negativistic as well as nonaffectionate and avoidant of their mothers. They lacked enthusiasm and persistence for the tasks and generally had a poor quality experience in this interactive situation with their mothers. In preschool, when they were 4 and 5 years of age these children lacked self-control and continued to be noncompliant and to express a great deal of negative affect. These children had adjustment problems, as reflected on the Preschool Behavior Questionnaire.

Hostile/verbal abuse group. Children whose mothers were verbally abusive (hostile, rejecting) exhibited behavior much the same as children in the physical abuse group. In view of considerable overlap between the groups this is not surprising; only four children in this group were not experiencing physical abuse. (Because of the small number in the verbal without physical abuse group, that group is omitted from Table 20.1.) These children did not differ significantly from the control group through 18 months of age. However, several of the children classified as B's in the Strange Situation at 12 and 18 months (Tables 20.2, 20.3) actually did not present a secure pattern of attachment, but rather presented a mixture of behaviors that made them difficult to classify. Thus, these children with a history of hostile/verbal abuse were less competent at 12–18 months than the figures in these tables imply.

On the BSID at 24 months, this group obtained a mean score of 90, compared to 107 for the control group. In the tool-using tasks at 24 months, they were frustrated, angry, and noncompliant, expressing less positive and more negative affect than children who were not maltreated. In the barrier box task alone at 42 months of age, children in the verbal abuse group expressed negative affect, showed a lack of ego control, and were judged to be low in self-esteem. In the teaching tasks, also at 42 months, these children were less persistent and displayed less enthusiasm for the task than did nonmaltreated children. Their interaction with their mothers was characterized by negativity, noncompliance, lack of affection, and a high degree of avoidance. In general, their experience in the teaching tasks was unpleasant. (Preschool data were available for too few children from this group to allow statistical analyses.)

Neglected children. As with the other maltreatment groups, neglected infants did not differ from the control group in the 3-month feeding situation, but at 6 months they displayed less social behavior during feeding than nonmaltreated children. On the Bayley Scales of Infant Development at 9 months, neglected children did not differ significantly from the control group. However, by 24 months, neglected children (regardless of being physically abused or not) differed markedly from nonmaltreated children ($\overline{X}$ = 81 for the total group; $\overline{X}$ = 78 for children who were neglected but not physically abused).

At both 12 and 18 months, neglected children were more likely than nonmaltreated children to be anxiously attached. At 12 months two-thirds of the neglected children were anxiously attached, with equal numbers of *A*s and *C*s. By 18 months, more were securely attached and there was a move away from the anxious–resistant (C) pattern, particularly for children who were neglected but not physically abused.

At 24 months of age neglected children demonstrated poor coping strategies in the tool-using tasks with their mothers. They lacked enthusiasm and they were angry, frustrated, and noncompliant, displaying more negative and less positive affect than nonmaltreated children. In the Barrier Box task alone at 42 months neglected children showed poor impulse control, were inflexible and uncreative in their approach to the problem, and were judged to be low in self esteem. They were extremely distractible and often withdrew from the task. Of all the maltreated children, the neglected appeared the most unhappy, presenting the most negative and the least positive affect of all groups. With their mothers in the teaching tasks these children differed significantly from the control group on all variables. They showed little persistence or enthusiasm for the tasks. They were avoidant of their mothers, nonaffectionate, angry and noncompliant, yet highly reliant on their mothers for help and support. In preschool, when they were 4 to 5 years of age, children with a history of neglect were observed to have poor impulse control, to be extremely dependent on their teachers for support and nurturance, and generally to have adjustment problems. Even when physical abuse was separated out and children who were neglected but not physically abused were compared to nonmaltreated children, the results were nearly the same. Significant differences on so many variables, despite the small size (n = 11) of this subgroup of children who were neglected but not physically abused, provides strong evidence of the extensive negative consequences of neglect during these early years.

Psychologically unavailable group. Although the outcomes for all groups of maltreated children in our sample were severe, the consequences of psychologically unavailable patterns of parenting were most striking. Children whose mothers were psychologically unavailable showed a notable decline in competence during the early years of life. Children in this group actually looked more robust than nonmaltreated infants at 3 months of age. At 6 months in feeding and play situations and at 9 months on the Bayley Scales of Infant Development, there were no differences between this group and the control group.

At 12 months of age approximately 44% of these children were securely attached, but by 18 months only 29% were secure. Most of the children in the psychologically unavailable group were classified as anxious–avoidant. This was true also for the children in this group who did not experience physical abuse. In fact, there were no C's in that subgroup.

At 24 months, children whose mothers were psychologically unavailable (regardless of whether they also were physically abused or not) were angry, noncompliant, extremely frustrated, and expressed little positive affect. Perhaps the most dramatic finding for these children was their marked decline in performance on the Bayley Scales of Infant Development from 9 to 24 months. At 9 months of age, the mean score for this group was 120, but by 24 months the mean score was only 84. (For children in this group who were not physically abused, scores dropped from 118 to 87.)

At 42 months of age children whose mothers were psychologically unavailable lacked creativity in the Barrier Box task, but otherwise did not differ from the control group in this situation. However, at the same age in interaction with their mothers they differed from nonmaltreated children on nearly all variables. They lacked persistence and enthusiasm for the tasks and they showed little affection toward their mothers, either avoiding them or being negativistic and noncompliant with them. Fewer differences were found when physical abuse was separated out, but these children still were negativistic, nonaffectionate, and generally had a poor experience with their mothers in the teaching tasks.

In preschool those children whose mothers were psychologically unavailable were noncompliant, negativistic, and lacked impulse control. They were highly dependent on their teachers for help and support and presented many behavior problems in the preschool, including nervous signs, self-abusive behavior, and other behaviors that may be considered particularly potent indicators of developing psychopathology (Egeland, Sroufe, and Erickson, 1983). Those children whose mothers were unavailable but not physically abusive also presented many adjustment problems in preschool and were extremely dependent and lacking in self-control. Generally, these children with unavailable mothers appeared to be poorly adjusted both in situations with their mothers and in the preschool in interaction with teachers and peers.

Conclusions of earlier studies. To summarize these earlier findings, children who experienced any form of maltreatment functioned poorly in a variety of situations from infancy through the preschool period. Varied maladaptive behaviors were apparent within each maltreatment group. There was a relatively high incidence of anxious attachment among all groups of maltreated children. As noted earlier in this chapter, we and other researchers have found anxious attachment to predict subsequent maladaptation (see, for example, Erickson, Sroufe, & Egeland, 1985). The psychologically unavailable pattern of maltreatment seemed especially detrimental to the child's development during these early years. These findings led us to conclude:

The sharp decline in the intellectual functioning of these children, their attachment disturbances and subsequent lack of social/emotional competence in a variety of situations is cause for great concern. The consequences of this form of maltreatment are particularly disturbing when considered in light of the fact that this is probably the least likely pattern of maltreatment to be detected. These findings must lead us to a careful reexamination of our society's definition of child abuse and a consideration of means for early identification and intervention to help prevent the cumulative malignant effects of this form of maltreatment. (Egeland and Erickson, 1987)

Maltreatment groups at six years

As described by Pianta, Egeland, and Erickson elsewhere in this volume, we again evaluated the quality of caretaking the children in our sample were receiving, based upon information collected when the children were 4 to 6 years of age. (The groups described on the preceding pages were identified during the toddler period based on information collected throughout infancy.) Between the preschool and early school years some parents were added to the maltreating groups and others were deleted. Maltreatment groups included physically abusive ($n = 16$), neglectful ($n = 17$), and psychologically unavailable ($n = 16$). Also, for the first time, we identified a group of children who had been the victims of sexual abuse ($n = 11$). Two of those children were sexually abused by their mothers, five by older male family members, and four by teenage males. As described in our other chapter in this volume, there were some children who experienced more than one type of maltreatment; thus the groups overlap slightly. As before, we identified a control group of good caretakers ($n = 65$) from this same high-risk sample. Then, by assessing the cognitive ability of these children, their behavior in an age-appropriate laboratory situation designed to capture the quality of the child's adaptation, and by following the adjustment of these children in school, we addressed several major questions: How do maltreated children compare to nonmaltreated children from the same high risk sample? What are the developmental sequelae of various types of maltreatment? Are the consequences different for specific patterns of maltreatment? Do consequences differ depending on the chronicity and/or the age of onset of maltreatment? Specifically, are there differences among groups of children who (a) have been subjected to chronic maltreatment from infancy through age 6; (b) experienced maltreatment early in life but for whom maltreatment did not continue; and (c) did not experience maltreatment until later in the preschool years?

Outcome measures; fifty-four months through kindergarten

As before, we selected outcome measures that best captured the way the child was negotiating salient issues during this period of development. At 54 months of age children were videotaped in the Curiosity Box situation. Following Banta's (1970) procedure, children were placed in a room with a brightly painted, attractive box containing a number of manipulative elements, peepholes, and interior chambers that can be explored. The child's adaptation to this highly novel situation requires a certain degree of engagement of the elements of the box and a degree of organization imposed by the child on these elements. Qualitative ratings were made of the degree to which the child was involved, engaged in symbolic play, was dependent on the observer, was impulsive, exhibited positive or negative affect, projected effectiveness in interacting with the box, and maintained self-esteem. It is the qualitative aspects of the child's ability to autonomously engage a novel stimulus, control affect and behavior, and maintain self-esteem in the face of ambiguity that is considered to reflect competence in this situation. In order to obtain an estimate of the child's intellectual functioning at 64 months the following subtests from the Wechsler Preschool and Primary Scale of Intelligence (Wechsler, 1967) were administered: vocabulary, comprehension, animal house, and block design.

A major developmental task at this stage is adaptation to the social environment and task demands of school. To assess how the child was coping with this new situation, information was gathered from teachers during spring of the kindergarten year. In addition to being interviewed about the child's adjustment and success in school, teachers completed two standardized behavior rating scales: The Devereux Elementary School Behavior Rating Scale (Spivack and Swift, 1967) and the Child Behavior Checklist–Teacher's Report Form (Achenbach and Edelbrock, 1980). On the Devereux measure teachers rate 47 behavioral items on a five-point scale. Factor analysis of this measure yields five major factors: externalizing, inattentiveness, competence and involvement, closeness to teacher, and anxiety. On the Child Behavior Checklist teachers rate 113 items on a three-point scale. This measure yields the following scales: anxiety, social withdrawal, unpopularity, self destruction, obsession/compulsion, inattentiveness, nervous overactivity, aggression, "other problems," externalizing, and internalizing.

In addition to these standard measures, teachers rated the child on four seven-point rating scales developed by our staff: self-control (how the child monitored impulses and modulated his or her responses to stimuli in the school environment); positive affect; and negative emotional tone. Teachers also were asked to rank order all the students in their class on two dimensions: emotional health and social competence.

Adaptation of maltreated children: fifty-four months through kindergarten

This section will summarize the social and emotional consequences for children identified as being maltreated at ages 4 to 6. Results are based on comparisons of each maltreatment group to a control group of children receiving adequate care at ages 4 to 6 (presented in Table 20.4); comparisons of each possible pair of maltreatment groups; and chi-square analyses of maltreatment groups by (a) groups of children who were and were not referred for special intervention (i.e., Special Education, Chapter I) and (b) groups presenting varying patterns and levels of social-emotional competence in kindergarten (based on a cluster analysis of data provided by classroom teachers).

Physically abused children. Nine boys and seven girls were identified at age 6 as being physically abused. In the Curiosity Box Situation these children were more impulsive, expressed more negative affect, and were more dependent than the control group. On the WPPSI, physically abused children earned lower scores on the block design, vocabulary, and comprehension subtests and on the total for the four subtests administered than did children in the control group. Physically abused children's scores did not differ significantly from scores of children in the other maltreatment groups.

Behavior rating scales completed by kindergarten teachers revealed many significant differences between physically abused children and children in the control group. On the Devereux School Behavior Rating Scale teachers rated physically abused children extremely high on classroom disturbance and low on comprehension. Physically abused children were impatient, reliant, and more likely to make irrelevant responses. On the Achenbach Child Behavior Checklist physically abused children were rated by their teachers as extremely inattentive, unpopular, aggressive, and overactive. They were more likely than children in the control group to engage in self-destructive and obsessive–compulsive behavior. Physically abused children scored higher on the externalizing scale of this measure, as well as on the total score for the entire behavior checklist, but not as high as children in the neglect group. When teachers were asked to rank order the children in their classrooms on dimensions of social competence and emotional health, physically abused children ranked lower on social competence and much lower on emotional health than children in the control group. On seven-point rating scales developed by our staff, teachers rated physically abused

Table 20.4. *Comparisons between controls and maltreatment groups on outcome measures from 54 months through kindergarten*

Variables	Control group versus			
	Physical abuse	Neglect	Psychologically unavailable	Sexual abuse
Curiosity Box (54 months)				
Involvement			C > U*	
Quality of play				
Dependency	P > C*	N > C*		S > C**
Impulsivity	P > C**	1		S > C**
Negative affect	P > C*			
WPPSI (64 months)				
Block design	C > P**		C > U*	C > S*
Vocabulary	C > P**	C > N**		
Comprehension	C > P*	C > N***		
Animal house		C > N**		
Total (4 subtests)	C > P**	C > N***		
Kindergarten assessments:				
Devereux Elementary School Behavior Rating Scale				
Classroom disturbance	P > C***	N > C**		S > C*
Impatience	P > C*	N > C*		
Disrespect		N > C*	U > C*	
External blame				
Achievement anxiety		N > C*		
External reliance	P > C*	N > C**		
Comprehension	P > C**	N > C***		S > C**
Inattentive–withdrawn		N > C**		
Irrelevant responses	P > C*	N > C*		S > C*
Creative initiative		C > N**		
Needs closeness				S > C*
Factor 1 – Uninvolvement		N > C**		S > C*
Factor 2 – Disturbing behavior	P > C*		U > C*	
Factor 3 – Defensiveness				
Factor 4 – Creative initiative		N > C**		
Factor 5 – Needs closeness				S > C***
Achenbach Child Behavior Checklist				
Anxious		N > C**		S > C*
Socially withdrawn		N > C**		S > C**
Unpopular	P > C**	N > C**	U > C**	S > C**
Self-destructive	P > C*	N > C***		
Obsessive–compulsive	P > C*	N > C*		S > C**
Inattentive	P > C***	N > C***		S > C***
Nervous–overactive	P > C**	N > C***	U > C*	S > C***
Aggressive	P > C**	N > C**	U > C**	S > C**
Other problems		N > C***		S > C***

Table 20.4. *(cont.)*

Variables	Control group versus			
	Physical abuse	Neglect	Psychologically unavailable	Sexual abuse
Internalizing scale		N > C***		S > C***
Externalizing scale	P > C**	N > C**	U > C**	S > C**
Total score	P > C**	N > C***	U > C**	S > C***
Rank order				
Social competence	C > P*	C > N***	C > U*	
Emotional health	C > P***	C > N**		
7-point rating scales				
Agency		C > N*		
Self control	C > P**			
Positive affect	C > P*	C > N**		C > S*
Negative emotion				
Interview with kindergarten teacher				
Needs approval		N > C***		S > C***
Seeks help				S > C**
Overall social–emotional adjustment	C > P*	C > N***		C > S*
Overall academic performance		C > N***	C > U*	
Work habits (composite score)	C > P**	C > N***		
Independent work	C > P**	C > N**		
Leadership	C > P**	C > N***		
Cooperation	C > P**	C > N*		
Reading skills		C > N**		
Follows directions		C > N*		
Expresses self		C > N*		
Needs encouragement		N > C***		
Sensitive, empathic		C > N**		
Sense of humor		C > N**		

$*P < .05$
$**P < .01$
$***P < .001$

children low on positive affect and extremely low on self-control compared to children in the control group from our sample. In an interview, kindergarten teachers described physically abused children as low on work habits, not working independently, lacking leadership, being uncooperative, and generally being low on overall social–emotional health.

Of 16 physically abused children, 7 (44%) were referred for special help in kindergarten. This compares to 21% of the children in the control group.

Based on a cluster analysis using data collected from kindergarten teachers, 9 of the 16 physically abused children (56%) were in the least competent group (compared to 27% of control group children). Of those 9, 1 child was described best as withdrawn, 5 were characterized as overly anxious, and 3 were distractible. In general, the school adjustment of physically abused children in this sample is poor, with many of them creating classroom disturbance and having difficulty following through with the work required in school.

Neglected children. At 6 years of age, nine boys and eight girls were identified as being neglected. Interestingly, in the Curiosity Box Situation, neglected children were more dependent than children in the control group, but otherwise did not differ significantly from the control group nor from children in other maltreatment groups. However, on all other outcome measures this group stood out as having more varied and more severe problems than children in all other groups. On the WPPSI these neglected children earned much lower scores on the comprehension, vocabulary, and animal house subtests as well as on the total for the four administered subtests. Neglected children's scores were also significantly lower than children in the psychologically unavailable group and in the sexually abused group.

These children presented dramatic problems in their adjustment to school. On the Devereux measure kindergarten teachers rated neglected children as having much more difficulty comprehending the day-to-day school work than children in the control group. Neglected children also were rated as extremely inattentive, uninvolved, reliant, and lacking creative initiative. They were impatient, disrespectful, expressed anxiety about their school achievement, and were more likely to make irrelevant responses in the classroom when compared to children in the control group. On the Achenbach Child Behavior Checklist, neglected children received much higher scores on both the internalizing and externalizing scales, as well as on the total measure, than children in the control group. Neglected children were self-destructive, inattentive, and nervous and overactive. They also were rated by their teachers as anxious, withdrawn, unpopular, aggressive, and obsessive–compulsive. Not only did neglected children present far more problems than children in the control group, but neglected children also presented more problems than children in the physical abuse group and were rated as more anxious and higher on the internalizing scale than were children in the psychologically unavailable maltreatment group. When kindergarten teachers rank-ordered children in their classroom on dimensions of social competence and emotional health, neglected children showed poorer emotional health and far less social competence than children in the control group. On our seven-point behavior rating scales teachers rated the neglected children as being very low in positive affect and lower on agency (confident self-assertion). Interviews with kindergarten teachers indicated that neglected children need much more approval and encouragement than do children receiving adequate care. Neglected children present poorer overall social and emotional and academic functioning. These children have extremely poor work habits, do not work independently, and are low in reading. Teachers rated them on the interview as lacking leadership skills, lacking a sense of humor, and showing little sensitivity and empathy. Neglected children also were judged by their teachers to be less cooperative and to be poorer at following directions and expressing themselves when compared to children in the control group.

Of 17 neglected children, 11 (65%) were referred for special help in kindergarten. And of these 17, 9 (53%) were in the most incompetent group based on a cluster analysis of kindergarten data. Three of those 9 were withdrawn, 3 were anxious, and 3 were distractible. In general, these neglected children showed a marked deficit in cognitive functioning and severe and varied problems in school, raising serious concern about their ability to function successfully in the school environment.

Children of psychologically unavailable mothers. The mothers of nine boys and seven girls were judged to be psychologically unavailable to their children when the children were 4 to 6 years of age. Whereas children in the psychologically unavailable group identified when they were 2 years old had shown a marked decline in functioning over the preschool years, children in this group identified at age 6 did not differ as significantly from control group children as we might have expected. There were, however, some significant differences between children whose mothers were psychologically unavailable and children in the control group. In the Curiosity Box Situation, children in the psychologically unavailable group were less involved than children in the control group. On the WPPSI they earned lower scores on the block design subtest and tended ($p = .06$) to earn lower total scores on the four subtests administered. In the kindergarten classroom these children presented a fairly consistent pattern of aggression and classroom disturbance, reflected on both the Devereux and Achenbach measures. They were rated higher than children in the control group on the classroom disturbance scale of the Devereux measure and on disrespect and classroom disturbance factors (based on our own factor analysis). On the Achenbach Child Behavior Checklist children in the psychologically unavailable group were rated as aggressive, unpopular, nervous, and overactive, earning much higher scores on the externalizing scale and on the total Achenbach measure. Teachers' ranking of children with their peers showed that children in the psychologically unavailable group were lower on social competence than were children in the control group. And interviews with the teachers revealed that these children were lower in overall academic performance.

Six of the 16 children (37%) in this group were referred for help in kindergarten. Cluster analysis placed 9 of these 16 (56%) in the least competent group among our sample. Of these 9, 4 were in a group described as anxious and 5 were in a group characterized by distractibility. In general, although there were relatively few significant differences between this group and other groups, children with psychologically unavailable mothers do appear to present significant problems in the classroom, particularly aggressive, acting-out kinds of behavior patterns.

Sexually abused children. Identified for the first time when the children were 6 years of age were seven girls and four boys who were victims of sexual abuse by an older person (see Pianta, Egeland, and Erickson, this volume, for criteria for identification of this group). In the Curiosity Box Situation sexually abused children were far more dependent and impulsive than were children in the control group. On the WPPSI these children earned lower scores than the control group only on the block design subtest.

Teachers' ratings in kindergarten of these children revealed a number of important differences between sexually abused children and the other children in our sample. On the Devereux measure sexually abused children received much higher scores on the need for closeness scale compared to children in both the control and in all other maltreatment groups. Sexually abused children demonstrated poor comprehension of the day-to-day school tasks, were rated as being more disturbing in the classroom, less involved, and more likely to make irrelevant responses in class, when compared to the control group. On the Achenbach measure, sexually abused children were far less attentive, more nervous and overactive, and presented more "other problems" than children in the control group. They earned much higher scores on the internalizing scale and on the total Achenbach measure than did the control group. Sexually abused children also were significantly more socially withdrawn, unpopular, obsessive–compulsive, and aggressive, and earned significantly higher scores on the externalizing scale of the Achenbach. They also were rated as more anxious than children in the control group. There were no significant differences between sexually abused children and children in other groups on the rank orders done by kindergarten teachers. Of the seven-point rating scales used, positive affect was the only one on which sexually abused children differed from the control group, with sexually abused children displaying less positive affect than controls. Teacher interviews revealed a strong need for approval among sexually abused children, far more help-seeking behavior, and poorer overall social-emotional adjustment, when compared to children in the control group.

Of 11 sexually abused children, 5 (45%) were referred for special intervention in kindergarten. Six (55%) were in the least competent group, based on cluster analysis, with 4 of those in the group described as anxious, 1 withdrawn, 1 distractible. In summary, sexually abused children in our sample present varied problems, but are most notable for their anxious, inattentive patterns of behavior and for their strong need for closeness. In school these children are strikingly dependent on adults for help and approval.

Chronicity of abuse

To address the question of whether consequences differ depending on the chronicity of abuse and/or the age at which maltreatment occurs, comparisons were made on all outcome measures between each possible pair among the following groups: children who were maltreated only during the first years of life; those whose maltreatment began later in the preschool years; and those who were maltreated from infancy through age 6. Because of the small number of cases within each group, the four maltreatment groups (physical abuse, neglect, psychologically unavailable, and sexual abuse) were combined for these analyses.

These comparisons revealed relatively few significant differences (no doubt some differences were obscured by the necessary combining of the maltreatment groups), but some interesting patterns were apparent. WPPSI scores indicated that children who had been maltreated *early* in life, regardless of whether that maltreatment still was occurring, were not functioning as well cognitively as children whose maltreatment had begun more recently. Children who had been maltreated early in life also demonstrated less confidence and assertiveness and less creative initiative than children whose maltreatment began later, as rated by teachers on our 7-point agency rating scale and the Devereux. Children who *currently* were being maltreated, regardless of whether maltreatment had started in infancy or more recently, were rated by their teachers as having a greater need for closeness than children who no longer were being maltreated.

When compared to children whose maltreatment began more recently, children who were maltreated early in life (but no longer were maltreated) were rated on the Devereux as being more inattentive and withdrawn, they were ranked lower on social competence, and they were rated on our 7-point rating scale as showing less positive affect. A somewhat surprising finding was that children whose maltreatment had stopped looked worse on some measures than children whose maltreatment continued. Specifically, these children were judged in the Barrier Box Situation to have lower self-esteem and were ranked by their teachers as having poorer emotional health.

Although these findings must be viewed as tentative at best, overall they suggest that maltreatment in infancy has a particular impact on cognitive development and on the child's development of initiative and the self-confidence to act assertively in the school environment. Children who currently are being maltreated are likely to be overtly dependent on their teachers.

Keeping in mind that the findings are tentative, it appears that the earlier the maltreatment occurs, the more severe the consequences. Even for those children who were maltreated starting in infancy but for whom the maltreatment appeared to stop, the consequences at 64 months and kindergarten were severe. We believed that the maltreatment had stopped; however, the poor functioning of the children suggests that perhaps it had not or, alternatively, that the consequences of having been maltreated during the first two years of life are extremely difficult to reverse even though the caretaking improves.

Summary and discussion

The findings described in this chapter, based on comparisons of children experiencing various types of maltreatment and a control group of nonmaltreated children from the same high-risk sample, provide evidence that children who are maltreated have significant social and emotional problems above and beyond the problems related to low socioeconomic background. And, although children within each maltreatment group presented a variety of problems, some specific patterns of behavior tended to be associated with particular patterns of maltreatment.

Among children who were identified at ages 4 to 6 as being physically abused, aggressive, noncompliant, acting-out behavior was prevalent at ages 5 to 6. (This was similar to the angry, noncompliant behavior observed earlier in the preschool years and toddlerhood among children who had been identified at age 2 as being physically abused.) Alone in the Curiosity Box Situation, faced with a task designed to tap the quality of the child's adaptation at 4½ years of age, these children did not organize their behavior effectively. They were impulsive and expressed considerable negative affect, and they were quick to seek help or attention from the examiner. Physically abused children also were functioning more poorly on cognitive tasks, both in a formal testing situation with examiners from the project and in the kindergarten classroom as reported by their teacher. Their school behavior was disturbing; they lacked both the social and work skills necessary to make a successful adjustment to kindergarten. Consequently, almost half of the physically abused children in this sample had been referred either for special intervention or retention by spring of their kindergarten year.

As reported in earlier publications and summarized elsewhere in this chapter, when children whose mothers were psychologically unavailable during infancy were followed from infancy through the preschool years, they showed a dramatic decline in cognitive and social-emotional functioning and their behavior was cause for great concern. Children whose mothers were judged to be psychologically unavailable when the children were 4 to 6 years old did not stand out as being so extremely deviant; however, this group still did appear to be significantly less well-adapted than children who were receiving adequate care at ages 4 to 6. When observed alone in a laboratory situation, they were relatively uninvolved with the task at hand. In kindergarten, both on academic tasks and in social situations, these children were functioning more poorly than children in the control group. Their aggression and disruptive behavior in the classroom was similar to the behavior of children who were physically abused.

The fact that the effects of this pattern of maltreatment were not as dramatic at this age might lead us to speculate that emotional neglect is more devastating if it occurs in infancy. That hypothesis has intuitive appeal and we would not discard it. However, such a simple interpretation does not necessarily fit the complexity of our data – particularly in view of the overlap among the different subtypes of maltreatment and the overlap of the earlier and later groups. For example, among 16 children in the current psychologically unavailable group, 10 had been in one or more maltreatment groups at the earlier time (6 in the psychologically unavailable group). Six children, to the best of our knowledge, had not been maltreated earlier in life. Interestingly, while the mothers of those 6 children were described by home visitors as extremely unavailable to their children, in each of those cases the child's father, stepfather, and/or grandparents were involved, providing stable, loving care. It may be these protective factors or "buffers" (Schneider-Rosen, et al., 1985) that modify the effects of the mother's psychological unavailability.

The maltreatment group presenting the most severe and varied problems at ages 5 to 6 was the neglected group. These children performed far more poorly on cognitive assessments than did children in the control group, the psychologically unavailable group, or the sexual abuse group. In the classroom they were anxious, inattentive, failed to comprehend their academic work, lacked initiative, and relied heavily on the teacher for help, approval, and encouragement. In social situations they exhibited both aggressive and withdrawn behavior and, understandably, they were not popular with peers. These neglected children were not cooperative with adults, nor were they sensitive or empathic with peers. They rarely expressed positive affect or a sense of humor. (This lack of joy was consistent with the sadness we observed in preschool among the children who had been identified as neglected in infancy.) By spring of their kindergarten year 65 percent of the neglected children already had been referred either for special intervention or retention. Given their inability to handle academic tasks, far more of these children might be expected to be referred for special help in later grades as more focused, attentive behavior is demanded. The neglected children were well below the other maltreatment groups and the total sample on academic achievement.

It is quite possible that the teachers were more familiar and aware of these children due to their academic problems and as a consequence tended to rate them low in all areas of school adjustment. It is also quite possible that they were rated low because they dressed poorly and were dirty and unkempt. In many instances, the teacher as well as the other children in the class reacted negatively to the neglected children because of their physical appearance. One child in this group was encopretic and would often come to school with soiled and dirty clothes. This child was rejected by the teacher and was not accepted by the other children in the class. Dirty clothes and unkempt appearance are less likely to have a negative effect on the project staff's observations and ratings of the child in structured situations during the period of infancy through preschool. Thus, the neglected children tended not to look as bad as the other maltreatment groups at the earlier periods of assessment. Their appearance may not be as likely to be tolerated by the teacher or the other children.

A major reason for the poor functioning of neglected children is that they have a history of deprivation in social and emotional areas as well as in those pertaining to cognitive and language development. In addition to overall poor-quality care and chaotic and disruptive living conditions, these children received little stimulation. Prior to going to school, they did not have much contact with other children, nor did they have many play materials or educationally stimulating experiences. The effects of this deprivation became more obvious as academic demands were made on the child. Most could not print their name and had not acquired other basic skills possessed by most of their kindergarten classmates.

Sexually abused children in our sample, identified for the first time at age 4 to 6, also presented varied problems. Within-group variability is not surprising considering the variability in terms of what constituted maltreatment in this group. For example, in a number of cases the actual sexual abuse was not committed by the caregiver. (However, in most cases the caregiver could be considered partly responsible for allowing the abuse to occur.) We have not looked systematically at who the perpetrator was, the specific nature of the abuse, the degree of force, or how continuous the abuse was, and the size of this group is too small to allow statistical analysis of these variables. And whereas with other patterns of maltreatment we usually can see clear evidence of the maltreatment during home visits and on videotape, with sexual abuse we must rely mostly on maternal report and indirect evidence.

Nevertheless, there were some patterns of behavior that were particularly characteristic of this group. Sexually abused children were impulsive and dependent when observed alone in the laboratory at age 4½. Their school performance suffered due to marked anxiety, inattentiveness, and failure to comprehend what was expected of them. The social behavior of these sexually abused children ranged from withdrawn to aggressive, and they were not well-liked by their peers. Perhaps the most striking characteristic of these children was their dependency on adults, evident in their strong need for approval and closeness and their frequent help-seeking in the classroom. The passive, dependent nature of their behavior in school seems consistent with their victim role at home.

Theorists often have suggested, and recent empirical evidence (e.g., Crittenden, 1985b) indicates that maltreated children behave in ways that maintain their maltreatment. Some of the behavior observed among the children in our study might be expected to increase their susceptibility to continued maltreatment. It is not difficult to imagine, for example, how the angry, disruptive behavior of the physically abused children in our sample would provoke further abuse. And the extreme dependency of the sexually abused children might render them vulnerable to continued exploitation by adults. This makes sense within the framework of attachment theory (Bowlby, 1969, 1973, 1980), which has guided much of our research. This theory proposes that children develop expectations of self and others based on their early experience with their primary caregiver(s). The problematic behavior of maltreated children might be viewed within that framework as representing their negative expectations of self and others. These children have histories that lead them to expect that they will not be cared for and/or that they will be hurt or taken advantage of, and they have learned to expect that they are not worthy of being treated otherwise. Thus, they behave in ways that perpetuate those expectations.

There are notable similarities among our maltreatment groups: all manifest anxiety in some form (e.g., inattentiveness, preoccupation, fidgety behavior, difficulty comprehending directions); all seem to have an abiding anger; all are unpopular; and all have difficulty functioning independently to meet even the minimal demands of kindergarten. Those common problems all can be tied to the lack of nurturance central to all patterns of maltreatment.

We would hope that school might provide the support, structure, and stability that could help the children move toward greater competence. Unfortunately, however, even in kindergarten these children often are facing failure likely to increase their anxiety and anger and lower their self-esteem. They present learning and behavior problems with which their teachers feel unable to cope adequately. It probably would require special, intense, long-term efforts to begin to counteract the effects of early maltreatment and an inadequate home environment and to alter the expectations the child has formed. Few schools are equipped to provide such service. Furthermore, many of the children in our sample change schools often and have little opportunity to establish long-term relationships with peers or teachers. They are unlikely to have a chance to avail themselves of the help a school might provide.

In some respects, the behavior we have observed in maltreated children is similar to the behavior patterns of their maltreating mothers. For example, the aggressiveness of the physically abused children, the uninvolvement of the children whose mothers are psychologically unavailable, and the generally disorganized, incompetent behavior of the neglected children in our sample might be seen as reflecting the similar patterns of behavior that led to the identification of their mothers as maltreating. (Other researchers have noted similarities in behavior – e.g., Hoffman-Plotkin and Twentyman, 1984; Main and Goldwyn, 1984 – or social-cognitive style – e.g., Barahal, Waterman, and Martin, 1981 – of maltreated children and their parents.) Again, this is coherent with attachment theory and related notions regarding the way early experience in relationships influences subsequent behavior. Elsewhere in this volume (Pianta, Egeland, and Erickson) we have discussed the concept, drawn from attachment theory, that children incorporate both roles of a primary infant–caregiver relationship, that both roles reside within the child and are carried forward as the child enters new situations and relationships (Sroufe and Fleeson, 1986). This would lead us to expect that maltreated children would learn both the role of victim and victimizer; thus some behavioral similarity between child and parent would not be surprising.

Crittenden (1985a) examined parent and child behavior among maltreating families within a representational model based on power and coercion. She proposes that abused children would be expected to show submissive behavior in the presence of a powerful caregiver and aggressive behavior in the absence of a person so powerful. Neglected children, on the other hand, would be expected to be consistently withdrawn from other people. This model allows for behavior to change from one situation to another while remaining consistent with the child's representational models. Although this makes sense theoretically, our data presented here do not support Crittenden's hypothesis regarding neglected children. Neglected children in our sample were described by teachers as both withdrawn and aggressive.

Our findings regarding the behavior of children who were maltreated early in life but who no longer were being maltreated at the age of 6 were very tentative, but nevertheless they raise some interesting questions regarding the course of their interactions with their caregivers. Crittenden (1985a) noted that children may predict the parent's hostility, learn to inhibit the angry behavior that provokes the parent's hostility, and thus protect themselves from further abuse. Although this may be adaptive in the immediate situation, such denial of strong emotions may be maladaptive in the long run in terms of the child's mental health. We cannot tell from the data currently available, but that could be the case for some of the quiet, withdrawn kindergartners in our group of children whose maltreatment stopped by the time they were 6. Those children might be less likely to provoke maltreatment, but their behavior certainly would not be considered healthy or conducive to school success. This is not to say that children *cause* their own maltreatment or are responsible for soliciting appropriate care. But they *are* part of a system and they behave in ways that influence interactions within that system. Schneider-Rosen et al. (1985) make a similar point in their discussion of "alternate pathways" to resolving salient developmental issues. They describe, for example, how an infant's avoidance of the caregiver may represent a reasonable adaptation to the caregiver's behavior, an "alternate pathway" to felt security and resolution of attachment issues. Yet that avoidant behavior may be maladaptive in middle-class society and may lead to problems in subsequent cognitive, linguistic, or socioemotional development.

Overall, our evaluation of the development of maltreated children from birth through kindergarten reveals that problems for children in each maltreatment group seem to vary and become more or less apparent in different situations and at different ages. This highlights the importance of a longitudinal design and leads us to be cautious about overgeneralizing results based on any specific measure at a particular age or in a particular situation. The consequences of psychologically unavailable parenting were dramatic in the early years as children showed a decline in cognitive functioning and presented a wide range of behavior problems. Upon school entrance, neglected children present the most severe and varied problems. Perhaps the task demands of the relatively structured school environment tap the particular organizational and social skills that these children have failed to develop. It seems plausible that demands at later stages of development may bring out greater problems in other groups. For example, the aggression of the physically abused children and the dependency of the sexually abused children may pose particular problems in adolescence, if those patterns of behavior persist.

References

Aber, J. L., and Cicchetti, D. (1984). The social-emotional development of maltreated children: An empirical and theoretical analysis. In H. Fitzgerald, B. Lester, and M. Yogman (Eds.), *Theory and research in behavioral pediatrics.* New York: Plenum.

Achenbach, T., and Edelbrock, C. (1980). *Child Behavior Checklist – Teacher's Report Form.* Burlington: University of Vermont.

Ainsworth, M. D. S., Blehar, M., Waters, E., and Wall, S. (1978). *Patterns of attachment.* Hillsdale, NJ: Erlbaum.

Arend, R., Gove, F., and Sroufe, L. A. (1979). Continuity of individual adaptation from infancy to kindergarten: A predictive study of ego-resiliency and curiosity in preschoolers. *Child Development, 50,* 950–959.

Banta, T. J. (1970). Test for the evaluation of early childhood education: The Cincinnati Autonomy Test Battery (CATB). In J. Hellmuth (Ed.), *Cognitive studies.* New York: Brunner/Mazel.

Barahal, R. M., Waterman, J., and Martin, H. P. (1981). The social-cognitive development of abused children. *Journal of Consulting and Clinical Psychology, 40,* 508–516.

Bayley, N. (1969). *The Baylay Scales of Infant Development.* New York: The Psychological Corporation.

Behar, L., and Stringfield, S. (1974). A behavior rating scale for the preschool child. *Developmental Psychology, 10* (5), 601–610.

Benward, J., and Densen-Gerber, J. (1973). Incest as a causative factor in antisocial behavior: An exploratory study. *Contemporary Drug Problems, 4,* 322–340.

Blanchard, M., and Main, M. (1979). Avoidance of the attachment figure and social–emotional adjustment of day-care infants. *Developmental Psychology, 15,* 445–446.

Bowlby, J. (1951). Maternal care and mental health. *Bulletin of the World Health Organization, 31,* 355–533.

Bowlby, J. (1969). *Attachment and loss,* Vol. 1, *Attachment.* New York: Basic Books.

Bowlby, J. (1973). *Attachment and loss,* Vol. 2, *Separation.* New York: Basic Books.

Bowlby, J. (1980). *Attachment and loss,* Vol. 3, *Loss, sadness, and depression.* New York: Basic Books.

Cicchetti, D., and Rizley, R. (1981). Developmental perspectives on the etiology, intergenerational transmission, and sequelae of child maltreatment. In R. Rizley and D. Cicchetti (Eds.), *New directions for child development: Developmental perspectives on child maltreatment.* San Francisco: Jossey-Bass, pp. 31–55.

Crittenden, P. M. (1985a). *Children's strategies for coping with adverse home environments: Abuse and neglect.* Paper presented at the meeting of the Society for Research in Child Development, Toronto, Canada, April 25–28.

Crittenden, P. M. (1985b). Maltreated infants: Vulnerability and resilience. *Journal of Child Psychology and Psychiatry, 26* (1), 85–96.

DeMause, L. (Ed.) (1974). *The history of childhood.* New York: Psychohistory Press.

Egeland, B., and Erickson, M. F. (1987). Psychologically unavailable caregiving. In M. Brassard, B. Germain, and S. Hart (Eds.), *Psychological maltreatment of children and youth.* New York: Pergamon.

Egeland, B., and Sroufe, L. A. (1981). Developmental sequelae of maltreatment in infancy. In R. Rizley and D. Cicchetti (Eds.), *New directions for child development: Developmental perspectives in child maltreatment.* San Francisco: Jossey-Bass.

Egeland, B., Sroufe, L. A., and Erickson, M. F. (1983). Developmental consequence of different patterns of maltreatment. *Child Abuse and Neglect, 7* (4), 459–469.

Elmer, E. (1977). A follow-up study of traumatized children. *Pediatrics, 59* (2), 273–314.

Erickson, M. F., and Egeland, B. (1981). *Behavior problem scale technical manual.* University of Minnesota, unpublished manuscript.

Erickson, M. F., Sroufe, L. A., and Egeland, B. (1985). The relationship between quality of attachment and behavior problems in preschool in a high-risk sample. In I. Bretherton and E. Waters (Eds.), *Monographs of the Society for Research in Child Development, 50* (1–2), pp. 147–166.

Finkelhor, D. (1979). *Sexually victimized children.* New York: The Free Press.

Gaensbauer, T. J., Mrazek, D., and Harmon, R. J. (1980). Affective behavior patterns in abused and/or neglected infants. In N. Frude (Ed.), *The understanding and prevention of child abuse: Psychological approaches.* London: Concord Press.

Galdston, R. (1971). Violence begins at home. *Journal of the American Academy of Child Psychiatry, 10,* 336–350.

Garbarino, J., and Vondra, J. (1987). Psychological maltreatment: Issues and perspectives. In M. Brassard, B. Germain, S. Hart (Eds.), *Psychological maltreatment of children and youth.* New York: Pergamon.

Gardner, L. I. (1972). Deprivation dwarfism. *Scientific American, 227,* 76–82.

Gersten, M., Coster, W., Schneider-Rosen, K., Carlson, V., and Cicchetti, D. (1986). The socio-emotional bases of communicative functioning: Quality of attachment, language development, and early maltreatment. In M. E. Lamb, A. L. Brown, and B. Rogoff (Eds.), *Advances in developmental psychology* (Vol. 4). Hillsdale, NJ: Erlbaum.

George, C., and Main, M. (1979). Social interactions of young abused children: Approach avoidance and aggression. *Child Development, 50,* 306–318.

Giaretto, H. (1976). Humanistic treatment of father–daughter incest. In R. Helfer and H. Kempe (Eds.), *Child abuse and neglect.* Cambridge, MA: Ballinger Publications.

Harlow, H. F. (1961). The development of affectional patterns in infant monkeys. In B. M. Foss (Ed.), *Determinants of infant behaviour* (Vol. 1). New York: Wiley.

Herman, J., and Hirschman, L. (1981). Families at risk for father–daughter incest. *American Journal of Psychiatry, 138,* 967–970.

Hoffman-Plotkin, D., and Twentyman, C. T. (1984). A multimodal assessment of behavioral and cognitive deficits in abused and neglected preschoolers. *Child Development, 55,* 794–802.

Hufton, I. W., and Oates, R. K. (1977). Non-organic failure to thrive: A long-term follow-up. *Pediatrics, 59,* 73–77.

Isaacs, S. (1930). *Intellectual growth in young children.* London: Routledge & Kegan Paul.

James, J., and Meyerding, J. (1977). Early sexual experiences as a factor in prostitution. *Archives of Sexual Behavior, 7,* 31–42.

Kempe, C. H., Silverman, F. N., Steele, B. F., Droegemueller, W., and Silver, H. K. (1962). The battered-child syndrome. *Journal of the American Medical Association, 181* (17), 17–24.

Kempe, R., and Kempe, C. H. (1978). *Child abuse.* London: Lontana/Open Books.

Kinard, E. M. (1980). Emotional development in physically abused children. *American Journal of Orthopsychiatry, 50,* 686–695.

Lamb, M. F., Gaensbauer, T. J., Malkin, C. M., and Schultz, L. A. (1985). The effects of child maltreatment on security of infant–adult attachment. *Infant Behavior and Development, 8,* 35–45.

Lorenz, K. (1952). *King Solomon's ring: New light on animal ways.* New York: Thomas Y. Crowell.

Lynch, M. (1985). Child abuse before Kempe: An historical literature review. *Child Abuse and Neglect, 9* (1), 7–15.

MacCarthy, D. (1979). Recognition of signs of emotional deprivation: A form of child abuse. *Child Abuse and Neglect, 3,* 423–428.

Main, M., and Goldwyn, R. (1984). Predicting rejection of her infant from mother's representation of her own experience: Implications for the abused–abusing intergenerational cycle. *Child Abuse and Neglect, 8,* 203–217.

Main, M., and Weston, D. (1981). The quality of the toddler's relationship to mother and father. *Child Development, 52,* 932–940.

Martin, H. P., and Beezley, P. (1977). Behavioral observations of abused children. *Developmental Medicine in Child Neurology, 19,* 373–387.

Martin, H. P., Beezley, P., Conway, E. F., and Kempe, C. H. (1974). The development of abused children. In I. Schulman (Ed.), *Advances in pediatrics 21.* Chicago: Year Book, pp. 25–73.

Matas, L., Arend, R., and Sroufe, L. A. (1978). Continuity of adaptation in the second year: The relationship between quality of attachment and later competence. *Child Development, 49,* 547–556.

Meiselman, K. (1980). Personality characteristics of incest history, psychotherapy patients: A research note. *Archives of Sexual Behavior, 9,* 195–197.

Morse, W., Sahler, O. J., and Friedman, S. B. (1970). A three-year follow-up study of abused and neglected children. *American Journal of Diseases of Children, 120,* 439–446.

Newberger, E. H. (1973). The myth of the battered child syndrome. In R. Bourne and E. H. Newberger (Eds.), *Critical perspectives on child abuse.* Lexington, MA: Lexington Books.

Newson, J., and Newson, E. (1974). Cultural aspects of childrearing in the English-speaking world. In M. P. M. Richards (Ed.), *The integration of a child into a social world.* London: Cambridge University Press.

Patton, R. G., and Gardner, L. I. (1962). Influence of family environment on growth: The syndrome of "maternal deprivation." *Pediatrics, 30,* 957–962.

Piaget, J. (1952). *The origins of intelligence in children.* New York: International Universities Press.

Polansky, N. A., Chalmers, M. A., Buttenweiser, E., and Williams, D. P. (1981). *Damaged parents: An anatomy of child neglect.* Chicago: University of Chicago Press.

Reidy, T. J. (1977). Aggressive characteristics of abused and neglected children. *Journal of Clinical Psychology, 33,* 1140–1145.

Rosenfeld, A. (1977). Sexual misuse and the family. *Victimology: An International Journal, 2,* 226–235.

Sandgrund, A., Gaines, R., and Green, A. H. (1974). Child abuse and mental retardation: A problem of cause and effect. *American Journal of Mental Deficiency, 79,* 327–330.

Schneider-Rosen, K., Braunwald, K. G., Carlson, V., and Cicchetti, D. (1985). Current perspectives in attachment theory: Illustration from the study of maltreated infants. In I. Bretherton and E. Waters (Eds.), *Monographs of the Society for Research in Child Development, 50* (1–2), pp. 194–210.

Schneider-Rosen, K., and Cicchetti, D. (1984). The relation between affect and cognition in maltreated infants: Quality of attachment and the development of visual self-recognition. *Child Development, 55,* 648–658.

Spitz, R. A. (1945). Hospitalism: An inquiry into the genesis of psychiatric conditions of early childhood. *Psychoanalytic study of the child, 1,* 53–74.

Spivack, G., and Swift, M. (1967). *Devereux elementary school behavior rating scale.* Devon, PA: The Devereux Foundation.

Sroufe, L. A. (1983). Infant–caregiver attachment and patterns of adaptation in preschool: The roots of maladaptation and competence. In M. Perlmutter (Ed.), *Minnesota symposium in child psychology* (Vol. 16). Hillsdale, NJ: Erlbaum.

Sroufe, L. A., and Fleeson, J. (1986). Attachment and the construction of relationships. In W. Hartup and Z. Rubin (Eds.), *Relationships and development* (pp. 51–72). Hillsdale, NJ: Erlbaum.

Sroufe, L. A., Fox, N., and Pancake, V. (1983). Attachment and dependency in developmental perspective. *Child Development, 54* (6), 1615–1627.

Steele, B. F. (1977). *Psychological dimensions of child abuse.* Paper presented to the American Association for the Advancement of Science, Denver, CO, February.

Steele, B. F., and Pollack, C. B. (1968). A psychiatric study of parents who abuse infants and small children. In R. E. Helfer and C. H. Kempe (Eds.), *The battered child.* Chicago: University of Chicago Press.

Summit, R., and Kryso, J. (1978). Sexual abuse of children. *American Journal of Orthopsychiatry, 48* (2), 237–251.

Tsai, M., and Wagner, N. N. (1978). Therapy groups for women sexually molested as children. *Archives of Sexual Behavior, 7* (5), 417–427.

Tyler, A. H. (1983). A comparison of child-abusing and non-abusing fathers on measures of: Marital adjustment, life-stress, and social support. Unpublished doctoral dissertation, University of Utah.

Waters, E., Wippman, J., and Sroufe, L. A. (1979). Attachment, positive affect and competence in the peer group: Two studies in construct validation. *Child Development, 50,* 821–829.

Wechsler, D. (1967). *Wechsler preschool and primary scale of intelligence.* New York: The Psychological Corporation.

Wolock, I., and Horowitz, B. (1984). Child maltreatment as a social problem: The neglect of neglect. *American Journal of Orthopsychiatry, 54,* 530–543.

21 Troubled youth, troubled families: the dynamics of adolescent maltreatment

James Garbarino

Abuse and neglect are embedded in a wide range of adolescent problems – delinquency, parricide, running away, and prostitution, to name but four that are mentioned frequently in research and clinical reports – with the degree of coincidence being in excess of 65 percent in some samples. These links provide an important aspect of the context within which we must understand and intervene in adolescent maltreatment. A second aspect of that context is public and professional stereotypes about adolescents.

Some of the most prominent observers of adolescence in the 1950s and 1960s saw negative stereotypes of youth as both the cause and effect of adolescent alienation from the adult world. Classics such as Paul Goodman's *Growing Up Absurd* (1956), Edgar Friedenberg's *The Vanishing Adolescent* (1959), and *The Dignity of Youth and Other Atavisms* (1965) explored this theme. Goodman's title is self-explanatory. Friedenberg emphasized the way adults often regard adolescents in general with fear and contempt, with high schools as the principal arena in which adult society plays out this theme:

They are problem-oriented and the feelings and needs for growth of their captives and unenfranchised clientele are the least of their problems; for the status of the "teenager" in the community is so low that even if he rebels, the school is not blamed for the conditions against which he is rebelling. What high school personnel become specialists in, ultimately, is the *control* of large groups of students. (Friedenberg, 1965, pp. 92–93)

Twenty years later, as controlling school crime and meeting basic scholastic requirements have become dominant issues, Friedenberg's analysis remains timely.

The author acknowledges the assistance of Andrew Kelley, Wendy Gamble, Janet Sebes, and Cynthia Schellenbach in the research and literature review upon which the chapter is based.

Based in part upon an invited address to Division 37 (Children, Youth, and Families) of the American Psychological Association annual convention, August 25, 1984, Toronto, Canada.

In her excellent book, *Children Without Childhood* (1983), Marie Winn speaks of "The Myth of the Teenage Werewolf":

A pervasive myth has taken hold of parents' imagination these days, contributing to their feeling of being powerless to control the fates of their children: the myth of the teenage werewolf. Its message is that no matter how pleasant and sweet and innocent their child might be at the moment, how amiable and docile and friendly, come the first hormonal surge of puberty and the child will turn into an uncontrollable monster. (p. 14)

This monstrous imagery is not without precedent. Consider this view of adolescents discovered in a 1972 book by Leonard Wolf entitled *A Dream of Dracula: In Search of the Living Dead:*

Adolescents recognize him at once. (His bad breath, his red, red lips.) If he kissed you once, will he kiss you again? They lie in the torpor of their pupa stage, waiting for something better to happen to them, dreaming about transformations. Pimpled, gawky, swollen with blood and other juices they do not quite understand, they know about being loathed, and loathing. . . .
Blood surges in and soils the young. Hearing the word "suck," they look about warily, in the grip of strange confusions: they know what all those films are about – ego, power, parasitism, loneliness, immortality, youth, youth, youth and thirty-eight kinds of sex. The living-dead. Finally it comes down to this: When Dracula's lips approach the delicate throat of the beautiful girl on the screen, *they* know. (p. 17)

These images of adolescence contribute to the context in which the dynamics of adolescent maltreatment take place. They find their professional parallel in the widely held image of adolescence as necessarily "stormy and stressful" ("Sturm and Drang") (Garbarino, Kelley, and Schulenberg, 1985; Kelley and Garbarino, 1985). In this view, adolescents experience conflict and turmoil as a *normal* part of their development. Many who hold this view most strongly have studied or worked professionally with disturbed adolescents engaged in deviant behavior.

Along these lines, Anna Freud (1958) wrote of the difficulty of distinguishing normality from psychopathology in adolescence:

Adolescence constitutes by definition an interruption of peaceful growth which resembles in appearance a variety of other emotional upsets and structural upheavals. The adolescent manifestations come close to symptom formation of the neurotic, psychotic or dissocial order and merge almost imperceptibly into borderline states, initial, frustrated or fully fledged forms of almost all the mental illnesses. Consequently, the differential diagnosis between the adolescent upsets and true pathology becomes a difficult task. (p. 267)

Anna Freud viewed adolescence as a developmental disturbance derived from the reawakening of libidinal impulses that marks the movement from the latency period into the pubertal period. Teenagers experience psychic conflict as they try to balance their Oedipal impulses with what society dictates as correct behavior. Childhood defenses (repression, rationalization, and projection) keep these Oedipal desires from awareness, and thereby permit escape from uncomfortable and threatening turmoil. As the individual matures, this defensive balance ("preliminary and precarious" as it is) becomes more and more inappropriate. It can't handle the powerful sexual drives that are resurgent in adolescence. Adolescents must overthrow their old systems and build new ones. This process results in the rebellion, the ups and downs, and the dramatic changes that Anna Freud saw as being typical of adolescence.

This "period of upheaval" is a healthy, normal expression of development, but during it adolescents will reject their parents (in response to the unacceptable desire to possess the opposite sex parent), and enter into a series of intense but brief romantic involvements with their peers (as they learn to accept and adapt to their new-found sexuality). This behavior, perceived as "rebellion," provides a theoretical explanation for the stereotyped view of adolescents as being necessarily "rebellious." It is interesting to recall what Anna Freud (1958) wrote concerning what is occurring when such "structural upheavals" and "rebellious" activities do *not* occur.

> We all know individual children who as late as the ages of 14, 15, or 16 show no such outer evidence of inner unrest. They remain, as they have been in dealing with the latency period, "good" children, wrapped up in their family relationships, considerate sons of their mothers, submissive to their fathers, in accord with the atmosphere, ideas, and ideals of the childhood background. Convenient as this may be, it signifies a delay of normal development and is, as such, a sign to be taken seriously. . . . These are children who have built up excessive defenses against their drive activities and are now crippled by the results, which act as barriers against the normal maturational processes of phase development. They are, perhaps more than any others, in need of therapeutic help to remove the inner restrictions and clear the path for normal development, however 'upsetting' the latter may prove to be. (p. 265)

From A. Freud's psychoanalytic perspective, the exhibition of "storm and stress" in the form of conflict with parents is not only a *natural* experience but it is also a *necessary* occurrence for normal adolescent development to occur. The "upholding of a steady equilibrium during the adolescent process is in itself abnormal" (A. Freud, 1958, p. 275). This undermines the validity of adolescent acting out behaviors as indicators of disrupted development, family conflict, or psychopathology. As such it may undermine our ability to intervene in adolescent maltreatment by casting its results as "just a phase," when in fact it is a genuine crisis.

But is this view correct? Anthropologists such as Margaret Mead and Ruth Benedict challenged it on the basis of their observations in other cultures. Survey research in the United States indicates that, although adolescence is usually a time of family challenge, *adolescents are not normally either crazy or highly rebellious.*

The first research systematic evidence that teenagers in modern Westernized societies do not necessarily experience major problems of adjustment was presented by two sociologists, Westley and Elkin (1956). Their small sample of middle-class adolescents in Montreal, Canada, reported little turmoil. Instead, they presented a picture of relative calm and stability. Douvan and Adelson (1966) conducted a study in which they extensively interviewed over 3,000 adolescents. The sample was constructed in such a way as to be representative of the entire United States population of boys and girls facing adolescence, although it was restricted to teenagers in school and somewhat underrepresented low income and racial minority youth. In this broad, more representative sample, there also was little evidence of *major* turmoil and conflict. In fact, their data presented a picture of the "typical" adolescent as a somewhat conservative and conforming individual (to which Anna Freud might respond that this only shows how widespread is the problem of abnormal placidity).

> The adolescent at the extremes responds to the instinctual and psychosocial upheaval of puberty by disorder, by failures of egosynthesis, and by a tendency to abandon earlier values and object attachments. In the normative response to adolescence, however, we more commonly find an avoidance of inner and outer conflict, premature identity consolidation, ego and ideological constriction, and a general unwillingness to take psychic risks. The great advantage of the survey technique is that it allows us to study these adolescents who make up the middle majority, who evoke neither grief nor wonder, and who all too often escape our notice. (p. 351)

Douvan and Adelson's study has been criticized for the fact that their interviewers were not mental health professionals (and thus presumably were more likely to miss signs of distress), but subsequent studies that *have* employed mental health professionals interviewing nonpatient populations have confirmed the finding that the majority of adolescents do *not* show overt signs of disorder. (Of course, the psychoanalytically oriented could respond that this shows that most adolescents suffer from the "problem" of no problems.)

One of the most extensive studies of adolescent normality was the Normal Adolescent Project carried out by Daniel Offer and his colleagues (Offer, 1969; Offer and Offer, 1973, 1974, 1975). Offer directed an eight-year project using a sample of 73 typical middle-class, male teenagers in the midwestern United States. The boys were assessed at various times from their freshman through senior years of high school. The assessment procedure consisted of parent interviews, psychological tests, and psychiatric interviews. In addition, 61 of the original 73 subjects were assessed in the same manner during their four years of college (and this reference to college attendance indicates the relative affluence of the sample).

Offer and his colleagues identified three major patterns of growth for these adolescents. "Continuous growth" refers to a gradual, smooth transition from adolescence to young adulthood, free from the turbulence and turmoil predicted by the "storm and stress" theorists. "Surgent growth" refers to a less gradual developmental pattern, where growth occurs in "spurts," between which development appears arrested. Most of the teenagers in this study developed in one of these two modes, experiencing little or no stress and discomfort on their way to normal, adaptive adjustment to adulthood. A third pattern of growth was termed "tumultuous growth," and corresponds to the kind of inner turmoil and crisis pattern the storm and stress hypothesis predicts for all adolescents. Twenty-one percent of the sample evidenced this kind of developmental process – a large enough minority to show that there are sufficient troubled adolescents to sustain the professional stereotype of storm and stress, but too few to validate the claim that it is the typical adolescent pattern.

In another study, Rutter, Graham, Chadwick, and Yule (1976) studied a large representative sample of all of the 14- to 15-year-olds on the Isle of Wight (in Great Britain). They found only a very slight increase in psychopathology from middle childhood to adolescence and a very low incidence of rejection or relationship difficulties between adolescents and parents. Interestingly, however, they found that about 22 percent of their sample reported that they *often* felt miserable or depressed and were having trouble sleeping. This is almost the exact percentage that reported this pattern in the studies by Offer (1973, 1974, 1975). (About 44 percent reported feeling miserable and depressed *at times*.) We should note that in Rutter, Graham, Chadwick, and Yule's study (1976), the incidence of psychopathology (as assessed by a formal psychiatric interview) was 16.3 percent among their sample, so that there is a difference between reporting depression and being considered clinically depressed.

Therefore, we have evidence from two fairly large-scale studies that about 20 percent of nonpatient adolescents report experiencing serious turmoil as they grow up. This is far short of the majority predicted by storm and stress theorists, and it tells us that we should be alert to families that are experiencing a high level of conflict, for it is not typical or "normal" to do so. In a survey of college students, Balswick and Macrides (1975) found that only 22 percent reported that they had been rebellious as teenagers.

In their study of middle-class families of adolescent boys, Bandura and Walters (1959) also found little evidence of storm and stress. When teenagers did exhibit aggressive behavior, such as fighting physically with their parents, it was found that these kids had presented the same problems as children – but only when they became bigger and stronger could they overpower their parents, a finding to which we will return. Bandura and Walters concluded: "Our findings suggest ... that the behavioral characteristics exhibited by children during the so-called adolescent stage are lawfully related to, and consistent with, pre-adolescent behavior" (Bandura and Walters, 1963, p. 196).

The general conclusion that profound conflict and turmoil across all life's domains is not the typical pattern of development for adolescents receives support from other studies of nonclinical populations (Grinker, Grinker and Timberlake, 1962; Hamburg, Coelho, and Adams, 1974; Oldham, 1978; Weiner, 1982). It seems fairly well established, then, that when one looks at the data, the typical adolescent is *not* one who is experiencing far-reaching psychic disturbance as a matter of predetermined developmental course. Keep in mind also, that no period in the human life course is totally free from stress and conflict. Adolescents certainly have no monopoly on storm and stress – no more so than toddlers or middle agers. All this tells us that seriously troubled youth should be taken seriously, and that the behaviors often identified as symptoms of adolescent maltreatment are usually indicators of genuinely serious problems, often problems of family breakdown associated with the special challenges of adolescence.

But why do negative stereotypes of adolescence continue? Why is the myth of the teenage werewolf so durable? We do not know for sure, but several hypotheses are plausible. From a psychoanalytic perspective, we can hypothesize that the negative stereotype serves an important function for adults. It may act as a kind of defense mechanism by transferring onto adolescents responsibility for the envy that the no-longer-young feel for the sexuality and freedom of the young. It may also serve to justify the structures of social control that adults impose in schools and in families.

From a more ecological perspective, these negative stereotypes are part of the larger macrosystems that rationalize and organize social relations. In this view, negative stereotypes of adolescence reflect a combination of factors: resistance to change in power dynamics, naive overgeneralization from the behavior of the "tumultuous" minority to the "continuous" majority of teenagers, and a lack of empathy and absence of self-understanding on the part of adults who do not see the parallels between adolescent and adult behavior.

Whatever the source of these negative stereotypes, they exist, and they contribute to the problems of troubled youth in troubled families. They justify unresponsive parenting and exacerbate family conflict of the serious variety. And they color and interpret the normal challenges to the family system that *do* inhere in adolescence in modern societies.

The challenge of being parent to an adolescent

What does adolescence mean for the family as a whole? For one thing, it means adjusting patterns of authority and interaction to incorporate a new person. Developmental psychologist John Hill (1980) has looked at the research on this matter, and he concludes that:

> Studies where family interaction is directly observed suggest that there may be a period of temporary disequilibrium in early adolescence while the family adjusts to having a "new person" in the household – "new" in stature, "new" in approaching

reproductive capability, "new" in cognitive competence – but this disequilibrium in no way approaches the shoot-out that many parents are led to expect from media reports. Instead, in most families, there appears to be a period of adaptation to the primary changes, a period when both parents and their newly adolescent children work out – often not consciously – what these changes mean for their relationships. (1980, p. 33)

At its heart, the task of being parent to an adolescent (and adolescent to a parent) is substantially different from the parent–child relationship in several ways, each of which has implications for the origins and impact of adolescent maltreatment (Garbarino and Gilliam, 1980).

The adolescent's power is much greater than the child's. This includes physical power, of course, including the capability for physical retaliation if assaulted by a parent. It goes beyond this, however, to include the power to stimulate and influence family conflict, to leave the family situation, to harm self and others, to embarrass the parents, to compare parents with other adults, and to help oneself and others. This enhanced power that comes with adolescence is often a destabilizing force, particularly when parents and/or adolescents have little motive or facility for flexible negotiation and compromise.

The adolescent has a broader field of other significant individuals with whom the parents must come to terms. Autonomous relationships with other adults and with peers increase, including sexual relationships that many parents may perceive as threatening. This broader field is a special challenge for parents who seek and expect social isolation.

The adolescent's cognitive abilities are likely to be more advanced than are the child's. Adolescents tend to reason much more like adults, and this injects a new element of complexity into the parent's task. It may also increase the relevance of cognitive sophistication for harmonious family relationships. In some ways, parents can "get away with more" in their interactions with young children than in their treatment of adolescents. The latter have a broader base of experience with which to compare parental actions. If treated badly, teenagers are more likely than young children to perceive the deviance of their treatment and to report it to someone outside the family (Garbarino and Gilliam, 1980). Adolescents have developed both the mental capacity to enable them better to understand flaws in parental reasoning and character and the physical capacity to do something about them.

Adolescents are likely to be a financial drain. U.S. Department of Agriculture figures indicate that the yearly cost of maintaining a teenager is about 140 percent that for a young child. This increased cost is stressful for many families, and may be a source of family conflict, particularly in families where the increased financial demands of adolescence are not matched by increasing income.

When these features are taken all together, it is little wonder that surveys such as that done by Pasley and Gecas (1983) report that a majority of parents say that the adolescent years are the most difficult ones for childrearing. They found that ages 14–18 were ranked most difficult, followed by the 10- to 13-year-old period. One reason for this is the pressure to rearrange family power relationships and adjust to new actors in the child's social field.

Many parents may feel rejected by the natural shift of attention and affection away from them to others (Dreyfus, 1976). Some may be specially vulnerable to this feeling because of their own life histories and contemporary needs (Pelcovitz, Kaplan, Samit, Krieger, and Cornelius, 1983). During this period, the power and affectional fabric in the family may be torn. This situation is particularly unfortunate because it occurs at a time when adolescents may most need parental support. On their side, parents need adolescent support if the parents are facing mid-life crisis or "midolescence" (McMorrow, 1977). Russell (1979) has developed a model of family functioning that seems useful in understanding why families differ in their ability to respond effectively to the challenge of adolescence. He views families along two dimensions: adaptability and cohesion. Extremes of either reduce the family's effectiveness. Too much cohesion is termed "enmeshed"; too little, "detached." Too much adaptability is "chaotic"; too little is "rigidity." As we shall see, this approach to characterizing the family *system* is useful in understanding what places a family at-risk for destructive parent–child relations in adolescence, particularly when coupled with an analysis of affection and modes of discipline.

Offer (1969) has described families with adolescents as being in a state of "transitional crisis characterized by confusion." The family reaches a time when there is a need for adjustment and accommodation. It is a difficult time; there are few clear-cut answers as to how much control parents should seek to maintain and how much freedom they should grant the adolescent. Diana Baumrind (1979) contends that in the current climate, in which "the rights of youth" are emphasized, parents have all the obligations but few rights. She believes that the current emphasis on the rights of children and adolescents leads to narcissistic, selfish behavior in adolescents, behavior that can precipitate crisis in some families. Baumrind holds that while adolescents depend upon their parents economically and socially it is unwise to grant them the full freedom and independence accorded to truly independent individuals. As Baumrind sees it, adolescents lack the natural limits imposed by society that arise from the experience of supporting oneself, and therefore develop unrealistic expectations concerning the future. This exemplifies how broad social influences can shape the family, and how the meaning of specific parental behavior depends upon the context in which it occurs.

The manner in which parents respond to the adolescent quest for autonomy depends partly upon the type of family structure present, as defined by cohesion, flexibility, authority, and affection (Gamble & Garbarino, 1985). In authoritarian homes there is little or no allowance for freedom on the adolescent's part. If authoritarian parents are unwilling to divest themselves of any power, and continue trying to maintain their dominance over the adolescent, they run the risk of facing a combination of rebellion and dependency on the adolescent's part (Balswick and Macrides, 1975; Douvan and Adelson, 1966; Nye, 1958). If adolescents are successful in challenging parental authority, they may become rebellious; if parental discipline has been severe and unjust without much love and affection, teenagers may become overtly aggressive and hostile (Weiner, 1970). The adolescent may leave home and become involved in delinquent activities (Nye, 1958). On the other hand, if children are completely dominated and have no success in challenging parental authority, they may become meek and conform to the parents' dictates. Both usually show some emotional difficulty (Weiner, 1970), and have trouble proceeding to mature identity.

Conflict of all kinds during adolescence is found more frequently in authoritarian or permissive homes than in authoritative homes. There is more conflict over spending money, friends, social life and activities outside of the home, and home chores (Edwards and Brauburger, 1973). The autocratically controlled adolescent is likely to harbor resentfulness toward the parents, and is less likely to identify with them (Flacks, 1971). Receiving little or no acceptance at home, the adolescent children of authoritarian parents may be driven outside the home for assurance. They may seek it from other adults or become peer dependent. In an effort to garner attention, they may become disruptive and antisocial. They may seek peer acceptance, sociability, and attention from membership in a delinquent gang (Martin, 1975). Thus, for authoritarian parents unwilling to adjust to the adolescent need for independence, attention and affection, the period of adolescence is likely to be conflict-ridden and stressful. It is, in fact, a vicious cycle: The teenager's wild behavior seems to justify the parents' treatment, and vice versa.

Permissive parents who cater to every need may engender resentment in the adolescent if they are viewed as being overly protective or overly indulgent, or overly detached (all of which are likely as part of a "permissive" approach). Adolescents may resent this babying ("infantilizing") approach as their contact with the world beyond the family increases. Adolescents sometimes complain that their parents are sticking too close, trying to be their "best friend" (Daly, 1963). Such "smothering" behavior can produce conflict when the adolescent finally does establish competing relationships, especially sexual ones. The adolescent may also feel confused and resentful at the lack of direction in the home. Or the adolescent who has experienced permissiveness as benign neglect may cause problems from both lack of supervision and a feeling of having been rejected.

Authoritative parents have the best relationships with their adolescents –

at least in families in the mainstream of North American, middle-class society (Balswick and Macrides, 1975; Devereux, Bronfenbrenner, and Rodgers, 1969; Baumrind, 1975). They are willing to grant their children sufficient autonomy to engender the development of self-governorship and ego control, but not so much responsibility that it would lead to feelings of omnipotence and social irresponsibility. Their lifelong experience with negotiation and shared control prepares them for adolescence in settings away from home as well as in the family.

With the emergence of the period of formal operational thought, many adolescents have the capacity to evaluate parental directions, and become increasingly aware of alternatives. Parents are then in the position of having to defend their points of view – a position the authoritative parent has already adopted and become used to. Baumrind (1975) has concluded that parents of adolescents will find the use of power assertion ineffectual; "She (the authoritative mother) makes limited use of power to settle parent–child differences, and then primarily to guard her personal interests or to break a stalemate when the adolescent's objection is based, not on principle, but on pique" (p. 143). Authoritative parents have the advantage during adolescence, because they can "state and defend their own thesis vigorously, and yet will not limit the freedom of the adolescent to express and argue for his antithesis" (Baumrind, 1975, p. 143). The job of being a parent, particularly parent to an adolescent, requires flexibility, the ability to adapt general principles (e.g., "be supportive") and techniques (e.g., "reward positive behavior") to the specifics of a particular adolescent.

Adolescent maltreatment: an overview

For all its importance, and the attention given to it in the public and professional press, the transmission of abuse from generation to generation is not the only pertinent developmental consideration in the issue of domestic violence. A more sophisticated developmental approach proceeds to investigate changes in the meaning, causes, correlates, and effects of mistreatment as a function of development and maturation (Cicchetti and Rizley, 1981). The issues for school-age children differ from those for infants, or for 3-year-olds, for that matter. The infant can do virtually nothing to protect itself from abuse and is totally defenseless against neglect. The battered baby is victimized in direct proportion to the parent's impulses and the presence of internal and external constraints (which are often few). The infant experiences neglect in exact proportion to the parent's failure to provide care, thus being liable to nonorganic failure to thrive. What is more, the infant's capacity to signal its plight to others is limited and largely unconscious. School-age children, on the other hand, have better resources. They can adapt to the parent to minimize abuse by assuming whatever role will appease the parent, for example, by being extremely compliant, innocuous, or responsible. They can counteract neglect by fending for themselves to some degree. Their ability to communicate their plight is greater because of language skills, and attending school offers many opportunities to do so. Finally, they are likely to have larger independent social networks from which to draw nurturance, support, and protection. This sort of developmental contrast is essential when we consider adolescent maltreatment.

These factors and others come together to shift the standards that guide appropriate behavior in family relationships when a child reaches adolescence. Some forms of behavior by parents toward their offspring that were appropriate (if not particularly wise) in childhood may become abusive in adolescence. For example, the psychological connotations and behavioral response to spanking a 3- or 4-year-old ("control through force") are usually different from those of spanking a 15-year-old. Likewise, a permissive policy of "control through indulgence" that is possible in response to the *child's* relatively benign impulses may become untenable in adolescence, for even the most permissive parent cannot fully indulge the more powerful impulses of the adolescent. Also, managing every detail of a 4-year-old's daily existence ("control through intrusion") may be acceptable, but the same intrusiveness with a teenager would be entirely inappropriate and is likely to produce a strong adverse reaction leading to family conflict.

These factors are crucial because observational research (Reid, 1984) shows that abusive families are behaviorally differentiated from nonabusive families in their handling of the 5 to 10 percent of parent–child interactions that are negative. Nonabusive families are able to conclude (or at least terminate) these negative interactions quickly. Abusive families are ineffective and become enmeshed in escalating conflict. It is possible that some of the families using the strategies enumerated earlier (control through force, indulgence, or intrusion) become abusive in adolescence because these approaches are no longer sufficient to prevent or put the lid on negative exchanges and prevent the escalation of conflict.

Adolescents typically demand a more nearly equal role in family decision making (Steinberg and Hill, 1980). Observational research presents a picture of the youth challenging the parents (particularly the father) for a more active role in leading family discussions and decision making.

These factors, combined with differences in our culture's view of adolescents (with suspicion) and in our institutional treatment of them (with little compassion), predict the phenomenon of how destructive parent–child relations in adolescence will differ from child maltreatment. In fact, as we shall see, in their interpersonal dynamics and cultural interpretation, such destructive relations may more closely resemble spouse abuse than the mistreatment of children, and efforts to understand adolescent maltreatment may serve as a bridge to constructing a much needed, general life-course theory of domestic violence.

Consider a circular continuum of maltreatment relating abused children, adolescents, wives, and elders. The central issue is power, the ability to determine one's own behavior and influence the actions of others. Children and the frail elderly are nearly powerless (though their behavior can have a significant effect on what happens to them). Teenagers gain power because of increases in the ability to think, argue, and act that adolescence brings. Just as wives in a patriarchal and sexist society are powerful enough to threaten the authority of husbands, teenagers challenge parental authority. Paradoxically, because children and the elderly are powerless, they are perfect victims – for two reasons. First, they are easily victimized. Second, they elicit sympathy once they are abused. Teenagers are closer to wives in being imperfect victims, in both respects. One evidence of the greater power of abused teens and wives is the fact they sometimes are involved in reciprocal assault. Obviously, children and the elderly cannot match the strength of the parent generation, but abuse has been identified as a contributing factor in many assaults by adolescents, from relatively minor incidents to parricide (Garbarino and Gilliam, 1980). Likewise, wives who murder their husbands do so often in retaliation for abuse, usually as the culmination of a long period of mutual assault in which wives are the chronic losers (Straus, Gelles, and Steinmetz, 1980). Straus et al. reported assault by youth against their parents in some 10 percent of American families. The likeness between adolescent and wife abuse extends beyond these power dynamics, of course. The two groups are likely to face similar psychodynamic issues, including ambivalence about dependency and separation in their relationships with family authority figures.

Research on adolescent maltreatment

Research on adolescent maltreatment is limited to a handful of small-scale studies and several major surveys. The surveys are the National Incidence Study (Burgdorff, 1980), the American Humane Association's annual tabulation (1982), and the national probability sample assessed for domestic violence by Straus, Gelles, and Steinmetz (1980). The small-scale studies include clinical and questionnaire studies of identified or suspected cases of adolescent maltreatment (e.g., Berdie, Berdie, Wexler, and Fisher, 1983; Farber and Joseph, 1985; Garbarino and Gilliam, 1980; Garbarino, Sebes, and Schellenbach, 1984; Libby and Bybee, 1979; Lourie, 1977; Pelcovitz et al., 1984).

The National Incidence Study (Burgdorff, 1980) collected data on suspected abuse and neglect occurring in a sample of 26 U.S. counties located in 10 states. In addition to child protective service agencies, other local agencies were surveyed (including schools, hospitals, police, and courts). This resulted in the identification of what would be projected nationally to be approximately 650,000 distinct cases. Olsen and Holmes (1983) undertook an analysis of these data contrasting child (11 and younger) with adolescent victims (12–17 years of age). The American Humane Association's National Study of Child Abuse and Neglect Reporting tabulates and analyzes cases reported to (and "accepted" by) official child protective service agencies, as compiled on a state by state basis (with approximately 80 percent of the states participating in the program). Straus, Gelles, and Steinmetz (1981) undertook to assess the level of violence in a national sample of more than 1000 U.S. families (containing two parents and at least one child 3 years of age or older).

Berdie and her colleagues (1983) studied 163 families (from two separate samples) being served by specialized adolescent maltreatment programs after having been identified as cases of adolescent abuse. Farber and his colleagues (Farber and Joseph, 1985; Farber, McCoard, Kinast, and Falkner, 1984) studied 77 families in which an adolescent was being served by an adolescent maltreatment demonstration treatment project. These adolescents had been identified by a local protective service agency (40% of the sample), a runaway youth center (31%), a hospital abuse team (20%), or some other agency (9%). Garbarino and his colleagues (Garbarino and Gilliam, 1980; Garbarino, Schellenbach, Sebes, and Associates, 1986; Garbarino, Sebes, and Schellenbach, 1984) studied two samples: 209 cases of maltreatment (100 of which involved adolescents) reported to a local child protective service agency and 61 families representing a spectrum of adolescent adjustment problems (22 of whom were later judged to have experienced maltreatment). Libby and Bybee (1979) studied 25 cases of adolescent abuse – all such cases reported to a local child protection agency over a ten-month period (but excluding all sexual abuse cases from the analysis). Lourie (1977) surveyed 258 cases and conducted an in-depth clinical assessment of 70 of these cases of confirmed adolescent abuse reported to a local child protection agency. Pelcovitz and his colleagues (1984) studied 33 adolescents (from 22 families) reported to a local child protective service agency and referred to a hospital-based treatment program.

Much of the existing body of research on abuse and neglect is based on hospital and protective service samples. This has biased designs and findings against adolescent victims who are less likely to be identified and served by these agencies. One finding of the National Incidence Study was that adolescent abuse cases were less likely to be reported to the protective services system than were cases involving abuse of other age groups (76% for children versus 39% for adolescents). An analysis conducted by the American Humane Association (Trainor, 1984) indicates, however, that the likelihood of adolescents receiving services once reported to protective services has risen as professional awareness of the problem has grown (from 33% receiving services in 1976 to 55% receiving some services in 1982). Adolescent maltreatment tends to be associated with problematic acting-out behavior of the teenager or dysfunction within the family, and to be dealt with as such by agencies other than protective services. These cases may often be buried under the labels of "dysfunctional families," "school adjustment problems," "running away," "acting out," or "marital problems," even when there is no apparent difference in the level of abuse experienced (Farber et al., 1984). This has implications for sampling in studying adolescent maltreatment, as we shall see.

Research-based conclusions and hypotheses for further study

Drawing upon the available research, we are in a position to put forth a series of conclusions and hypotheses concerning adolescent maltreatment. Each reflects an attempt to critically synthesize existing findings and highlight issues for further study.

The incidence of adolescent maltreatment equals or exceeds the incidence of child maltreatment (Burgdorff, 1980). The National Incidence Study indicates that, despite public and professional emphasis on *child* abuse and neglect, adolescent maltreatment accounts for some 47% of the known cases of maltreatment (42% according to Holmes and Olsen's analysis, which eliminated all "unsubstantiated" cases), although teenagers account for only 38% of the population under the age of 18. The American Humane Association cites a figure of 23% of all reported cases of abuse. As noted earlier, adolescent cases are less likely to be reported, and this is the presumable source of this discrepancy. Studies confined to specific localities (and thus varying on the basis of both local reporting/definitional practices and ecological factors) vary between the National Incidence Study and the American Humane Association figures (e.g., Morgan, 1977).

Adolescent maltreatment includes all forms of abuse and neglect, but psychological and sexual abuse appear to be particularly prevalent. Psychological maltreatment includes "terrorizing," "rejecting," and "isolating" (Garbarino and Vondra, 1987). The sexual abuse data reflect the fact that minors are neither fully capable of giving nor free to give informed consent in sexual relationships with adults – particularly authority figures like parents and guardians (Finkelhor, 1979). The National Incidence Study reports that adolescents receive less severe physical injuries, more psychological maltreatment, and experience more sexual abuse than do children (Olsen and Holmes, 1983). The small-scale studies present a mixed picture with respect to this hypothesis. The significance of these discrepancies is difficult to establish, however. Some studies are explicitly limited to physical abuse (e.g., Libby and Bybee, 1979); others seem to depend upon selective referral that may distort the relative proportion of each type of maltreatment (e.g., Berdie et al., 1983; Pelcovitz et al., 1984). At this point, it seems wise to accept the National Incidence Study's findings as the best report on this matter, namely, that physical assault constitutes smaller proportions for adolescents (42% versus 52%), whereas psychological abuse accounts for a larger proportion for adolescents (32% for adolescents versus 25% for children).

Females appear more likely to be abused as they pass through adolescence than they are in childhood, whereas risk for males peaks early and generally declines through adolescence. This is evident in the National Incidence Study, in which female adolescents outnumber males 2 to 1 (Olsen and Holmes, 1983). Small-scale studies tend to confirm this: 65% female (Farber and Joseph, 1985); 72% female (Lourie, 1977); 64% female (Libby and Bybee, 1979); 55% female (Garbarino, Schellenbach, Sebes, and Associates, 1986), with few exceptions (e.g., 45% in Pelcovitz et al., 1984). We cannot be sure as yet that these observed sex differences are more than artifacts of institutional definition. Male and female adolescents tend to be "treated" in different settings – in part because of differences in the form of their acting-out behaviors, in part because of direct sexual discrimination. Boys are more likely to be dealt with in court-related correctional and detention facilities in which the diagnosis of abuse may be less readily forthcoming.

Some cases of adolescent maltreatment are simply the continuation of abuse and neglect begun in childhood; others represent the deterioration of unwise patterns of child rearing or the inability of a family that functioned well in childhood to meet new challenges in adolescence. The relative proportion of adolescent maltreatment cases in each category varies from study to study (based in part, it seems, on differences in definition and/or sampling). Lourie (1977) concluded that 90% of the adolescent abuse cases begin in adolescence. In Libby and Bybee's study (1979) 80% were so described. Garbarino and Gilliam (1980) report a 50–50 split. Pelcovitz et al. (1984) report a 57% adolescent onset. Farber and Joseph (1985) report 29% displayed adolescent onset, whereas 51% began in childhood but became qualitatively more severe in adolescence, and 21% were severe through childhood into adolescence. Berdie and her colleagues concluded that 24% of their adolescent cases began in adolescence (Berdie et al., 1983). There can thus be little doubt that a distinctly *adolescent* maltreatment phenomenon exists, although its relative magnitude is not yet clear.

Unlike families at high risk for child maltreatment, families at high risk for destructive parent–adolescent relations are socioeconomically equivalent to low-risk families – although a perception of strain on resources associated with larger family size may play a role (Vondra, 1986). The big social class differences found to characterize *child* maltreatment cases are largely absent (or at least are attenuated).

This is evident in the National Incidence Study. Families with adolescent abuse cases were half as likely as those with child maltreatment cases to be earning less than $7,000 per year, and three times as likely to be earning $15,000 per year or more. Nonetheless, 66% of the adolescent maltreatment cases had family incomes below $15,000 – with 25% below $7,000 and 33% above $15,000 (Olsen and Holmes, 1983). Berdie and her colleagues (1983) reported that about 51% of the families in her study had incomes less than $15,000. Garbarino and Gilliam (1980) reported findings consistent with the National Incidence Study. What is more, when they compared adolescent-onset with childhood-onset adolescent maltreatment cases they found even more striking differences, with the adolescent onset cases being about half as likely to be in the poverty group than the child onset (and child maltreatment) cases. In that protective-service-based sample, adolescent onset families were four times as likely to have incomes in excess of $11,000 (in 1978 dollars): 42% versus 11%. Garbarino and his colleagues (1986) report no difference in family income between families judged abusive and families judged nonabusive, with about half of each group of families having incomes of nearly $20,000 (in 1982 dollars).

Several studies have used measures of social class other than income. The National Incidence Study reports higher educational levels for parents of maltreated adolescents than for maltreated children (Olsen and Holmes, 1983). Farber and Joseph (1985) report that their families were predominantly lower class (average Hollingshead Index of 53). Pelcovitz and his colleagues report that 59% of their families were classified in the two top socioeconomic groups (5 point Hollingshead Index). Libby and Bybee (1979) indicate that only 12% of their families were located in the lowest (of 8) socioeconomic status categories. Garbarino and his colleagues (1986) report no difference between families judged to be abusive and comparable, nonabusive families on a Hollingshead Index.

Families at high risk for maltreatment in adolescence are more likely to contain stepparents. A variety of analyses point to the stepparent–adolescent relationship as a very risky one, particularly among families in which adolescents exhibit developmental pathology (cf., Burgess and Garbarino, 1983; Daly and Wilson, 1981; Kalter, 1977). Research on adolescent maltreatment tends to confirm this. Libby and Bybee (1979) report that 28% of their families were stepfamilies and an additional 8% were adoptive. Berdie and her colleagues (1983) reported that 25% of their families were step and 31% had no father-figure in the home. Olsen and Holmes's (1983) analysis of the National Incidence Study data revealed that 40% of the adolescent maltreatment cases contained a stepparent. Garbarino and colleagues (1986) found that 41% of the families judged to be abusive were stepfamilies (versus 0% judged nonabusive). Farber and Joseph (1985) reported that only 30% of their adolescents were living with both biological parents. The processes linking maltreatment to stepfamilies are genuine as well as artifactual. The complicated dynamics of parent–adolescent relations appear to become even more challenging in the step-context. What is more, the attenuations of incest taboos raises the risk of sexual abuse, as do the developmentally disruptive effects of the marital conflict that caused the divorce that predates the step-family arrangement. Of course, artifactual elements play a role in these results as well. In contrast to young children, adolescents are more likely to be in families that have experienced the entire divorce–remarriage pattern.

Adolescents at high risk for maltreatment are less socially competent and exhibit more developmental problems than their peers. Most studies comment upon the aversive and/or dysfunctional character of the adolescent victim of maltreatment. Libby and Bybee (1979) report that in more than 90% of the cases they studied, specific abusive incidents were preceded by negative adolescent behavior (such as disobeying or arguing). Berdie and her colleagues (1983) report that 49% of their adolescent maltreatment victims exhibited significant clinical indicators of depression and that problems such as "nervous habits," "isolation," "poor social skills with peers," "lethargy," "low self-esteem," "low frustration tolerance," "temper outbursts," and "stubbornness" characterized from 45% to 70% of the adolescents (depending upon which problem is being considered in the analysis).

Garbarino and his colleagues (1986) used the Achenbach Child Behavior Checklist to assess the presence of problems in abused adolescents. (Note that this study used parental and adolescent self-ratings of adolescent problems and thus suffers from lack of independent evaluation.) Having selected a sample to maximize the presence of such problems (the overall group's score is at the 85th percentile on such problems), the important finding is in the contrast between maltreated and nonmaltreated youth. The abused group was significantly more problem ridden (the 90th versus the 80th percentiles), evidencing between 50% and 100% more problems (depending upon the type of problems being considered and the source of the report). The difference was greater for externalizing problems (acting-out) than for internalizing problems (e.g., somatic complaints, obsessive–compulsive behavior, withdrawal). Of course, all these studies are problematic with respect to the cause/effect relations between social incompetence and maltreatment. They do not permit us to determine if social incompetence preceded or resulted from maltreatment. Even in studies of *child* maltreatment this is difficult to determine conclusively.

Families characterized as high risk for adolescent maltreatment are also at high risk on the dimensions of adaptability, cohesion, support, discipline, and interparental conflict. Lourie's (1977) model of family functioning offered three categories of adolescent abuse: (1) families that continued a childhood pattern, (2) families that escalated from harsh (though nonabusive by community standards) punishment in childhood to abuse in adolescence, and (3) families that functioned normally in childhood but in which the transition to adolescence precipitated abuse. This early formulation figures permanently in many subsequent analyses of family functioning in adolescent maltreatment.

Libby and Bybee (1979) reported that 13 of their 25 cases could be characterized as "reasonably well-functioning families who had recently been under stress." The other 12 cases were characterized by "psychopathology or disturbed behavior by either the adolescent or parents." Few cases seemed to be attributable to the high stress/social isolation syndrome characteristic of many child maltreatment families. In contrast, Berdie and her colleagues (1983) concluded that "adolescent maltreatment families, like many child maltreatment families, are multi-problem families with high rates of divorce and separation, financial stresses and family conflict." Farber and Joseph (1985) do not comment directly on family functioning, but do report that an analysis of adolescent problems did not find differences based upon Lourie's classification of maltreatment types (with its implicit classification of families).

Pelcovitz and his colleagues (1984) conducted a clinical analysis of their 22 adolescent maltreatment families. They classified cases into childhood and adolescent onset. The eight childhood onset families (14 adolescents) were characterized in the multiproblem child abuse mode – intergenerational abuse, spouse abuse, developmentally inappropriate demands – all the elements of what Helfer and Kempe (1976) termed "the world of abnormal rearing." The 14 adolescent onset families (19 adolescents) fell into two categories (on the basis of multiple, independent clinical assessments): seven "authoritarian" and seven "overindulgent."

The authoritarian families were characterized by paternalistic, harsh, rigid, domineering styles of childrearing. This was coupled with denial: denial of parental feelings toward each other and about the family system. Abuse typically arose from adolescent challenge (acting-out and testing behavior) that was met with overwhelming force. The high priority placed upon control provided the foundation for high levels of force.

In contrast, the overindulgent families were characterized by parental efforts to compensate for the emotional deprivation they had experienced in their own childhood (12 of the 14 parents had lost one or both of their parents during childhood). These families made few demands upon their children, set few limits, and desired a high level of emotional gratification from them. When the children reached adolescence and both sought to form primary attachments outside the home and began to act impulsively in important social settings, the overindulgent parents reacted with excessive force.

Garbarino and his colleagues (1984, 1986) have assessed the family system of families judged to be abusive in contrast to families judged to be nonabusive. They used an assessment of family adaptability and cohesion (FACES) to assess the overall interaction. Abusive families tended to score high in the "chaotic" and "enmeshed" categories (on adaptability and cohesion, respectively). Nonabusive families scored lower on these scales, putting them in the more normal "flexible" and "connected" range. On a measure of interparental conflict, adolescents in the abusive families tended to rate their parents as evidencing more conflict. This average difference (of 368 versus 252) masks the fact that some abusive families evidenced extremely high conflict, whereas others evidenced extremely low conflict. Adolescents in the abusive families tend to describe their parents as being much more punishing. This is also found in an assessment of attitudes and values concerning punishment that measures risk for abuse (Sebes, 1983). This Adolescent Abuse Inventory taps parental commitment to abusive versus nonabusive responses to adolescent problem behavior. An analysis that defined any family with at least one parent in the top quartile of risk (based upon AAI score) correctly classified as abusive or nonabusive 100% of the families based upon the adolescent's description of the family as either abusive or nonabusive (Sebes, 1983), and 85% using the description of outside observers. An assessment of stressful life changes (A-FILE) indicated 50% more recent changes in the lives of adolescents in abusive families than in nonabusive families.

Adolescent abuse is less likely to be transmitted intergenerationally than is child abuse. Pelcovitz and his colleagues report that 75% of the parents in families with childhood onset of abuse had themselves been abused in childhood, as opposed to 25% of the parents in the adolescent onset group. Garbarino and his colleagues (Garbarino and Gilliam, 1980) reported that 21% of the childhood onset cases (being served by child protective services) had a parental history of abuse versus 10% for the adolescent onset group. Berdie and her colleagues (1983) report a trend in this direction. It may well be that the intergenerational transmission of maltreatment is less strong in the case of adolescent maltreatment because the more complex dynamics involved implicate a somewhat different segment of the population as at risk than in child abuse.

Conclusion

In conclusion, it seems clear that our understanding of the meaning, origins, and impact of adolescent maltreatment is progressing. We can see that it does seem to represent a set of phenomena that differentiate it from child maltreatment. With the preceding hypotheses as a guide we can proceed with research and clinical efforts – particularly in the area of dealing with the patterns of childrearing, child development, family resources and system characteristics, and community context that seem to set the stage for the onset of maltreatment in adolescence.

References

American Humane Association (1982). Annual Report of the National Study of Child Abuse and Neglect Reporting. Denver, CO: American Humane Association.

Balswick, J. O., and Macrides, C. (1975). Parental stimulus for adolescent rebellion. *Adolescence, 10,* 253–266.

Bandura, A., and Walters, R. H. (1959). *Adolescent aggression.* New York: Ronald.

Bandura, A., and Walter, R. H. (1963). *Social learning and personality development.* New York: Holt, Rinehart, & Winston.

Baumrind, D. (1975). Early socialization and adolescent competence. In S. Dragastin and G. H. Elder, Jr. (Eds.), *Adolescence in the life cycle: Psychological change and social content.* New York: Wiley.

Baumrind, D. (1979). A dialectical materialists' perspective on knowing social reality. *New Directions in Child Development, 2,* 61–82.

Berdie, J., Berdie, M., Wexler, S., and Fisher, B. (1983). *An empirical study of families involved in adolescent maltreatment.* San Francisco: URSA Institute.

Burgdorff, K. (1980). *Recognition and reporting of child maltreatment: Findings from the National Incidence and Severity of Child Abuse and Neglect.* Prepared for the National Center on Child Abuse and Neglect, Washington, DC, December, 1980.

Burgess, B., and Garbarino, J. (1983). Doing what comes naturally? An evolutionary perspective on child abuse. In D. Finkelhor, R. Gelles, G. Hataling, and M. Straus (Eds.), *The dark side of families.* Beverly Hills, CA: Sage.

Cicchetti, D., and Rizley, R. (1981). Developmental perspectives on the etiology, intergenerational transmission, and sequelae of child maltreatment. *New Directions for Child Development, 11,* 31–52.

Daly, M., and Wilson, M. (1981). Child maltreatment from a sociobiological perspective. *New Directions for Child Development,* Number 11, 93–112.

Daly, S. J. (1963). *Questions teenagers ask.* New York: Dodd, Mead.

Devereux, E. C., Bronfenbrenner, U., and Rodgers, R. R. (1969). Child-rearing in England and the United States. *Journal of Marriage and the Family, 31,* 257–270.

Douvan, E., and Adelson, J. (1966). *The adolescent experience.* New York: Wiley.

Dreyfus, E. A. (1976). *Adolescence: Theory and experience.* Columbus, OH: Charles E. Merrill.

Edwards, J. N., and Brauburger, M. B. (1973). Exchange and parent–youth conflict. *Journal of Marriage and the Family, 35,* 101–107.

Farber, E., and Joseph, J. (1985). The maltreated adolescent: Patterns of physical abuse. *Child Abuse and Neglect, 9,* 201–206.

Farber, E., McCoard, W. D., Kinast, C., and Falkner, D. (1984). Violence in the families of adolescent runaways. *Child Abuse and Neglect, 8,* 295–300.

Finkelhor, D. (1979). *Sexually victimized children.* New York: The Free Press.

Flacks, R. (1971). *Youth and social change.* Chicago: Markham.

Friedenberg, E. Z. (1959). *The vanishing adolescent.* Boston: Beacon Press.

Friedenberg, E. Z. (1965). *The dignity of youth and other atavisms.* Boston: Beacon Press.

Freud, A. (1958). Adolescence. *Psychoanalytic Study of the Child, 13,* 255–278.

Gamble, W., and Garbarino, J. (1985). Families and their adolescents. In J. Garbarino and Associates (Eds.), *Adolescent development: An ecological perspective.* Columbus, OH: Charles E. Merrill.

Garbarino, J., and Gilliam, G. (1980). *Understanding abusive families.* Lexington, MA: Lexington Books.

Garbarino, J., Kelley, A., and Schulenberg, J. (1985). Adolescence: An introduction. In J. Garbarino and Associates, *Adolescent development: An ecological perspective.* Columbus, OH: Charles E. Merrill.

Garbarino, J., Schellenbach, C., Sebes, J., and Associates. (1986). *Troubled youth, troubled families.* New York: Aldine Publishing Co.

Garbarino, J., Sebes, J., and Schellenbach, C. (1984). Families at-risk for destructive parent–child relations in adolescence. *Child Development, 55,* 174–183.

Garbarino, J., and Vondra, J. (1988). The psychological maltreatment of children: Issues and perspectives. In M. Brassard, R. Germain, and S. Hart (Eds.), *The psychological maltreatment of children and youth.* New York: Pergamon.

Goodman, P. (1956). *Growing up absurd.* New York: Vintage.

Grinker, R. R., Sr., Grinker, R. R., Jr., and Timberlake, J. (1962). A study of mentally healthy young males (homoclites). *Archives of General Psychiatry, 6,* 405–453.

Hamburg, D. A., Coelho, G. V., and Adams, J. E. (1974). Coping and adaptation: Steps toward a synthesis of biological and social adaptation. In G. V. Coelho, D. A. Hamburg, and J. E. Adams (Eds.), *Coping and adaptation.* New York: Basic Books.

Helfer, R., and Kempe, C. H. (1976). *Child abuse and neglect: The family and the community.* Cambridge, MA: Ballinger.

Hill, J. P. (1980). The family. In M. Johnson (Ed.), *Seventy-ninth yearbook of the national society for the study of education.* Chicago: University of Chicago Press.

Kalter, N. (1977). Children of divorce in an outpatient psychiatric population. *American Journal of Orthopsychiatry, 47,* 40–51.

Kelly, A., and Garbarino, J. (1985). Adjustment problems in adolescence. In J. Garbarino and Associates (Eds.), *Adolescent development: An ecological perspective.* Columbus, OH: Charles E. Merrill.

Libby, P., and Bybee, R. (1979). The physical abuse of adolescents. *Journal of Social Issues, 35,* 101–126.

Lourie, I. (1977). The phenomenon of the abused adolescent: A clinical study. *Victimology, 2,* 268–276.

Martin, B. (1975). Parent–child relations. In F. O. Horowitz (Ed.), *Review of child development research:* Vol. 4. Chicago: University of Chicago Press.

Martin, H. (1976). *The abused child.* Boston, MA: Ballinger.

McMorrow, F. (1974). *Midolescence: The dangerous years.* New York: Strawberry Hills Publishing Co.

Morgan, R. (1977). The battered adolescent: A developmental approach to identification and intervention. *Child Abuse and Neglect, 1,* 343–348.

Nye, F. I. (1958). *Family relationships and delinquent behavior.* New York: Wiley.

Offer, D. (1969). *The psychological world of the teenager: A study of normal adolescent boys.* New York: Basic Books.

Offer, D., and Offer, J. D. (1973). Normal adolescence in perspective. In J. C. Schoolar (Ed.), *Current issues in adolescent psychiatry.* New York: Brunner/Mazel.

Offer, D., and Offer, J. D. (1974). Normal adolescent males: The high school and college years. *Journal of the American College Health Association, 22,* 209–215.

Offer, D., and Offer, J. D. (1975). *From teenager to young manhood: A psychological study.* New York: Basic Books.

Offer, D., Ostrov, E., and Howard, K. I. (1981). The mental health professional's concept of the normal adolescent. *Archives of General Psychiatry, 38,* 149–152.

Oldham, D. G. (1978). Adolescent turmoil: A myth revisited. In S. C. Feinstein and P. L. Gioracchini (Eds.), *Adolescent psychiatry,* Vol. VI.

Olsen, L., and Holmes, W. (1983). *Youth at risk: Adolescents and maltreatment.* Boston, MA: Center for Applied Social Research.

Pasley, K., and Gecas, U. (1984). Stresses and satisfactions of the parental role. Personnel and guidance journal, *62*, 400–404.

Pelcovitz, D., Kaplan, S., Samit, C., Krieger, R., and Cornelius, P. (1984). Adolescent abuse: Family structure and implications for treatment. *Journal of Child Psychiatry, 23*, 85–90.

Reid, J. (1984). Social interactional patterns in families of abused and non-abused children. In C. Waxler and M. Radke-Yarrow (Eds.), *Social and biological origins of altruism and aggression.* Cambridge: Cambridge University Press.

Russell, C. S. (1979). Circumplex model of marital and family systems III: Empirical evaluation with families. *Family Process, 18*, 29–45.

Rutter, M., Graham, P., Chadwick, O. F. D., and Yule, W. (1976). Adolescent turmoil: Fact or fiction? *Journal of Child Psychology and Psychiatry, 17*, 35–56.

Sebes, J. M. (1983). *Determining risk for abuse in families with adolescents: The development of a criterion measure.* Unpublished doctoral dissertation, Pennsylvania State University, 1983.

Steinberg, L., and Hill, J. (1980). Family interaction patterns during early adolescence. In R. Muuss (Ed.), *Adolescent behavior and society: A book of readings* (3rd ed.). New York: Random House.

Straus, M., Gelles, R., and Steinmetz, S. (1980). *Behind closed doors.* New York: Doubleday.

Trainor, C. (1984). *A description of officially reported adolescent maltreatment and its implications for policy and practice.* Denver, CO: American Humane Association.

U.S. Department of Agriculture (1982). *Costs of raising children.* Washington, DC: U.S. Government Printing Office.

Vondra, J. (1986). *The socioeconomic context of parenting.* Unpublished masters thesis, Pennsylvania State University.

Weiner, I. B. (1970). *Psychological disturbance in adolescence.* New York: Wiley.

Weiner, I. B. (1982). *Child and adolescent psychopathology.* New York: Wiley.

Westley, W. A., and Elkin, F. (1956). The protective environment and adolescent socialization. *Social Forces, 35*, 243–249.

Winn, M. (1983). *Children without childhood.* New York: Penguin Books.

Wolf, L. (1972). *A dream of Dracula: In search of the living dead.* Boston: Little, Brown.

22   Child abuse, delinquency, and violent criminality

Dorothy Otnow Lewis, Catherine Mallouh,
and Victoria Webb

Most physically abused children do not become violent delinquents – at least as far as we know. However, a high proportion of delinquents, particularly violent delinquents, have been severely abused. Indeed, many, perhaps most, violent adult criminals have histories of extraordinary abuse in childhood. Thus, there is clearly an association of childhood abuse and subsequent antisocial, aggressive acts. The purpose of this chapter is to explore the relationship of these phenomena and consider some additional factors that seem to influence whether physical abuse in childhood will be followed by violence in youth and adulthood.

Estimates of the extent of delinquency in the general population vary widely, depending on sources of data and criteria for delinquency. Obviously more delinquent acts are performed than ever reach the attention of the police, much less the juvenile justice system. A study in 1974 (Corbett and Vareb, 1974), using census figures, estimated that fewer than 3.75% of all children in the United States were involved with juvenile court systems in that year. A more recent study (Griffin and Griffin, 1978) estimated that, although 90% of youngsters at some time commit delinquent acts, approximately 34% are taken into police custody, and only 3% are adjudicated delinquent. Poulin and colleagues (Poulin, Levitt, Young, and Pappanfort, 1980) estimated that in the mid 1970s approximately 1.3% of juveniles were admitted to detention centers and/or adult jails annually. Those admitted to such institutions constitute a minority of those apprehended. These data provide some baseline against which to assess the relative prevalence of delinquency in youngsters known to have been abused.

In a small follow-up study of 34 child abuse victims in Washington, D.C., Silver and colleagues (Silver, Dublin, and Loure, 1969) found that 20% had come to the attention of the juvenile court system as delinquents within a four-year period, In a larger, follow-up study of 5392 children referred to the state agency in Arizona because of abuse, 14% were brought to the attention of juvenile authorities within five years of follow-up (Bolton, Reich, and Gutierres, 1977). By the time 10 years had passed, 32% had been adjudicated delinquent (Gray, 1984). Alfaro (1978, 1981) reported similar findings in his lengthy follow-up study of 3637 child victims of abuse and neglect from eight counties in New York State. Of this group, 19% were subsequently known to juvenile authorities for delinquent or ungovernable behavior. Notably, counties differed greatly in outcome: Figures for delinquency in abused boys ranged from 8% to 32% and for abused girls from 2% to 24%. Alfaro reported that in one particular county, although only 2% of children in that county became court involved in a given period, 10% of abused or neglected children came into conflict with the law. Abuse alone does not usually lead to a career of violence. It would seem either that something peculiar about certain kinds of abuse promotes violence, or that additional factors interact with abuse and together with it contribute to the development of antisocial, often aggressive behaviors.

Although only about 20% of abused children go on to become delinquent, retrospective studies indicate that surprisingly high percentages of delinquents were previously abused, neglected, or both. This situation is analogous to the epidemiology of many diseases. For example, few people who eat clams develop hepatitis, however high percentages of hepatitis victims have a history of having eaten clams. The United States Department of Health and Human Services has estimated that approximately 3.4 children per 1,000 per year are physically abused. If sexual and emotional abuse are included, the estimate rises to 5.7 per thousand. These proportions provide some measure with which to compare the prevalence of a history of abuse in delinquents.

Whereas follow-up studies of abused children are relatively rare, retrospective studies of delinquents are more numerous, undoubtedly because they are easier to conduct. To cite but a few of the more recent studies: (1) In a study of 100 juvenile offenders in a Denver detention center whose statements could be verified, 84% had been abused or neglected before age 6 years (Steele, 1976); (2) In a study of 100 juvenile offenders in Philadelphia, 82% had been abused or neglected (Steele, 1976); in a study of 191 juvenile delinquents in residences in Oregon, 58% had been abused by their fathers and 40% had been abused by their mothers (Rhoades and Parker, 1981); Kratkoski (1982) reported that 26% of 863 incarcerated delinquents in Ohio had been abused; Sandberg (1983) reported that 66% of 150 court-referred delinquents to a private residential treatment program had been abused; Lewis and colleagues (Lewis, Shanok, Pincus, and Glaser, 1979) reported that 75% of violent incarcerated male delinquents, and 33% of less violent incarcerated male delinquents, had histories of severe abuse.

The question arises whether these reportedly high percentages of abused delinquents reflect exaggerated accounts by youngsters seeking sympathy.

There have been a few studies that have avoided this methodological problem by using case records to document abuse. For example, Alfaro (1978, 1981) found that of a sample of 1963 delinquent or ungovernable children in New York State in 1971–1972, 21% of the boys and 29% of the girls had previously been reported to authorities as having been abused or neglected. In our own study comparing hospital records of matched samples of delinquents and nondelinquents, 9% of delinquents had been treated for injuries secondary to abuse, compared with 1% of nondelinquents (Lewis and Shanok, 1977). Our study of the medical hospital records of 81 incarcerated delinquents revealed a documentation of abuse in 15% of these cases (Lewis and Shanok, 1981).

These figures from hospital records probably reflect only the most serious episodes of abuse. Our own clinical observations suggest that, rather than exaggerate experiences of abuse, delinquent children are more likely to minimize or deny such experiences. In one instance, a boy who had actually killed his abusing parents denied any mistreatment at their hands. Only after the examiner revealed that she was aware of some of the treatment the boy had experienced did he show her a deep scar on his scalp inflicted by his mother. He then went on to recount how his mother attempted to suture the scalp wound herself rather than take him to a hospital. It would seem that in many cases a combination of fear, shame, and even loyalty prevents delinquent youngsters from revealing the nature and extent of abuse suffered at the hands of family members.

In 1963, shortly after the battered child syndrome was first described by Kempe (Kempe, Silverman, Steele, Droegemueller, and Silver, 1962), Curtis (1963) published a brief article in the *American Journal of Psychiatry* in which he speculated on the effects of battering upon child development.

It is important that the psychological implications of such extreme treatment of children be kept in mind. One might expect the sequelae would be varied. . . . However, it may be useful to re-emphasize one possible consequence which is overt, obvious, and of great public concern and social consequence in its own right; namely, the probable tendency of children so treated to become tomorrow's murderers and perpetrators of other crimes of violence. (Curtis, 1963, p. 368)

Given the importance of the question raised by Curtis, there have been remarkably few studies focusing on the relationship of severe abuse to violent delinquency. Of those who have examined this question, most have reported an association between the degree of violence expressed by delinquents and a history of abuse. In a longitudinal study of 411 boys followed from age 8 years onward, Farrington (1978) and West (1969; West and Farrington, 1973) found that by age 18 years, 27 boys had been convicted of violent offenses, and 98 boys had been convicted of nonviolent offenses. Of the violent boys, 62% had been exposed to harsh parental discipline compared to 33% of the nonviolent offenders and 7% of the nondelinquent boys in the sample. Similarly, Welsh (1976), in his study of 58 court-referred boys, found a significant relationship to exist between severity of corporal punishment and degree of aggressiveness by delinquents. Alfaro (1978) reported that in his study of almost 2,000 delinquents from New York State, those delinquents who had been victims of either abuse or neglect were far more likely than their nonabused delinquent counterparts to have engaged in violent delinquent acts.

Studies of abused children have also pointed to the effects of abuse on aggressive behaviors in general. Kent (1976), in his study comparing abused with neglected children, found that the abused group was more aggressive and disobedient. His finding suggested "that one of the sequelae of physical assault on children is an increase in problems in managing their own aggression" (p. 298).

In his comparison of abused, neglected, and normal children, using both the Thematic Apperception Test and observations of play, Reidy (1977) also found abused children to be more aggressive in their play than neglected or normal children and to have significantly more aggressive fantasies in response to the TAT cards. Our own studies comparing more and less violent delinquents (Lewis, Shanok, Pincus, and Glaser, 1979) indicated a significant difference in histories of abuse between the more violent youngsters and their less aggressive counterparts. Indeed 75 percent of the more violent youths had been the victims of extraordinary physical abuse. For example, one child's father chained him to the bed and burned his feet; one child's mother broke all his fingers; one child's father flung him across the room into his crib when he was an infant, and his mother subsequently broke his leg with a broom handle.

We are currently in the process of conducting a follow-up study of this sample of 97 incarcerated delinquent boys. Our findings suggest that a childhood history of severe abuse and of witnessing family violence is significantly associated with ongoing violent behaviors in adulthood.

The findings of others have been equivocal. For example, Bolton and his colleagues (Bolton, Reich, and Gutierres, 1977) in a comparison of 774 abused delinquents and 900 nonabused delinquents, reported that the abused were less likely than the nonabused to engage in violent acts. They were far more likely to engage in truancy and runaway behavior. Subsequent follow-up of this group, however, suggested that these distinctions no longer existed, and that the abused youngsters were as likely as their nonabused counterparts to behave in aggressive ways. In a retrospective study using files of delinquent youths incarcerated in four Ohio institutions for serious offenders, Kratkoski (1982) found similar histories of violence in abused and nonabused incarcerated male delinquents. As they observed, however, a history regarding abuse was not obtained routinely and had to be gleaned from a variety of clinical reports. Given the reluctance of many delinquents to reveal histories of abuse when asked, much less to volunteer such information, there exists a good possibility that abuse in this sample was underestimated.

The most violent of delinquent or criminal acts is murder. Thus, the association of physical abuse to murderous behavior is of special interest. As early as 1940, Bender and Curran highlighted the importance of early severe physical abuse in the histories of child and adolescent murderers. Easson and Steinhilber (1961) described eight murderous boys. In two cases they found a clear history of recurrent brutal beating by parents, and in three additional cases there were indications that abuse had occurred. Our own follow-up study of nine youngsters who, subsequent to psychiatric evaluation, committed murder (Lewis, Moy, Jackson, Aaronson, Restifo, Serra, and Simos, 1985), revealed that a history of physical abuse was present in almost every case. One mother beat her child while he was naked with belt buckles, cords, and wire hangers; one father tried to kill the subject and his brother; and another father not only beat his son, but also beat his wife so severely that he was jailed for the attack.

There is good evidence that adult violent criminality is associated with a history of severe child abuse. McCord (1979) found that home atmosphere, including parental aggression and conflict, was related to later criminal behavior in terms of the numbers and types of crimes committed. Smith asserted that child abuse and other factors such as modelling, brain damage, and parental psychopathology could lead to adult violence (Canadian Subcommittee on Health, Welfare and Science, 1979). Few studies have addressed specifically and in depth the issues of child abuse in the backgrounds of murderers. Duncan and colleagues (Duncan, Frazier, Litin, Johnson, and Barron, 1958), in case studies of six adult murderers, found that four of these subjects had been victims of severe physical brutality. Similarly, Satten, Menninger, Rosen, and Mayman (1960) reported extreme violence in the background of four murderers. In a study of 54 homicidal offenders, Tanay (1969) found that 67 percent had histories of severe corporal punishment. In contrast to these findings, Langevin and colleagues (Langevin, Paitich, Orchard, Handy, and Russon, 1983), using questionnaires of case records, found no differences in family violence between murderers and nonviolent offenders.

One might hypothesize a relationship between the intensity of parental brutality toward a child and the severity of that child's subsequent violent behaviors. Just as there are degrees of criminal behavior, so there are degrees of parental abuse, the most extreme manifestation of which is filicide. Surprisingly little work has been done on the possible association of having been the victim of attempted murder and, subsequently, becoming the perpetrator. Studies have attempted to define the characteristics of filicidal parents (D'Orban, 1979; Hussain and Daniel, 1984; Resnick, 1969), but have ignored the long-term effects on children of having been the victims of attempted filicide. It was, therefore, of great interest to find that, among 15 death row inmates awaiting execution for murder, 8 had been the victims of potentially filicidal assaults (Feldman, Mallouh, and Lewis, 1986).

For example, one mother shot at her son with a gun as he tried to get away from her. She threatened him with a knife, kicked him, and whipped him all over his body with horse whips, ironing cords, sticks, and belts. When she tied him to a water heater and horsewhipped him, police were called to intervene. One father held his son outside a car at age 4 as it sped down a highway. Both parents frequently beat the boy all over his body. One mother burned her son on the chest with a hot iron and tried to choke him. She also held him outside the window of a moving car when he was an infant and attempted to throw him out. The child's father restrained her. Another subject's mother tried to choke him; his father knocked him unconscious, slashed him with a metal slide, hit him in the head with 2×4 boards, and strapped him with belt buckles. One father on several occasions threatened the subject and his siblings with a shotgun. He also forced them at gunpoint to watch him beat their mother. Other times, he tied his children to the bed and whipped them. He also threw an axe at the subject, injuring the boy's ankle. In addition to the subjects who were the victims of potentially filicidal acts, four subjects were brutally assaulted to a point considered by raters to be short of actual attempted murder. Thus, of the 15 death row subjects, there was evidence of extraordinary abuse in 12 cases. Did extraordinary, almost filicidal, abuse lead to the creation of murderers?

Of the 12 physically abused subjects, 4 also had been the victims of sexual abuse, and one subject, who had not been otherwise physically abused, had been sexually abused throughout childhood. Examples of sexual abuse are as follows: One mother forced her son to sleep with her throughout his childhood and forced him to stimulate her orally and to fondle her breasts. Another subject was fondled and forced by a parent and several close relatives to have sexual intercourse throughout childhood; a neighbor also brutally forced oral sex on this subject. One subject's mother played half-naked on her bed and teased the subject by placing hot dogs in her panties. She lay naked with legs spread and had her son fondle her. This subject was also raped by a male cousin. One subject's father inserted objects into the subject when the subject was a small child, forced penetration when the subject reached adolescence, and continued to force sexual relations with this child until the child left home at 18 years of age.

The question remains unanswered whether or not specific kinds of abuse are associated with specific kinds of violent delinquent or criminal acts. In three of the four cases in which the murderers had been sexually victimized themselves, their own murderous acts included sexual assaults. In two instances, the murders occurred during rapes. In the third case, the condemned person had been sexually abused since early childhood by a father who inserted objects into the subject's rectum and actually forced penetration when the subject reached adolescence. This subject was found guilty of having imprisoned an adolescent girl, thumb cuffing and toe cuffing the victim, inserting objects into the victim's rectum and vagina, and performing a variety of other bizarre sexual acts prior to what may well have been accidentally murdering of the victim.

Our studies of violent juveniles, especially our recent study of those who go on to commit murder and our studies of adult murderers (Lewis, Pincus, Feldman, Jackson, and Bard, 1986) indicate, however, that a history of abuse is but one important factor associated with violent behaviors. As mentioned in the beginning of this chapter, most abused children do not become delinquents, much less violent delinquents. Other neuropsychiatric factors seem to combine with a history of abuse to influence aggressive delinquent outcomes.

Whether intrinsic vulnerabilities in the child, such as brain dysfunction or hyperactivity, elicit abuse from parenting figures, or whether it is abuse itself that causes the kinds of central nervous system impairments that are so frequently found in delinquents, remains a question. Such characteristics as prematurity (Duncan et al., 1958; Elmer and Gregg, 1967; Friedrich and Boriskin, 1976), mental retardation (Brandwein, 1973; Elmer, 1967, 1977; Martin, Beezley, Conway, and Kempe, 1974; Morse, Sahler, and Friedman, 1970), neurological dysfunction (Nichamin, 1973), and a variety of atypical physical and behavioral attributes (Gil, 1970; Johnson and Morse, 1968; Klein and Stern, 1971) are reported to be more prevalent in abused children than in other children. Because abuse often occurs early in infancy, and because the behavioral, intellectual, and neurological manifestations of early abuse are often indistinguishable from the central nervous system abnormalities secondary to prematurity or traumatic delivery, it is rarely possible to determine whether childhood atypicality antedated abuse or resulted from it.

Perinatal difficulties and childhood head trauma are commonly found together in the medical histories of individual delinquents. Whatever the etiology of central nervous system vulnerabilities, current research suggests the existence of a high prevalence of such disorders in the delinquent population (Lewis and Shanok, 1977, 1981; Shanok and Lewis, 1981).

In our own study of 97 incarcerated delinquents (Lewis et al. 1979), among the most significant clinical factors distinguishing the most violent youngsters from their less violent counterparts was the existence of major and minor neurological impairment. For example, the more violent group was more likely to have had an abnormal electroencephalogram or a history of seizures and to have had a multiplicity of minor signs such as choreiform movements, inability to skip, and problems in coordination. The more violent group also had significantly more serious learning disabilities, especially in the area of reading. These findings are especially relevant to issues of delinquency and abuse because the prevalence of a history of extreme abuse in the more violent group was 75 percent compared with a prevalence of 33 percent in the less violent, less neurologically impaired group.

In what ways do these kinds of neurological and cognitive vulnerabilities contribute to delinquency, especially violent delinquency? Central nervous system dysfunction is often associated with irritability, difficult concentration, short attention span, poor social skills, and impaired impulse control. The existence of learning disabilities makes academic work frustrating and ungratifying. Children with such disorders disturb classrooms, fight with peers and others, and experience defeat in every area of functioning. They rarely experience the positive reinforcement of receiving a good grade, much less a good report card. They are easily drawn into fights, and once involved often cannot stop of their own accord. These youngsters, by virtue of their maladaptive behaviors, invite ridicule, in response to which they often lash out.

Because of their social and academic problems, these multiply handicapped youngsters drop out of school early and are left with vast amounts of free time at a developmental stage when they are too immature to be able to organize their lives effectively. Notably, the developmental stages in which delinquents suffer the greatest numbers of adverse medical events are between birth and 4 years of age and between 14 and 16 years of age (Lewis and Shanok, 1977).

In order to understand these phenomena, it is important to consider the characteristics of many of the families from which these delinquents come. Our previously cited statistics indicate that many delinquents, especially those who are most violent, come from abusive families. But abuse is only part of the picture of violence within the families of aggressive delinquents. The preponderance of studies document an association of early victimization and subsequent aggressive behaviors, but few address specifically the effects on a child of violence between parents. Lystad (1975) discussed studies on violence between husbands and wives and noted that the effects on children have not really been explored. Levine (1975) studied 50 families with interparental violence, distinguishing those families in which violence was restricted to the parents from those in which violence was beginning to be expressed toward children. In all cases, the children were affected. They displayed psychiatric and behavioral problems including aggression. In his study of 19 families that abused their children, Stratton (1985) found a 61 percent prevalence of interparental violence. Thus, it would seem that child abuse is but one aspect of family violence.

Our own studies of the families of juvenile and adult violent offenders reveal the existence of extraordinary interparental violence. When children were not themselves victimized, they were often witnesses to assaultive acts between their parents or parent surrogates. For example, in our study of family characteristics of 15 death row inmates, we found that the majority of subjects came from families in which parents or stepparents threatened each other as well as relatives and acquaintances with extreme violence. In six of these cases, these acts were homicidal. For example, one subject's mother tried to stab his father with a knife. Another father threatened his wife with a gun and she threatened him with a butcher knife. Another father was jailed for assaulting his wife. In one case, the subject was brought up by a single, violent mother who threatened a man with a gun in the presence of the subject. Thus, in 12 of the households there was extraordinary violence between adults.

In the histories of violent individuals, abuse is rarely a circumscribed, time-limited event in the individual's life. A careful history will usually reveal that severe abuse interspersed with times of indifference or complete abandonment characterized the individual's household experiences until he or she could leave home.

The study of the 15 death row inmates provided a unique opportunity to observe abuse and neglect carried into adulthood. We wondered what, if any, family support was offered to our subjects. Though this was difficult to quantify, we were able to count the number of actual contacts each subject had with family members while he or she was incarcerated.

Nine subjects received no visits at all. Of those six who did receive visits while on death row, one received no visits from parents, both of whom were alive, but was visited weekly by a daughter. Another subject's parents were both dead and he was visited once in the ten years he was on death row by an aunt. She visited him just before he was scheduled to be executed. One subject's father was dead, but he was visited occasionally by his mother and siblings, who lived in another state. Two subjects, whose parents were both dead, were visited by siblings. In one of these cases, the subject's siblings visited once on the day before his execution and once six years earlier. For one subject the frequency of visits could not be determined.

Thus, with the exception of one subject who received frequent visits by a young daughter, the inmates received few or no visits – five received occasional visits and nine received no visits at all.

Not only did most of these individuals lack supportive family testimony at their trials for purposes of mitigation, but in several cases family members actually assisted in the prosecution. For example, one psychotic mother wrote to the judge requesting that her son be condemned to death. In two cases, parents testified against the subjects. Another family encouraged the subject to plead guilty because it was too expensive to hire a lawyer. In this case, the subject's cousin testified against him.

Family members often concealed the history of abusive behavior, although revelation of such behaviors might have influenced mitigation and saved the lives of some of the subjects. One prisoner who had been brutally sexually assaulted by several family members, and who revealed these facts during psychiatric interviews, went to execution refusing to permit revelation of this family secret. These sexually abusive family members were still alive and urged the subject not to reveal this information even though it could have influenced commutation of the death sentence.

From these data one might readily conclude that filicidal attitudes continued through childhood, into adulthood, and in some cases even influenced the fact that some of the subjects were sentenced to death.

It has been common practice, until recently, to look upon the parents of delinquents as merely sociopathic, irresponsible, violent, and alcoholic. These adjectives do not begin to define the quality of psychopathology within these families. Indeed, these pejoratives obfuscate underlying psychiatric disorders that make many parents of delinquents inadequate to the tasks of childrearing and more likely than others to strike out in abusive ways when stressed beyond their coping skills. In the course of our clinical work with delinquents and their families, we were impressed with the numbers of parents who, themselves, suffered from psychotic, organic, and/or intellectual disorders that affected their parenting abilities. Our epidemiological studies indicated that the parents of delinquents were significantly more likely than members of the general population to have been psychiatrically hospitalized (Lewis and Balla, 1976). What is more, psychiatrically hospitalized mothers were likely to be married to psychiatrically hospitalized and/or criminal fathers.

Our clinical and epidemiological findings suggest that the violence and abuse to which many delinquents are subjected are manifestations of life within households in which one or both parents are significantly psychiatrically impaired. Contrary to the studies suggesting that physically abusive parents are not seriously psychiatrically disturbed, the abusive parents of the delinquents we studied gave ample evidence of disturbances that were often of psychotic proportions. For example, one father, recently discharged from a psychiatric hospital, threw his infant son across the room into his crib; another chained his son and burned his feet; one mother broke all of her son's fingers; and one psychotic aunt in whose custody a child was left had her lovers hold his arms and legs while she wet down his back and beat him with a cord.

In the case of the 15 death row inmates it was impossible to ascertain the degree of psychopathology in their parents and stepparents because of lack of clear documentation; however, there were indications that severe psychopathology existed in 10 cases. For example, one father would experience episodic rages lasting a week at a time during which he brutalized his hunting dogs, stomping on their heads. Another extremely brutal father was idosyn-cratically religious, setting up a shrine in the woods, at which he would pros-trate himself and pray regularly. One mother was so suspicious that she thought that the investigator for the defense was an escaped convict coming to kill her. She therefore called the FBI to check the validity of the defense counselor's letters. Two subjects' mothers were psychiatrically hospitalized. Several parents showed severe symptoms of mood disorders. Seven of the 16 subjects had at least one alcoholic parent.

The fact that many abusive parents of delinquents and violent criminals are at times psychotically disturbed sheds further light on the association of abuse and violent delinquency and criminality. Many subsequently violent individuals are raised in conditions of extreme irrationality as well as vio-lence. The physical abuse that they experience is but one aspect of the vio-lence they witness at home. They see fathers and mothers attack each other with fists and weapons. When they are not victims of parental aggression they often feel the need to try to protect one parent from the other. In doing so, they too become the targets of violence.

Furthermore, many of the delinquent youngsters who come from families in which one or both parents is psychotic are themselves especially vulner-able to distorted thought processes. Such vulnerabilities to thought disor-ders undoubtedly make these youngsters less able than normal children to tolerate abuse and exposure to violence without becoming violent them-selves. As in the case of neurological impairment, it is usually impossible to tell whether a delinquent who suffers from psychotic symptoms such as paranoid episodes was originally vulnerable to distortion of reality, or whether life within a psychotic household engendered the psychiatric con-dition. It may be that those 50 percent to 80 percent of abused children who do not become violent themselves are more psychiatrically and neurologi-cally intact to begin with than those abused children who later do become delinquent and violent. The evidence cited suggests that abuse alone, although an important factor, is not usually sufficient in and of itself to cause delinquency.

Our findings indicate that severe physical abuse is most likely to be asso-ciated with violent delinquency and criminality when one or more of the following additional factors is present: The child suffers from some sort of central nervous system dysfunction that impairs his ability to modulate his emotions and control his responses; the child suffers from some form of psychiatric disturbance that impairs his reality testing at times so that he misperceives his environment and feels needlessly and excessively threat-ened; the child is exposed to extraordinary household violence between par-ents or caretakers.

How might one conceptualize the relationship of severe abuse to the development of violence? First, abuse toward a child functions as an example of behavior. Whether one calls this effect "modeling," "identification with the aggressor," or simply "imitation," is irrelevant. What is important is that children copy parent behaviors. Second, child abuse itself often results in central nervous system injury. This kind of brain injury is often manifested clinically by emotional lability, extremes of anger, and difficulty controlling behavior. There is also evidence that indicates that early central nervous system insults can be associated with subsequent psychotic disturbances in vulnerable youngsters who otherwise might not have become psychotic (Pollin and Stabenau, 1968). As stated, psychotic misperceptions and misinterpretations of a paranoid nature are commonly found in the violent delinquent population and often account for some ostensibly motiveless or precipitous violent acts. Finally, although it is difficult to measure origins or degrees of anger, it is reasonable to suspect that the mindless, irrational, extreme abuse to which many delinquents have been exposed engenders extraordinary rage. This rage, though occasionally expressed toward abusive parents, more often is displaced onto others in the environment – teachers, police, other authority figures, and even peers.

Abuse alone does not usually create violent youngsters. It would seem that abuse, family violence, and neuropsychiatric vulnerabilities in the child together engender violence. Unfortunately, this combination of factors is prevalent in our society today.

The recognition that extraordinary violence is often, perhaps usually, the result, at least in part, of having been the victim of extreme abuse raises theoretical, moral, and legal questions. Among the questions raised are the following:

1. To what extent is physical abuse alone responsible for the development of violent behaviors?
2. Is the degree or nature of physical abuse experienced by the victim proportional to the degree and nature of violence perpetrated by the abused individuals?
3. Can emotional or verbal abuse lead to the same degree of violence as actual physical abuse?
4. How powerful is the effect of witnessing violence?
5. Are there particularly vulnerable developmental periods during which physical or emotional abuse is most likely to lead to violence?
6. Can the potentially detrimental effects of abuse be reversed and, if so, how?
7. To what extent does an intrinsic vulnerability (e.g., central nervous system dysfunction, psychosis, retardation) increase the individual's susceptibility to the violence-inducing effects of abuse and witnessing violence?

Fortunately, in a free, principled society, these kinds of questions do not lend themselves to the kind of scientific experimentation that might answer them clearly. This situation, however, does not mean that they cannot be addressed. They must be studied, however, by observing closely and systematically those natural experiments that occur within societies. We know that probably everyone, under certain circumstances, is capable of violence. The question is, simply, what kinds of stresses on what kinds of vulnerabilities and for what duration of time make violent behavior a probability – even a certainty – rather than an unlikely possibility?

This basic theoretical question raises a moral and, therefore, legal question. To what extent is a violently abused individual responsible for his or her own violent behaviors? We know that human beings are remarkably resilient; however, this is compromised when the central nervous system is disordered by virtue of injury, psychosis, retardation, or the myriad of other factors that affect its functioning. Thus, society wrestles with the question of just how much control the physically and mentally traumatized individual has over the expression of rage. It is at this cynosure of psychology, medicine, morality, and law that research on the relationship of abuse to violence must focus.

References

Alfaro, J. D. (1978). *Report on the Relationship Between Child Abuse and Neglect and Later Socially Deviant Behavior.* Albany, NY: New York State Assembly.

Alfaro, J. D. (1981). Report on the relationship between child abuse and neglect and later socially deviant behavior. In R. J. Hunner and Y. E. Walker (Eds.), *Exploring the Relationship Between Child Abuse and Delinquency,* Montclair, NJ: Allanheld, Osman.

Bender, L., and Curran, F. (1940). Children and adolescents who kill. *Criminal Psychol., 1,* 297–322.

Bolton, F. G., Reich, J. W., Gutierres, S. E. (1977). Delinquency patterns in maltreated children and siblings. *Victimology, 2,* 349–357.

Brandwein, H., (1973). The battered child: A definite and significant factor in mental retardation. *Ment. Retard., 11,* 50–51.

Canadian Subcommittee on Health, Welfare and Science (1979). Proceedings of the Subcommittee on Childhood Experience as Causes of Criminal Behavior. Testimony by Selwyn Smith, Issue No. 7 (Feb. 9).

Corbett, J., and Vareb, T. S. (1974). *Juvenile Court Statistics* (Department of Justice Grant Nos. 76–JN–99–0006 and 76–DF–99–0034). Washington, DC: Office of Juvenile Justice and Delinquency Prevention.

Curtis, G. C. (1963). Violence breeds violence. Perhaps? *Am. J. Psychiatry, 120,* 386–387.

D'Orban, P. T. (1979). Women who kill their children. *Brit. J. Psychiatry, 134,* 560–571.

Duncan G. M., Frazier, S. H., Litin, E. M., Johnson, A. M., Barron, A. J. (1958). Etiological factors in first-degree murder. *J.A.M.A., 168* (13), 1755–1958.

Easson, W. M., and Steinhilber, R. M. (1961). Murderous aggression by children and adolescents. *Arch. Gen. Psychiatry, 4,* 27.

Elmer, E. (1967). *Children in Jeopardy: A Study of Abused Minors and Their Families.* Pittsburgh, PA: University of Pittsburgh Press.

Elmer, E. (1977). A follow-up study of traumatized children. *Pediatrics, 59,* 273–279.

Elmer, E., and Gregg, G. S. (1967). Developmental characteristics of abused children. *Pediatrics, 40,* 596.

Farrington, D. P. (1978). The family backgrounds of aggressive youths. In L. A. Hersov and M. Berger (Eds.), *Aggression and Antisocial Behavior in Childhood and Adolescence.* Book supplement to *J. Child Psychol. Psychiat.,* (No. 1). New York: Pergamon.

Feldman, M. Mallouh, C., and Lewis, D. O. (1986). Filicidal abuse in the histories of 15 condemned murderers. *Bull. Am. Acad. Psychiat. Law., 14* (4), 345–352.

Friedrich, W. N., and Boriskin, J. A. (1976). The role of the child in child abuse: A review of literature. *Am. J. Orthopsychiat., 46* (4), 580–590.

Gil, D. G. (1970). *Violence Against Children: Physical Child Abuse in the United States.* Cambridge, MA: Harvard University Press.

Gray, E. (1984), *Child Abuse: Prelude to Delinquency?* Final report of a research conference conducted by the National Committee for the Prevention of Child Abuse. Washington, DC: Office of Juvenile Justice and Delinquency Prevention.

Griffin, B. S., and Griffin, C. T. (1978). *Juvenile Delinquency in Perspective.* New York: Harper and Row.

Gutierres, S. E., and Reich, J. W. (1981). A developmental perspective on runaway behavior: Its relationship to child abuse. *Child Welfare, 60,* 89–94.

Husain, A., and Daniel, A. (1984). A comparative study of filicidal and abusive mothers. *Canadian J. Psychiatry, 29,* 596–598.

Johnson, B., and Morse, H. (1968). Injured children and their parents. *Children, 15,* 147–152.

Kempe, C. H., Silverman, F. N., Steele, B. F., Droegemueller, W., and Silver, H. K. (1962). The battered child syndrome, *J.A.M.A., 181,* 17–24.

Kent, J. (1976). A follow-up study of abused children. *J. Pediat. Psychol., 1,* 25–31.

Klein, M., and Stern, L. (1971). Low birth weight and battered child syndrome. *Am. J. Dis. Child., 122,* 15–18.

Kratkoski, P. C. (1982). Child abuse and violence against the family. *Child Welfare, 61,* 435–444.

Langevin, R., Paitich, D., Orchard, B., Handy, L., and Russon, A. (1983). Childhood and family background of killers seen for psychiatric assessment: A controlled study. *Bulletin Am. Acad. Psychiat. Law, 11* (4), 331–341.

Levine, M. B., (1975). Interparental violence and its effect on the children. A study of 50 families in general practice. *M. Science Law, 15* (3), 172–176.

Lewis, D. O., and Balla, D. A. (1976). The parents: Clinical and epidemiological findings. In their *Delinquency and Psychopathology.* New York, San Francisco, London: Grune and Stratton.

Lewis, D. O., Moy, E., Jackson, L. D., Aaronson, R., Restifo, N., Serra, S., and Simos, A (1985). Biopsychosocial characteristics of children who later murder: A prospective study. *Am. J. Psychiatry, 142* (10), 1161–1167.

Lewis, D. O., Pincus, J. H., Feldman, M., Jackson, L., and Bard, B. (1986). Psychiatric, neurological and psychoeducational characteristics of 15 death row inmates in the United States. *Am. J. Psychiatry, 143* (7), 838–845.

Lewis, D. O., and Shanok, S. S. (1977). Medical histories of delinquent and nondelinquent children: An epidemiological study. *Am. J. Psychiatry, 134,* 1020–1025.

Lewis, D. O., and Shanok, S. S. (1981). Perinatal difficulties, head and face trauma, and child abuse, in the medical histories of seriously delinquent children. *Am. J. Psychiatry, 136* (4A), 419–423.

Lewis, D. O., Shanok, S. S., Pincus, J. H., and Glaser, G. H. (1979). Violent juvenile delinquents: Psychiatric, neurological, psychological, and abuse factors. *J. Am. Acad. Child. Psychiat., 18,* 307–319.

Lystad, M. H. (1975). Violence at home: A review of the literature. *Am. J. Orthopsychiat., 45* (3), 328–345.

Martin, H. P., Beezley, P., Conway, E. F., and Kempe, C. H. (1974). The development of abused children. *Adv. Pediatrics, 21,* 23–73.

McCord, J. (1979). Some child-rearing antecedents of criminal behavior in adult men. *J. Personality Social Psychology., 37* (9), 1477–1486.

Morse, C. W., Sahler, O. J., and Friedman, S. B. (1970). A three year follow-up study of abused and neglected children. *Am. J. Dis. Child., 120,* 439–446.

Nichamin, S. (1973). Battered child syndrome and brain dysfunction. *J.A.M.A., 223,* 1390.

Pollin, W., and Stabenau, J. R. (1968). Biological, psychological, and historical differences in a series of monozygotic twins discordant for schizophrenia. In D. Rosenthal and S. S. Kety (Eds.), *The Transmission of Schizophrenia*, Oxford: Pergamon.

Poulin, J. E., Levitt, J. L., Young, T. M., Pappanfort, D. M. (1980). *Juveniles in Detention Centers and Jails* (GPO Report No. 1980–0311–379/1413). Washington, DC: Office of Juvenile Justice and Delinquency Prevention.

Reidy, T. J. (1977). The aggressive characteristics of abused and neglected children. *J. Clin. Psychology*, (33), 1140–1145.

Resnick, P. J. (1969). Child murder by parents: A psychiatric review of filicide. *Am. J. Psychiatry, 126*, 325–334.

Rhoades, P. W., and Parker, S. L. (1981). *The Connections Between Youth Problems and Violence In The Home* (DHHS Grant No. 10–4–1–80101). Portland: Oregon Coalition Against Domestic and Sexual Violence.

Sandberg, D. N. (1983). *The Relationship Between Child Abuse and Juvenile Delinquency*. Testimony submitted to the Senate State Subcommittee on Juvenile Justice, Oct. 19.

Satten, J., Menninger, K., Rosen, I., and Mayman, M. (1960). Murder without apparent motive: A study in personality disorganization. *Am. J. Psychiatry, 117*, 48–53.

Shanok, S. S., and Lewis, D. O. (1981). Medical histories of abused delinquents. *Child Psychiat. Hum. Developm., 11*, 222–231.

Silver, L. B., Dublin, C. C., and Lourie, R. S. (1969). Does violence breed violence? Contributions from a study of the child abuse syndrome. *Am. J. of Psychiatry., 126*, 404–407.

Steele, B. (1976). Violence within the family. In R. E. Helfer and C. H. Kempe (Eds.), *Child Abuse and Neglect: The Family and The Community*. Cambridge, MA: Ballinger.

Stratton, C., (1985). Comparison of abusive and nonabusive families with conduct-disordered children. *Am. J. Orthopsychiat., 55* (1), 59–69.

Tanay, E. (1969). Psychiatric study of homicide. *Am. J. Psychiatry., 125* (9), 1252–1258.

Welsh, R. S. (1976). Severe parental punishment and delinquency: A developmental theory. *J. Clin. Child Psychology., 5*, 17–21.

West, D. J. (1969). *Present Conduct and Future Delinquency: First Report of the Cambridge Study in Delinquent Development*. New York: International Universities Press.

West, D. J., and Farrington, D. P. (1973). *Who Becomes Delinquent? Second Report of the Cambridge Study in Delinquent Behavior*. London: Heinemann.

23   The prevention of maltreatment

David L. Olds and Charles R. Henderson, Jr.

Introduction

During the last 20 years, public concern about child abuse and neglect has grown dramatically (Garbarino and Stocking, 1980; Gerbner, Ross, and Zigler, 1980; Kempe, Silverman, Steele, Droegemuller, and Silver, 1962). Within the past decade, a National Center on Child Abuse and Neglect has been established by the federal government, a National Committee for the Prevention of Child Abuse has been created in the private sector, and the media routinely convey the message that abuse and neglect are preventable. Two recent surveys have suggested a sharp increase in child abuse and neglect reports in the last six years (American Humane Association, 1985; National Center on Child Abuse and Neglect, 1981). These reports indicate that hundreds of thousands of children and families are in crisis and emphasize the importance of preventive programs and research efforts in this area (U.S. Senate, 1983). In view of these developments, it is disturbing that little is known about the prevention of maltreatment (Helfer, 1982).

A variety of program models and community strategies have been proposed, including the enhancement of parent–newborn contact and interac-

This chapter is based on an article that was originally published in *Pediatrics*, 1986, *78*, 65–78, and coauthored with R. Chamberlin and R. Tatelbaum. We are indebted to them for significant contributions to this work. The research upon which this chapter is based was supported by grants from the Bureau of Community Health Services (HHS–MCR–360403–06), the Robert Wood Johnson Foundation (Grant No. 5263), and the W. T. Grant Foundation (Grant No. 0723–809).

We wish to thank Karen Hughes, Jean Thom, Janice Sheppard, and Elizabeth Bement for their help with preparing the manuscript and processing the data; Urie Bronfenbrenner, Vicki Carlson, Dante Cicchetti, Robert Cole, Jim Garbarino, Zorika Petic Henderson, Robert Hoekelman, Howard Foye, Gregory Liptak, Elizabeth McAnarney, Ingrid Overacker, Joannie Pinhas, Martha Sandler, and Cassie Stevens for offering helpful comments on the manuscript; John Shannon for his administrative support of the project; and Elizabeth Chilson, Diane Farr, Georgianna McGrady, Jacqueline Roberts, and Lyn Scazafabo for their outstanding work with the families enrolled in the program.

tion (Garbarino, 1980; Klaus and Kennel, 1982), parenting education (Gelles and Cornell, 1985), telephone hotlines (Johnston, 1976), crisis or respite care of the child (Cohn, 1981), the provision of home-health visitors (Kempe, 1976), the enhancement of natural community helpers (Collins, 1981; Pancoast, 1981), the provision of increased employment opportunities and a guaranteed minimum income (Gil, 1974), the reduction of society's acceptance of violence (Gelles, 1984), as well as more comprehensive, multifaceted programs based on ecological theory (Lutzker and Rice, 1984; Lutzker, Frame, and Rice, 1982). Most of these proposals remain untested with carefully constituted comparison or control groups, however, so the prospects for their success are unclear. Three of these preventive interventions (early contact between parents and newborns, home visitation, and respite care) have been examined in studies that employed appropriate control groups (Lealman, Haigh, Phillips, Stone, and Ord-Smith, 1983; Gray, Cutler, Dean, and Kempe, 1979; O'Connor, Vietze, Sherrod, Sandler, and Altemeier, 1980; Siegel, Bauman, Schaefer, Saunders, and Ingram, 1980). They are reviewed below. Those other proposals that have not been tested within the context of controlled trials should be reviewed, nevertheless, from the standpoint of both their theoretical and empirical underpinnings. In this way, we can determine whether they deserve the enormous investment that is required to carry out carefully controlled trials.

Analysis of selected prevention proposals

As the other chapters in this volume indicate, no single causal factor can explain maltreatment. It is a multiply determined event or series of events – the product of parents' own childrearing histories, their current psychological resources, the levels of stress with which they have to contend (including the difficulty of the child's temperament), the degree to which violence is accepted in parents' social groups, and the quality of parents' social support – that can best be understood from the standpoint of ecological theory (Belsky, 1980). Many proposed preventive interventions are predicated on the notion that abuse or neglect will be reduced if the correlated risk factor is reduced. Ecological theory leads one to question this assumption.

Parents who abuse or neglect their children, for example, are frequently identified as being socially isolated (Garbarino and Crouter, 1978), leading some to propose the enhancement of informal social support as a preventive strategy (Collins, 1981; Pancoast, 1981). The close involvement of friends and neighbors is thought to reduce the risk of maltreatment through the provision of emotional and material support and through processes of social control and sanctioning (Garbarino, 1980). Social isolation may play little direct role in abuse or neglect, however, and instead may reflect a more fundamental deficiency in parents' abilities to form relationships, one outgrowth of which may be dysfunctional childrearing. Efforts to decrease child abuse and neglect by trying to enhance families' social networks may be less effective than one might predict from the correlational data, because parents at risk for maltreatment may lack the social skills to take advantage of the social support made available to them, and because their social isolation may be more of a symptom than a cause of maltreatment. In spite of this, the enhancement of informal social support may be a useful objective (as the support and control that result from participation in social networks are potentially powerful forces), as long as this tactic is part of a more comprehensive effort that helps parents improve their self-confidence and their social skills and that addresses other factors that place parents at risk for maltreatment.

Similar kinds of problems can be found with other single-variable interventions. Parents who have abused their children, for example, often overestimate their children's abilities (Spinetta and Rigler, 1972). On the basis of this and other related evidence, some workers have recommended providing parent education classes for new parents so they might learn about normal child development and about what to expect from their children at specific ages. This kind of preventive intervention is probably not well suited for most parents at risk for maltreatment, though, because they are often reluctant to attend parent-group meetings. One randomized trial of paraprofessional home-visitation and parent group sessions for high-risk parents had to eliminate the group sessions from the study because so few of the parents attended (vanDoorninck, Dawson, Butterfield, and Alexander 1980). Moreover, even if they attended, one must question the extent to which simply providing high-risk parents with information about child development and childrearing would have a discernible impact on the quality of care that they provide to their children. Such parents are often buffeted by overwhelming stresses that can interfere with their efforts to turn their knowledge into appropriate caregiving activities. Education about children's needs and competencies is undoubtedly an essential component of an overall strategy to prevent maltreatment, but efforts also need to be directed toward reducing some of the pressing problems that can interfere with parents' caregiving efforts.

In light of the association between social class and maltreatment (Gil, 1970; Light, 1973) and the role that unemployment plays in maltreatment (Gil, 1971; Steinberg, Catalano, and Dooley, 1981), some workers have suggested that child abuse and neglect will not be reduced significantly unless major changes are made in the social and economic structure of the society so that all families are guaranteed jobs and a minimum income (Gil, 1971, 1977, 1978). These same proposals have been made on behalf of families by the Carnegie Council on Children in their consideration of a wide range of child health and developmental outcomes (Keniston, 1977).

Given the pervasive influence of unemployment and inadequate income on most dimensions of family functioning, it seems reasonable that such reforms would reduce the incidence of maltreatment. But because the influence of increased income and employment on maltreatment may be indirect, and may take a considerable length of time (perhaps generations) to work, the extent of its impact on maltreatment is difficult to predict. Although such reforms are attractive on many grounds, including their promotion of social and economic equality, it is unlikely that they will be undertaken in the foreseeable future. As a result, it makes sense for preventive programs to try to improve the employment and financial context in which the family is functioning, but to do so on a case-by-case basis, because changing the larger socioeconomic conditions of the society is virtually impossible for the planners and providers of health and human services.

Because the acceptance of violence in the society contributes to child abuse (Alvy, 1975; Gil, 1970; Strauss, 1974), other workers have proposed public information campaigns and educational programs in the schools in order to increase community awareness of the destructive force of violence on family life. Again, it is reasonable to direct efforts in this direction, but in the absence of other changes in personal and family conditions that contribute to abuse and neglect, these efforts are likely to have limited impact; this is especially true when conditions that create stress and frustration for parents (such as unemployment, racism, and sexism) continue at current levels, and conditions that sustain family life (such as two-parent households and the extended family) are deteriorating.

As this short analysis suggests, the most promising approaches to prevention are those programs that are multifaceted and capable of simultaneously addressing the numerous factors that create contexts for maltreatment. Unfortunately, comprehensive preventive services have not been studied with research designs that employed appropriate control groups, so it is difficult to estimate their effectiveness. Several of the less comprehensive interventions for preventing maltreatment listed above (enhancing parent–newborn contact, home visitation, and respite care) have been tested in four investigations that employed control groups. The conclusions that can be drawn from these studies are less clear than one might expect, however, because the results are inconsistent.

Controlled trials of maltreatment prevention

The first 2 trials grew out of the ethological work of Klaus and Kennel (1982) on the influence of early and extended parent–newborn contact on the formation of attachment and "bonding" (O'Connor et al., 1980; Siegel et al., 1980). This work has been advanced on the observation that among certain species there is a sensitive period after birth during which separation of the offspring from its mother can significantly alter subsequent maternal behavior. Klaus and Kennell's work has been devoted to exploring whether there is an analog to this pattern from other species in the impact of modern hospital maternity care (which until recently has routinely separated mothers and newborns) on the quality of maternal caregiving behavior. Two studies out of a series of at least 19 investigations in this area have examined child abuse and neglect as an outcome.

One investigation studied the impact of extended postpartum contact (rooming-in) between mothers and newborns on subsequent caregiving dysfunction (O'Connor et al., 1980). The sample consisted of 301 low-income mother–child pairs in which the mothers were all primiparous. The extended contact group received up to eight hours of extra contact per day (once the baby was at least 7 hours old) for two days postpartum. The control group was provided routine hospital care (a glimpse of the baby immediately after delivery, separation for at least two hours postpartum, and thereafter together for feedings). By the time the infants were 17 months of age, ten (7 percent) of the control families and two (1.5 percent) of the extended contact families displayed evidence of caregiving inadequacy (reports of physical abuse, nonorganic failure to thrive, abandonment, abnormal development, or repeated hospitalization).

In a second investigation, the effect of early and extended contact was compared to home visitation and a no-treatment control with a sample of low-income multiparous women (Siegel et al., 1980). The early and extended contact consisted of at least 45 minutes of mother–newborn contact during the first three hours immediately after delivery plus at least five hours each day during the mothers' and newborns' stay in the hospital. The home-visitation program was carried out by highly trained and well-supervised paraprofessionals who first visited mothers in the hospital and then paid nine home visits during the first three months postpartum. The goal of the home visitation program was to promote mother–infant attachment and to help mothers cope with situational stresses in their lives. No differences were detected between the early- and extended-contact, home-visited, and control group in reports of child abuse and neglect and health care utilization patterns. There were indications, however, that the group provided early and extended contact displayed improvements in some aspects of mother–infant interaction (such as maternal acceptance and consoling of the infant). Maternal background characteristics (age, race, education, parity, and housing) explained a much larger portion of the variance in their measures of attachment than did early and extended contact. In general, it seems unrealistic to expect a few extra minutes or hours of contact between high-risk parents and their newborns to inoculate them from the frequently stressful life circumstances that will characterize their lives during the days, months, and years following their discharge from the hospital.

The failure of the home-visit program examined in the second study, according to the home visitors themselves, may be connected to its inception postnatally. The home visitors reported that they might have been more successful if they had visited the families during pregnancy, when they might have been able to establish rapport with parents more effectively. The relatively short duration of the program (three months) also should be considered. Given the myriad stresses with which low-income families frequently must contend, it is not surprising that a three month program of nine home visits showed no effect on the incidence of child abuse and neglect. In principle, home visitation has the potential (if properly designed and executed) to address the factors that lead to abuse and neglect, but we are not provided sufficient detail about this program to determine whether it indeed addressed those factors in an intensive and systematic way. Home-visitation programs vary considerably along a variety of dimensions, including their frequency of contact, duration, educational content, structure, sensitivity to parental needs, and emotional supportiveness. In order to interpret the presence or absence of program effects, it is essential that a detailed description of the program be provided. From the standpoint of research design, it is unfortunate that no attempt was made in this study to determine whether treatment effects were present or intensified for higher risk groups within their sample. An intensification of program effects for higher risk families has been reported in one study of early contact that did not examine child abuse and neglect as an outcome (Anisfeld and Lipper, 1983).

In a third controlled trial, from Bradford, England, a group of families at risk for childrearing dysfunction was judged to be unaffected by the provision of preventive services (Lealman et al., 1983). The study does not provide a fair test of preventive services, however, because the intervention had a limited theoretical basis for affecting the quality of caregiving. The services consisted of a contact by the project social worker after mothers' and newborns' discharge from the hospital, the creation of a drop-in center for mothers and babies (respite care) that was open one day a week, and, in case mothers were having difficulty, giving them the project secretary's phone number to call for help. Obviously, this set of services was not capable of affecting the complex, interrelated factors that undermine parents' capacities to care for their children. In light of its limited chances for success, one must question the wisdom of having invested in the study of this intervention.

The fourth study examined the effects of providing intensive pediatric consultation plus home visitation to a sample of women at risk for child abuse and neglect (Gray et al., 1979). Families were assessed with pre- and postnatal interviews as well as observations of mothers and newborns in the delivery room, and then classified into high- and low-risk groups. The high-risk group was randomly assigned to either a treatment or control condition. Those in the treatment were provided intensive well-child care from a single pediatrician who provided extra phone contact and office visits in which she counseled parents on nutrition, accident prevention, and discipline, and attempted to promote maternal attachment to the newborn. Those in the treatment group also received weekly home visits by public health nurses. A lay health visitor assessed the health of the child, provided emotional support to the family, and served as a liaison with professional health-care providers. A randomly selected subsample of half of the children and parents in each group was assessed when the children were between 17 and 35 months of age. The assessments consisted of Denver Developmental Screening Tests (DDSTs), home observations, and interviews to assess medical and social functioning. A review of the State Child Abuse Registry was carried out on the entire sample. In contrast to the high-risk controls, the high-risk intervened group had fewer hospitalizations for serious injury. There were no significant differences in the incidence of verified cases of child abuse and neglect or other indicators of abnormal parenting practice; but there were trends for the intervened group to have a higher number of child abuse reports (which may be due to increased reporting on the part of the health-care providers who were so closely involved with the families) and a higher number of failed DDST items ($p < .10$ for both findings). Because of these inconsistent findings and because most evaluations were carried out on only half of the sample, the findings of this study should be viewed with caution.

It is evident that a variety of problems with research and program design make it difficult to estimate the extent to which abuse and neglect are indeed preventable. Even though home visitation has been postulated as a potent means of preventing maltreatment (Kempe, 1976; Olds, 1981, 1982, 1983), as the studies outlined above indicate, at the time the current study was designed, its potential had not been sufficiently explored. In the present study, my colleagues and I tried to construct a powerful home-visiting program, grounded in ecological theory (Bronfenbrenner, 1979; Olds, 1981, 1982, 1983), and aimed at improving many aspects of maternal and child functioning, including abuse and neglect.

Design and method

The study design consisted of a randomized clinical trial. Families were assigned at random to one of the four treatment conditions outlined in Table 23.1.

Treatment conditions

Treatment 1. Families in the first condition served as a control. During pregnancy, no services were provided through the research project. When the babies turned 1 and 2 years of age, an infant specialist hired by the research project screened them for sensory and developmental problems.

Table 23.1. *Services provided in each of the 4 treatment groups*

	Treatment group			
Services provided	1 $n = 90$	2 $n = 94$	3 $n = 100$	4 $n = 116$
Sensory and developmental screening at the children's 12th and 24th month of life	+	+	+	+
Free transportation to regular prenatal and well-child visits		+	+	+
Nurse home visitation during pregnancy			+	+
Nurse home visitation during the child's first 2 years of life				+

Suspected problems were referred to other specialists for further evaluation and treatment.

Treatment 2. Families in the second condition were provided free transportation for regular prenatal and well-child care at local clinics and physicians' offices through a contract with a local taxicab company. Sensory and developmental screening, as in Treatment 1, was provided when the babies turned 1 and 2 years of age.

Treatment 3. In the third condition, families were provided a nurse home visitor during pregnancy in addition to the screening and transportation services. The nurses visited families approximately once every two weeks and made an average of nine visits during pregnancy, each of which lasted approximately 1 hour and 15 minutes.

Treatment 4. Families assigned to the fourth condition received the same services as those in Treatment 3, but, in addition, the nurse continued to visit until the child was 2 years of age. For 6 weeks following delivery, the nurses visited families every week; from 6 weeks to 4 months, every 2 weeks; from 4 to 14 months, every 3 weeks; from 14 to 20 months, every 4 weeks; and from 20 to 24 months, every 6 weeks. Under predetermined crisis conditions, they visited weekly. As during pregnancy, the visits lasted approximately 1 hour and 15 minutes.

The home-visitation program

The home-visitation program was designed to systematically address those factors that have been directly implicated in child abuse and neglect (Olds,

1981), but it also was designed to promote the health and wellbeing of the mother and child in a variety of other areas, including the mothers' own life-course development (completing their educations, finding work, and reducing the number of subsequent pregnancies), birth outcomes (reducing preterm delivery, low birthweight, and newborn complications), the child's developmental status, the incidence of selected childhood illnesses associated with qualities of caregiving and stress, accidents and ingestions, and the child's physical growth and nutritional status. The nurses' efforts to prevent maltreatment need to be understood in the context of their efforts to improve these other aspects of maternal and child functioning.

Prenatal inception. We began the program during pregnancy and continued it into infancy because these periods were considered highly labile phases in the life cycle of families during which the potential for helping parents and children was unusually strong. It was our judgment that beginning the program during pregnancy was crucial for developing an effective, caring relationship with parents. Women would be more likely to accept support when they were going through the profound biological, psychological, and social changes produced by pregnancy, and they would be less defensive, we reasoned, if help was offered during a time when all first-time parents, regardless of their income or personal situations, have questions and special needs. Offering help once the baby was born, on the other hand, might have been interpreted as an indication that we thought parents had made mistakes or were incapable of caring for their children. Moreover, because some of our objectives, such as the prevention of low birthweight and prematurity, would have to be accomplished by the time of the child's birth, assistance had to begin during pregnancy at the latest.

During their prenatal home visits, the nurses began carrying out three major activities that formed the basis of the program and were continued through the second year of the child's life: (1) parent education regarding influences on fetal and infant development; (2) the involvement of family members and friends in the pregnancy, birth, early care of the child, and in the support of the mother; and (3) the linkage of family members with other formal health and human services. A central aspect of the nurses' approach was to emphasize the strengths of the women and their families.

Parent education. In their home-based education program, the nurses provided parents with information on fetal and infant development, with the ultimate objective of improving parental health habits and behaviors that theoretically affect the child's well-being. The nurses also encouraged parents to complete their own formal educations and to make decisions for themselves about eventually finding employment and bearing additional children.

During pregnancy, specific educational objectives covered by the nurses included improving women's diets; helping women monitor their weight gain and eliminate the use of cigarettes, alcohol, and drugs; teaching parents to identify the signs of pregnancy complication; encouraging regular rest, appropriate exercise, and good personal hygiene related to obstetrical health; and preparing parents for labor, delivery, and early care of the newborn. After delivery, specific educational objectives included improving parents' understanding of the infant's temperament, especially crying behavior and its meanings; the infant's socioemotional and cognitive needs – including his or her need for responsive caregiving and for progressively more complex motor, social, and intellectual experiences; the infant's physical health-care needs, such as dietary requirements and bathing, taking the baby's temperature and managing common health problems, and fulfilling the infant's need for a physically safe environment, routine health care, and immunizations. The nurses used a detailed curriculum to guide their educational activities, but tailored the content of their visits to the individual needs of each family.

A central aspect of the nurses' educational activities was to encourage parents to clarify their plans for completing their education, returning to work, and bearing additional children. The nurses emphasized that the decision to return to school or seek employment after delivery should be made after parents fully considered what was in their own and their babies' best interest. Beginning toward the end of pregnancy and following throughout the first two years postpartum, if the women were interested, the nurses helped them find appropriate educational and vocational-training services, helped them make concrete plans for child care, and advised them in methods of finding jobs and interviewing. The advantages of different methods of birth control were discussed and birth control devices were presented. The discussions of family planning were carried out in the context of the women's desires for their continued education, work, and achieving what they considered to be their optimal family size.

Enhancing informal support. The second major activity of the nurses was to enhance the informal support available to the women during pregnancy, birth, and the period of early childrearing. The nurses encouraged the women's close friends and relatives to participate in the home visits, to help with household responsibilities, to accompany the women to the hospital at the time of delivery, to be present for the birth, to aid in the subsequent care of the child, and to reinforce the advice of the nurses in their absence. They were encouraged to be sensitive to the mother's needs and to help her follow appropriate health behaviors – without nagging and finding fault. The women's husbands and boyfriends especially were encouraged to participate in the home visits, as they were believed to play decisive roles in determining the extent to which the women would be successful in accomplishing their goals. Grandmothers and other family members were encouraged to participate as well, especially in the discussions of mothers' health habits, desires to finish their educations, finding work, securing appropriate child care, and the needs of the child. They were not always involved in the discussions of family planning, however, because many young mothers and grandmothers were uncomfortable talking with one another about sex in the presence of the nurse. In order to facilitate the involvement of friends and family members, the nurses paid weekend and evening visits to accommodate their work schedules.

Two cases illustrate the value of involving other family members and friends. One mother was having a hard time controlling her excessive weight gain. The nurse's advice to replace cookies and Coke with nutritional snacks went unheeded until the woman's younger sister was asked to encourage her. Another young woman found it difficult to cut down on smoking until the nurse enlisted the help of the young woman's friends to remind her of the harmful effect of smoking on the fetus. Unfortunately, the involvement of other family members is sometimes limited by institutional barriers. At the beginning of the study, for instance, only husbands were allowed to enter the delivery room with the mother at one of the two local hospitals.

Linkage with formal services. The nurses also connected families with formal health and human services. Parents were urged to keep prenatal and well-child care appointments and to call the physician's office when a health problem arose, so that the office staff might help them make decisions as to whether sick or emergency-room visits were necessary. The nurses sent two regular reports of their observations regarding medical, social, and emotional conditions to the private physicians who provided the mothers' and babies' care. In this way, the physicians and office nurses could provide more informed and sensitive care in the office and, by communicating regularly with the mother's and babies' primary health care providers, the nurses could clarify and reinforce physicians' recommendations in the home. When necessary, parents were referred to other services such as Planned Parenthood, mental-health counseling, legal aid, and the nutritional supplementation program for women, infants, and children (WIC). Thus, to the extent possible, the resources of the formal health and human service system were summoned to meet the needs of the families visited by the nurse.

An integrative approach to the prevention of maltreatment. A central focus of the nurses' work was to systematically assess the family, beginning during pregnancy, according to its vulnerabilities that put the child at risk for maltreatment. This assessment was organized around the following questions:

> Does either parent report having experienced a childhood characterized by violence, deprivation, or lack of nurturance?

Do the parents have realistic expectations about the baby and the demands of childcare?

Does either parent appear to have any emotional difficulties, especially poor impulse control?

Are there any factors in the home that may create later stresses for parents and undermine their control of impulses (for example, unemployment, overcrowded housing, marital problems)?

Do the parents appear to be isolated from sources of support such as family, friends, or neighbors?

Do the parents' friends, neighbors, and relatives condone violence toward children and substandard caregiving?

Information on these topics was used by the nurses to plan future home visits and to develop ways to employ community resources in aiding the family. In two cases, the nurses became so concerned during pregnancy about the mothers' eventual capacity to care for their children that, after thorough review with other nurses and members of the program team, they discussed the case with workers from the local child protective service unit and, in concert with other human service providers in the community, encouraged these mothers to give up their children for adoption at birth. The two cases involved enduring histories of psychopathology on the part of the mother, with strong indications that they would not be able to protect and care for themselves or the baby. It should be emphasized that this approach was taken only after careful review of the case to determine the likelihood of harm to the child upon discharge from the hospital.

As part of the enhancement of informal support, all mothers were encouraged toward the end of pregnancy to identify friends or relatives who might provide additional support to them if they had temperamentally difficult babies. Having a reliable, trustworthy friend or relative to help with an irritable or colicky baby or to provide periodic relief from the demands of full-time parenting was considered especially important in relieving parental stresses that might lead to maltreatment. Not all informal social networks, however, served constructive purposes for the child and family. One young pregnant woman in the pilot study, who as a young child had been practically tortured for bed-wetting, was living at home in a large extended family in which members commonly disciplined their children by slapping them, often on the face. In spite of this young woman's integration into a social network, the norms and feedback of that network with respect to childrearing made abuse on her own part more likely. The nurse's task in this case was thus complicated by the need to counteract these prevailing standards for caregiving. In this particular case, the nurse was able to arrange for the young woman and her newborn child to spend several weeks after delivery with a stable, nurturant neighbor whom the mother thought of as a grandmother. Once mother and baby were functioning adequately together they moved into an apartment on their own. The neighbor continues to serve as a "lifeline" source of support for this young woman in times of crisis.

Helping families find formal community services to help with pressing personal problems is one of the other ways the nurses relieved some of the stresses that often create a background for maltreatment. With these stresses reduced, we reasoned that parents eventually would be able to devote more time and energy to their baby. For instance, two of the women in the pilot study who themselves had been mistreated as children displayed such inadequate emotional functioning, including poor impulse control and low self-esteem, that their nurses recommended mental health counseling, a suggestion that the families accepted surprisingly well. One of the young women requested that her nurse attend the first session with her. Her nurse agreed but explained that she would go only the first time. After counseling began, the nurse reported an improvement in communication between herself and the mother. We have no way of knowing whether counseling itself improved the mother's communication skills, but this experience suggests that the effectiveness of the nurse was enhanced by other formal services.

The potential for the program to prevent maltreatment also must be analyzed in terms of the other activities of the nurse that were not focused directly on this outcome. Because prematurity and low birthweight have been implicated in maltreatment (Hunter, Kilstrom, Kraybill, and Luda, 1978; Lynch, 1975), the prevention of prematurity and low birthweight may indirectly prevent maltreatment.

Similarly, to the extent that women reduce the number of subsequent pregnancies, the stresses of caring for additional children are reduced, and the chances for subsequent maltreatment diminished accordingly (Light, 1973; Vesterdal, 1977; Young, 1964).

Thus, each of the program components – parent education to improve pregnancy outcomes, childrearing, and maternal lifecourse development; the enhancement of informal support; and the linkage of families with formal health and human services – was designed to work in an integrated, complementary way to promote the health and well-being of mothers and children from socially disadvantaged families and to prevent maltreatment. Detailed record-keeping systems and regular case reviews were used to ensure that the home-visit protocol was followed by each nurse. Detailed descriptions of the program are provided elsewhere (Olds, 1981, 1982, 1983).

The setting

The study was carried out in a small, semirural county of approximately 100,000 residents in the Appalachian region of New York State. At the time the study was initiated, the community was well served from the standpoint of both health and human services. Prenatal care was available through nine private obstetricians and a free antepartum clinic sponsored by the health department. Pediatric care was provided by two sophisticated pediatric practices (with a total of 11 pediatricians) and eight physicians in family practice. A variety of social services was available for children and families. In spite of an abundance of health and human services, the community has consistently exhibited the highest rates of reported and confirmed cases of child abuse and neglect in the state (New York State Department of Social Services, 1973–1982). Moreover, in 1980 the community was rated the worst Standard Metropolitan Statistical Area in the United States in terms of its economic conditions (Boyer and Savageau, 1981).

The sample

Because we were interested in preventing a wide range of maternal and child health problems, we used general criteria (risk factors) for the identification of the families most likely to benefit from the service. At the time that we designed the study, the literature suggested that being a teenager, being unmarried, and being poor all increased the likelihood of poor health and developmental outcomes on the part of the child and arrested personal development on the part of the mother (Birch and Gussow, 1970; Card and Wise, 1978; Lawrence and Merritt, 1981; McAnarney, 1978). Because the literature was not clear on which of these factors was most important in predicting poor outcomes, we decided to recruit women who had any one of these three risk characteristics. We reasoned that women having first children would be more receptive to the nurses' offers of help, that the skills and resources that women developed in coping with their first pregnancies and children would be carried over to subsequent childbearing and childrearing experiences, and that reducing future pregnancies and returning to school and work would be more feasible if we limited the program to women having first children. By limiting the program to first-time parents, we reasoned that we would increase the long-term impact of the program and its potential cost-effectiveness. Because we also were interested in creating a program that was not stigmatized as being exclusively for the poor or for parents at risk for maltreatment, we allowed anyone bearing a first child to be enrolled, regardless of their risk status. By eliminating the label of being at risk for maltreatment, I think that we increased the willingness of women to participate. By creating sample heterogeneity through the enrollment of these non-risk women, we also were able to determine the extent to which the effects of the program were greater for families at higher risk.

Consequently, women were actively recruited if, at intake, they had no previous live births and had any one of the following characteristics: (1) young age (<19 years), (2) single-parent status, (3) low socioeconomic status, but anyone bearing a first child was allowed to register. All women were enrolled prior to the 30th week of pregnancy. They were recruited through the health department antepartum clinic, the offices of private obstetricians, Planned Parenthood, the public schools, and a variety of other health and human service agencies. Approximately 10 percent of the target population was missed due to late registration for prenatal care. An additional 10 percent was missed because some eligible women from the offices of private obstetricians were not referred. Between April 1978 and September 1980, 500 women were interviewed and 400 enrolled. There were no differences in age, marital status, or education between those women who participated and those who declined. Ninety-four percent of the nonwhites (mostly blacks) enrolled as opposed to 80 percent of the whites ($p = .02$). At registration, 47 percent of the participating women were under 19 years of age, 62 percent were unmarried, and 61 percent came from families in Hollingshead's social classes IV and V (semiskilled and unskilled laborers) (Hollingshead, 1976). (Hollingshead's index was adapted slightly to accommodate the variety of household compositions found in our sample.) Eighty-five percent of the women met at least one of the age, marital status, or SES criteria, and 23 percent possessed all three risk characteristics.

Forty-six nonwhites were removed from the analyses reported here because the sample of nonwhites was too small to crossclassify race with other variables of importance in the statistical analyses. Results for these nonwhite cases are presented elsewhere (Olds, Henderson, Birmingham, Chamberlin, and Tatelbaum, 1983).

This statistical profile of the sample does not fully reveal its risk status. From the nurses' reports, we learned that a substantial number of the nurse-visited families lived under unbearably stressful circumstances, such as households with open sewers, caving-in roofs, bedrooms located in a dirt basement, no running water or cooking facilities, and households where violence, alcoholism, and drug abuse were common. One young woman was mysteriously beaten unconscious during pregnancy and had no recollection of the incident. Another was jailed for holding up a local establishment with a knife, and had to be visited by her nurse in the county jail. Histories of women having been abused as young children were common. Although we have no comparable anecdotal data on the women not visited by nurses, the living conditions and life histories of many were undoubtedly equally wretched.

Treatment assignment

Every effort was made to ensure that those families assigned to the program would be essentially equivalent to those assigned to the comparison conditions. Families enrolled in the program were stratified by marital status, race, and seven geographic regions within the county (based on census tract boundaries), and then randomly assigned to one of the four treatment conditions in table one. At the end of the intake interview, the women drew their treatment assignments from a deck of cards. The stratification was executed by using separate decks for the groups defined by the women's race, marital status at intake, and, for whites, the geographic region in which they resided. In order to ensure reasonably balanced subclasses, the decks were reconstituted periodically to overrepresent those treatments with smaller numbers of subjects, a procedure similar to Efron's biased-coin designs (Efron, 1971). Women in Treatments 3 and 4 subsequently were assigned on a rotating basis, within their stratification blocks, to one of five home visitors.

There were two deviations from the randomization procedure. First, in six cases, women who enrolled were living in the same household as other women already participating in the study. In order to avoid potential horizontal diffusion of the treatment in the case of different assignment within households, the six new enrollees were assigned to the same treatment as their housemates.

Second, during the last 6 months of the 30-month enrollment period, the number of cards representing Treatment 4 was increased in each of the decks in order to enlarge the size of that group and to enhance the statistical power of the design to compare the infancy home-visiting program with Treatments 1 and 2 on infant health and developmental outcomes. Analysis of selected dependent variables confirmed that this slight confounding of treatments with time did not alter the pattern of treatment effects reported here.

Data collection

Interviews and infant assessment procedures relevant for this report were carried out at registration (prior to the 30th week of pregnancy), and at 6, 10, 12, 22, and 24 months of the infant's life. Medical records were abstracted for the infant's first 2 years of life, and the records of child abuse and neglect registries for 15 states in which families had lived were reviewed. Reliability of the medical-record review procedure was checked on a systematic and regular basis and was found to be acceptable (Olds et al., 1983).

Except in a small number of cases where participating women inadvertently disclosed their treatment assignments, all interview and medical-record data were collected by staff members who were unaware of the families' treatment assignments. The workers who reviewed the child abuse and neglect registries did not know whether families were nurse-visited.

At registration, prior to their assignment to one of the treatment conditions, the women were interviewed to determine their family characteristics, psychological resources, health conditions, health habits, availability of informal support, and childhood histories.

During infancy, the babies were brought to the project office at 6, 12, and 24 months for weighing and measuring. The infants also were administered developmental tests in the project offices, using the Bayley scales at 12 months and the Cattell scales at 24 months. At each of these assessments, the mothers were interviewed concerning common infant behavioral problems, such as feeding difficulties and crying, and how the mothers responded to these problems. At the sixth month of life, the mothers were administered an infant temperament Q-sort procedure (Pedersen, Anderson, and Cain, 1976).

At the infant's tenth and twenty-second months of life, the mothers were interviewed in their homes, and the Caldwell Home Observation checklist and interview procedure was completed. The Caldwell procedure evaluates qualities of the home environment and parental caregiving according to six dimensions, including the mother's avoidance of restriction and punishment and the provision of appropriate play materials (Caldwell and Bradley, 1979). Rates of inter-observer agreement for the Caldwell procedure on individual items ranged from 82 to 100 percent (Olds et al., 1983).

A list containing the names of all participating women and their children, their children's ages, and their addresses was given to state department of social service workers, who thoroughly reviewed the department records for the presence of "indicated" (i.e., verified) cases of abuse or neglect. Verified cases consisted of those that were reported for abuse or neglect and investigated by a department caseworker who determined that an episode of abuse or neglect, as defined by state law, had indeed occurred. Those cases were then reviewed by department workers to abstract standard information such as age of the child at the time of the first confirmed report, the specific type of abuse and neglect, the alleged perpetrator, and source of the maltreatment report. The names of children and parents who moved to 15 other states during the investigation were sent for review. Fourteen states cooperated, leaving only one case (a nurse-visited nonrisk family with no indication of maltreatment from the local records) that had to be omitted from the sample because of incomplete data.

Statistical model and methods of analysis

For all analyses, a core statistical model was derived that consisted of a 3 × 2 × 2 × 2 factorial structure (leading to 24 subclasses): treatments (1 and 2 versus 3 versus 4) × maternal age (<19 versus ≥19 years) × marital status × social class (Hollingshead classes IV and V versus I, II, and III). Two covariates measured at registration (maternal sense of control and reported husband/boyfriend support) also were included in the model for most analyses in order to adjust for chance differences between treatment groups for certain at-risk subsamples and to reduce error variance.

Treatments 1 and 2 were combined for purposes of analysis after it was determined that there were no differences between these two groups in their use of routine prenatal and well-child care, the primary means by which transportation was hypothesized to affect pregnancy and infancy outcomes. We refer to the combination of Treatments 1 and 2 as the comparison group and to Treatment 4 as the nurse-visited group. In the tables, Treatment 3 is labeled "NV pregnancy" and Treatment 4 is labeled "NV infancy." Planned comparisons focused on the contrast of the nurse-visited versus the comparison group for the whole sample and for those subsamples defined as being at risk: the teenagers (<19 years), the unmarried, the poor, and the group with all three risk characteristics.

Dependent variables for which a normal distribution was assumed were analyzed in the general linear model, the one dichotomous outcome (presence or absence of abuse and neglect) in the logistic–linear model (assuming a binomial distribution), and low-incidence outcomes in the form of counts (number of emergency-room visits), in the log-linear model (assuming a Poisson distribution). No formal tests of distributional assumptions were performed. Estimates and tests were adjusted for all covariates, classification factors, and interactions. Analysis was by our own computer programs, except that in the logistic- and log-linear cases the model-fitting algorithm of GLIM (Baker and Nelder, 1978) was invoked as a subroutine. These programs have been developed over many years and have been subjected to rigorous accuracy tests.

The means presented correspond directly to the tests: they are equally weighted averages of the 24 smallest-subclass means, adjusted for the covariates. In the logistic- and log-linear cases, means are given in incidence form because this corresponds more closely to the presentation of general linear model results than would, for example, log odds ratios. Hypothesis tests are unaltered by the form of presentation.

A thorough investigation was carried out for each covariate to determine whether its relationship with the dependent variable was the same for contrasting groups defined by levels of the classification factors – that is, whether the slopes were parallel (the regressions were homogeneous). Non-homogeneous regressions represent an interaction between the covariate and one or more categorical variables, and certain tests of means depend on the covariate in that a different test exists for each value of the covariate (Henderson, 1982).

For tests that depend on the covariate, the situation can be shown pictorially by plotting the separately estimated regression lines for the groups being compared. With the effects of other covariates and relevant subclasses subsumed in the intercept of the equation, the vertical distance between the lines represents the estimated mean difference at a given covariate value. A test of the mean difference can be carried out for any specified value, or alternatively, a region can be computed within which means differ statistically. Because the region provides information about a continuum of covariate values, the use of simultaneous statistical inference is appropriate (Johnson and Neyman, 1936; Miller, 1966; Potthoff, 1964).

In the current analysis, we extended these methods to dependent variables with binomial and Poisson error distributions. As seen in Figures 23.1 and 23.2 (pp. 749–50), the relationship between certain outcomes (child abuse or neglect and emergency-room visits) and maternal sense of control differed depending on whether the women were nurse-visited or assigned to the comparison group. For these dependent variables, results are first presented without adjustment for maternal sense of control; then the regions of significant treatment differences, delimited by values of this covariate, are shown. We used a significance level of .10 in computing these regions. It sometimes is suggested that a significance level higher than the conventional .05 be used in simultaneous inference, where achieving significance is more difficult (e.g., Scheffé, 1959); as a comparison, we also present the value of sense of control at which treatments differ at the .05 level for a single test.

Results

Preintervention equivalence of treatment conditions

The treatment conditions were examined carefully to determine their equivalence at registration. Table 23.2 shows that the nurse-visited and comparison-group women were equivalent on all standard sociodemographic characteristics. On psychological and social support variables, however, in contrast to their comparison-group counterparts, there was a trend for the nurse-visited women to expect less accompaniment to labor and delivery (p = .10); the unmarried women assigned a nurse had a significantly greater sense of control over their lives (p = .04); and the poor, unmarried teenagers assigned a nurse reported greater support from their boyfriends (p = .03). Because sense of control and husband/boyfriend support were related more consistently to the outcomes of this study than was expected accompaniment to labor and delivery, the potential bias created by this initial nonequivalence was handled by including the two former variables in the statistical model as covariates.

Attrition

During the first 2 years of the children's lives, the rates of attrition varied from 15 to 21 percent, and there were no differences across treatments in

Table 23.2. *Preintervention treatment differences and 95 percent confidence intervals for maternal background characteristics*

		Sample			
		Whole		Poor unmarried teenagers (<19 years at registration)	
Dependent variable	Treatment group	$\bar{x}$	n	$\bar{x}$	n
Proportion in	Comparison	0.61	(165)	1.00	(32)
Hollingshead's	NV pregnancy	0.62	(90)	1.00	(19)
social classes IV	NV infancy	0.60	(99)	1.00	(23)
and V	Comparison – NV infancy	0.01 ± 0.12		0.00 ± 0.24	
Proportion	Comparison	0.57	(165)	1.00	(32)
unmarried	NV pregnancy	0.59	(90)	1.00	(19)
	NV infancy	0.60	(99)	1.00	(23)
	Comparison – NV infancy	−0.03 ± 0.12		0.00 ± 0.24	
Proportion less than	Comparison	0.41	(165)	1.00	(32)
19 years of age	NV pregnancy	0.47	(90)	1.00	(19)
	NV infancy	0.49	(99)	1.00	(23)
	Comparison – NV infancy	−0.08 ± 0.12		0.00 ± 0.24	
Proportion with no	Comparison	0.17	(165)	0.00	(32)
risk characteristics	NV pregnancy	0.14	(90)	0.00	(19)
	NV infancy	0.14	(99)	0.00	(23)
	Comparison – NV infancy	0.03 ± 0.09		0.00 ± 0.18	
Maternal education	Comparison	11.25	(165)	9.78	(32)
(years completed)	NV pregnancy	11.58	(90)	10.16	(19)
	NV infancy	11.32	(99)	9.87	(23)
	Comparison – NV infancy	−0.07 ± 0.32		−0.09 ± 0.62	
Maternal sense of	Comparison	12.21	(165)	11.93	(32)
control[a]	NV pregnancy	12.31	(90)	12.47	(19)
	NV infancy	12.44	(99)	12.48	(23)
	Comparison – NV infancy	−0.23 ± 0.41		−0.55 ± 0.78	
Number of people/	Comparison	5.30	(165)	4.75	(32)
helping network	NV pregnancy	5.16	(90)	3.95	(19)
	NV infancy	5.01	(99)	4.87	(23)
	Comparison – NV infancy	0.29 ± 0.66		−0.12 ± 1.26	
Number of intimates/	Comparison	1.75	(165)	1.56	(32)
helping network	NV pregnancy	2.08	(90)	1.79	(19)
	NV infancy	1.57	(99)	1.39	(23)
	Comparison – NV infancy	0.18 ± 0.40		0.17 ± 0.81	
Number of kin/	Comparison	3.42	(165)	2.69	(32)
helping network	NV pregnancy	3.09	(90)	1.84	(19)
	NV infancy	3.09	(99)	1.96	(23)
	Comparison – NV infancy	0.33 ± 0.51		0.73 ± 0.97	

Table 23.2. *(cont.)*

Dependent variable	Treatment group	Whole $\bar{x}$	Whole n	Poor unmarried teenagers (<19 years at registration) $\bar{x}$	Poor unmarried teenagers (<19 years at registration) n
Expected	Comparison	9.66	(165)	9.30	(32)
accompaniment to	NV pregnancy	9.36	(90)	9.50	(19)
labor and delivery	NV infancy	9.04	(99)	8.68	(23)
	Comparison – NV infancy	0.62 ± 0.74(*)		0.62 ± 1.46	
Husband/boyfriend	Comparison	0.85	(165)	−5.22	(32)
support[b]	NV pregnancy	1.55	(90)	−2.41	(19)
	NV infancy	0.34	(99)	−0.94	(23)
	Comparison – NV infancy	0.51 ± 2.03		−4.28 ± 3.87*	
Grandmother	Comparison	0.12	(165)	4.37	(32)
support[c]	NV pregnancy	−1.07	(90)	−2.22	(19)
	NV infancy	−0.07	(99)	3.62	(23)
	Comparison – NV infancy	0.19 ± 1.45		0.75 ± 2.79	
Predicted positive	Comparison	0.61	(165)	0.41	(32)
parenting[d]	NV pregnancy	0.57	(90)	0.37	(19)
	NV infancy	0.54	(99)	0.48	(23)
	Comparison – NV infancy	0.07 ± 0.10		−0.07 ± 0.19	

[a] Scale measuring extent to which women felt control over their life circumstances using a short-form variant of Rotter's locus of control instrument (Rotter, 1966).
[b] Scale characterizing availability, contact, and anticipated help with pregnancy and childrearing from the women's husbands or boyfriends.
[c] Scale characterizing availability, contact, and anticipated help with pregnancy and childrearing from the women's own mothers.
[d] Scale derived from discriminant analysis to predict quality of caregiving, based on weighted sum of mother's reports of being yelled at, spanked, and treated restrictively in her own childhood; the level of psychosocial stress in her family of origin; her level of ego development; her prepregnant level of smoking; the economic status of her current household; and a housing-crowdedness index.
(*)$p < .10$
*$p < .05$

the proportion of subjects with completed assessments. In the nurse-visited condition, however, the women who discontinued tended to have a greater sense of control than those who discontinued the comparison group ($p = .06$). An examination of the reasons for these women's discontinuation showed that they had either moved or miscarried. Because women with greater sense of control were more likely to discontinue the nurse-visited group than the comparison group, the preintervention treatment difference for unmarried women in sense of control was not significant in the sample available for assessment at the child's second birthday. The treatment conditions remained essentially equivalent after attrition.

Child abuse and neglect

Table 23.3 shows that during the first 2 years of the children's lives, 19 percent of the comparison group at greatest risk (the poor, unmarried teens) and 4 percent of their nurse-visited counterparts had abused or neglected their children ($p = .07$). (There also was a trend ($p = .07$) for the nurse-visited teens to have fewer confirmed reports of abuse and neglect than the teenagers in the comparison group. Because there was little corroborating evidence to support the interpretation that the program was effective with all teenagers, irrespective of their marital status and poverty, we have not emphasized this finding in the remainder of the report.) Although the treatment contrasts for the groups at lower risk did not reach statistical significance, it is important to note that virtually all of the contrasts were in the expected direction. Moreover, in the comparison condition the incidence of abuse and neglect increased as the number of risk factors accumulated, but in the nurse-visited condition, the incidence of abuse and neglect remained relatively low, even in those groups at higher risk. It also is important to note that the incidence of maltreatment in Treatment 3 (NV pregnancy) in general, fell in between the infancy nurse-visited and comparison conditions. (This pattern, in which the means of the NV pregnancy group fell in between the other two groups, as indicated below, also held for most of the other outcomes.)

A qualitative review of the eight cases of abuse and neglect among the poor, unmarried teens in the comparison condition indicated that four of the eight cases consisted of neglect alone, whereas the remaining four involved a combination of abuse and neglect. In five of the eight cases the mother was the sole perpetrator; in the three remaining cases the mother and father shared responsibility for the incidents. Five of the eight families were reported by nonmandated sources (e.g., neighbors, family members), and the remaining three were reported by mandated sources (professionals required by law to report suspected maltreatment). The one nurse-visited case consisted of a combination of abuse and neglect in which both the mother and her boyfriend were the perpetrators. This case was reported by a mandated source. Because the child abuse finding was only marginally significant and subject to potential reporting bias, it was important to determine the extent to which the finding was corroborated by other evidence.

Table 23.3. *Treatment differences and 95 percent confidence intervals for child abuse and neglect: Adjusted for husband/boyfriend support*

Treatment group	Sample[a]																	
	Whole		Nonrisk		Nonpoor		Married		Older (≥19 yrs)		Poor		Unmarried		Teenager (<19 years)		Poor unmarried teenagers	
	$\bar{x}$	n	$\bar{x}$	n	$\bar{x}$	n	$\bar{x}$	n	$\bar{x}$	n	$\bar{x}$	n	$\bar{x}$	n	$\bar{x}$	n	$\bar{x}$	n
Comparison	0.10	(161)	0.05	(27)	0.08	(62)	0.10	(69)	0.05	(94)	0.12	(99)	0.10	(92)	0.15	(67)	0.19	(32)
NV pregnancy	0.08	(86)	0.00	(11)	0.00	(31)	0.09	(35)	0.10	(45)	0.17	(55)	0.08	(51)	0.07	(41)	0.18	(18)
NV infancy	0.05	(95)	0.00	(14)	0.04	(40)	0.04	(38)	0.06	(48)	0.07	(55)	0.06	(57)	0.05	(47)	0.04	(22)
Comparison NV infancy	0.05 ± 0.09		0.05 ± 0.10		0.04 ± 0.06		0.06 ± 0.13		−0.01 ± 0.12		0.05 ± 0.08		0.04 ± 0.07		0.10 ± 0.11(*)		0.15 ± 0.16(*)	

[a]For the whole sample, the teenagers, the poor, the unmarried, and the group for which all three risk characteristics were present, the comparisons of treatments were planned. The tests shown in this table are not independent, and are not to be interpreted as individual findings, but are presented to illustrate in detail the pattern of results.

(*)$p < .10$

Reports of infant temperament and behavioral problems, and maternal concern, conflict, scolding, and spanking

Table 23.4 shows that, in contrast to women assigned to the comparison condition, nurse-visited women reported that their babies had more positive moods (happier, less irritable dispositions) ($p = .04$), but that their babies had more frequent episodes of resisting eating ($p = .01$). There was a trend for the nurse-visited poor, unmarried teens to report that their babies cried less frequently ($p = .07$). In response to their 6-month-old's behavioral problems, nurse-visited women, irrespective of their risk status, reported greater concern ($p = .05$), and there were trends for the nurse-visited poor, unmarried teens to report less conflict with and scolding of their babies than their comparison-group counterparts ($p = .06$ and $p = .09$ respectively).

The provision of appropriate play materials and the avoidance of restriction and punishment

Table 23.5 shows that within the group at greatest risk (the poor, unmarried teens), the nurse-visited women were observed in their homes at the 10th and 22nd months of the child's life to punish and restrict their children less frequently than were their counterparts in the comparison group ($p = .02$ and $p = .04$ respectively). Similarly, the nurse-visited poor, unmarried teens

Table 23.4. *Treatment differences and 95 percent confidence intervals for reports of infant temperament, behavioral problems, and maternal reaction to behavioral problems at 6 months of age – adjusted for husband/boyfriend support and maternal sense of control*

		Sample			
		Whole		Poor unmarried teenagers	
Dependent variable	Treatment group	$\bar{x}$	n	$\bar{x}$	n
Positive mood[a]	Comparison	2.29	(135)	2.12	(28)
	NV pregnancy	2.34	(64)	2.20	(13)
	NV infancy	2.40	(74)	2.32	(14)
	Comparison – NV infancy	-0.11 ± 0.10*		-0.20 ± 0.20 (*)	
Crying (number of episodes last 2 weeks)	Comparison	3.93	(107)	4.51	(22)
	NV pregnancy	4.05	(57)	4.22	(12)
	NV infancy	3.44	(56)	3.53	(11)
	Comparison – NV infancy	0.49 ± 0.59		0.98 ± 1.17 (*)	

Table 23.4. (*cont.*)

Dependent variable	Treatment group	Sample			
		Whole		Poor unmarried teenagers	
		$\bar{x}$	n	$\bar{x}$	n
Resist eating	Comparison	1.72	(107)	1.88	(22)
(number of	NV pregnancy	2.01	(57)	1.83	(12)
episodes last 2 weeks)	NV infancy	2.29	(56)	1.89	(11)
	Comparison – NV infancy	-0.57 ± 0.45**		-0.01 ± 0.90	
Night awake	Comparison	2.83	(107)	3.43	(22)
(number of	NV pregnancy	3.25	(57)	3.15	(12)
episodes last 2 weeks	NV infancy	2.69	(56)	3.44	(11)
	Comparison – NV infancy	0.14 ± 0.66		-0.01 ± 1.30	
Worry or concern	Comparison	0.54	(107)	0.52	(22)
(sum of positive	NV pregnancy	0.61	(57)	0.34	(12)
responses for behavioral problems)	NV infancy	0.83	(56)	0.84	(11)
	Comparison – NV Infancy	-0.29 ± 0.28*		-0.32 ± 0.55	
Conflict (sum of	Comparison	0.25	(107)	0.68	(22)
positive	NV pregnancy	0.27	(57)	0.50	(12)
responses for behavioral problems)	NV infancy	0.29	(56)	0.28	(11)
	Comparison – NV Infancy	-0.04 ± 0.20		0.40 ± 0.40 (*)	
Yell or scold	Comparison	7.90	(103)	8.45	(22)
(number of	NV pregnancy	7.56	(48)	10.48	(10)
times last 2 weeks)	NV infancy	3.99	(56)	0.70	(10)
	Comparison – NV Infancy	3.91 ± 5.00		7.75 ± 8.82(*)	
Spank or hit	Comparison	1.09	(103)	1.89	(22)
(number of	NV pregnancy	1.71	(48)	2.00	(10)
times last 2 weeks)	NV infancy	0.19	(56)	-0.02	(10)
	Comparison – NV infancy	0.90 ± 1.75		1.91 ± 3.10	

[a]One of five dimensions of infant temperament measured. The others include adaptability, approach, activity level, and rhythmicity.
(*)$p < .10$
*$p < .05$
**$p < .01$

Table 23.5. *Treatment differences and 95 percent confidence intervals for avoidance of restriction and punishment and provision of play materials at 10 and 22 months of age – adjusted for husband/boyfriend support and maternal sense of control*

Dependent variable	Treatment group	Sample			
		Whole		Poor unmarried teenagers	
		$\bar{x}$	n	$\bar{x}$	n
Avoidance of	Comparison	5.60	(123)	5.06	(27)
restriction and	NV pregnancy	5.77	(61)	5.63	(10)
punishment[a]	NV infancy	5.40	(68)	6.26	(16)
10th month					
	Comparison – NV infancy	0.20 ± 0.46		-1.20 ± 0.87**	
Provision of	Comparison	7.26	(128)	5.94	(28)
appropriate	NV pregnancy	7.45	(67)	6.70	(11)
play materials[b]	NV infancy	7.36	(73)	7.35	(16)
10th month					
	Comparison – NV infancy	-0.10 ± 0.56		-1.41 ± 1.08**	
Avoidance of	Comparison	6.28	(115)	5.28	(24)
restriction and	NV pregnancy	5.53	(56)	6.12	(8)
punishment[a]	NV infancy	5.82	(65)	6.45	(15)
22nd month					
	Comparison – NV infancy	0.46 ± 0.60		-1.17 ± 1.11*	
Provision of	Comparison	8.65	(126)	7.76	(26)
appropriate	NV pregnancy	8.66	(64)	8.35	(11)
play materials[b]	NV infancy	8.68	(72)	8.59	(15)
22nd month					
	Comparison – NV infancy	-0.03 ± 0.26		-0.83 ± 0.52**	

[a]Scale consisting of sum of 8 yes/no items observed in home (e.g., mother does not shout at child during visit; mother neither slaps nor spanks child during visit).
[b]Scale consisting of sum of 9 yes/no items (e.g., child has one or more muscle toys or pieces of equipment; child has push or pull toys).
*$p < .05$
**$p < .01$

provided their children with a larger number of appropriate play materials than did the poor, unmarried teens in the comparison group ($p = .01$ and $p = .002$ respectively).

Developmental quotient

As illustrated in Table 23.6, at 12 and 24 months of life there were trends for the babies of poor, unmarried teens assigned to the nurse-visited con-

Table 23.6. *Treatment differences and 95 percent confidence intervals for infant developmental quotients at 12 and 24 months of life – adjusted for husband/boyfriend support and maternal sense of control*

		Sample			
		Whole		Poor unmarried teenagers	
Dependent variable	Treatment group	$\bar{x}$	n	$\bar{x}$	n
Bayley Mental	Comparison	109.94	(131)	104.13	(26)
Development Index	NV pregnancy	105.44	(68)	105.86	(13)
12 month	NV infancy	111.23	(73)	115.01	(15)
	Comparison – NV infancy	-1.29 ± 5.53		-10.88 ± 11.12 (*)	
Cattell	Comparison	106.49	(122)	101.94	(25)
24th month	NV pregnancy	105.73	(64)	96.02	(12)
	NV infancy	109.34	(71)	110.56	(16)
	Comparison – NV infancy	-2.83 ± 5.23		-8.62 ± 9.64 (*)	

(*)$p < .10$

Table 23.7. *Treatment differences and 95 percent confidence intervals for emergency-room visits (total and for accidents and ingestions) for the first and second years of life – adjusted for husband/boyfriend support*

		Sample			
		Whole		Poor unmarried teenagers	
Dependent variable	Treatment group	$\bar{x}$	n	$\bar{x}$	n
Number of ER visits, 1st year of life	Comparison	1.02	(136)	1.66	(29)
	NV pregnancy	1.12	(69)	1.27	(13)
	NV infancy	0.74	(87)	0.95	(21)
	Comparison – NV infancy	0.28 ± 0.20*		0.71 ± 0.64*	
Number of ER visits for accidents	Comparison	0.06	(136)	0.12	(29)
and ingestions, 1st year of life	NV pregnancy	0.12	(69)	0.07	(13)
	NV infancy	0.12	(87)	0.09	(21)
	Comparison – NV infancy	-0.06 ± 0.14		0.03 ± 0.18	
Number of ER visits, 2nd year of life	Comparison	1.09	(121)	1.27	(27)
	NV pregnancy	1.04	(64)	1.19	(12)
	NV infancy	0.74	(75)	0.90	(16)
	Comparison – NV infancy	0.35 ± 0.28**		0.37 ± 0.67	
Number of ER visits for accidents	Comparison	0.34	(121)	0.33	(27)
and ingestions, 2nd year of life	NV pregnancy	0.32	(64)	0.23	(12)
	NV infancy	0.15	(75)	0.26	(16)
	Comparison – NV infancy	0.19 ± 0.17*		0.07 ± 0.42	

*$p < .05$
**$p < .01$

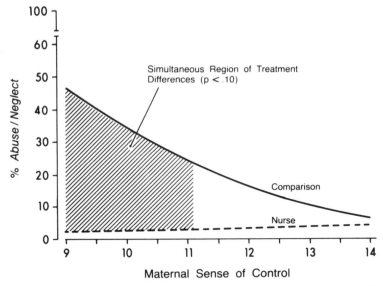

Figure 23.1. Estimated regression lines of abuse/neglect on maternal sense of control among poor, unmarried teens for nurse-visited and comparison-group women.

dition to have higher developmental quotients than the babies of their counterparts assigned to the comparison group ($p = .06$ and $p = .08$, respectively).

Emergency-room visits

Table 23.7 shows that, during the first year of life, the babies of nurse-visited women, especially the babies of poor, unmarried teenagers, were seen in the emergency room fewer times than their counterparts in the comparison group ($p = .04$ for both contrasts). A detailed review of the medical records revealed that these differences were explained by a reduction in visits for upper respiratory infections. During the second year of life, the babies of nurse-visited women were seen in the emergency room fewer times ($p = .01$) and presented with fewer accidents and ingestions than their counterparts in the comparison condition ($p = .03$).

Maternal sense of control as a conditioner of treatment effects

Figure 23.1 shows that among the poor, unmarried teenagers, the treatment difference in child abuse and neglect was greater at lower levels of maternal sense of control. For the comparison group, the incidence of maltreatment increased as maternal sense of control declined ($p = .005$), but among the

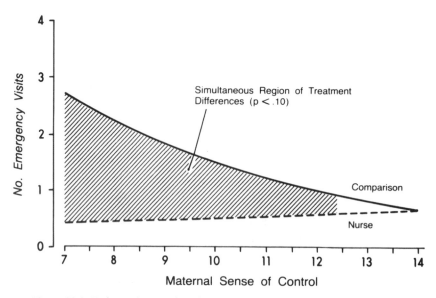

Figure 23.2. Estimated regression lines of number of second-year emergency-room visits on maternal sense of control for nurse-visited and comparison-group women–whole sample.

nurse-visited women, a decline in maternal sense of control did not lead to an increase in abuse and neglect ($p = .75$). The test of the difference between the 2 regression lines produced a probability of .11, a level low enough to have a significant effect on the interpretation of treatment mean differences (Henderson, 1982). The shaded area of the figure shows the simultaneous region of treatment differences in abuse and neglect ($p < .10$), allowing statements to be made over a continuum of covariate values. (At the single sense-of-control value of 11.5, the difference between the nurse-visited and comparison groups was significant at $p = .05$.)

Figure 23.2 shows the estimated regressions of number of emergency-room visits during the second year of life on the women's reported sense of control – for all nurse-visited and comparison-group women, irrespective of their sociodemographic risk status. For the comparison group, the incidence of emergency-room visits increased as maternal sense of control declined ($p = .004$); but among the nurse-visited women, there was no such relation ($p = .53$). The difference between these regression lines was significant ($p = .02$). The shaded area of this figure shows the region of treatment differences ($p < .10$) in incidence of emergency-room visits. (At the single sense-of-control value of 12.5, the treatment difference in number of emergency-room visits was significant at $p = .05$.) A nearly identical pattern (not shown) emerged for the regression of number of second-year emergency-room visits for accidents and ingestions on women's sense of control.

Discussion

The pattern of results from this investigation provides evidence that nurse home visitors are capable of preventing a number of caregiving dysfunctions, including child abuse and neglect. The positive effects of the program were concentrated on those women at greatest risk for caregiving dysfunction, and the picture of abuse and neglect prevention comes from a variety of sources: department of social service records, maternal reports of child behavior and maternal caregiving, observations of maternal caregiving, the children's developmental tests, and emergency-room records.

As coherent as these results appear to be, they must be viewed with caution for two reasons. First, the nurse-visited unmarried women reported greater sense of control over their lives at the start of the study than did their counterparts in the comparison group. The intensification of treatment effects for the child maltreatment and emergency-room outcomes among women with decreasing sense of control over their lives may be a product of this initial nonequivalence.

It should be noted, nevertheless, that these preintervention differences were attenuated, because women with greater sense of control were more likely to discontinue the nurse-visited condition than the comparison condition. Moreover, it is theoretically coherent that the positive effects of the program would intensify as the vulnerability of the population increases. It was only in the case of the dichotomous and low-frequency count data (the abuse and neglect and emergency room outcomes) that we encountered non-homogeneous regressions by treatments – an intensification of the treatment effect on the given outcome as maternal sense of control declined. This intensification occurred, in large part, because the incidence of these adverse outcomes was relatively infrequent in the nurse-visited group, whereas the incidence increased among comparison-group women who had little sense of control over their lives. For other caregiving outcomes, the regressions on maternal sense of control were homogeneous for treatments. Thus, tests of treatment differences could be made with conventional adjustments for biasing background characteristics.

The presence of treatment differences for reports of infant crying behavior, positive mood, maternal conflict with and scolding of the child, play materials, and observations of punishment and restriction (variables for which there is no interaction of treatments with sense of control) increases our confidence that the treatment differences for child abuse and emergency-room visits are products of the nurse intervention.

Moreover, it should be emphasized that we were unable to detect any other preintervention treatment differences in a careful examination of the sample on a wide range of theoretically important background characteristics that predispose to caregiving dysfunction. A scale was constructed, for example, to predict the extent to which women would provide optimal care for their children. It included data on the women's own childrearing histories (including information related to their having been abused and neglected), their current level of psychological functioning, their prenatal health habits, and the level of stress in their current household. There were no preintervention treatment differences on this measure (Table 23.2).

The second reason for caution in interpretation is that these findings may be the result of systematic reporting bias. For each of the sources of data, one can construct an alternative explanation for specific findings. For example, the nurse-visited women may have been taught by the nurses to give more socially desirable answers and to behave more appropriately in front of the interviewers. Their friends, neighbors, and relatives may have been more reluctant to report them for abuse and neglect than in the case of women in the comparison group. The picture of superior caregiving for the highest risk nurse-visited women over their comparison-group counterparts comes from a variety of sources, however, and it is unlikely that each of these sources could have its own idiosyncratic bias and still produce the same pattern of results overall. Assuming that the treatment differences observed are truly a reflection of the nurse's work, how do these pieces of evidence fit together?

It is noteworthy that the nurse-visited women reported less crying and fussiness on the part of their babies. Because reports of temperament and behavioral problems may be just as much a reflection of the mother's characteristics as the child's (Sameroff, Seifer, and Elias, 1982; Vaughn, Taraldson, Crichton, and Egeland, 1981), we interpret reports of excessive crying and irritability as a problem in the parent–child relationship. One previous intervention study, which focused on adolescent parents of high-risk newborns, found more favorable reports of infant temperament as a result of intervention (Field, Widmayer, Stringe, and Ignatoff, 1980). It is not surprising that we detected treatment differences in parents' reports of their infants' temperaments and crying behavior in the present study, because the nurses spent a considerable portion of their prenatal and postpartum visits helping parents appreciate and manage differences in the temperaments of young infants. Beginning during pregnancy and following with a Brazelton examination (Brazelton, 1973) after delivery, the nurses encouraged parents to anticipate and recognize differences in infant temperament, especially crying behavior, so that they might not misinterpret the babies' cries as either caregiving failure on their own part or as an indication that the infants were intentionally trying to disrupt their lives. We suspect that the nurse-visited poor, unmarried teenagers were able to interpret their infants' cries more correctly and respond more appropriately, thus forming the basis for secure attachments, which may protect the child from abuse and neglect (Ainsworth, 1980; Egeland and Sroufe, 1981; Schneider-Rosen and Cicchetti, 1984).

This interpretation is supported by the pattern of results derived from the interviewers' assessments of the highest risk mothers' treatment of their children and the provision of appropriate play materials during the tenth- and twenty-second-month interviews. In the extreme, restriction and punishment are abusive, and the absence of appropriate play materials is a form of neglect.

Additional corroboration for the nurses' prevention of child abuse and neglect is provided by the reduction in emergency-room visits. Although the treatment difference in emergency-room visits during the first year of life was attributable to the comparison-group mothers taking their babies more frequently for upper respiratory infections, the more appropriate use of the emergency room on the part of nurse-visited women can be viewed as indirect corroboration, as it shows that the program was working as intended. Moreover, the reduction in emergency-room visits for accidents and ingestions for nurse-visited women during the second year of life provides more direct corroboration of the child abuse and neglect finding, as accidents and ingestions are tied more closely to the quality of parental care (Miller, Court, Walton, and Knox, 1960; Newberger, Reed, Daniel, Hyde, and Kotelchuck, 1977; Wheatley, 1973).

Although there clearly is some overlap, the underlying factors leading to child maltreatment and excessive utilization of the emergency room, even for accidents and ingestions, in many cases are quite different. Overuse of the emergency room, in large part, probably reflects heightened parental concern about the child's well-being and little knowledge about where to turn for help, factors that are likely to be present in a broad portion of the socially disadvantaged population. Abuse and neglect, on the other hand, appear to be the products of converging psychological, material, and social risks, factors that are limited to a much smaller segment of that population. This probably explains why the treatment difference in abuse and neglect was concentrated on the highest risk subsample, whereas the teratment difference in emergency-room visits was present for the whole sample. That we observe treatment differences consistent with these general models of risk, as well as with the objectives of the program, lends credibility to the pattern of results overall.

Finally, the improved intellectual functioning of 9 to 11 points on the developmental tests for children from the highest risk families, although only marginally significant statistically, is of clinical importance. Treatment effects in this range are consistent with those obtained for children of this age enrolled in intensive early childhood intervention programs aimed specifically at enhancing cognitive development (Ramey and Campbell, 1977).

Implications for the design of preventive programs

Even though it could be argued that other preventive strategies may be as effective as the present program, with the exception of the study carried out by Siegel and associates, comparing the effectiveness of early contact with home-visiting (Siegel et al., 1980), there are no studies in the literature that systematically compare the effectiveness of different maltreatment prevention strategies. It therefore is useful to consider whether, theoretically, the present program model has any advantages as a means of preventing maltreatment.

Home visitation. Home visitation has a number of characteristics that make it particularly well-suited for the prevention of maltreatment. It provides a means of reaching out to parents who lack self confidence and trust in formal service providers – those least likely to show up for other services, such as parent-group meetings. If properly carried out, home visitation can eventually increase parents' confidence and help them feel more comfortable expressing themselves among other parents and with other service providers. It has been our experience that the special attention provided by one caring, nonjudgmental professional can eventually bolster parents' self-confidence to the point where seeking other formal services and attending meetings are no longer threatening.

Unless the program has a major home-visitation component, it is likely that a significant portion of the families who need the sevice the most will not receive it, unless the preventive intervention consists of changing institutional procedures, such as hospitals promoting early contact and rooming-in following delivery, in which case the population is virtually captive. This is not to suggest that home-visitation is the answer to the lack of participation on the part of insecure, distrustful parents (parents can refuse to answer the door or can conveniently not be at home). A greater portion of high-risk parents are likely to receive the service, however, if they are enrolled in a home-visitation program than if they are enrolled in a program they must make the effort to attend.

Another significant advantage is that the home-visitor can acquire a more accurate and complete understanding of all of the factors in the home and family that interfere with parents' efforts to create optimal conditions for pregnancy and early childrearing. By assessing the home environment, the home-visitors can provide more sensitive, informed services themselves and can help other service providers do the same. Because socially disadvantaged, high-risk parents may not always articulate their needs clearly and completely, it helps to have a sensitive home-visitor spend time getting to know the parents, and simultaneously assess the home and family, so that appropriate services can be rendered. In this way, the potential of the home-visitation model can be realized.

Even though there are significant advantages to home-visitation, there are drawbacks as well. In many of our large urban areas, especially where many families in need of this kind of service live in housing projects, it is often

unsafe for home-visitors. Consequently, community health nurses sometimes have to be accompanied by security guards, which increases the cost
of the program, and has an unknown but probably deleterious impact on
the home-visitor's ability to establish rapport with the family. In addition,
if home-visitors are not carefully selected, trained, and supervised, they may
inadvertently interfere with families' natural coping mechanisms, and may
actually undermine rather than enhance family functioning (Olds, 1983). (In
the present program, we assessed whether such negative side-effects
occurred and found no such intrusiveness but, given the nature of the intervention, this is a potential problem that should be explicitly considered in
the design and evaluation of any home-visitation program.)

Program content. In order to maximize the potential of the home-visitation
model, we have concluded that the service should be based on an ecological
theoretical framework, a position that is promoted for all types of programs
for children and families in a recent report from the National Research
Council (Travers and Light, 1982). Based on our experience in the present
program, it is our judgment that parent education, without improvements
in those aspects of the home environment that work against behavioral
change, is likely to be of limited success; likewise, an improvement in the
social and material conditions in the home, without a focused and individualized educational program, will have a limited impact on parents' treatment of their children. The simultaneous provision of education and social
support are essential.

By approaching pregnancy and early childrearing from an ecological
framework, the nurses were able to achieve considerable leverage in improving pregnancy outcomes (Olds, Henderson, Tatelbaum, and Chamberlin,
1986a) and maternal life-course development (Olds et al., 1983) in addition
to qualities of maternal caregiving, outcomes that had a synergistic effect on
one another. By calling attention to the deleterious effects of smoking and
inadequate weight gain on the part of the mother during pregnancy on fetal
development, for example, the nurses helped women change those health
behaviors that lead to preterm delivery and fetal growth retardation, but
also helped them begin to appreciate how their behavior affected their children's well-being later in life. Moreover, as indicated above, the prevention
of prematurity in itself may reduce the incidence of subsequent maltreatment. In a similar way, by involving other family members in the pregnancy, birth, and early care of the child, the nurses helped increase the social
resources for the mother herself and for her baby, an outcome important on
its own, but also important for the prevention of maltreatment.

Correspondingly, by linking parents with other health and human services, the nurses can help reduce many of the stresses that can lead to maternal depression (Fergusson, Hons, Horwood, and Shannon, 1984; Hall, Wil-

liams, and Greenberg, 1985; Hopkins, Marcus, and Campbell, 1984) and interference with caregiving (Belle, 1982). By helping young women find ways to continue their education, find work, and plan future pregnancies more effectively, the nurses helped them increase their financial resources, and reduce the stresses associated with caring for several young children simultaneously. These aspects of the program, although important in their own right, undoubtedly contributed to its success in reducing the rate of maltreatment.

Finally, the mere presence of the nurse in the home served as a visible and regular reminder to parents that excessive punishment and neglect of children in our society are not condoned. Although this monitoring function was not an explicit feature of the program, its impact on the parents' qualities of caregiving cannot be overlooked.

Target population

Based on the evidence of the current study, one might conclude that nurse home-visitation services should be focused on poor, unmarried teenagers, because it was with this group that the program was most effective in preventing maltreatment. Evidence from subsequent studies (Olds, Lombardi, and Henderson, 1986c) using the same data base, has shown that nurse-visited poor unmarried *older* women also benefited (although in other ways), especially in terms of their finding employment after delivery. Because there is a substantial payback to the government in the form of reduced public assistance payments for those women who find jobs (and because there also were corresponding but less dramatic improvements in the quality of caregiving on the part of nurse-visited poor unmarried older women), we have decided that the most judicious allocation of these services would be to concentrate them on all poor unmarried women bearing first children, irrespective of their age.

In general, the results of the present study suggest that, rather than attempting to focus preventive services on parents suspected of being at risk for maltreatment per se, it makes more sense to focus limited health and human-service resources on a broader population that is at risk for a whole range of health and caregiving disorders, and to design the intervention in a way that tries to enhance many of those aspects of functioning simultaneously. Because efforts to predict maltreatment suffer from fundamental flaws in screening, especially by producing too many false positives, which can lead to inappropriate intervention on the part of government agencies (Newberger et al., 1977), identifying groups at more general risk for a variety of difficulties by virtue of their life circumstances (e.g., being pregnant, unmarried, poor) avoids the problems of labeling and puts the program in a more positive, constructive light. By making these services available to all women having first children in impoverished health-service catchment areas, for example, one could concentrate the services on poor unmarried women (by virtue of the high concentrations of poverty and unmarried parents in the targeted areas).

Service providers. The central service providers in the present program were nurses. Although some workers claim that paraprofessionals are able to deliver this kind of service equally well, while minimizing some of the class and cultural barriers that sometimes separate nurses from the families they visit, the advantages of paraprofessionals are overstated, especially if nurses are carefully selected to include only those who are compassionate and sensitive to differences in life style and childrearing methods but who can be assertive when necessary. Indeed, there are reasons to believe that nurses can carry out this work more effectively than paraprofessionals. Nurses have educational backgrounds and experiences that orient them to the content of the program, which minimizes the amount of training and supervision that must take place. Their professional role helps them obtain the respect of the families they visit, and it helps them communicate effectively with physicians and other health and human service providers caring for the family. Moreover, it has been reported that parents are sometimes reluctant to reveal personal matters to indigenous workers from the neighborhood because of a fear of loss of privacy (Thomas, 1986), a problem that is reduced when parents communicate with professionals.

One of the other advantages of employing nurses as home-visitors is that nurse home-visitation is a public health activity that has a long history in this country, and that has an institutional base in home-health agencies and public health departments. Consequently, carrying out the program would not require the establishment of a new institution or the adoption of the home-visitation program by an institution with which it is not suited. Unfortunately, financial support for community health nursing has been cut deeply during the past two decades, so that today virtually every large city in the country lacks adequate financial support for community home-health nursing for pregnant women and babies (Chavigny and Korske, 1983; Coyner, 1985).

Alternative and complementary prevention strategies

In spite of the success of the present program in improving many different aspects of maternal, child, and family functioning, it is important to note that it was not completely successful. The rate of maltreatment, although substantially reduced in the nurse-visited condition, was still 4 to 5 percent – a rate too high by any standard. It would be useful to determine why the nurses were unable to prevent the more intractable cases of maltreatment, but our data do not provide any clues. The cases of maltreatment among the nurse-visited women (unlike the cases of maltreatment in the comparison group) were distributed without a consistent pattern across all age, marital status, and poverty subgroups; and decreasing maternal psychological resources (at least as indicated by maternal locus of control) was not associated with an increase in maltreatment in the nurse-visited sample. In the end, the nurses were able to shift the early life streams for most of the families they visited in more favorable directions, but were unable to eliminate a small number of treacherous, unpredictable whirlpools into which some families were drawn.

Because there is no empirical pattern to the failure of the program to prevent certain cases of maltreatment, it is useful to examine the limitations of the program on purely theoretical grounds. Although the present program was designed to address those underlying emotions and cognitions that play an important role in caregiving, it seems reasonable that a long history of abuse or neglect in mother's own childhood, in certain cases, would continue to influence her ability to form relationships and her quality of caregiving, even in the presence of a two-and-a-half-year, comprehensively designed intervention. It is increasingly clear that, although there are notable exceptions to the pattern, the intergenerational transmission of caregiving dysfunction does take place and that it can be explained, at least in part, by disorders of attachment (Main and Goldwyn, 1984; Ricks, 1985). Because of this, it makes sense to complement home-visitation with comprehensive therapy for the parent- and child-victims of maltreatment. To the extent that comprehensive, therapeutic treatment is able to create safe, secure, and nurturant environments for child victims, they may begin to establish a sense of trust, interpersonal skill, and mastery over their lives that will lead to more favorable life-course development and successful parenting on their own part. Thus, the sensitive and comprehensive treatment of child victims and their families becomes an important long-range preventive strategy, in addition to being of immense importance in its own right.

Even though the nurses in the present program tried to moderate the effects of poverty on family life by linking parents with needed services in the community (including vocational training and employment services), ultimately there are structural constraints limiting what is possible with this kind of intervention. Communities with high rates of unemployment, drug abuse, and other conditions antithetical to productive living exert powerful, insidious forces that work against the influence of the nurse. In light of this, it is not unreasonable for the nurses to fail in their efforts to prevent maltreatment in certain cases. Thus, in contrast to preventive approaches that focus on the individual, policy-makers and investigators need to consider the preventive effects of reducing inequities in the social and economic structures of our society (Gelles, 1984). Public policies that in the long run increase educational and employment opportunities and that reduce racial and sex discrimination are likely to reduce the stresses and frustrations that lead to drug abuse and alcoholism and that interfere with parents' own personal accomplishments as well as their functioning as caregivers (Gil, 1978).

Other structural, community-wide factors need to be considered as well. Even though the nurses tried to imbue parents with an appreciation for the importance of nonviolent childrearing methods, their efforts were counteracted by the acceptance of physical punishment as a method of discipline on the part of many families that they visited. When questioned about their disciplinary methods during the research interviews, a surprisingly large number of parents in the present study apologized for not spanking their children *more* frequently. In light of the widespread acceptance of physical violence and psychological denigration as methods of disciplining children (Alvy, 1975; Garbarino, Guttman, and Seeley, 1986; Gil, 1970), it makes sense to complement the nurse home-visitation strategy with community education campaigns aimed at promoting more positive methods of childrearing.

In spite of its limitations, the results of the present investigation provide a basis for considerable hope that the incidence of abuse and neglect can indeed be reduced with home-visitation services. Before these findings are used as a basis for a major public-policy initiative, however, it is important to replicate the present findings with different nurses and with families living in different circumstances. If the findings of the present study are replicated, it would appear that, when combined with the systematic, comprehensive treatment of the child victims and the kinds of social and economic changes outlined above, this kind of program may produce significant reductions in the incidence of caregiving dysfunction.

Because of its service intensity, however, this home-visitation program is more expensive than most other public services for families, leading some to question its feasibility on a wide-scale basis. Preliminary cost-benefit analyses suggest that a major portion of the cost for home visitation can be offset by avoided foster-care placements, hospitalizations, emergency-room visits, and child-protective service worker time incurred during the same period that the home-visiting program is provided. Short-range projections (through the child's sixth year of life) of cost-savings to the government resulting from the nurse-visited, unmarried women's returning to the work force and reducing the number of subsequent children show even greater cost-savings (Olds, Lombardi, and Henderson, 1986c). Given the association between early maltreatment and subsequent psychosocial dysfunctions, such as juvenile delinquency (Garbarino and Plantz, 1986) and violent behavior (Lewis, Shanok, and Balla, 1979), the long-range financial savings to the community are in all likelihood substantially greater, as is the reduction in human suffering.

References

Ainsworth, M. Attachment and child abuse. In G. Gerbner, C. Ross, and E. Zigler (Eds.), *Child abuse: An agenda for action*. New York: Oxford University Press, 1980.

Alvy, K. Preventing child abuse. *American Psychologist*, 1975, *30*, 921–928.

American Humane Association. *Annual report, 1983: Highlights of official child neglect and abuse reporting*. Denver, CO: American Humane Association, 1985.

Anisfeld, E., and Lipper, E. Early contact, social support, and mother–infant bonding. *Pediatrics*, 1983, *72*, 79–83.

Baker, R., and Nelder, J. *The GLIM system – release three: Generalized linear interactive modeling*. Oxford, Eng.: Numerical Algorithms Group, 1978.

Belle, D. (Ed.) *Lives in stress: Women and depression*. Beverly Hills, CA: Sage Publications, 1982.

Belsky, J. Child maltreatment: An ecological integration. *American Psychologist*, 1980, *35*, 320–335.

Birch, H., and Gussow, H. *Disadvantaged children: Health, nutrition, and school failure*. New York: Harcourt, Brace, and World, 1970.

Boyer, R., and Savageau, D. *Places rated almanac*. New York: Rand McNally, 1981.

Brazelton, T. B. *Neonatal behavioral assessment scale. Clinics in developmental medicine*. Philadelphia: Lippincott, 1973, No. 50.

Bronfenbrenner, U. *The ecology of human development: Experiments by nature and design*. Cambridge, MA: Harvard University Press, 1979.

Caldwell, B., and Bradley, R. *Home observation for measurement of the environment*. Little Rock, AK: University of Arkansas, 1979.

Card, J. J., and Wise, L. L. Teenage mothers and teenage fathers: The impact of early childbearing on the parents' personal and professional lives. *Family Planning Perspectives*, 1978, *10*, 199–205.

Chavigny, K., and Korske, M. Public health nursing in crisis. *Nursing Outlook*, 1983, *31*, 312–316.

Cohn, A. H. *An approach to preventing child abuse*. Chicago: National Committee for Prevention of Child Abuse, 1981.

Collins, A. H. Helping neighbors intervene in cases of maltreatment. In J. Garbarino (Ed.), *Protecting children from abuse and neglect*. San Francisco: Jossey-Bass, 1981.

Coyner, A. Home visiting by public health nurses: A vanishing resource for families and children. *Zero to Three: Bulletin of the National Center for Clinical Infant Programs*, 1985; *VI*, 1–13.

Efron, B. Forcing a sequential experiment to be balanced. *Biometrika*, 1971, *58*, 403–417.

Egeland, B., and Sroufe, A. Attachment and early maltreatment. *Child Development*, 1981, *52*, 44–52.

Fergusson, D. M., Hons, B. A., Horwood, L. J., and Shannon, F. T. Relationship of family life events, maternal depression, and child-rearing problems. *Pediatrics*, 1984, *73*, 773–776.

Field, T., Widmayer, S., Stringe, S., and Ignatoff, E. Teenage, lower-class, black mothers and their preterm infants: An infant and developmental follow-up. *Child Development*, 1980, *51*, 426–436.

Garbarino, J. An ecological perspective on child maltreatment. In L. Pelton (Ed.), *The social context of child abuse and neglect*. New York: Human Sciences Press, 1980.

Garbarino, J., and Crouter, K. Defining the community context of parent–child relations: The correlates of child maltreatment. *Child Development*, 1978, *49*, 604–616.

Garbarino, J., Guttman, E., and Seeley, J. *The psychologically battered child*. San Francisco: Jossey-Bass, 1986.

Garbarino, J., and Plantz, M. C. Child abuse and juvenile delinquency: What are the links? In J. Garbarino, C. Schellenbach, J. Sebes, and Associates (Eds.), *Troubled youth, troubled families*. New York: Aldine, 1986.

Garbarino, J., and Stocking, S. (Eds.). *Protecting children from abuse and neglect.* San Francisco: Jossey-Bass, 1980.

Gelles, R. *Applying our knowledge of family violence to prevention and treatment: What difference might it make?* Paper presented to the Second National Conference for Family Violence Researchers, Durham, New Hampshire, August 7–10, 1984.

Gelles, R. J., and Cornell, C. P. *Intimate violence in families.* Family Studies Text Series 2. Beverly Hills, CA: Sage Publications, 1985.

Gerbner, G., Ross, C., and Zigler, E. (Eds.). *Child abuse: An agenda for action.* New York: Oxford University Press, 1980.

Gil, D. G. *Violence against children: Physical child abuse in the United States.* Cambridge, MA: Harvard University Press, 1970.

Gil, D. Violence against children. *Journal of Marriage and the Family,* 1971, *33,* 639–648.

Gil, D. A holistic perspective on child abuse and its prevention. *Journal of Soc and Soc Welfare,* 1974, *2,* 110–125.

Gil, D. Child abuse: Levels of manifestation, causal dimensions, and primary prevention. *Victimology,* 1977, *2,* 186–194.

Gil, D. A holistic perspective on child abuse and its prevention. In R. Bourne, and E. Newberger (Eds.), *Critical perspective in child abuse.* Lexington, MA: Health, 1978.

Gray, J., Cutler, C., Dean, J., and Kempe, C. Prediction and prevention of child abuse and neglect. *Journal of Social Issues,* 1979, *35,* 127–139.

Hall, L., Williams, C., and Greenberg, R. Support, stressors, and depressive symptoms in low-income mothers of young children. *American Journal of Public Health,* 1985, *75,* 518–522.

Helfer, R. A review of the literature on the prevention of child abuse and neglect. *Child Abuse and Neglect,* 1982, *6,* 251–261.

Henderson, C. Analysis of covariance in the mixed model: Higher level, nonhomogeneous, and random regressions. *Biometrics,* 1982, *38,* 623–640.

Hollingshead, A. B. *Four-factor index of social status.* Unpublished manuscript. New Haven, CT, Yale University, 1976.

Hopkins, J., Marcus, M., and Campbell, S. Postpartum depression: a critical review. *Psychological Bulletin,* 1984, *95,* 498–515.

Hunter, R. S., Kilstrom, N., Kraybill, E. N., & Luda, F. Antecedents of child abuse and neglect in premature infants: A prospective study in a newborn intensive care unit. *Pediatrics,* 1978, *161,* 629–635.

Johnson, P. O., and Neyman, J. Tests of certain linear hypotheses and their application to some educational problems. *Statistical Research Memoirs,* 1936, *1,* 57–93.

Johnston, C. A. *The art of the crisis line: A training manual for volunteers in child abuse prevention.* Oakland, CA: Parent Stress Service, Inc., 1976.

Kempe, C. Approaches to preventing child abuse: The health visitor concept. *American Journal of Diseases of Children,* 1976, *130,* 941–947.

Kempe, C. H., Silverman, F. N., Steele, B. F., Droegemueller, W., and Silver, H. K. The battered child syndrome. *Journal of the American Medical Association,* 1962, *181,* 17.

Keniston, K. *All our children: The American family under pressure.* New York: Carnegie Corporation, 1977.

Klaus, M. H., and Kennel, J. H. *Parent–infant bonding.* St. Louis: C. V. Mosby Company, 1982, 2nd ed.

Lawrence, R. A., and Merritt, T. A. Infants of adolescent mothers: Perinatal, neonatal, and infancy outcome. *Seminars in Perinatology,* 1981, *5,* 19–32.

Lealman, G., Haigh, D., Phillips, J., Stone, J., and Ord-Smith, C. Prediction and prevention of child abuse – An empty hope? *Lancet,* 1983, *1,* 1423–1424.

Lewis, D. O., Shanok, S. S., and Balla, D. A. Perinatal difficulties, head and face trauma, and child abuse in the medical histories of seriously delinquent children. *American Journal of Psychiatry,* 1979, *136,* 419–423.

Light, R. Abused and neglected children in America: A study of alternative policies. *Harvard Educational Review,* 1973, *43,* 556–598.

Lutzker, J. R., Frame, R. E., and Rice, J. M. Project 12-Ways: An ecobehavioral approach to the treatment and prevention of child abuse and negelct. *Education and Treatment of Children,* 1982, *5,* 141–155.

Lutzker, J. R., and Rice, J. M. Project 12-Ways: Measuring outcome of a large in-home service for treatment and prevention of child abuse and neglect. *Child Abuse and Neglect,* 1984, *8,* 519–524.

Lynch, M. A. Ill-health and child abuse. *Lancet,* 1975, *2,* 317–319.

Main, M., and Goldwyn, R. Predicting rejection of her infant from mother's representation of her own experience: Implications for the abused–abusing intergenerational cycle. *Child Abuse and Neglect,* 1984, *8,* 203–217.

McAnarney, E. R. Adolescent pregnancy – A national priority. *Am J Dis Child,* 1978, *132,* 125.

Miller, F., Court, S., Walton, W., and Knox, E. *Growing up in Newcastle upon Tyne.* London: Oxford University Press, 1960.

Miller, R. G., Jr. *Simultaneous statistical inference.* New York: McGraw Hill, 1966.

National Center on Child Abuse and Neglect (NCCAN). National study of the incidence and severity of child abuse and neglect. U.S. Department of Health and Human Services, DHHS Publication No. (OHDS) 81–30325, 1981.

Newberger, E. H., Reed, R. B., Daniel, J. H., Hyde, J. N., and Kotelchuck, M. Pediatric social illnesses: Toward an ediologic classification. *Pediatrics,* 1977, *60,* 178–185.

New York State Department of Social Services. *Annual report of Child Protective Services in New York State.* Albany: New York State Department of Social Services, 1973–1982.

O'Connor, S., Vietze, P., Sherrod, K., Sandler, H., and Altemeier, W. Reduced incidence of parenting inadequacy following rooming-in. *Pediatrics,* 1980, *66,* 176–182.

Olds, D. Improving formal services for mothers and children. In J. Garbarino and S. Stocking (Eds.), *Protecting children from abuse and neglect: Developing and maintaining effective support systems for families.* San Francisco: Jossey-Bass, 1981.

Olds, D. The prenatal/early infancy project: An ecological approach to prevention of developmental disabilities. In J. Belsky (Ed.), *In the beginning.* New York: Columbia University Press, 1982.

Olds, D. An intervention program for high-risk families. In R. Hoekelman (Ed.), *Minimizing high-risk parenting.* Media, PA: Harwal Publishing Company, 1983.

Olds, D., Henderson, C., Birmingham, M., Chamberlin, R., and Tatelbaum, R. Final report to The Maternal and Child Health and Crippled Children's Services Research Grants Program, Bureau of Community Health Services, HSA, PHS, DHHS, Grant No. MCJ–36040307, November 1983.

Olds, D., Henderson, C., Tatelbaum, R., and Chamberlin, R. Improving the delivery of prenatal care and outcomes of pregnancy: A randomized trial of nurse home visitation. *Pediatrics,* 1986a, *77,* 16–28.

Olds, D., Henderson, C., Tatelbaum, R., and Chamberlin, R. Preventing child abuse and neglect: A randomized trial of nurse home visitation. *Pediatrics,* 1986b, *78,* 65–78.

Olds, D., Lombardi, J., Birmingham, M. T., and Henderson, C. *Prenatal/Early Infancy Project: A follow-up evaluation at the third and fourth years of life.* Final report to the William T. Grant Foundation, Grant Number 840723–80, July 1986c.

Pancoast, D. L. Finding and enlisting neighbors to support families. In J. Garbarino (Ed.), *Protecting Children from Abuse and Neglect.* San Francisco: Jossey-Bass, 1981.

Pedersen, F., Anderson, F., and Cain, R. L., Jr. *A methodology for assessing parent perception of infant temperament.* Presented at the Fourth Biennial Southeastern Conference on Human Development, Nashville, TN, April 1976.

Potthoff, R. F. On the Johnson-Neyman technique and some extensions thereof. *Psychometrics,* 1964, *29,* 241–256.

Ramey, C., and Campbell, F. The prevention of developmental retardation in high-risk children. In P. Mittler (Ed.), *Research to practice in mental retardation,* Vol. 1, *Care and Intervention.* Baltimore, Maryland: University Park Press, 1977.

Ricks, M. H. The social transmission of parental behavior: Attachment across generations. In
   I. Bretherton and E. Waters (Eds.), *Growing points of attachment theory and research.*
   Monographs of the Society for Research in Child Development, 1985, *50,* 211–227.
Rotter, J. B. Generalized expectancies for internal versus external control of reinforcement.
   Psychological Monographs: General and Applied, 1966, *80* (1), 1–28.
Sameroff, A., Seifer, R., and Elias, P. Sociocultural variability in infant temperament ratings.
   Child Development, 1982, *53,* 164–173.
Scheffé, H. *The analysis of variance.* New York: Wiley, 1959.
Schneider-Rosen, K., and Cicchetti, D. The relationship between affect and cognition in mal-
   treated infants: Quality of attachment and the development of visual self-recognition.
   Child Development, 1984, *55,* 648–658.
Siegel, E., Bauman, K., Schaefer, E., Saunders, M., and Ingram, D. Hospital and home support
   during infancy: Impact on maternal attachment, child abuse and neglect, and health care
   utilization. *Pediatrics,* 1980, *66,* 183–190.
Spinetta, J., and Rigler, D. The child-abusing parent: A psychological review. *Psychological*
   Bulletin, 1972, *77,* 296–304.
Steinberg, L. D., Catalano, R., and Dooley, D. Economic antecedents of child abuse and
   neglect. *Child Development,* 1981, *52,* 975–985.
Strauss, M. Cultural and social organizational influences on violence between family members.
   In R. Prince and D. Barried (Eds.), *Configurations: Biological and cultural factors in sex-*
   uality and family life. Lexington, MA: Health, 1974.
Thomas, J. Children's Hospital National Medical Center, Washington, DC. Personal commu-
   nication, April 1986.
Travers, J., and Light, R. (Eds.). *Learning from experience: Evaluating early childhood dem-*
   onstration programs. Washington, DC: National Academy Press, 1982.
U.S. Senate. Child abuse prevention and treatment and adoption reform amendments of 1983.
   Report from the Committee on Labor and Human Resources (to accompany S. 1003).
   Report No. 98–246. Washington: U.S. Government Printing Office, 1983.
vanDoorninck, W. J., Dawson, P., Butterfield, P. M., and Alexander, H. I. Parent–infant sup-
   port through lay health visitors. Final report submitted to the Bureau of Community
   Health Services. U.S. Public Health Service, National Institute of Health, Department of
   Health, Education, and Welfare, 1980.
Vaughn, B., Taraldson, B., Crichton, L., and Egeland, B. The assessment of infant tempera-
   ment: A critique of the Carey Infant Temperament Questionnaire. *Infant Behavior and*
   Development, 1981, *4,* 1–17.
Vesterdal, J. Handling of child abuse in Denmark. *Child Abuse and Neglect,* 1977, *1,* 193–198.
Wheatley, G. M. Childhood accidents 1952–1972: An overview. *Pediatric Annals,* 1973, *2,* 10–
   30.
Young, L. *Wednesday's children: A study of child neglect and abuse.* New York: McGraw-Hill,
   1964.

Name index

Subject index

781